Handbook of Experimental Pharmacology

Volume 101

Biochemical Pharmacology of Blood and Bloodforming Organs

Contributors

K. Agrawal, Barbara S. Beckman, R.L. Capizzi
Marion Dugdale, A.C. Eaves, C.J. Eaves, J.W. Fisher
G.A. FitzGerald, R.A. Joyce, D.M. Kerins, R.D. Lange
M. Mason-Garcia, T.P. McDonald, D.C.B. Mills
J. Nakashima, P.J. Quesenberry, J.B. Smith
L.R. Solomon, J.L. Spivak

Editor

James W. Fisher

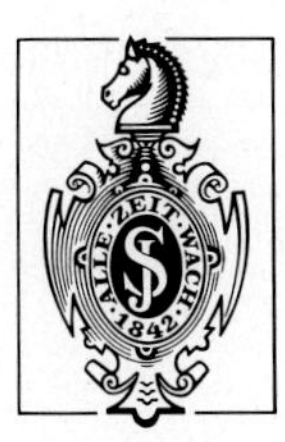

Springer-Verlag
Berlin Heidelberg New York London Paris
Tokyo Hong Kong Barcelona Budapest

JAMES W. FISHER, Ph.D.

Regents Professor and Chairman
Tulane University School of Medicine
Department of Pharmacology
1430 Tulane Avenue
New Orleans, LA 70112
USA

With 64 Figures and 47 Tables

ISBN 3-540-52844-X Springer-Verlag Berlin Heidelberg New York
ISBN 0-387-52844-X Springer-Verlag New York Berlin Heidelberg

Library of Congress Cataloging-in-Publication Data Biochemical pharmacology of blood and blood-forming organs/contributors, K. Agrawal . . . [et al.]; editor, James W. Fisher. p. cm. — (Handbook of experimental pharmacology; v. 101) Includes bibliographical references and index. ISBN 3-540-52844-X. — ISBN 0-387-52844-X 1. Hematopoiesis. 2. Hematopoietic growth factors. 3. Erythropoietin. I. Agrawal, K. (Krishna) II. Fisher, James W. (James William), 1925– . III. Series. [DNLM: 1. Anemia—blood. 2. Anemia—drug effects. 3. Blood—drug effects. 4. Hematopoiesis—drug effects. 5. Hematopoietic Cell Growth Factors—pharmacology. W1 HA51L v. 101/WH 140 B6143] QP905.H3 vol. 101 [QP92] 615′.1 s—dc20 [612.4′1] DNLM/DLC for Library of Congress 91-5014 CIP

Typesetting: Best-set Typesetter Ltd., Hong Kong
27/3130-543210 – Printed on acid-free paper

List of Contributors

Agrawal, K., Department of Pharmacology, Tulane Medical Center, School of Medicine, Tulane University, 1430 Tulane Avenue, New Orleans, LA 70112, USA

Beckman, Barbara S., Department of Pharmacology, Tulane Medical Center, School of Medicine, Tulane University, 1430 Tulane Avenue, New Orleans, LA 70112, USA

Capizzi, R.L., Executive Vice President US Bioscience Inc., One Tower Bridge, 100 Front Street, West Conshohocken, PA 19428. Formerly, Director, comprehensive Cancer Center of Wake Forrest University, Winston-Salem, NC 27103, USA

Dugdale, Marion, University of Tennessee Hemophilia Clinic, Division of Hematology/Oncology, The University of Tennessee, College of Medicine, 3 N. Dunlap, Memphis, TN 38163, USA

Eaves, A.C., Terry Fox Laboratory, B.C. Cancer Agency, 601 West 10th Avenue, Vancouver, B.C., Canada V5Z 1L3, and Department of Medicine and Pathology, University of British Columbia, Vancouver, B.C., Canada

Eaves, C.J., Terry Fox Laboratory, B.C. Cancer Agency, 601 West 10th Avenue, Vancouver, B.C., Canada V5Z 1L3 and Department of Medical Genetics, University of British Columbia, Vancouver, B.C., Canada

Fisher, J.W., Department of Pharmacology, Tulane Medical Center, School of Medicine, Tulane University, 1430 Tulane Avenue, New Orleans, LA 70112, USA

FitzGerald, G.A., Center for Cardiovascular Science, Department of Medicine and Experimental Therapeutics, University College Dublin, Water Hospital, 41 Eccles St., Dublin 7, Ireland

Joyce, R.A., Cancer Institute, Baptist Medical Center, Jacksonville, FL 32207, USA

Kerins, D.M., Center for Cardiovascular Science, Department of Medicine and Experimental Therapeutics, University College Dublin, Water Hospital, 41 Eccles St., Dublin 7, Ireland

Lange, R.D., Department of Medical Biology, The University of Tennessee Medical Center at Knoxville, 1924 Alcoa Highway, Knoxville, TN 37920-6999, USA

Mason-Garcia, M., Department of Anatomy, Tulane Medical Center, School of Medicine, Tulane University, 1430 Tulane Avenue, New Orleans, LA 70112, USA

McDonald, T.P., Department of Animal Science, University of Tennessee, College of Veterinary Medicine, P.O. Box 1071, Knoxville, TN 37901-1071, USA

Mills, D.C.B., Thrombosis Research Center, Temple University Health Sciences Center, 3400 North Broad Street, Philadelphia, PA 19140, USA

Nakashima, J., Department of Pharmacology, Tulane Medical Center, School of Medicine, Tulane University, 1430 Tulane Avenue, New Orleans, LA 70112, USA

Quesenberry, P.J., Division of Hematology/Oncology, Department of Medicine, University of Virginia School of Medicine, Box 502, Charlottesville, VA 22908, USA.

Smith, J.B., Department of Pharmacology, Temple University Medical School, 3420 North Broad Street, Philadelphia, PA 19140, USA

Solomon, L.R., The Connecticut Hospice, Inc., 61 Burban Drive, Branford, CT 06405, USA

Spivak, J.L., Hematology Division, Department of Medicine, The Johns Hopkins Hospital, 600 N. Wolfe Street, Baltimore, MD 21205, USA

Preface

A large number of chemical agents are known which affect blood and blood-forming organs. The purpose of this volume is to review the significant advances made over the past several years regarding such chemical agents. The purification, biological action, and therapeutic implications of several widely used hematopoietic growth factors such as interleukin 3 (IL-3 or multi-CSF), granulocyte/macrophage colony stimulating factor (GM-CSF), granulocyte colony stimulating factor (G-CSF), colony stimulating factor (CSF-1 or M-CSF), thrombopoietin, and erythropoietin are included in this volume. These factors are important in regulating several hematopoietic cell lines such as neutrophils, monocytes, eosinophils, macrophages, megakaryocytes, platelets, and erythrocytes.

People are exposed daily to numerous toxic chemical substances present in our environment which produce a suppression of erythropoiesis, myelopoiesis, lymphocytopoiesis, and megakaryocytopoiesis. Attempts have been made in this volume to assess the therapeutic role of some of the hematopoietic factors such as erythropoietin in the anemia of end stage renal disease, as well as colony stimulating factors in other hematopoietic abnormalities. In addition, some of the chemical factors in our environment which suppress major hematopoietic lineages stimulated by erythropoietin, macrophage colony stimulating factor, granulocyte colony stimulating factor, interleukin 1-alpha, interleukin 1-beta, and interleukins 2, 3, 4, 5, 6, 7, and 9 are also included. An updating of the mechanism of action of each of these factors on the major hematopoietic lineages is covered.

Erythropoietin is currently enjoying widespread use in the treatment of the anemia of end stage renal disease, and the work included on it can provide practicing hematologists and nephrologists with updated information on the mechanism of production and sites of action of erythropoietin. Other uses of erythropoietin are the enemia of AIDS, cancer and cancer therapeutic agents, rheumatoid arthritis, and autologous blood donors. This volume also includes sections on the effects of arachidonic acid and its metabolites on erythroid cell proliferation, iron deficiency and megaloblastic anemia mechanisms and therapy; the humoral control of thrombocytopoiesis; arachidonic acid, its metabolites, and other chemical agents which influence platelets in thromboembolic diseases; an updated section on anticoagulant, antithrombotic, and thrombolytic agents in disease processes; chemical agents which suppress myelopoiesis; and finally an updated chapter on drugs which are useful in the chemotherapy of acute leukemias. It is hoped that this volume will prove useful to investigators in the fields of pharmacology, physiology, nephrology, urology, hematology, pathology, endocrinology, biochemistry, and molecular and cell biology.

I gratefully acknowledge the technical assistance of Mr. Jesse Brookins, Mr. Eugene Maulet, and Ms. Judy Wigginton for their assistance in the preparation of this book. This volume is dedicated to my loving wife, Mrs. Carol B. Fisher, who has over the years been patient with me in the time that I have had to sacrifice away from my family in the preparation of this work.

New Orleans JAMES W. FISHER

Contents

CHAPTER 4

The Mechanism of Action of Erythropoietin: Erythroid Cell Response

CHAPTER 5

The Arachidonic Acid Cascade and Erythropoiesis

CHAPTER 6

Iron Deficiency and Megaloblastic Anemias
L.R. SOLOMON. With 6 Figures 137

CHAPTER 7

Erythropoietin in the Anemia of End-Stage Renal Disease

CHAPTER 8

Humoral Control of Thrombocytopoiesis

CHAPTER 9

Arachidonic Acid Metabolism Platelets and Thromboembolic Disease
D.M. KERINS and G.A. FITZGERALD. With 6 Figures 299

CHAPTER 10

Chemical Agents That Inhibit Platelet Aggregation
J.B. SMITH and D.C.B. MILLS. With 4 Figures 353

CHAPTER 12

Granulocyte-Macrophage Growth Factors

CHAPTER 13

Chemical Agents Which Suppress Myelopoiesis: Agranulocytosis and Leukemia

CHAPTER 1

Introduction

J.W. Fisher

Significant advances have been made over the past several years which have led to a better understanding of the mechanism of the effects of drugs on blood and blood-forming organs. A very important advance has been made in the purification of several growth factors, such as erythropoietin and several colony stimulating factors, which are important in regulating the production of red blood cells, leukocytes, megakaryocytes, and platelets. Numerous toxic chemical substances in our environment, to which people are exposed daily, also produce suppression of erythropoiesis, myelopoiesis, and megakaryocytopoiesis. It is the purpose of this volume to provide an update on the mechanisms of action, therapeutic uses, and toxic manifestations of chemical agents which affect blood and blood-forming organs. The first part includes an introductory chapter on the fundamental mechanism involved in the control of hematopoiesis, covering the responsible growth factors and describing the major hematopoietic lineages stimulated by factors such as erythropoietin, macrophage colony stimulating factor (CSF), granulocyte CSF, IL-1α, β, 2, 3, 4, 5, 6, 7, and 9. Major consideration is also given to clonigenic progenitors which affect the normal human adult marrow such as erythroid (CFU-E, BFU-E) and granulocytic-macrophage (CFU-GM) colony stimulating factors.

The second part details the effects of chemical agents on erythropoietin production and erythropoiesis. A chapter is devoted to the regulation of kidney production of erythropoietin which includes a model for the role of external messenger substances in its hypoxic stimulation. Several chemical messengers are discussed which are released during hypoxia such as adenosine, eicosanoids, β_2-adrenergic agonists, and oxygen-derived metabolites, all of which activate adenylate cyclase to increase erythropoietin generation. The primary focus is on adenosine which may be a key autacoid here. A section on the mechanism and sites of action of erythropoietin in the erythroid cell compartment is also included which covers the erythropoietin gene, the physicochemical characterization of erythropoietin itself, the target erythroid cells (BFU-E and CFU-E), a model system for the interaction of erythropoietin with erythroid progenitor cells, the erythropoietin receptor, and the characteristics of binding of erythropoietin to its receptor. The relationship of other growth and developmental factors with erythroid progenitors, gene expression during erythroid cell differentiation, and signal transduction in erythroid progenitor cells are also covered in this section. The delineation of the kinetics of the interaction of erythropoietin with its receptors on erythropoietin-responsive cells is considered to be one of the most important advances in erythropoietin research during the past few years. A very important new finding, which is covered in the section on erythropoiesis, is the involvement of the arachidonic acid cascade in erythroid cell proliferation. Attention is paid to the prostaglandins generated through the cyclooxygenase pathway and their participation in the CFU-E response to erythropoietic factors. Prostaglandins, thromboxane, and the leukotrienes, which are the metabolites of arachidonic acid generated through the lipoxygenase pathway, are considered. The eicosanoids produced from arachidonic acid, their blockade with cyclooxygenase inhibitors, such as meclofenamate, indomethacin, and aspirin, production of erythropoietin and the effects of erythropoietin on the erythroid cell compartment are described. The kinases, e.g., protein kinase C, are included in a model for the actions of erythropoietin involving leukotrienes on erythroid progenitor cells. The area of drug-induced suppression of hematopoiesis is also depicted and covers the effects of drugs on three cell lines: erythropoietic, myelocytic, and megakaryocytic. Drugs which are useful in the treatment of iron deficiency and megaloblastic anemias are listed. The role of vitamin B_{12} and folic acid metabolism in megaloblastic anemias and the present day mechanisms of megaloblastosis are also covered. An up-to-date model of the erythron involving iron metabolism, mucosal transport of iron, and the role of the reticuloendothelial system and the hepatocyte in iron metabolism is presented. A current model for the role of folic acid and vitamin B_{12} in intermediary metabolism and the mechanism of vitamin B_{12} absorption from the intestine are delineated. A section of the book covering the mechanism of the anemia of end-stage renal disease includes a comparison of the biologic and radioimmuno-assays for erythropoietin, the pathogenesis of the anemia of chronic renal failure, kidney production of erythropoietin, and the use of purified recombinant erythropoietin in the therapy of renal anemia. The use of erythropoietin is one of the most significant advances in the therapy of anemia during the past few years. It was only possible to provide this recombinant erythropoietin after erythropoietin had been purified to homogeneity, the amino acid sequence elucidated, the gene for erythropoietin cloned, and a transfected cell line developed for the large-scale production of recombinant erythropoietin. The clinical use of erythropoietin in other types of anemia is being vigorously explored at the present time.

The third part of the book deals with thrombopoiesis and blood coagulation. A chapter covering the humoral control of thrombocytopoiesis presents a model for megakaryocytopoiesis and the factors which are involved in the regulation and control of megakaryocytopoiesis and thrombopoietin production. This section includes a detailed historical background on thrombopoietin, its assay and standardization, site of production, purification, antibodies to it, its effects on megakaryocyte colony formation, the potentiation of megakaryocyte CSF (MegCSF), and its effects on thrombocytopoiesis. Stimulation of megakaryocytopoiesis by erythropoietin, IL-3, and GM-CSF is also considered. A section on arachidonic acid metabolism, platelets, and thromboembolic disorders is given, covering the cyclooxygenase, lipoxygenase, and hepoxygenase pathways and sites of action of antiplatelet pharmacologic agents. Thromboembolic diseases and the implications of pharmacologic agents in the treatment of unstable angina and acute myocardial infarction are discussed. The use of antiplatelet drugs in coronary by-pass procedures and other manipulations, such as prosthetic valves and coronary angioplasty, are described. Specific chemical agents that inhibit platelet aggregation and their mechanism of action, especially the involvement of cyclic AMP and cyclic GMP, are included. A model for the mechanisms involved in platelet activation, the regulation of platelet function by agents which act on the cyclic AMP and cyclic GMP systems, and a consideration of drugs that inhibit platelet activation and are useful clinically are presented. The pharmacology of antithrombotic agents such as dextrans, physical methods, defibrotide and brinase, low molecular weight heparins, streptokinase, tissue plasminogen activator, acyl plasminogen streptokinase activation complex (APSAC), urokinase, vitamin K, and warfarin is listed.

A fourth part on myelopoiesis considers CSF-1, GM-CSF, and the interleukins. The biologic actions of CSF-1, GM-CSF, and several interleukins and their actions on cell proliferation are described. A detailed chapter on chemical agents which suppress myelopoieis, e.g., those which produce agranulocytosis, is included. The selectivity of the activity of these compounds on purine and pyrimidine biosynthesis is considered. Drug-induced myeloid suppression with compounds such as ethanol, phenothiazines, anticoagulants, anti-inflammatory agents, antiviral substances, H_2 receptor antagonists as well as idiosyncratic neutropenias induced by analgesics, antibiotics, cardiovascular and diuretic agents, thyrostatic drugs, sulfonamides, and agents which produce secondary leukemias are represented. A final chapter in this part is devoted to an overview of the chemotherapy of acute leukemias. This section assesses the relative value of a number of antileukemia agents which have been demonstrated over the past few years to be most useful therapeutically.

The number of chemical agents which produce anemia, agranulocytosis, or changes in blood coagulation and platelet aggregation is overwhelming. Therefore, it is not possible to include an update on all chemical agents which have toxic effects on blood formation or those used for the treatment of diseases of the blood-forming organs. I apologize for any new or old compounds that have been overlooked and for any seeming overlap of the material in some of the chapters.

CHAPTER 2

Fundamental Control of Hematopoiesis

C.J. EAVES and A.C. EAVES

A. Introduction

Blood cells have been a major target of scientific investigation and clinical interest throughout the history of medicine. This focus reflects in part the unique properties of mature blood cells, which continue to command the attention of biophysicists, membrane biologists, geneticists, immunologists, and developmental biologists, as well as clinicians. In addition, many of the functions of blood cells, e.g., oxygen delivery to the peripheral tissues, maintenance of hemostasis, and infection control, are key to survival itself, and the crucial roles of these cells rapidly manifest themselves whenever the process of blood cell production is compromised or aberrant.

Because of the ease of obtaining mature blood cells in pure form, a great deal has been learned about their molecular make-up, including many of the specialized gene products whose synthesis represents the final expression of the various blood cell differentiation programs. Some of these are cell-specific structural molecules, e.g., erythroid cell spectrin, ankyrin, etc.; others, e.g. globin, myeloperoxidase, etc., relate to the unique metabolic functions of the mature blood cell types in which they are found. Thus, one of the hallmarks of terminal blood cell differentiation is the rapid synthesis of a large amount of protein which, not surprisingly, is preceded by the appearance in the cytoplasm of a large amount of RNA. This sequence of biochemical events together with the nuclear changes that occur during the maturation of most of the different types of blood cells results in a series of gross morphological changes that can be readily visualized at the cellular level under standard light microscopy and used to define the final stages of mature blood cell development. With the aid of DNA labelling studies, it has been possible to assign each of these morphologically defined stages to specific terminal cell divisions, as illustrated in Fig. 1 for the red cell pathway. A hierarchy of differentiative divisions at the end of each of the hematopoietic pathways is thus now a familiar concept and provides an important framework for visualizing how each differentiative division may serve as a control point for regulation of terminal cell output.

Erythropoietin (Ep), a hormone that controls the output of terminally differentiating erythroid cells, was the first growth regulator of blood cell production to be recognized (ERSLEV and CARO 1983). Its identity was

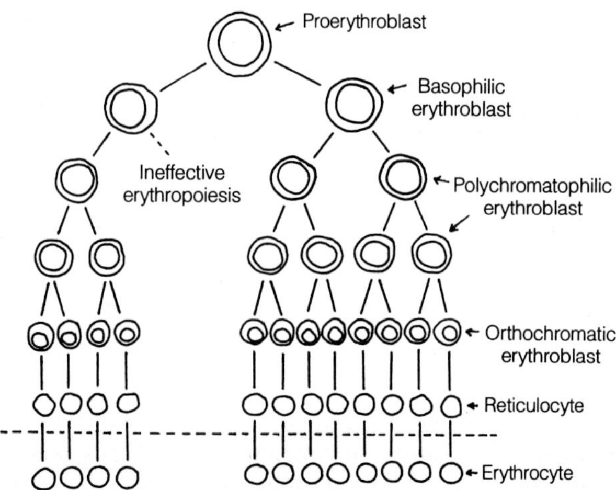

Fig. 1. Terminal stages of erythroid cell differentiation recognized by morphological assessment

initially established by experiments in which Ep-containing samples were injected into animals whose hematocrits had been artificially elevated by red cell transfusions. Raising the hematocrit causes all recognizable erythroid cells in the marrow and reticulocytes in the blood to disappear. The bioactivity of the injected Ep could thus be detected by its ability to induce the rapid appearance of new erythroblasts in the marrow or the subsequent release of new erythrocytes into the blood. Later, erythroid cell culture systems were developed that enabled this erythropoietic bioactivity to be detected in vitro with greater precision. This facilitated biochemical characterization of the active molecule, which was finally isolated in pure form in 1977 (Miyake et al. 1977) Amino acid sequence data led to the subsequent cloning of the Ep gene in 1985 (Jacobs et al. 1985) and its expression to yield an active recombinant product.

In contrast to erythrocytes which have a relatively long lifespan after being released into the circulation, the half-life of most of the other mature blood cell types is very short. Therefore, in vivo manipulation of the output of these cells could not be achieved by an analogous approach, and the physiological mechanisms regulating their production remained obscure for a much longer time. However, as cell culture methodology improved in the early 1960s, conditions that supported the growth and differentiation of colonies of granulopoietic cells in vitro were discovered (Pluznik and Sachs 1965; Bradley and Metcalf 1966; Senn et al. 1967). This led, in turn, to the recognition of specific factor requirements of granulopoietic cells developing in these cell culture systems and the subsequent use of these cultures as quantitative assays for the identification and purification of what eventually proved to be a large family of hematopoietic growth factors (Table 1).

Table 1. List of cloned hematopoietic growth factors

Name	Abbreviations	Other common names	Major hematopoietic lineage stimulated
Erythropoietin	EPO, Ep		Erythroid
Macrophage colony-stimulating factor	M-CSF, CSF-1	MGI-IM	Monocyte/macrophage
Granulocyte colony-stimulating factor	G-CSF, CSF-β	Pluripoietin, MGI-IG	Neutrophil
Granulocyte-macrophage colony-stimulating factor	GM-CSF, CSF-α	Pluripoietin-alpha, MGI-IGM	Neutrophil/macrophage
Interleukin-1α	IL-1α	Hemopoietin-1, lymphocyte activating factor	Co-stimulator of early cells, T cells
Interleukin-1β	IL-1β		Co-stimulator of early cells, T cells
Interleukin-2	IL-2	T-cell growth factor	T cells
Interleukin-3	IL-3	Multilineage colony stimulating factor, persisting cell factor, hemopoietin-2, hemopoietic cell growth factor, mast cell growth factor	Most myeloid lineages
Interleukin-4	IL-4	B-cell stimulating factor-1, B-cell differentiation factor, IgG induction factor	B cells, T cells
Interleukin-5	IL-5	T cell replacing factor, B-cell growth factor-2, B-cell differentiation factor, eosinophil differentiation factor	
Interleukin-6	IL-6	B-cell stimulating factor-2, hybridoma growth factor, plasmacytoma growth factor	B cells, costimulator of early cells
Interleukin-7	IL-7	–	Pre-B cells, T cells
Interleukin-9	IL-9	P40, mast cell growth enhancing activity	Early erythroid, mast cells

Seiler and Schwick (1988); Donahue et al. (1989); Goodwin et al. (1989); Hultner et al. (1989); Yang et al. (1989).

With the advent of recombinant DNA technology, progress in understanding the role of these growth factors in the regulation of hematopoiesis has greatly accelerated. Initially, being able simply to establish firmly the separate identities of various similar "activities" at both the DNA and protein level was by itself an important step forward. Later, with the production of large amounts of pure factor of defined identity, precise definition of target cell responsiveness became possible, and mechanism of action studies began. These have already shown that many factors have a much broader range of target cell specificity than previously anticipated, including effects on mature blood cells as well as their precursors (SEILER et al. 1988) and extending in many instances to actions on cells that are ontologically unrelated to hematopoietic cells (DEDHAR et al. 1988; BUSSOLINO et al. 1989).

The production of Ep by recombinant methods also introduced a new era of hematopoietic growth factor therapy in which the clinical potential of many of the hematopoietic growth factors has only just begun to be recognized. Ep "replacement" therapy for the treatment of the anemia of chronic renal failure became the first success story in this area (ESCHBACH et al. 1987). The results of these studies also showed that the deficient erythropoiesis seen in this disease is exclusively due to a failure of Ep production. In vivo effects of the hematopoietic colony-stimulating factors (CSFs) and interleukins under a variety of conditions are also now being catalogued. These studies have led to the identification of new therapeutic possibilities and at the same time have confirmed the important role these factors can play in regulating various parts of the complex process of hematopoiesis in vivo.

Over the past 30 years there has also been considerable progress in defining the developmental organization of the hematopoietic system. We now know that the most primitive hematopoietic cells are individually capable of regenerating all blood cell lineages following transplantation into histocompatible, marrow-ablated recipients and that this is accomplished by an extensive series of differentiation steps during which proliferative potential progressively declines. The intermediate stages that define the cell types undergoing these changes are, like the most primitive pluripotent cells, rare and morphologically similar to one another. However, these intermediate cells have now been well characterized by assays that detect their ability to proliferate and give rise to colonies of mature end cells within a few days or weeks in vitro. Studies using in vitro colony assays have also provided much information about how hematopoiesis may be normally regulated at a number of levels and how this may be altered under various pathologic conditions. Nevertheless, many fundamental processes such as the mechanism of lineage determination still remain largely a mystery. Clonogenic assay procedures have thus not only become part of the modern capability for investigating a variety of routine clinical diagnostic problems, they also continue to serve as a springboard for exploring aspects of hematopoiesis not yet understood.

B. Hierarchical Organization of Hematopoietic Cells

Figure 2 presents a schematic outline of the general hierarchy of hematopoietic progenitor populations that are now recognized. Each developmental stage in this lineage map corresponds to a different assay procedure. However, some overlap in the cells detected by different assays almost certainly exists, and there are a number of other aspects of this scheme that are still rather vague, particularly in regard to the hematopoietic stem cell compartment. The most primitive hematopoietic stem cell depicted in this scheme possesses both lymphoid and myeloid differentiation potential and is capable of sustaining the production of all lineages of cells in both of these systems for several months. Extensive data from murine studies using various genetic marking strategies in combination with bone marrow transplantation have established the existence of totipotent lymphomyelopoietic cells in the bone marrow of adult mice (Wu et al. 1968; Abramson et al. 1977; Dick et al. 1985; Keller et al. 1985; Lemischka et al. 1986). The presence of cells with similar properties in adult human marrow has been inferred for many years from studies of the different lineages represented in the neoplastic clone in patients with various hematopoietic malignancies (Whang et al. 1963; J.T. Prchal et al. 1978; Raskind and Fialkow 1987). Perhaps the best known example is chronic myeloid leukemia (CML), in which the presence of the Philadelphia chromosome (the hallmark of CML) in erythroid, megakaryo-

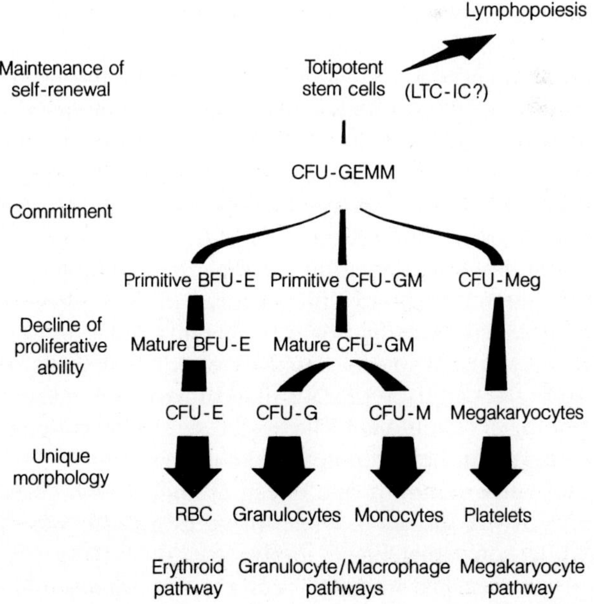

Fig. 2. Hierarchical organization of hematopoietic cell differentiation as defined by currently available clonogenic assays. *LTC-IC* long-term culture-initiating cells, described under Sect. E

cytic, and some B-lymphoid cells as well as granulocytes and macrophages has been documented, implying that the Philadelphia chromosome and hence of the disease originates in a pluripotent stem cell (RASKIND and FIALKOW 1987). More recently, evidence that a lymphomyeloid repopulating cell normally exists in adult human marrow has also been obtained (TURHAN et al. 1989).

However, even amongst primitive hematopoietic cells with the properties of pluripotentiality, transplantability, and extensive proliferative capacity, some hierarchical organization appears to exist. Evidence for hierarchy at this level has, again, been derived largely from studies of murine cells, in which the definition and selective isolation of distinct subpopulations of pluripotent cells have been possible. Such subpopulations appear to vary in the rapidity with which they give rise to detectable numbers of mature progeny and as to whether the production of such progeny is sustained or self-limited. Even amongst those that are capable of regenerating hematopoiesis in the long term, selectivity in recruitment in vivo can be consistently revealed by competitive repopultion assays in which the progeny of mixed grafts of repopulating cells are evaluated. Presumably, these parameters have a biologic basis at the cellular level, although as yet we have no molecular handles on what the mechanisms might be.

Another issue not well addressed by the scheme shown in Fig. 2 concerns the nature and timing of the process by which commitment to a single hematopoietic cell differentiation lineage normally occurs in vivo. Related to this is the question of whether the process of lineage restriction can be directly influenced by exposure of pluripotent cells to extrinsic factors. Analyses of the number of daughter pluripotent cells produced by individual pluripotent parent cells as well as the number and types of unipotent (committed) progenitor cells each may give rise to (either in vivo or in vitro) have revealed extensive heterogeneity in all of these measurements of stem cell behavior (TILL et al. 1964; GREGORY and HENKELMAN 1977; HUMPHRIES et al. 1981; OGAWA et al. 1984; LIM et al. 1984; SUDA et al. 1984; LEARY and OGAWA 1987). Similarly, maintenance of both "unrestricted" differentiation and proliferation potential, even under apparently similar (exogenous) conditions, has been found to exhibit features of a stochastically regulated process, i.e., one best described by a probability function (TILL et al. 1964; SUDA et al. 1984), suggesting the involvement of undefined influences (perhaps intrinsic to the cell itself) rather than of extrinsic factors at least under normal physiologic conditions. The exact sequence of lineage-restricting events that pluripotent hematopoietic cells undergo to reach unipotency can also vary apparently randomly and does not appear to be dictated normally by the specific growth factors to which the cells may be exposed.

It should be noted that Fig. 2 implies that each of the various hematopoietic cell pathways has a finite, reproducible, and similar "length" as measured by the number of cell divisions intervening between commitment and the final appearance of the mature end cell. This concept has served as a convenient framework for much useful experimentation, although many of the details have obviously not been vigorously tested. The pathway lengths shown are based on the demonstrated range of proliferative *potentialities* expressed by different lineage-restricted clonogenic progenitors exposed to conditions of "maximal" stimulation in vitro. It is then assumed that under such conditions, the size a colony achieves will be limited only by the innate proliferative capacity of its progenitor. Differently sized colonies will thus reflect the activation of distinct progenitor subpopulations with varying proliferative capacities. This interpretation is now supported by a large body of data indicating that progenitors of differently sized colonies can be physically and biologically separated (e.g., Bol and Williams 1980; Eaves and Eaves 1985; Long et al. 1986).

If hematopoiesis in the normal adult involved the exponential expansion of cells from the earliest clonogenic cell detectable, then one would expect the relative sizes of sequential compartments in vivo to correspond to the number of divisions separating them. However, examination of the proportion of clonogenic cells in S-phase for many of the compartments indicated in Fig. 2 shows that in the normal adult this proportion decreases dramatically in the more primitive populations (Becker et al. 1965; Iscove et al. 1970; Fauser and Messner 1979; Eaves and Eaves 1987). Such kinetics would thus allow large variations in the numbers of very primitive hematopoietic cells from those predicted by an exponential expansion model, consistent with the concept of a large stem cell "reserve."

Control of hematopoiesis, in terms of extrinsic factors, may thus be viewed as a problem of defining which molecules allow or promote (or prevent) the amplification of hematopoietic cells as they differentiate. Most of our concepts of which factors are important are based on studies of the effects of single (or combinations of) growth factors on the plating efficiency of different types of clonogenic cells in vitro. For example, it was recognized early on that Ep must be added to any culture in which erythroid colony formation from normal erythropoietic cells was sought because, without it, terminal erythroid cell differentiation does not occur. However, Ep alone is neither necessary nor sufficient to support the proliferation of the most primitive erythropoietic cells, which require other hematopoietic growth factors (Aye 1976). Thus, to detect primitive erythropoietic cells which have the potential to form very large erythroid colonies, the separate factor requirements of both the earliest and the latest stages of erythropoiesis must be met. Now that various cloned factors have been examined specifically for this activity, it has become apparent that there are a number that can stimulate early erythropoietic cells in both mouse and man. From this, one might infer that the regulation of the viability and proliferation of primitive erythropoietic cells may be relatively flexible, with the possibility of considerable variation in the number of early progenitor cells even amongst normal individuals. One would then also expect the imposition of a very stringent regulatory mechanism during the last few erythroid cell divisions.

This appears to fit well with what we know about the feedback control and actions of Ep. Thus, the system appears designed to accommodate variations in primitive cell numbers without compromising the maintenance of a tightly controlled hematocrit. Less is understood about the role of specific growth factors in the regulation of other pathways in vivo, although the concept of alternative regulators and synergy between two or more factors has become an increasingly common theme (Table 1).

C. Assay and Characterization of In Vitro Clonogenic Cells

All clonogenic assays used to detect and quantitate hematopoietic progenitor cells in vitro depend on the provision in the culture medium of an appropriate combination and amount of certain soluble growth factors. These must be sufficient to support the proliferation and differentiation to maturity of isolated progenitor cells suspended at low cell density in a semisolid matrix that limits cell movement and hence allows individual clones of mature progeny to be recognized and counted. In order for interpretable data to be obtained, a number of other conditions must also be met. First, it must be established that the number of colonies produced is linearly related to the number of cells plated under the conditions to be used. For applications in which the objective is to quantitate progenitors in different populations, the composition of the culture is ideally one that achieves a constant and preferably maximal plating efficiency of the particular progenitor of interest, regardless of the number or type of cells coexisting in the suspension to be assayed. This can be checked by confirmation of a linear relationship between the concentration of cells in the assay culture and the number of colonies produced (at least over the range of cell concentrations to be employed). Second, conditions must be identified that support all developmental stages through which the cells must pass to reach maturity. Third, the kinetics of clonal growth and maturation must be understood so that scoring is undertaken at an appropriate time and valid criteria are used for the recognition of separate and distinct types of colonies. Finally, since each colony is assumed to represent the independent proliferative activity of a single progenitor in the original cell suspension assayed, the quality of that suspension is an important consideration, as is the use of plating densities that avoid significant overlap between adjacently developing colonies or that may result in an inhibition of colony development due to overcrowding.

For each of the major myeloid pathways, the assay methodologies now most commonly used have been validated with respect to each of the above considerations. The two most commonly employed support systems (to make the cultures semisolid) for the detection of clonogenic erythropoietic cells are methylcellulose (EAVES et al. 1984) and plasma or fibrin clots (MCLEOD et al.

1974; NATHAN et al. 1978). Methylcellulose has the advantage that cultures can be readily maintained in appropriately humidified incubators for at least 3 weeks to allow adequate time for very primitive erythropoietic progenitors of human origin to generate mature progeny. Since mature erythroblasts are well hemoglobinized, they can usually be recognized directly by their red color without staining. (An exception to this are murine erythroid colonies whose tiny size and tight clustering of the maturing erythroblasts are sufficient for recognition in situ.) In contrast, plasma or thrombin clots are very difficult to keep for useful colony scoring beyond 2 weeks.

Secondly, methylcellulose has the advantage of being a thickening agent rather than a solidifying agent. Thus, methylcellulose cultures are really not semisolid but very viscous liquids, and, therefore, the cells within them can be readily removed using a micropipette, for example, for staining or cytogenetic analysis (DUBÉ et al. 1981; FRASER et al 1987). On the other hand, clotted cultures, like agar cultures, can be readily handled in their entirety because they are solid. This is more useful for staining entire colonies in situ and for the generation of permanent preparations to allow subsequent reevaluation or more flexibility in the time of scoring. Obviously, the method of choice depends on the particular application.

In our experience methylcellulose assays have proven more useful, reliable, and cost-effective for most routine experimental and clinical purposes. However, considerable training in colony evaluation is required because of the variation in morphology encountered in cultures established from different species or from individuals with different types of hematologic disorders. Agar has historically been more popular for studies of clonogenic granulopoietic cells and is still widely used for this purpose. However, for reasons not well understood, erythroid colonies develop poorly in agar cultures. Since optimization of erythropoietic and granulopoietic (and megakaryocyte) colony formation can be achieved simultaneously in methylcellulose cultures, this system has the additional advantage that assessment of different types of lineage-restricted as well as pluripotent clonogenic progenitors can be assayed simultaneously using a single procedure.

Figure 3 outlines the general procedure for quantitating human hematopoietic progenitors based on their ability to generate colonies of mature cells in what may now be considered "standard" methylcellulose assay cultures (GREGORY and EAVES 1977; EAVES and EAVES 1985). Standardization is achieved through the controlled use of culture reagents that give reproducible optimal plating efficiencies and internally validated scoring criteria. For the purposes of quantitating clonogenic progenitors from different sources or following varied treatments, all components are usually added at concentrations that are on the upper plateau of their respective dose-response curves for the type(s) of clonogenic cells to be evaluated, as determined from previous studies of colony formation in cultures, in which one component at a time is systematically made limiting. On the other hand, a frequent application of clonogenic culture assays is to determine whether the response

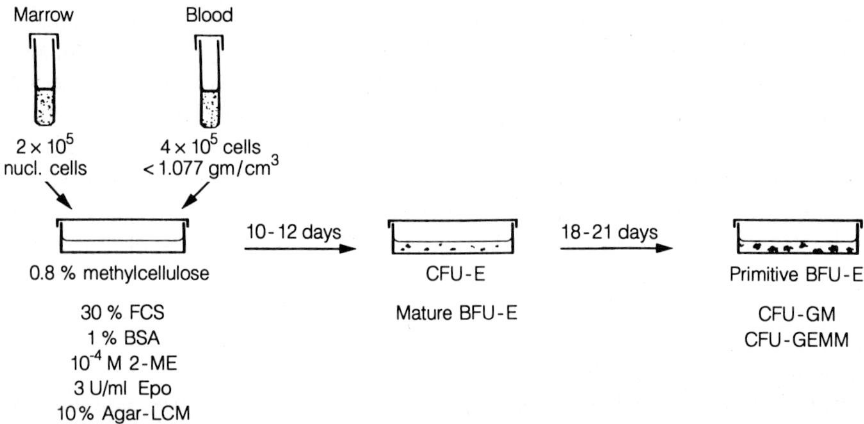

Fig. 3. Assay procedure for quantitating clonogenic progenitors. *FCS*, fetal calf serum; *BSA*, bovine serum albumin; *LCM*, leukocyte conditioned medium

of a given progenitor type to a known regulator (normally added as one of the culture components) has been altered. In this case, the number of cells added is then usually kept constant, and the amount of regulator is varied to generate a dose-response curve. It should be noted that many reagents including some impure growth factor preparations may contain substances that are toxic. It is therefore important to ensure that all components to be used give plating efficiencies equivalent to known standards at "optimal" concentrations. Even so-called pure preparations of growth factors now available commercially usually contain some protein additive (e.g., albumin) as a stabilizer that may not have been selected for lack of toxicity for in vitro colony assay applications.

Since the pioneering work of AYE (1976), who was the first to identify an additional hematopoietic growth factor requirement of cells passing through the early stages of erythroid progenitor cell development, it is now clear that several growth factors can have this effect. Perhaps the best documented are interleukin-3 (IL-3) and granulocyte-macrophage colony-stimulating factor (GM-CSF), although the latter, even at high concentrations, rarely stimulates all the primitive erythropoietic cells present. Standardization of culture conditions for early erythropoietic progenitors thus also depends on the standardization of this early stage growth factor requirement as well as the selection of an appropriate Ep preparation. We have found that crude conditioned medium prepared from normal human leukocytes under defined conditions which can be optimized for this application (EAVES and EAVES 1978) is a generally more effective all-purpose (and cheaper) reagent than IL-3 or GM-CSF for the stimulation of primitive human erythropoietic cells. Such conditioned media can be readily prepared, tested, and combined to give large batches of standardized, nontoxic material of reproducible activity. Moreover, concentrations that stimulate primitive erythropoietic cells maximally lie on the upper plateau of the dose-response curve for granulopoietic and multilineage (erythropoietic and granulopoietic) colony formation, although megakaryocyte progenitors require additional factors. Similarly, we have found that medium conditioned by pokeweed mitogen-activated murine spleen cells also prepared under conditions optimized for colony assay applications is a cheap and effective all-purpose reagent for assays of murine myeloid progenitors, in this case of all types, including pluripotent as well as lineage-restricted populations (Eaves et al. 1984).

The specific hematopoietic growth factor supplements used in colony assays have historically received the greatest attention because of interest in defining the factor responsiveness of different types of hematopoietic progenitors. Nevertheless, standardization of other "nutrient" requirements has also received considerable attention and is equally important for the establishment of reproducible assays to detect and quantitate progenitor cells on a routine basis. The components listed in Fig. 3 are those which we have found to be significant to obtain optimal plating efficiencies of erythropoietic progenitors of human (or mouse) origin; plating efficiencies may decrease if too much or too little of any of these is added. It is now clear that the "nutrient" requirements include provision of adequate levels of iron-transferrin, albumin, insulin (or insulinlike growth factor), and certain lipids (Guilbert and Iscove 1976; Sonoda and Ogawa 1988; Sawada et al. 1989). Although these may be sufficient for assays of murine cells, optimal plating efficiency of human erythroid progenitors may not be achieved when pure forms of these molecules are used to replace the requirements not met by erythropoietin and a serum-free source of IL-3 and/or GM-CSF. Thus, the use of selected "optimal" batches of fetal calf serum and solutions prepared from certain selected crude batches of bovine serum albumin are still recommended for most routine human progenitor measurements. In general, the growth requirements of granulopoietic progenitors are less stringent than those of erythropoietic cells. Thus, conditions suitable for the latter are also generally suitable for the former, but the reciprocal is not necessarily true.

In both methylcellulose and clotted culture systems, erythropoietic progenitors generate colonies that at the end of their growth appear to be made up of a multiplicity of smaller clusters of hemoglobinized erythroblasts. The initial recognition of this "clustering" phenomenon led to its rapid exploitation for the classification of different sizes of mature colonies. In conjunction with the simultaneous demonstration that erythroid colonies achieve their maximal size (at the time of their maturation) at various times (Gregory 1976; Gregory and Eaves 1977), it became possible to distinguish different categories of erythroid colonies. Subsequent experiments established that differently sized erythroid colonies obtained under optimal plating conditions were in fact derived from progenitors at sequential stages of differentiation along the erythroid pathway distinguishable in terms of a number of their physical, immunophenotypic, and kinetic properties (Eaves et al. 1979, 1984; Eaves and Eaves 1985).

The term CFU-E (colony-forming unit – erythroid) is conventionally used to refer to those cells that give rise to the smallest erythroid colonies readily visualized under light microscopy, that is colonies that consist of only one or two clusters of erythroblasts, each containing at least 8 cells at maturity. Such colonies are the first to become recognizable as erythroid (in assays of human cells on the basis of their content of readily detectable amounts of hemoglobin). Colonies derived from human CFU-E reach maximal numbers in methylcellulose assays 10–14 days after plating. Because the final mature erythroid cells produced are, like initially plated mature erythrocytes, unstable in regular culture media, the small CFU-E-derived erythroid colonies tend to lyze just as they complete their maturation. Hence, attempts to score them at later times may lead to a significant underestimation of their numbers. The progenitors of multiclustered erythroid colonies, or "bursts," are referred to as BFU-E (burst-forming unit – erythroid) and may be further subdivided into "mature" and "primitive" subpopulations that generate smaller (3–8 clusters per colony) and earlier maturing colonies as compared with larger (>8 clusters per colony) and later maturing erythroid colonies, respectively. In methylcellulose assays of human cells, the kinetics of erythroid colony growth and maturation makes it most convenient to score mature BFU-E-derived colonies at the same time that CFU-E-derived colonies are best counted. Cultures can then be returned to the incubator for another week at the end of which primitive BFU-E-derived colonies are best scored. The extra week's incubation allows maximal expression of the latter. It also minimizes potential confusion at earlier times with other types of colonies that are also usually present and are derived either from nonerythroid (primarily granulopoietic) progenitors or from pluripotent progenitors (with granulopoietic and/or megakaryocytic potential as well as late expressing erythropoietic potential, CFU-GEMM). By scoring all three of these at the later (3-week) time point, maximal distinction can be achieved.

Clonogenic granulopoietic progenitors defined by their ability to generate colonies of at least 20 (or by some groups 50) granulocytes and/or macrophages were in fact the first hematopoietic cells to be successively cultured in semisolid media (Pluznik and Sachs 1965; Bradley and Metcalf 1966; Senn et al. 1967). At that time, the full potentiality of these progenitors was not known, and the general term CFU-C (colony-forming unit – culture) was therefore coined. This term continued to be used until it became clear almost a decade later that the vast majority of all CFU-C actually represented a population of progenitors apparently restricted to the granulocyte and/or macrophage pathway of differentiation, and the terms CFU-G, CFU-M, and CFU-GM became established. Granulopoietic progenitors also vary in their proliferative capacity. Moreover, they show a similar relationship between this function and other changes associated with their position on the granulopoietic pathway, as is characteristic of erythropoietic cells at various stages of differentiation (Bol and Williams 1980). Although such distinctions have rarely offered profound new information and have therefore not been widely employed, the recent recognition that human CFU-GM with a proliferative capacity sufficient to generate colonies of at least 500–1000 cells are differently regulated than those with less proliferative capacity (Cashman et al. 1985) is relevant to the present discussion. These primitive CFU-GM, like primitive human BFU-E (Eaves et al. 1979) and CFU-GEMM (Fauser and Messner (1979) (the progenitors of mixed granulopoietic-erythroid-megakaryocytic colonies), are all populations in a vary slow state of turnover in normal adult marrow and share a common selective sensitivity to the inhibitory, albeit reversible, action of tumor growth factor-β (TGF-β) (Cashman et al. 1985).

Clonogenic progenitors capable of generating differently sized megakaryocyte colonies (CFU-Meg or CFU-Mk) have also been reported to exist in both murine and human marrow cell suspensions (Messner et al. 1982; Long et al. 1986). Because the terminal amplification of the megakaryocyte involves polyploidization, the minimum number of cells used to define the formation of a megakaryocyte colony is generally set at two. In unstained cultures, megakaryocytes are most readily confused with macrophages. Since the latter are prevalent in most assays, the use of a procedure for the unique identification of mature megakaryocytes (e.g., by staining for acetylcholinesterase in mouse assays or Factor VIII in assays of human cells) adds confidence to the data.

For additional descriptions of the properties and behavior of different types of clonogenic progenitors, the reader is also referred to other, more detailed reviews (Metcalf 1977; Levin 1983; Messner et al. 1985; Gewirtz and Hoffman 1990).

D. Use of In Vitro Clonogenic Cell Assays

Probably the most common use of in vitro assays for clonogenic cells is to monitor numerical changes of a given progenitor type. This may be part of an in vivo study in which an alteration in the size of the population of interest is anticipated, or it may be part of an in vitro study in which some experimental manipulation, either physical, biochemical, or biological, has been applied to the starting cell suspension prior to its assessment. In evaluating changes in progenitor numbers in vivo, the validity may be compromised by any one of a number of potentially confounding variables and will also depend on the quality of the available database for "control" values. Figure 4 illustrates the normal distribution of values expected from a series of measurements from a group of average adult humans. A test value is usually considered to be unusual if it lies at least two standard deviations above or below the mean of values determined for the control group. The

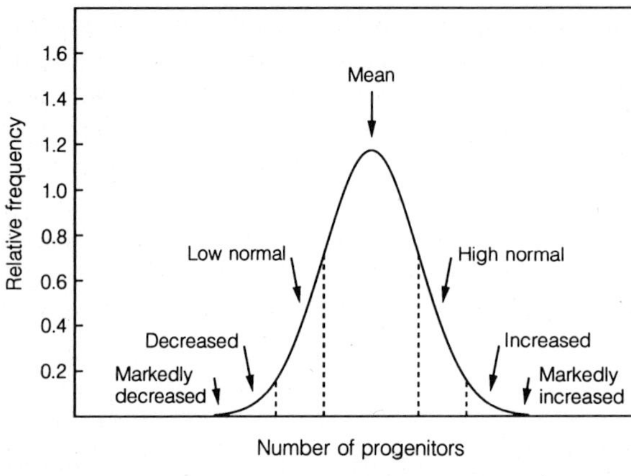

Fig. 4. Frequency distribution of normal progenitor values and the selection of criteria for the designation of "abnormal" values. *Inner set of dotted lines* indicates the range delimited by ±1SD on each side of the mean. *Next set* indicates the range delimited by ±2SD and the *final set* (barely visible) ±3SD

mean and range (i.e., ±2SDs) for hematopoietic clonogenic cells derived from a series of measurements made in our laboratory on normal adult human marrow and blood samples are listed in Table 2. It should be noted that the blood values are absolute. They are thus the most useful for in vivo comparisons. However, typically only a small fraction of the total clonogenic population is circulating, and the size of this fraction decreases even further for the more mature types of clonogenic cells. It is also likely that the proportion of progenitors which are circulating is not exclusively related to changes in their numbers (or concentration) in the bone marrow, since it is known that a variety of factors may influence the peripheral blood content of progenitors (e.g., the presence or absence of myelofibrosis). Therefore, interpretation of numerical changes in blood progenitor values must accommodate these possibilities.

Table 2. Numbers of clonogenic progenitors of various types in normal adult human blood and marrow

Progenitor	Marrow (per 2×10^5 buffy coat cells)	Blood (per ml)
CFU-E	194 (66–568)	16 (1–146)
BFU-E	92 (30–284)	134 (33–535)
CFU-GM	73 (12–412)	26 (4–147)

Values shown are means ± 2SD, from EAVES and EAVES (1984).

Interpretation of in vivo human marrow data is, unfortunately, also problematic. The most significant issue in this case is the nature of the specimen from which the data is derived. Although in some experimental situations, such as in studies of mice, absolute marrow progenitor measurements can be made (e.g., per femur), human marrow aspirates allow only the ratio of progenitors to total cells to be made (and hence values are expressed as progenitors per *n* cells, where *n* is the number of all nucleated cells in a defined sample). In addition, there is the problem that all marrow aspirates are diluted to some extent with peripheral blood, but the extent of dilution is virtually impossible to control or assess on a routine basis. Since the relative number of different types of progenitors is clearly different in marrow and blood (Table 2), the variable dilution of marrow aspirates with peripheral blood cells is a potentially important source of variability. Similarly, even without this problem, alterations in the relative number of mature cells or the presence of significant numbers of an abnormal population (e.g., leukemic blasts) can profoundly distort apparent progenitor concentrations, even when there may not necessarily be any change in the absolute size of the population.

These issues are of importance in the assessment of clonogenic progenitor numbers after various periods of maintenance of cell suspension in culture, for example, in the long-term marrow culture system (Dexter et al. 1980; Eaves et al. 1987). In this case, however, absolute changes in clonogenic progenitor numbers are easy to derive as long as a record is kept of the proportion of the long-term culture used to perform the clonogenic cell assay. Again, because the net change (up or down) in the total number of nonclonogenic cells present (e.g., fibroblasts, granulocytes, macrophages, lymphocytes) may be quite different from the change in clonogenic progenitor cell number, the relative concentration of the latter is unlikely to predict how absolute numbers have changed.

Table 3 lists the clinical conditions under which extensive progenitor measurements have been performed and the findings generally obtained. It can be seen that such measurements rarely reveal significant numerical changes. A notable exception are patients with CML, in whom a marked elevation in the peripheral blood content of all progenitor types is typical (Eaves et al. 1980; Eaves and Eaves 1987). Also, in patients with myelodysplasia (MDS) and acute myeloid leukemia (AML) at diagnosis or in relapse, CFU-GEMM, BFU-E, and CFU-E numbers in both blood and marrow appear significantly decreased but not necessarily absent, while normal CFU-GM are usually not detectable and are commonly replaced by varying numbers of progenitors that give rise to predominantly small colonies of

Table 3. Diseases for which erythropoietic clonogenic cells have been evaluated extensively for numerical changes

Disease	Effect on numbers of erythropoietic progenitors
Polycythemia vera	No change detectable
Essential thrombocytosis	No change detectable
Chronic myeloid leukemia	Increased
Idiopathic myelofibrosis	Increased in the circulation
Acute myeloid leukemia	Decreased
Myelodysplastic syndromes	Decreased

immature-appearing blasts (METCALF 1977; TILL et al. 1978; MESSNER 1984; GREENBERG 1986).

A diagnostically more powerful application of colony assay methodology has been to detect the presence in patient samples of erythropoietic cells that exhibit an abnormal (lack of a) requirement for Ep. The first indication of such cells in patients with polycythemia vera (PV) was provided by the initial suspension culture experiments of KRANTZ and colleagues (KRANTZ 1968). Using ^{59}Fe incorporation as an endpoint for in-vitro-stimulated erythroid precursors, they found that samples from patients with PV appeared to be able to differentiate in the absence of added Ep. This "Ep-independent erythropoiesis" was subsequently confirmed in colony assays and when subjected to quantitative dose-response curve analysis enabled the detection of a subset of cells within the neoplastic clone (PRCHAL and AXELRAD 1974; EAVES and EAVES 1978).

Surveys of large patient populations have now revealed that this ability of terminally differentiating erythroid cells to bypass the normal requirement for continuous contact with Ep may be seen under a variety of neoplastic conditions (EAVES et al. 1980). Its consistency in PV makes it the simplest diagnostic test to distinguish this myeloproliferative disorder from secondary erythrocytosis (EAVES et al. 1988). Detection of Ep-independent erythropoiesis is also an attractive laboratory test because it can be applied to peripheral blood samples as well as to bone marrow samples.

Although the presence of Ep-independent erythroid precursors is not exclusive to patients with PV, the presence of such cells in patients with any of the other myeloproliferative disorders occurs with greater variability. Ep-independent precursors have also been demonstrated in occasional patients with MDS or AML (ANDERSON et al. 1982; HOGGE et al. 1987; BRANDWEIN et al. 1990). This is not surprising in view of the possibility that the development of all of these diseases could share mutations that confer this phenotype. Interestingly, in experimental models it was shown that expression of a variety of viral oncogene products in murine erythroid precursors can also alter the normal Ep requirement (HANKINS et al. 1983). This suggests that interference with the Ep-stimulated signal transduction pathway by a variety of molecular mechanisms may be responsible for the naturally occurring state of Ep independence seen in neoplastic disorders of the human hematopoietic system.

E. Newer Assays for More Primitive Cells

The developmental properties that are thought to distinguish hematopoietic stem cells are pluripotentiality, self-renewal capacity, and very extensive proliferative potential. Accordingly, assays to detect and quantitate hematopoietic stem cells have historically relied on the use of conditions that support the expression of one or more of these functions. However, all are clearly difficult or cumbersome to assess on a routine basis, and associated end-points have therefore been adopted in most instances. For example, for many years enumeration of macroscopic colonies appearing on the surface of the spleen of supralethally irradiated mice injected intravenously at least 8 or 9 days previously with "test cells" of the same genotype (TILL and MCCULLOCH 1961) was assumed to quantitate the most primitive hematopoietic cell type. This was later challenged by the demonstration that most early appearing spleen colonies are pure (not multilineal) and are short-lived (disappear), and do not contain cells capable of generating new spleen colonies upon injection into secondary recipients (MAGLI et al. 1982). Even later appearing spleen colonies (12–14 days postinjection) may not necessarily be derived from pluripotent cells with the capacity to self-renew themselves, although this does appear to be the case when fresh bone marrow is assayed. Conversely, W/W^v mice clearly have functional, albeit defective, hematopoietic stem cells, and yet these do not form macroscopically visible spleen colonies (MCCULLOCH et al. 1964). Thus, macroscopic spleen colony formation, even if restricted to enumeration at later times after injection, is unreliable as an exclusive indicator of stem cell activity. In fact, several lines of evidence suggest that most cells detectable by standard spleen colony assays (and hence operationally defined as colony-forming units – spleen, CFU-S) may not be capable of long-term repopulation of hematopoietic tissues (BOGGS et al. 1982; PLOEMACHER and BRONS 1988; SZILVASSY et al. 1989b).

Another example of this situation may be that exemplified by cells capable of generating multilineage colonies in vitro (CFU-GEMM). In assays of murine cells, many CFU-GEMM produce colonies that achieve an enormous size ($>10^6$ cells) and contain daughter cells that can upon replating produce secondary, even tertiary, colonies of similar size and composition (HUMPHRIES et al. 1981; EAVES et al. 1981). Some can also be shown to contain CFU-S (HUMPHRIES et al. 1979, 1980) but not cells that can competitively repopulate mice in the long term (EAVES C.J., unpublished). Similarly, in the human system CFU-GEMM do not undergo extensive self-renewal under the conditions used to support expression of their multilineage differentiation potential (ASH et al. 1981; MESSNER 1984). These experiments do not exclude the possibility that some CFU-GEMM have the capacity for long-term self-maintenance since the requirements for maintenance of this function and expression of multilineage differentiation may be different. However, they do serve to highlight the fact that pluripotentiality and high self-renewal of that potential are not necessarily tightly associated properties. Thus, even where one stem cell property can be directly assessed as part of the end-point used to define a progenitor compartment, variable expression and/or association with other stem cell properties must be anticipated.

Because of these uncertainties, new approaches to stem cell quantitation applicable to both mouse and humans cells are badly needed. In the mouse, in which experimental transplants can be performed to evaluate long-term repopulation of the hematopoietic system, a method for quantitating lymphomyeloid repopulating cells based on limiting dilution methodology has been developed (Szilvassy et al. 1989b, 1990). To ensure detection of the most primitive hematopoietic cells with long-term repopulating potential and to enhance recipient survival (by provision of excess short-term repopulating cells), test cells are injected into supralethally irradiated recipients together with a large number of cells containing normal numbers of short-term repopulating cells (CFU-S) but reduced numbers of long-term repopulating cells (the latter being obtained by subjecting fresh marrow to two sequential cycles of transplantation and regeneration). Progeny of the test cells are distinguished by an innocuous genetic marker (e.g., Y-chromosome) and the number of competitive repopulating units (CRU) injected determined by assessment of the proportion of recipients showing detectable repopulation with test cells after a minimum of 5 weeks. Although obviously lengthy and cumbersome, this assay does have the advantage that the endpoint used is designed to detect stem cell activity.

In humans, such an assay is clearly not possible. However, since lymphomyeloid repopulating cells can be shown to persist and even proliferate in long-term marrow cultures established with mouse marrow (Fraser et al., 1990), it may be possible to identify some endpoint of the hematopoietic activity of long-term marrow cultures that is related to the number of CRU initially added. Recent experiments with long-term marrow cultures initiated with human cells suggest that the total clonogenic progenitor content after 5 weeks may provide such an endpoint (Sutherland et al. 1990). Certainly, this allows detection of a different and more primitive cell than the vast majority of cells detectable in standard in vitro colony assays (Winton and Colenda 1987; Sutherland et al. 1989; Andrews et al. 1989; Lansdorp et al. 1990; Udomsakdi et al., 1991). Moreover, the assay is quantitative and generally applicable, requiring only that standardized, preestablished, irradiated, normal marrow feeders be provided. The latter are absolutely necessary to support the generation of clonogenic cells from "long-term culture-initiating cells" (LTC-ICs) and therefore need to be removed as a variable in the assay, in much the same way as provision of an optimal concentration of CSFs is essential for the quantitation of colony-forming cells in semisolid assays.

Ideally, it would be preferable if LTC-ICs could be quantitated more directly by primary colony assays. Two approaches to the detection of colony-forming cell precursors ("blast colony-forming cells") have been reported, and both have been useful for characterizing primitive hematopoietic progenitor populations (Nakahata and Ogawa 1982a,b; Gordon et al. 1985, 1987a). However, these also require single colony replating studies for confirmation of the essential feature of each primary colony being typed. Thus, in practice, both of these "assays" are more cumbersome to carry out for analyses of test cell suspensions than the LTC-IC assay.

Moreover, the frequency of "blast colony-forming cells," like the frequency of LTC-ICs, in unseparated marrow (<1/10^4) makes it impossible to detect these cells in most hematopoietic cell suspensions without some major manipulation for removing or inhibiting the growth of the many CFU-GM, BFU-E, and CFU-GEMM also present.

F. Regulatory Mechanisms

Regulation of erythropoiesis by Ep appears to fit the classic concept of an endocrine feedback control loop readily monitored by assessing changes in serum Ep levels. Although very little has as yet been established concerning the molecular mechanisms that regulate the output of cells on other pathways, several principles have nevertheless emerged. First, it is now clear that the number of factors that can regulate the survival and/or proliferation of any single type of developing (or mature) hematopoietic cell either alone or in combination with another factor(s) appears to be large (see Table 1). Thus, although there seems to be some specificity of target cell action, simplistic models based on only one or two factors per lineage no longer seem realistic. Moreover, it now seems likely that many growth-factor-stimulated responses are determined by the nature of the target cell rather than by the particular factor to which the cell is exposed, although clearly some exceptions to this do exist. In addition, the list of factors thus far defined by sequence data is likely still incomplete. One might ask how murine fibroblasts support the maintenance of primitive human hematopoietic cells (SUTHERLAND et al., 1991).

Second, many of the hematopoietic growth factors can affect not only a broad range of target cells; they are also known to be produced by a multiplicity of cell types of both hematopoietic and nonhematopoietic origin. Growth-factor-producing cells in the latter category (e.g., fibroblasts, endothelial cells, astrocytes) coexist with hematopoietic cells in marrow tissue, which suggests they may exercise regulatory functions in the hematopoietic origins (CLARK and KAMEN 1987; MALIPIERO et al. 1990). However such cells are also present in other nonhematopoietic tissues. The situation is made even more complex by the fact that production of hematopoietic growth factors by most cells is, itself, generally a highly regulatable process, in many cases involving activation of the cell by another hematopoietic growth factor. As a result, it will likely prove very difficult to sort out direct and indirect effects of specific factors in the in vivo setting.

Third, there is now evidence that at least some of the hematopoietic growth factors can be bound to extracellular matrix components (GORDON et al. 1987; ROBERTS et al. 1988). This may well serve as an important mechanism for increasing and/or enhancing their effective concentration at localized sites of production. Similarly, other hematopoietic growth factors have been shown to exist as cell-bound forms (Rettenmier et al. 1987; Cerretti et al. 1988) with potentially the same result. Given the in vivo (McCulloch et al. 1965; Gidali and Lajtha 1972) and in vitro (Dexter et al. 1980; Cashman et al. 1985; Sutherland et al. 1990) findings suggesting that at least some aspects of hematopoiesis are locally regulated, such mechanisms may well prove to be of major importance.

Finally, it should be mentioned that there is growing evidence of "negative" regulators of hematopoiesis, i.e., molecules that can selectively arrest the proliferation of hematopoietic cells and even stimulate their death. Transforming growth factor (TGF-β) appears to have particular selectivity in this regard for very primitive hematopoietic cells (Keller et al. 1988; Cashmen et al. 1990) and lymphoid cells (Roberts and Sporn 1988). More recently, macrophage inflammatory protein-α (MIP-α) has also been shown to mimic TGF-β in its effect on primitive myelopoietic cells (Graham et al. 1990). Such effects are intriguing because of the known ability of these same cell types to enter a quiescent state reversibly. Thus, it may be essential to understand how competing and opposing signals influence hematopoietic cell behavior in order to describe how some populations are regulated.

G. Future Outlook

The development of clonogenic assays for murine and human progenitors in the mid-to-late 1960s introduced a new era in the characterization of the early stages of the hematopoietic cell differentiation process and its regulation by various hematopoietic growth factors. Many of these factors have now been isolated and expressed using recombinant DNA techniques in quantities sufficient for the initiation of clinical trials. In general, the use of these factors in vivo has borne out in vitro predictions and substantiated concepts of hematopoietic cell regulation which had been developed largely on the basis of data collected from clonogenic assays.

Much has thus been learned about the cellular anatomy of hematopoiesis from studies of cells with in vitro clonogenic potential. Colony assay procedures have also been found to play specific and valuable roles in the diagnostic armamentarium of tests available to the clinical hematologist. With time, it has become possible to develop standardized culture reagents that are commercially available. Hopefully, the further use of such reagents and the general adoption of more consistent scoring criteria will reduce discrepancies in results between laboratories. Moreover, as the surface phenotype of different classes of progenitors is analyzed in increasing detail, it may enable us to establish unique profiles for their direct distinction and enumeration. Thus, having had to abandon morphology in the 1960s to develop more powerful but increasingly cumbersome and indirect developmental strategies for the detection of primitive hematopoietic progenitor populations, perhaps we can now look forward to the use of such assays to define unique surface phenotype profiles of different types. We may thus anticipate the reemergence of a new era of morphology in which monoclonal antibodies replace metachromatic stains and multiparameter flow cytometric analysis replaces the use of the light microscope for the direct visualization and counting of primitive hematopoietic cells.

Also still at an early stage is our understanding of how growth factors elicit their various effects on the variety of target cells on which they are now known to act. An even greater problem is that of delineating which factors serve which regulatory functions in vivo both under conditions of normal and perturbed hematopoiesis. Cytokines of unknown identity or hematopoietic regulatory functions are still being discovered. Continued work to obtain this information should help to provide a better framework for predicting how growth factors might be most usefully exploited clinically and for approaching the exciting goal of large scale human blood cell production in vitro.

Acknowledgements. Some of the work described in this chapter was supported by the National Cancer Institute of Canada. We also thank Mrs. Lesley Reynolds for typing the manuscript. C.J. Eaves is a Terry Fox Cancer Research Scientist of the National Cancer Institute of Canada.

References

Abramson S, Miller RG, Phillips RA (1977) The identification in adult bone marrow of pluripotent and restricted stem cells of the myeloid and lymphoid systems. J Exp Med 145:1567–1579

Anderson WF, Beckman B, Beltran G, Fisher JW, Stuckey WJ (1982) Erythropoietin-independent erythroid colony formation in patients with erythroleukaemia (M6) and related disorders. Br J Haematol 52:311–317

Andrews RG, Singer JW, Bernstein ID (1989) Precursors of colony-forming cells in humans can be distinguished from colony-forming cells by expression of the CD33 and CD34 antigens and light scatter properties. J Exp Med 169:1721–1731

Ash RC, Detrick RA, Zanjani ED (1981) Studies of human pluripotential hemopoietic stem cells (CFU-GEMM) in vitro. Blood 58:309–316

Aye MT (1976) Erythroid colony formation in cultures of human marrow: effect of leukocyte conditioned medium. J Cell Physiol 91:69–78

Becker AJ, McCulloch EA, Siminovitch L, Till JE (1965) The effect of differing demands for blood cell production on DNA synthesis by hemopoietic colony-forming cells of mice. Blood 26:296–308

Boggs DR, Boggs SS, Saxe DS, Gress RA, Confield DR (1982) Hematopoietic stem cells with high proliferative potential. Assay of their concentration in marrow by the frequency and duration of cure of W/W^v mice. J Clin Invest 70:242–253

Bol S, Williams N (1980) The maturation state of three types of granulocyte/macrophage progenitor cells from mouse bone marrow. J Cell Physiol 102:233–243

Bradley TR, Metcalf D (1966) The growth of mouse bone marrow cells in vitro. Aust J Exp Biol Med Sci 44:287–300

Brandwein JM, Horsman DE, Eaves AC, Eaves CE, Massing BG, Wadsworth LD, Rogers PCJ, Kalousek DK (1990) Childhood myelodysplasia: suggested classification as myelodysplastic syndromes. Am J Pediatr Hematol Oncol 12:63–70

Bussolino F, Wang JM, Defilippi P et al. (1989) Granulocyte- and granulocyte-macrophage-colony stimulating factors induce human endothelial cells to migrate and proliferate. Nature 337:471–472

Cashman JD, Eaves AC, Eaves CJ (1985) Regulated proliferation of primitive hematopoietic progenitor cells in long-term human marrow cultures. Blood 66:1002–1005

Cashman JD, Eaves AC, Raines EW, Ross R, Eaves CJ (1990) Mechanisms that regulate the cell cycle status of very primitive hematopoietic cells in long-term human marrow cultures. I. Stimulatory role of a variety of mesenchymal cell activators and inhibitory role of TGF-β. Blood 75:96–101

Cerretti DP, Wignall J, Anderson D, Tushinski RJ, Gallis BM, Stya M, Gillis S, Urdal DL, Cosman D (1988) Human macrophage-colony stimulating factor: alternative RNA and protein processing from a single gene. Mol Immunol 25:761–770

Clark SC, Kamen R (1987) The human hematopoietic colony-stimulating factors. Science 236:1229–1237

Dedhar S, Gaboury L, Galloway P, Eaves C (1988) Human granulocyte-macrophage colony-stimulating factor is a growth factor active on a variety of cell types of nonhemopoietic origin. Proc Natl Acad Sci USA 85:9253–9257

Dexter TM, Spooncer E, Toksoz D, Lajtha LG (1980) The role of cells and their products in the regulation of in vitro stem cell proliferation and granulocyte development. J Supramol Struc 13:513–524

Dick JE, Magli MC, Huszar D, Phillips RA, Bernstein A (1985) Introduction of a selectable gene into primitive stem cells capable of long-term reconstitution of the hemopoietic system of W/W^v mice. Cell 42:71–79

Donahue RE, Yang YC, Paul S, Clark SC (1989) Human interleukin-9 (IL-9) is capable of stimulating erythroid colony formation in vitro. Blood 74 (suppl 1):116a

Dubé ID, Eaves CJ, Kalousek DK, Eaves AC (1981) A method for obtaining high quality chromosome preparations from single hemopoietic colonies on a routine basis. Cancer Genet Cytogenet 4:157–168

Eaves AC, Eaves CJ (1984) Erythropoiesis in culture. In: McCulloch EA (ed) Cell culture techniques – clinics in haematology. WB Saunders, Eastbourne, pp 371–391

Eaves AC, Henkelman DH, Eaves CJ (1980) Abnormal erythropoiesis in the myeloproliferative disorders: an analysis of underlying cellular and humoral mechanisms. Exp Hematol 8:235–245

Eaves AC, Cashman JD, Gaboury LA, Eaves CJ (1987) Clinical significance of long-term cultures of myeloid blood cells. CRC Crit Rev Oncol Hematol 7: 125–138

Eaves AC, Krystal G, Cashman JD, Eaves CJ (1988) Polycythemia vera: in vitro analysis of regulatory defects. In: Zanjani ED, Tavassoli M, Ascensao JD (eds) Regulation of erythropoiesis. PMA Publishing, New York, pp 523–535

Eaves CJ, Eaves AC (1978) Erythropoietin (Ep) dose-response curves for three classes of erythroid progenitors in normal human marrow and in patients with polycythemia vera. Blood 52:1196–1210

Eaves CJ, Eaves AC (1985) Erythropoiesis. In: Golde DW, Takaku F (eds) Hematopoietic stem cells. M Dekker, New York, pp 19–43

Eaves CJ, Eaves AC (1987) Cell culture studies in CML. In: Goldman JM (ed)

Bailliere's clinical haematology vol 1, no 4. Chronic myeloid leukaemia. Bailliere Tindall, London, pp 931–961

Eaves CJ, Humphries RK, Eaves AC (1979) In vitro characterization of erythroid precursor cells and the erythropoietic differentiation process. In: Stamatoyannopoulos G, Nienhuis AW (eds) Cellular and molecular regulation of hemoglobin switching. Grune and Stratton, New York, pp 251–273

Eaves CJ, Humphries RK, Eaves AC (1981) Self-renewal of hemopoietic stem cells: evidence for stochastic regulatory processes. In: Stamatoyannopoulos G, Nienhuis AW (eds) Hemoglobins in development and differentiation. Alan R Liss, New York, pp 35–44

Eaves CJ, Krystal G, Eaves AC (1984) Erythropoietic cells. In: Baum SJ (ed) Bibliotheca haematologica – current methodology in experimental hematology, vol 48. Karger, Basel, pp 81–111

Erslev AJ, Caro J (1983) Pathophysiology of erythropoietin. In: Dunn CDR (ed) Current concepts in erythropoiesis. John Wiley & Sons Chichester, pp 1–19

Eschbach JW, Egrie JC, Downing MR, Browne JK, Adamson JW (1987) Correction of the anemia of end-stage renal disease with recombinant human erythropoietin. Results of a combined phase I and II clinical trial. N Engl J Med 316:73–78

Fauser AA, Messner HA (1979) Proliferative state of human pluripotent hemopoietic progenitors (CFU-GEMM) in normal individuals and under regenerative conditions after bone marrow transplantation. Blood 54:1197–1200

Fraser C, Eaves CJ, Kalousek DK (1987) Fluorodeoxyuridine synchronization of hemopoietic colonies. Cancer Genet Cytogenet 24:1–6

Fraser CC, Eaves CJ, Szilvassy SJ, Humphries RK (1990) Expansion in vitro of retrovirally marked totipotent hematopoietic stem cells. Blood 76:1071–1076

Gewirtz AM, Hoffman R (1990) Human megakaryocyte production: cell biology and clinical considerations. Hematol Oncol Clin North Am 4(1):43–63

Gidali J, Lajtha LG (1972) Regulation of haemopoietic stem cell turnover in partially irradiated mice. Cell Tissue Kinet 5:147–157

Goodwin RG, Lupton S, Schmierer A, Hjerrild KJ, Jerzy R, Clevenger W, Gillis S, Cosman D, Namen AE (1989) Molecular cloning and growth factor activity on human and murine B-lineage cells. Proc Natl Acad Sci USA 86:302–306

Gordon MY, Hibbin JA, Kearney LU, Gordon-Smith EC, Goldman JM (1985) Colony formation by primitive haemopoietic progenitors in cocultures of bone marrow cells and stromal cells. Br J Haematol 60:129–136

Gordon MY, Riley GP, Greaves MF (1987a) Plastic-adherent progenitor cells in human bone marrow. Exp Hematol 15:772–778

Gordon MY, Riley GP, Watt SM, Greaves MF (1987b) Compartmentalization of a haematopoietic growth factor (GM-CSF) by glycosaminoglycans in the bone marrow microenvironment. Nature 326:403–405

Graham GJ, Wright EG, Hewick R, Wolpe SD, Wilkie NM, Donaldson D, Lorimore S, Pragnell IB (1990) Identification and characterization of an inhibitor of haemopoietic stem cell proliferation. Nature 344:442–444

Greenberg PL (1986) In vitro culture techniques defining biological abnormalities in the myelodysplastic syndromes and myeloproliferative disorders. Clin Haematol 15:973–993

Gregory CJ (1976) Erythropoietin sensitivity as a differentiation marker in the hemopoietic system: studies of three erythropoietic colony responses in culture. J Cell Physiol 89:289–301

Gregory CJ, Eaves AC (1977) Human marrow cells capable of erythropoietic differentiation in vitro: definition of three erythroid colony responses. Blood 49:855–864

Gregory CJ, Henkelman RM (1977) Relationships between early hemopoietic progenitor cells determined by correlation analysis of their numbers in individual spleen colonies. In: Baum SJ, Ledney GD (eds) Experimental hematology today. Springer, Berlin Heidelberg New York, pp 93–101

Guilbert LJ, Iscove NN (1976) Partial replacement of serum by selenite, transferrin, albumin and lecithin in haemopoietic cell cultures. Nature 263:594–595

Hankins WD, Kaminchik J, Luna J (1983) Transformation of adult and fetal hemopoietic tissues with RNA tumor viruses. In: Stamatoyannopoulos G, Nienhuis AW (eds) Globin gene expression and hemopoietic differentiation. Progress in clinical and biological research, vol 134. Alan R Liss, New York, pp 245–261

Hogge DE, Shannon KM, Kalousek DK, Schonberg S, Schaffner V, Zoger S, Eaves CJ, Eaves AC (1987) Juvenile monosomy 7 syndrome: evidence that the disease originates in a pluripotent hemopoietic stem cell. Leuk Res 11:705–709

Hultner L, Moeller J, Schmitt E, Jager G, Reisbach G, Ring J, Dormer P (1989) Thiol-sensitive mast cell lines derived from mouse bone marrow resond to a mast cell growth-enhancing activity different from both IL-3 and IL-4. J Immunol 142:3440–3446

Humphries RK, Jacky PB, Dill FJ, Eaves AC, Eaves CJ (1979) CFU-S in individual erythroid colonies derived in vitro from adult mouse marrow. Nature 279: 718–720

Humphries RK, Eaves AC, Eaves CJ (1980) Expression of stem cell behaviour during macroscopic burst formation in vitro. In: Baum SJ, Ledney GD, van Bekkum DW (eds) Experimental hematology today. Karger, New York, pp 39–46

Humphries RK, Eaves AC, Eaves CJ (1981) Self-renewal of hemopoietic stem cells during mixed colony formation in vitro. Proc Natl Acad Sci USA 78: 3629–3633

Iscove NN, Till JE, McCulloch EA (1970) The proliferative states of mouse granulopoietic progenitor cells. Proc Soc Exp Biol Med 134:33–36

Jacobs K, Shoemaker C, Rudersdorf R, Neill SD, Kaufman RJ, Mufson A, Seehra J, Jones SS, Hewick R, Fritsch EF, Kawakita M, Shimizu T, Miyake T (1985) Isolation and characterization of genomic and cDNA clones of human erythropoietin. Nature 313:806–810

Keller G, Paige C, Gilboa E, Wagner EF (1985) Expression of a foreign gene in myeloid and lymphoid cells derived from multipotent haematopoietic precursors. Nature 318:149–154

Keller JR, Mantel C, Sing GK, Ellingsworth LR, Ruscetti SK, Ruscetti FW (1988) Transforming growth factor β1 selectively regulates early murine hematopoietic progenitors and inhibits the growth of IL-3-dependent myeloid leukemia cell lines. J Exp Med 168:737–750

Krantz SB (1968) Response of polycythemia vera marrow to erythropoietin in vitro. J Lab Clin Med 71:999–1012

Lansdorp PL, Sutherland HJ, Eaves CJ (1990) Selective expression of CD45 isoforms on functional subpopulations of CD34+ hemopoietic cells from human bone marrow. J Exp Med 172:363–366

Leary AG, Ogawa M (1987) Blast cell colony assay for umbilical cord blood and adult bone marrow progenitors. Blood 69:953–956

Lemischka IR, Raulet DH, Mulligan RC (1986) Developmental potential and dynamic behavior of hematopoietic stem cells. Cell 45:917–927

Levin J (1983) Murine megakaryocytopoiesis in vitro: an analysis of culture systems used for the study of megakaryocyte colony-forming cells and of the characteristics of megakaryocyte colonies. Blood 61:617–623

Lim B, Jamal N, Messner HA (1984) Flexible association of hemopoietic differentiation programs in multilineage colonies. J Cell Physiol 121:291–297

Long MW, Heffner CH, Gragowski LL (1986) In vitro differences in responsiveness of early (BFU-Mk) and late (CFU-Mk) murine megakaryocyte progenitor cells. In: Levine RI (ed) Megakaryocyte Development and Function. Alan R Liss, New York, pp 179–186

Magli MC, Iscove NN, Odartchenko N (1982) Transient nature of early haematopoietic spleen colonies. Nature 295:527–529
Malipiero UV, Frei K, Fontana A (1990) Production of hemopoietic colony-stimulating factors by astrocytes. J Immunol 144:3816–3821
McCulloch EA, Siminovitch L, Till JE (1964) Spleen colony formation in anemic mice of genotype W/W^v. Science 144:844–846
McCulloch EA, Siminovitch L, Till JE, Russell ES, Bernstein SE (1965) The cellular basis of the genetically determined hemopoietic defect in anaemic mice of genotype Sl/Sl^d. Blood 26:399–410
McLeod DL, Shreeve MM, Axelrad AA (1974) Improved plasma culture system for production of erythrocytic colonies in vitro: quantitative assay method for CFU-E. Blood 44:517–534
Messner HA (1984) Human stem cells in culture. Clin Haematol 13:393–404
Messner HA, Jamal N, Izaguirre C (1982) The growth of large megakaryocyte colonies from human bone marrow. J Cell Physiol [Suppl]1:45–51
Messner HA, Solberg LA, Jamal N (1985) Human megakaryocytopoiesis in cell culture. In: Cronkite EP, Daniak N, McCaffrey RP, Palek J, Quesenberry PJ (eds) Hematopoietic stem cell physiology. Progress in clinical and biological research, vol 184. Aln R Liss, New York, pp 215–222
Metcalf D (1977) Hemopoietic colonies. In vitro cloning of normal and leukemic cells. Springer, Berlin Heidelberg New York
Miyake T, Kung CKH, Goldwasser E (1977) Purification of human erythropoietin. J Biol Chem 252:5558–5564
Nakahata T, Ogawa M (1982a) Identification in culture of a class of hemopoietic colony-forming units with extensive capability to self-renew and generate multipotential hemopoietic colonies. Proc Natl Acad Sci USA 79:3843–3847
Nakahata T, Ogawa M (1982b) Hemopoietic colony-forming cells in umbilical cord blood with extensive capability to generate mono- and multipotential hemopoietic progenitors. J Clin Invest 70:1324–1328
Nathan DG, Chess L, Hillman DG (1978) Human erythroid burst-forming unit: T-cell requirement for proliferation in vitro. J Exp Med 47:324–339
Ogawa M, Suda T, Suda J (1984) Differentiation and proliferative kinetics of hemopoietic stem cells in culture. In: Young NS, Levine AS, Humphries RK (eds) Aplastic anemia stem cell biology and advances in treatment. Alan R Liss, New York, pp 35–43
Ploemacher RE, Brons NHC (1988) Isolation of hemopoietic stem cell subsets from murine bone marrow: II. Evidence for an early precursor of day-12 CFU-S and cells associated with radioprotective ability. Exp Hematol 16:27–32
Pluznik DH, Sachs L (1965) The cloning of normal 'mast' cells in tissue culture. J Cell Physiol 66:319–324
Prchal JF, Axelrad AA (1974) Bone marrow responses in polycythemia vera. N Engl J Med 290:1382
Prchal JF, Adamson JW, Murphy S, Steinmann L, Fialkow PJ (1978) Polycythemia vera. The in vitro response of normal and abnormal stem cell lines to erythropoietin. J Clin Invest 61:1044–1047
Prchal JT, Throckmorton DW, Caroll AJ, Fuson EW, Gams RA, Prchal JF (1978) A common progenitor for human myeloid and lymphoid cells. Nature 274: 590–591
Raskind WH, Fialkow PJ (1987) The use of cell markers in the study of human hematopoietic neoplasia. Adv Cancer Res 49:127–167
Rettenmier CW, Roussel MF, Ashmun RA, Ralph P, Price K, Sherr CJ (1987) Synthesis of membrane-bound colony-stimulating factor 1 (CSF-1) and downmodulation of CSF-1 receptors in NIH 3T3 cells transformed by cotransfection of the human CSF-1 and c-*fms* (CSF-1 receptor) genes. Mol Cell Biol 7: 2378–2387
Roberts AB, Sporn MB (1988) Transforming growth factor β. Adv Cancer Res

51:107–145

Roberts R, Gallagher J, Spooncer E, Allen TD, Bloomfield F, Dexter TM (1988) Heparan sulphate bound growth factors: a mechanism for stromal cell mediated haemopoiesis. Nature 332:376–378

Sawada K, Krantz SB, Dessypris EN, Koury ST, Sawyer ST (1989) Human colony-forming units-erythroid do not require accessory cells, but do require direct interaction with insulin-like growth factor I and/or insulin for erythroid development. J Clin Invest 83:1701–1709

Seiler FR, Henney CS, Krumwieh D, Schulz G (1988) Colony stimulating factors – CSF. Behring Institute Mitteilungen, no 83. Medizinische Verlagsgesellschaft, Marburg

Senn JS, McCulloch EA, Till JE (1967) Comparison of colony-forming ability of normal and leukaemic human marrow in cell culture. Lancet 2:597–598

Sonoda Y, Ogawa M (1988) Serum-free culture of human hemopoietic progenitors in attenuated culture media. Am J Hematol 28:227–231

Suda T, Suda J, Ogawa M (1984) Disparate differentiation in mouse hemopoietic colonies derived from paired progenitors. Proc Natl Acad Sci USA 81:2520–2524

Sutherland HJ, Eaves CJ, Eaves AC, Dragowska W, Lansdorp PM (1989) Characterization and partial purification of human marrow cells capable of initiating long-term hematopoiesis in vitro. Blood 74:1563–1570

Sutherland HJ, Lansdorp PM, Henkelman D, Eaves AC, Eaves CJ (1990) Functional characterization of individual human hematopoietic stem cells cultured at limiting dilution on supportive marrow stromal layers. Proc Natl Acad Sci USA 87:3584–3588

Sutherland HJ, Eaves CJ, Lansdorp PM, Thacker JD, Hogge DE (1991) Differential regulation of primitive human hematopoietic cells in long-term cultures maintained on genetically engineered murine stromal cells. Blood 78:666–672

Szilvassy SJ, Fraser CC, Eaves CJ, Lansdorp PM, Eaves AC, Humphries RK (1989a) Retrovirus-mediated gene transfer to purified hemopoietic stem cells with long-term lympho-myelopoietic repopulating ability. Proc Natl Acad Sci USA 86:8798–8802

Szilvassy SJ, Lansdorp PM, Humphries RK, Eaves AC, Eaves CJ (1989b) Isolation in a single step of a highly enriched murine hematopoietic stem cell population with competitive long-term repopulating ability. Blood 74:930–939

Szilvassy SJ, Humphries RK, Lansdorp PM, Eaves AC, Eaves CJ (1990) Quantitative assay for totipotent reconstituting hematopoietic stem cells by a competitive repopulation strategy. Proc Natl Acad Sci USA 87:8736–8740

Till JE, McCulloch EA (1961) A direct measurement of the radiation sensitivity of normal mouse bone marrow cells. Radiat Res 14:213–222

Till JE, McCulloch EA, Siminovitch L (1964) A stochastic model of stem cell proliferation, based on the growth of spleen colony-forming cells. Proc Natl Acad Sci USA 51:29–36

Till JE, Lan S, Buick RN, Sousan P, Curtis JE, McCulloch EA (1978) Approches to the evaluation of human hematopoietic stem-cell function. In: Clarkson B, Marks PA, Till JE (eds) Differentiation of normal and neoplastic hematopoietic cells, vol 5. Cold Spring Harbor Laboratory, New York, pp 81–92

Turhan AG, Humphries RK, Phillips GL, Eaves AC, Eaves CJ (1989) Clonal hematopoiesis demonstrated by X-linked DNA polymorphisms after allogeneic bone marrow transplantation. N Engl J Med 320:1655–1661

Whang J, Frei E III, Tjio JH, Carbone PP, Brecher G (1963) The distribution of the Philadelphia chromosome in patients with chronic myelogenous leukemia. Blood 22:664–673

Winton EF, Colenda KW (1987) Use of long-term human marrow cultures to demonstrate progenitor cell precursors in marrow treated with 4-hydroperoxy-cyclophosphamide. Exp Hematol 15:710–714

Wu AM, Till JE, Siminovitch L, McCulloch EA (1968) Cytological evidence for a relationship between normal hemopoietic colony-forming cells and cells of the lymphoid system. J Exp Med 127:455–464

Yang Y-C, Ricciardi S, Ciarletta A, Calvetti J, Kelleher K, Clark SC (1989) Expression cloning of a cDNA encoding a novel human hematopoietic growth factor: human homologue of murine T-cell growth factor P40. Blood 74:1880–1884

CHAPTER 3

Kidney Regulation of Erythropoietin Production*

J.W. FISHER and J. NAKASHIMA

A. Introduction

Hypoxia is the fundamental stimulus for erythropoietin (Ep) production (FISHER 1983, 1988; KURZ et al. 1986). Our model for kidney Ep production postulates that an oxygen deficit initiates a cascade of events which lead to increased biosynthesis and secretion of Ep. The physiologic and pathophysiologic control involved is still not clearly understood. However, there is a primary oxygen-sensing reaction in the kidney which is triggered by a reduction in ambient partial pressure of oxygen (high altitude, hypobaria); a decreased passage of oxygen across the pulmonary endothelium (obstructive lung disease); a decrease in the oxygen-carrying capacity of hemoglobin (anemia); a decrease in oxygen utilization by the kidney (cobalt) (FISHER and BIRDWELL 1961); and a decrease in the flow of blood to the kidney (renal artery constriction, atherosclerosis, thrombosis).

B. Model for the Control of Erythropoietin Production

Our model for the control of Ep production is shown in Fig. 1. It seems most likely that several transducer substances released during hypoxia (adenosine, eicosanoids, catecholamines) and reoxygenation (oxygen-derived metabolites such as hydrogen peroxide) activate adenylate cyclase to generate cAMP, which in turn activates protein kinase A. The latter leads to the production of phosphoproteins which are involved in transcription and/or translation of the final 166-amino acid Ep molecule. These phosphoproteins may also be important in the release of Ep from the cell. Dibutyryl cAMP increases the secretion in Ep-producing renal carcinoma cells in culture (HAGIWARA et al. 1985; SHERWOOD et al. 1987) and leads to a rise in red cell mass when injected into mice (RODGERS et al. 1975a). An augmentation in renal cortical cAMP levels following cobalt administration in rats showed a temporal relationship with increases in plasma levels of Ep (RODGERS et al. 1975b).

* Supported by USPHS grant DK13211 and private funds.

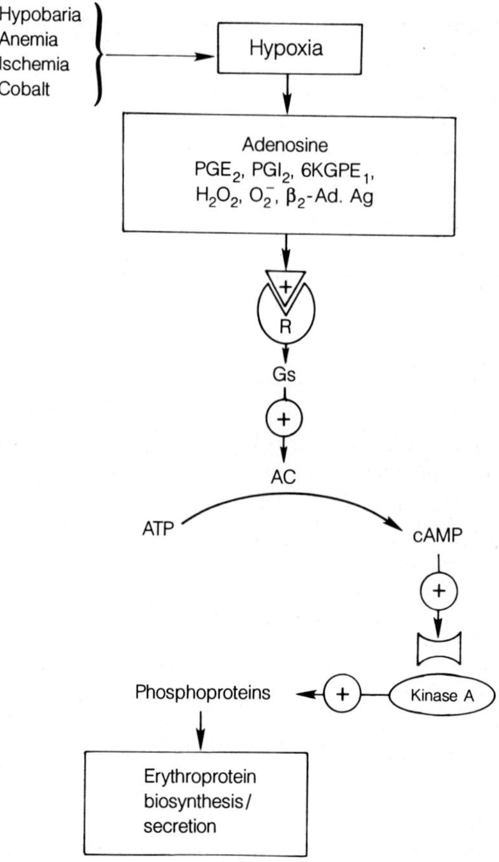

Fig. 1. Role of second messengers and hypoxia in the regulation of kidney production of erythropoietin. Erythropoietin biosynthesis/secretion can be switched on by hypoxia through the release of several chemical agents that activate receptors in the cell membrane to increase stimulatory G proteins (*Gs*): prostaglandin E_2 (*PGE_2*), prostacyclin (*PGI_2*), 6-ketoprostaglandin E_1 (*$6KPGE_1$*), hydrogen peroxide (*H_2O_2*), superoxide (*O_2^-*), and B_2-adrenergic agonists (*B_2-Ad. Ag*). Gs activates adenylate cyclase (*AC*), which increases cyclic 3′-5′-adenosine monophosphate (*cAMP*); cAMP activates kinase A to phosphorylate proteins (phosphoproteins), which are important in the transcriptional and/or translational stages of biosynthesis and/or secretion

The stimuli of Ep secretion that may act through adenylate cyclase are adenosine (UENO et al. 1988a; PAUL et al. 1988); the eicosanoids (prostaglandins), PGE_2, PGI_2, 6-keto-PGE_1 (NELSON et al. 1983); H_2O_2 which is generated from superoxide ion during hypoxia (TOLEDO-PEREYRA et al. 1974; SHAH 1984; MCCORD 1985); and β_2-adrenergic agonists (FINK et al. 1975; FINK and FISHER 1977). Therefore, we postulate that increased Ep production in response to hypoxia is most likely due to the release of several transducer molecules which may act in concert to increase Ep production, depending upon the severity of the hypoxic stimulus.

There are several possible negative feedback mechanisms in Ep production and/or secretion. Inositol trisphosphate (IP_3) increases the mobilization of intracellular calcium from the endoplasmic reticulum, providing the calcium for the activation of calcium calmodulin kinase. This activation may increase the level of an inhibitory phosphoprotein, thus resulting in a decrease in Ep secretion. It is quite possible that the reduction in IP_3 that was reported following ischemic hypoxia (STROSZNAJDER et al. 1987) could lead to a decrease in the mobilization of calcium from the endoplasmic reticulum, a decrease in the intracellular calcium pool, and therefore a decrease in the negative feedback on Ep secretion. Diacylglycerol levels are markedly increased in brain membranes following ischemic hypoxia (HUANG and SUN 1986) and may play a regulatory role by providing a negative feedback for Ep biosynthesis and/or secretion via activation of renal kinase C to increase the phosphorylation of inhibitory proteins (BERRIDGE 1984). Diacylglycerol and the phorbol ester 12-O-tetradecanaylphorbol-13-acetate (TPA) have been shown to inhibit secretion in an Ep-producing human renal carcinoma cell line (HAGIWARA et al. 1987). Diacylglycerol may be generated from a specific renal phosphodiesterase in response to hypoxia, and diacylglycerol lipase may increase the production of arachidonic acid. A rapid and specific biphasic liberation of arachidonic acid and stearic acid has been reported following cerebral ischemic hypoxia, which coincided with the time course for the decrease in brain ATP (YASUDA et al. 1985). Even though this arachidonic acid may be available for eicosanoid synthesis, most of it is due to the action of phospholipase A_2 on membrane phospholipids. The eicosanoids that are produced play a secondary role in increasing Ep production in response to hypoxia rather than being involved in a negative feedback mechanism (FISHER 1991).

Subcellular distribution studies (SMITH and FISHER 1976) as well as analyses of inhibitors of lysosomal hydrolytic and proteolytic enzymes (SMITH and FISHER 1976) indicate that an increase in these proteases in the lysosomal granules of the kidney correlates with rise in plasma levels of Ep during hypoxia or following cobalt injections. both cobalt and hypoxia have been reported to provoke a labilization of lysosomal membranes *in vivo*, as indicated by the discharge of lysosomal marker enzymes (SMITH and FISHER 1976). Injection of cobalt into rats produces significant increases in the activity of the renal proteases cathepsins A and B and plasma proteases (SMITH and FISHER 1976). The role of these lysosomal proteases in the cascade of events leading to increased Ep biosynthesis is not known. Earlier studies indicate that guanylate cyclase activity increases very early following cobalt adminstration (RODGERS et al. 1976) and generates cGMP, which activates protein kinase G and raises the levels of a phosphorylated protein. The function of these cGMP-generated phosphoproteins in Ep production is not clear.

C. Hypoxia and Erythropoietin Production

Hypoxia is considered to be the primary stimulus for Ep secretion both in vivo (NELSON et al. 1983) and in vitro (KURZ et al. 1986). A sensitive oxygen-sensor mechanism seems to be associated with the regulation of both renal and extrarenal Ep production. Hypoxia and cobalt treatment have been reported previously both to increase (GOLDBERG et al. 1987) and to decrease (NIELSEN et al. 1987) Ep biosynthesis in $HepG_2$ cells in culture depending on the concentration. It has been well documented that Ep production is controlled by the level of cAMP, either administered exogenously (HAGIWARA et al. 1985; SHERWOOD et al. 1987) or accumulated endogenously through the activation of adenylate cyclase. Forskolin has been reported to activate directly and reversibly the catalytic subunit of adenylate cyclase (SEAMON et al. 1981).

Studies were carried out to assess the effects of various concentrations of molecular oxygen and adenylate cyclase activation on Ep secretion in $HepG_2$ cell cultures. Figure 2 illustrates their exponential growth, with an approximate population doubling time of 1–2 days. Ep levels in the culture medium began to increase after the 2nd day in culture, and the cells reached confluency 4 days after seeding (2×10^5 viable cells/4.5-cm^2 well). This $HepG_2$ cell line has been reported to produce at least 17 major human proteins (KNOWLES et al. 1980); some of these, such as albumin and transferrin, could cause an enhancement of the in vitro bioactivity of Ep (GUILBERT and ISCOVE 1976).

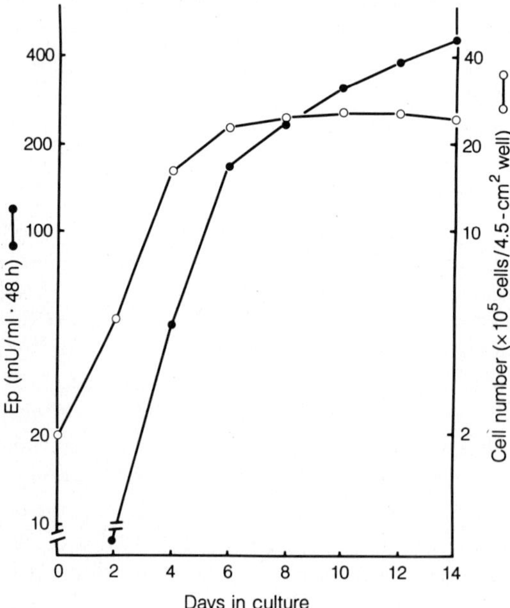

Fig. 2. Correlation between growth of $HepG_2$ cells (○) and erythropoietin levels (●) in 2-day spent culture medium determined by a sensitive radioimmunoassay

$HepG_2$ cells were incubated under several different oxygen tensions for 18 h (Fig. 3). Hypoxia (O_2 levels of 5% and 1%) enhanced Ep secretion in low-density ($<3.5\times10^6$ cells/25 cm^2) cells by 2.5- and 4-fold, respectively, when compared with normoxia (20% O_2) (10.63 ± 0.96 mU Ep/10^6 viable cells, n = 29 experiments). In contrast, hyperoxia (40% O_2) significantly reduced spontaneous Ep secretion (6.15 ± 0.53 mU/10^6 cells, n = 12 experiments). In no case was cell growth affected by treatment with 1%, 5%, 20%, and 40% oxygen. A similar inhibitory effect on Ep secretion was seen with 95% O_2, although this high level of oxygen inhibited cell growth by 10% (data not shown). As noted in Fig. 4, a significant dose-related increase in Ep secretion was produced when the cells were incubated for 12 h with cobaltous chloride in a concentration range of 2×10^{-6}–$2.5\times10^{-4}M$. These concentrations did not affect cell growth, whereas at higher concentrations ($>2.5\times10^{-4}M$) cobalt failed to enhance Ep secretion due to a marked reduction in cell viability.

$HepG_2$ cells were treated with forskolin (4×10^{-7}–$4\times10^{-5}M$) or cholera toxin (0.005–50 ng/ml) for 20 h under normoxic or hypoxic conditions. As shown in Figs. 5 and 6, these agents produced a significant ($P < 0.05$) increase in Ep secretion in hypoxic cells, whereas no increase was noted in the normoxic cells. 3-Isobutyl-1-methylxanthine (IBMX), a potent phosphodiesterase inhibitor, at a concentration of $10^{-4}M$ was added to all $HepG_2$ cell experiments in which cAMP was being measured to decrease the background phosphodiesterase activity. This concentration of IBMX did not affect basal levels of Ep in either normoxic or hypoxic cells. The growth of $HepG_2$ cells was not affected by any of the chemical agents tested, indicating that at the concentrations used these compounds did not produce a cytotoxic

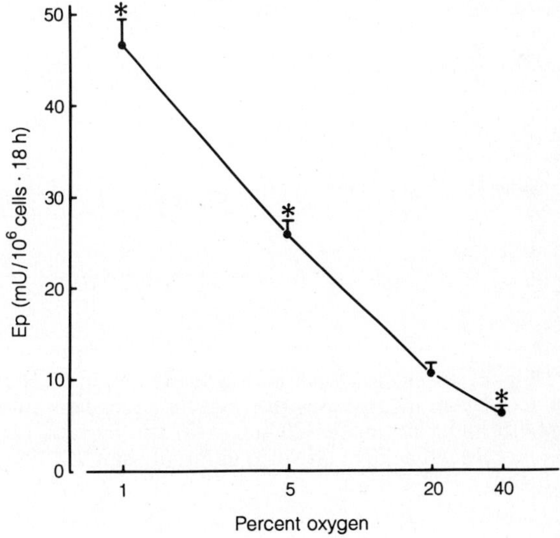

Fig. 3. Effects of hypoxia and hyperoxia on Ep secretion in $HepG_2$ cells. Cells were incubated at low density for 18 h at 37°C at O_2 concentrations between 1% and 40%. Cell count was usually $<3.5\times10^6$ cells/25 cm^2 after incubation and did not differ among the various O_2 concentrations. Each value represents mean ± SE of 12–29 samples. * Significantly different from 20% O_2 concentration ($P < 0.05$)

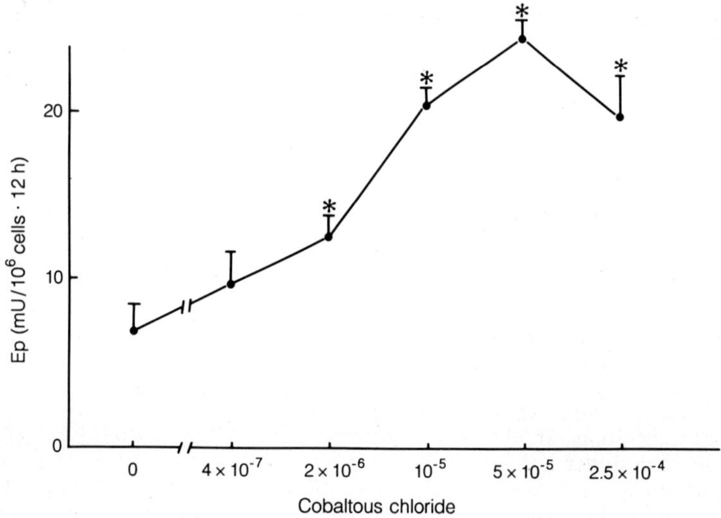

Fig. 4. Effects of cobalt on Ep secretion in $HepG_2$ cells. Cells were incubated at low density ($< 8 \times 10^5$ cells/4.5-cm^2 multiwell) for 12 h at 37°C. Each value represents mean ± SE of 8 samples. * Significantly different from control ($P < 0.05$)

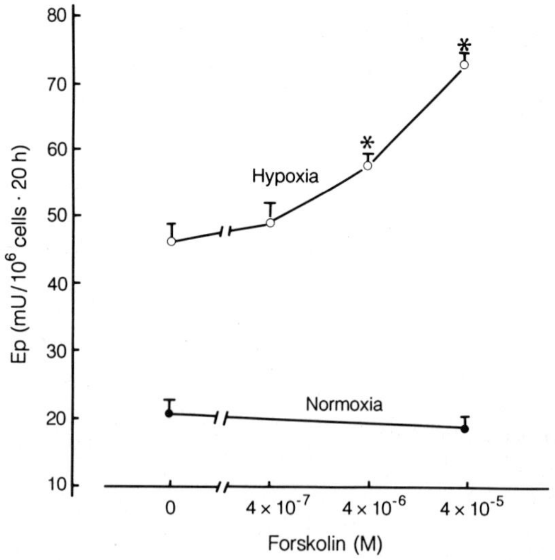

Fig. 5. Effects of forskolin on Ep secretion in $HepG_2$ cells in response to hypoxia. Cells were incubated with forskolin at concentrations of $4 \times 10^{-7} - 4 \times 10^{-5}$ *M* for 20 h under normoxic (20% O_2, ●) and hypoxic (1% O_2, ○) conditions. Each value represents mean ± SE of 6 different samples. * Significantly different from hypoxia alone ($P < 0.05$)

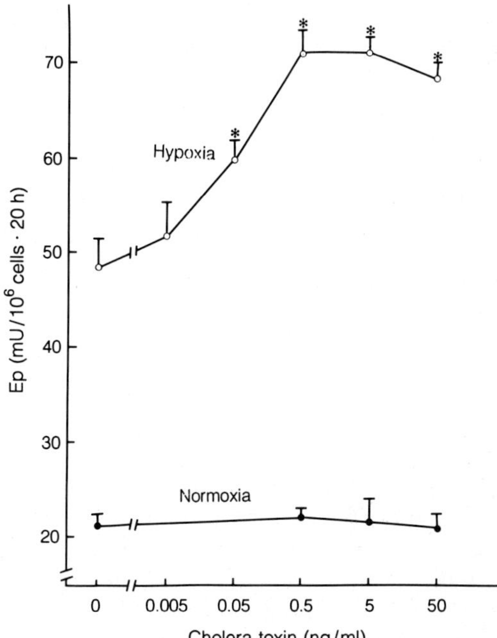

Fig. 6. Effects of cholera toxin on Ep secretion in $HepG_2$ cells in response to hypoxia. Cells were incubated with cholera toxin in concentrations of 0.005–50 ng ml for 20 h under normoxic (20% O_2, 5% CO_2, and 75% N_2) and hypoxic (1% O_2, 5% CO_2, and 94% N_2) conditions. Each value represents mean ± SE of 6 different samples. * Significantly different from hypoxia alone ($P < 0.05$)

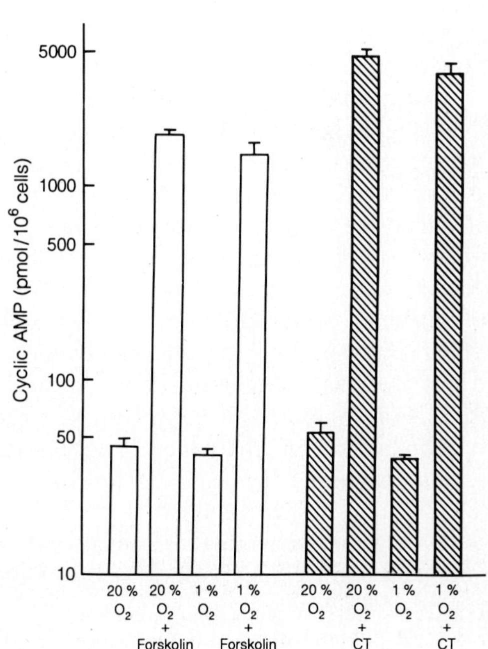

Fig. 7. Effects of 1-h treatment with $4 \times 10^{-5} M$ forskolin and 3-h treatment with 50 ng/ml cholera toxin (*CT*) on cAMP accumulation in $HepG_2$ cells under normoxic (20% O_2) and hypoxic (1% O_2) conditions. Incubations were carried out in presence of $10^{-4} M$ 3-isobutyl-1-methylxanthine. Each value represents mean ± SE of 3 different samples

effect. Figure 7 illustrates that a 1-h incubation with forskolin ($4 \times 10^{-5} M$) or a 3-h incubation with cholera toxin (50 ng/ml) produced a 45- and 90-fold enhancement of cAMP levels, respectively, under normoxic conditions. On the other hand, hypoxia (1% O_2) alone failed to increase cAMP levels in the $HepG_2$ cells when exposed overnight (data not shown). In addition, no synergistic action was seen when these cells were treated with forskolin or cholera toxin in the presence of hypoxia.

D. Adenosine and Erythropoietin Production

In order to study the relationship of our postulated primary external messenger adenosine on Ep production, it is necessary to have physiologic and/or pathophysiologic models. Ep is produced in the adult mammalian kidney, but in anephric subjects extrarenal production occurs primarily from the liver. Therefore, we employed two models for studies on the regulation of Ep production. The first is our in vivo model, radioiron incorporation in red cells of exhypoxic polycythemic mice, and the second is our in vitro model, a hepatocellular carcinoma cell line (Hep3B) producing Ep. The Hep3B cell line responds to both hypoxia and cobalt, two well-known stimuli of in vivo Ep production. We used exhypoxic polycythemic mice as the in vivo model for Ep production because it assesses the effects of hypoxia in the whole animal on both renal and extrarenal Ep production. A much more severe hypoxic stimulus is needed to switch on liver Ep production. Therefore, we postulate that most of the Ep being produced in vivo with the moderate hypoxic stimulus used in these studies is from renal sources.

Adenosine production by the kidney is significantly increased very early following ischemic hypoxia (MILLER et al. 1978). The primary oxygen-sensing reaction continues by triggering secondary biochemical changes such as a decrease in cellular ATP, increases in ADP and NADH, or stimulation of adenosine and hypoxanthine (JONES 1986). There are two independent routes for the production of extracellular adenosine. When the energy demand exceeds supply, cytoplasmic ATP is converted to ADP and AMP. Intracellular 5′-nucleotidase dephosphorylates AMP to yield adenosine, which is transported out of the cell by the symmetric nucleoside transporter. Adenosine has a ‘retaliatory’ action against stimuli that deplete intracellular ATP. For example, in many tissues it acts to improve energy supply by vasodilatation and stimulation of insulin-dependent glucose uptake. Extracellular adenosine can also be formed by a second route from the ATP released into the extracellular space by, for example, exocytosis of vesicles containing the nucleotide. Ectonucleotidases then degrade ATP to adenosine. This extracellular pathway acts to antagonize many of the extracellular effects of ATP.

Two subclasses of cell membrane adenosine receptors have been proposed (LONDOS et al. 1980; DALY 1982). They have been characterized physiologically and pharmacologically. A_1 adenosine receptors exhibit high affinity in binding studies (nanomolar) and are coupled to, and inhibit, adenylate cyclase. On the other hand, A_2 adenosine receptors exhibit lower affinity (micromolar) and are coupled to, but stimulate, adenylate cyclase. Adenosine could stimulate Ep production at high concentrations through A_2 receptor activation and could inhibit it at lower concentrations through A_1 receptor activation. A_1 receptor stimulation may lead to the activation of an inhibitory G protein which reduces adenylate cyclase activity, whereas A_2 receptor activation may stimulate a G protein which increases adenylate cyclase activity. Intracellular P binding sites for adenosine have also been identified (LONDOS and WOLFF 1988) which may be important in modulating its effects on biological processes. An increase in adenylate cyclase activity leads to the generation of cAMP, the activation of protein kinase A, and the phosphorylation of important nuclear proteins that may be active in the transcriptional and/or the translational stage of Ep biosynthesis in the kidney.

We have used our hepatocellular carcinoma cell line (Hep3B) which produces Ep spontaneously for in vitro studies on the role of adenosine in Ep production. Note in Fig. 8 that hypoxia (1% O_2, 5% CO_2, 94% N_2) produced an exponential increase in Ep secretion over a period of 16–24 h. These Hep3B cells were used at early confluency. The effects of N^6-cyclohexyladenosine (CHA), an adenosine analogue, on hypoxia-induced Ep secretion was studied (Fig. 9). A significant ($P < 0.05$) stimulatory effect of CHA on Ep secretion was noted at concentrations of 10^{-5} and $5 \times 10^{-5} M$,

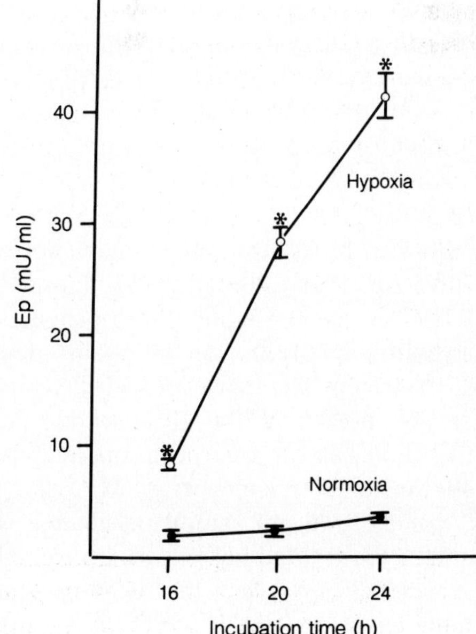

Fig. 8. Effects of hypoxia on Ep secretion in Hep3B cells. Cells were incubated at low density over a period of 16–24 h under normoxia (20% O_2, 5% CO_2, and 75% N_2, ●) and hypoxia (1% O_2, 5% CO_2, and 94% N_2, ○). Each value represents mean ± SE of 4 different samples. * Significantly different from the respective normoxic control ($P < 0.05$)

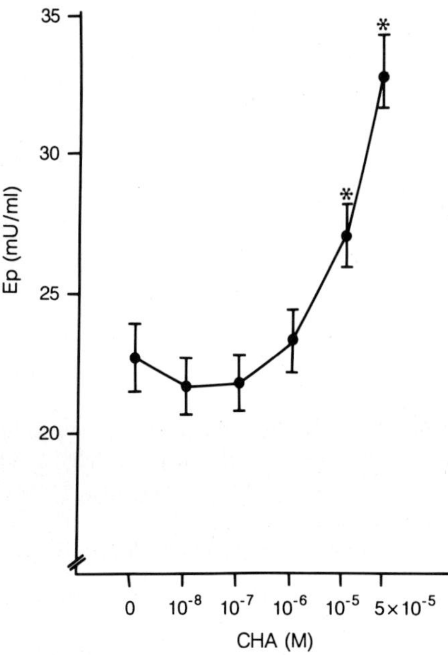

Fig. 9. Effects of N^6-cyclohexyladenosine (*CHA*) on Ep secretion in Hep3B cells under hypoxia. The cells were incubated with CHA in concentrations of 10^{-8}–5×10^{-5}*M* for 20 h under hypoxic conditions (1% O_2, 5% CO_2, and 94% N_2). Each value represents mean ± SE from 7 different experiments (6 replicate culture plates/experiment). * Significantly different from control ($P < 0.05$)

whereas a slight but not statistically significant inhibitory effect was seen at concentrations of 10^{-8}–10^{-7}*M*. No significant change in cell number was noted in these experiments. Thus, CHA seems to have a dose-dependent stimulatory effect on Ep secretion at higher concentrations and a slight inhibition effect at low concentrations.

With our in vivo model, the percentage of ^{59}Fe incorporation in red cells in exhypoxic polycythemic mice treated with adenosine (ADE) at concentrations of 400 and 1600 nmol/kg and exposed to 4 h of hypoxia was significantly ($P < 0.05$) increased to 12.26% ± 1.28% and 13.38% ± 1.53%, respectively, and significantly ($P < 0.05$) higher than vehicle controls (7.18% ± 0.67%) (Fig. 10). On the other hand, when the dose of ADE was increased to 6400 nmol/kg, the radioiron incorporation was not significantly elevated above the hypoxic controls. 5′-N-ethylcarboxamideadenosine (NECA), the A_2 agonist, also produced a significant ($P < 0.05$) increase in radioiron incorporation in a dose-dependent manner in a dose range of 25–100 nmol/kg. However, NECA produced much less of an augmentation at 200 nmol/kg than at 100 nmol/kg. NECA produced a significantly greater rise in radioiron incorporation than ADE but appeared to be toxic when administered in concentrations higher than 400 nmol/kg. In contrast, CHA did not produce a significant change in radioiron incorporation even when mice were treated with doses up to 1600 nmol/kg. It is possible that the test substances may affect the response to Ep or may protect Ep from degradation. Therefore, ADE and NECA were administered to mice along with Ep

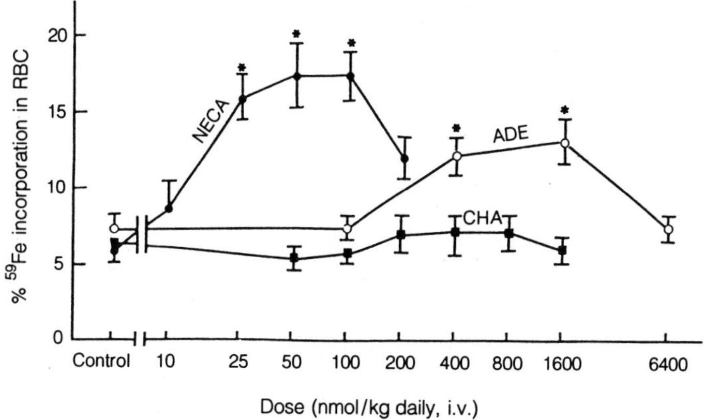

Fig. 10. Effects of ADE (●, 100–6400 nmol/kg daily, i.v.), CHA (■, 50–1600 nmol/kg daily, i.v.), and NECA (○, 10–200 nmol/kg daily, i.v.) on radioiron incorporation in red cells in response to 4 h of hypoxia on the 6th posthypoxic day. The control value is the radioiron incorporation for untreated mice exposed to reduced atmospheric pressure (0.42 atm) for 4 h on posthypoxic day 6. Each value represents the mean ± SE of 11–34 mice. * Significantly different from control ($P < 0.05$). Values in *parentheses* represent the hematocrits of mice in each group. The mean hematocrit for the control nonhypoxic mice was 60.5 ± 0.9 (n=35). The mean hematocrit values for all of the treatment groups ranged between 61.3–64.1 and were not significantly different

without exposure to 4 h of hypoxia on the 6th posthypoxic day. As noted in Table 1, the response to dosages of 0.2 and 0.8 units Ep was not significantly enhanced by ADE. However, a significant ($P < 0.05$) enhancement was seen with NECA when compared with the group receiving 0.2 units Ep alone. Therefore, it is unlikely that this increase in radioiron incorporation resulted from an effect of NECA on the response of mice to Ep since NECA alone significantly enhanced % ^{59}Fe incorporation.

Table 1. Effects of ADE and NECA on radioiron incorporation in response to erythropoietin (Ep)

Drugs[a]	Without Ep	Ep[b] (Units)	
		0.2	0.8
Saline	0.54 ± 0.06 (9)	5.48 ± 0.73 (9)	25.07 ± 1.46 (9)
ADE (1600 nmol/kg)	1.18 ± 0.61 (9)	7.18 ± 1.24 (10)	23.14 ± 1.13 (9)
NECA (100 nmol/kg)	2.33 ± 0.56 (8)*	9.55 ± 1.48 (9)*	24.14 ± 1.83 (8)

Each % ^{59}Fe incorporation value represents the mean ± SE.
[a] Drugs were administered i.v. on the 3rd, 4th, 5th, and 6th posthypoxic days.
[b] Ep was administered subcutaneously on the 6th and 7th posthypoxic days.
* Significantly different from control (saline) group ($P < 0.05$).
Numbers in parentheses indicate the number of mice.

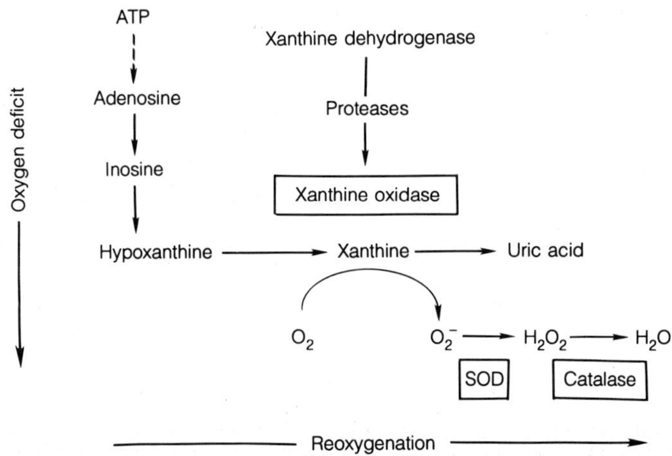

Fig. 13. A proposed mechanism for oxygen free radical production during hypoxia. Modification of model of McCORD (1985)

(BEAUCHAMP and FRIDOVICH 1970; DIONISI et al. 1975; OSSWALD et al. 1977; McCORD 1985). We postulate that adenosine is produced after a moderate to severe hypoxic stimulus, and the oxygen-derived metabolites H_2O_2 and superoxide (O_2) ion are produced following reperfusion (Fig. 13). Adenosine and perhaps H_2O_2 play a significant role in hypoxic stimulation of kidney production of Ep in vivo as renal blood flow waxes and wanes due to the regional redistribution of flow during intermittent hypoxia (UENO et al. 1988b). H_2O_2 enhances Ep production, perhaps through the activation of adenylate cyclase to generate cAMP, while superoxide ion produces a deleterious effect on the kidney to suppress Ep production. Superoxide dismutase may protect the kidney by converting superoxide ion to H_2O_2. The H_2O_2 generated may shield the kidney against injury and increase Ep secretion by decreasing the superoxide ion level or by increasing kidney Ep production directly.

References

Beauchamp C, Fridovich I (1970) A mechanism for the production of ethylene from methional: the generation of hydroxyl radicals by xanthine oxidase. J Biol Chem 245:4641

Berridge MJ (1984) Inositol triphosphate and diacylglycerol as second messengers. Biochem J 222:345–360

Daly JW (1982) Receptors: targets for future drugs. J Med Chem 25:197–207

Dionisi O, Galeotti T, Terranova T, Azzi A (1975) Superoxide radicals and hydrogen peroxide formation in mitochondria from normal and neoplastic tissues. Biochim Biophys Acta 403:292

Fink GD, Fisher JW (1977) Stimulation of erythropoiesis by beta adrenergic agonists. II. Mechanism of action. J Pharmacol Exp Ther 202:199–208

Fink GD, Paulo LG, Fisher JW (1975) Effects of beta-adrenergic blocking agents on erythropoietin production in rabbits exposed to hypoxia. J Pharmacol Exp Ther 193:176–181

Fisher JW (1983) Control of erythropoietin production. Proc Soc Exp Biol Med 173:289–305

Fisher JW (1988) Pharmacologic modulation of erythropoietin production. Annu Rev Pharmacol Toxicol 28:101–122

Fisher JW, Birdwell BJ (1961) The production of an erythropoietin factor by the in situ perfused kidney. Acta Haematol (Basel) 26:224–232

Fisher JW (1991) Regulation of erythropoietin (Ep) production. In: Handbook of renal physiology. Oxford University Press, New York (in press)

Goldberg MA, Glass A, Cunningham JM, Bunn HF (1987) The regulated expression of erythropoietin by two human hepatoma cell lines. Proc Natl Acad Sci USA 84:7972–7976

Guilbert LJ, Iscove NN (1976) Partial replacement of serum by selenite, transferrin, albumin and lecithin in haemopoietic cell cultures. Nature 263:594–595

Hagiwara M, Pincus SM, Chen I-L, Beckman BS, Fisher JW (1985) Effects of dibutyryl adenosine 3′–5′-cyclic monophosphate on erythropoietin production in human renal carcinoma cultues. Blood 66:714–17

Hagiwara M, Nagakura K, Ueno M, Fisher JW (1987) Inhibitory effects of tetradecanoylphorbol acetate and diacylglycerol on erythropoietin production in human renal carcinoma cell cultures. Exp Cell Res 173:129–136

Huang S, Sun GY (1986) Cerebral ischemia induced quantitative changes in rat membrane lipids involved in phosphoinositide metabolism. Neurochem Int 9:185–190

Jones DP (1986) Renal metabolism during normoxia, hypoxia, and ischemic injury. Annu Rev Physiol 48:33–50

Knowles BB, Howe CC, Aden DP (1980) Human hepatocellular carcinoma cell lines secrete the major plasma proteins and hepatitis B surface antigen. Science 209:497–499

Kurz AW, Jelkmann A, Pfuhl K, Malmstrom K, Bauer C (1986) Erythropoietin production by fetal mouse liver cells in response to hypoxia and adenylate cyclase. Endocrinology 118:567–572

Londos C, Wolff J (1988) Two distinct adenosine-sensitive sites on adenylate cyclase. Proc Natl Acad Sci USA 74:5482–5486

Londos C, Cooper DMF, Wolff J (1980) Subclasses of external adenosine receptors. Proc Natl Acad Sci USA 77:2551–2554

McCord JM (1985) Oxygen derived free radicals in postischemic tissue injury. N Engl J Med 312:159–163

Miller WL, Thomas RA, Berne RM, Rubia R (1978) Adenosine production in the ischemic kidney. Circ Res 43:390–397

Nelson JA, Drake S (1984) Potentiation of methotrexate toxicity by dipyridamole. Cancer Res 44:2493–2496

Nelson PK, Brookins J, Fisher JW (1983) Erythropoietin effects of prostacyclin (PGI_2) and its metabolite 6-keto-prostaglandin (PG_1) E. J Pharmacol Exp Ther 226:493–499

Nielsen OJ, Schuster SJ, Kaufman R, Erslev AJ, Caro J (1987) Regulation of erythropoietin production in a human hepatoblastoma cell line. Blood 70: 1904–1909

Osswald H, Schmitz HJ, Kemper R (1977) Tissue content of adenosine, inosine and hypoxanthine in the rat kidney after ischemia and post-ischemic recirculation. Pflugers Arch 371:45

Paul P, Rothmann SA, Meagher RC (1988) Modulation of erythropoietin production by adenosine. J Lab Clin Med 112:168–173

Rodgers GM, Fisher JW, George WJ (1975a) Increase in hematocrit hemoglobin and red cell mass in normal mice after treatment with cyclic AMP. Proc Soc Exp Biol Med 148:380–382

Rodgers GM, Fisher JW, George JW (1975b) The role of renal adenosine 3′,5′-monophosphate in the control of erythropoietin production. Am J Med 58:31

Rodgers GM, Fisher JW, George WJ (1976) Renal cyclic GMP and cholinergic mechanisms in erythropoietin production. Life Sci 17:1807–1814

Seamon KB, Padgett W, Daly JW (1981) Forskolin: unique diterpene activator of adenylate cyclase in membranes and in intact cells. Proc Natl Acad Sci USA 78:3363–3367

Shah SV (1984) Effect of enzymatically generated reactive oxygen metabolites on the cyclic nucleotide content in isolated rat glomeruli. J Clin Invest 74:393–401

Sherwood JB, Burns ER, Shouval D (1987) Stimulation by cAMP of erythropoietin secretion by an established human renal carcinoma cell line. Blood 69:1053–1057

Smith RJ, Fisher JW (1976) Neutral protease activity and erythropoietin production in the rat after cobalt administration. J Pharmacol Exp Ther 197:714–722

Spielman WS (1984) Antagonistic effect of theophylline on the adenosine-induced decrease in renin release. Am J Physiol 247:F246–F251

Strosznajder J, Wikiel H, Sun GY (1987) Effects of cerebral ischemia on [^{3}H] inositol lipids and [^{3}H] inositol phosphate of gerbil brain and subcellular fractions. J Neurochem 48:943–949

Toledo-Pereyra LH, Simmons RL, Najarian JS (1974) Effects of allopurinol on the preservation of ischemic kidneys perfused with plasma or plasma substitutes. Ann Surg 180:780–782

Ueno M, Brookins J, Beckman BS, Fisher JW (1988a) Effects of reactive oxygen metabolites on erythropoietin production in renal carcinoma cells. Biochem Biophys Res Commun 154:773–780

Ueno M, Brookins J, Beckman BS, Fisher JW (1988b) Effects of reactive oxygen metabolites on erythropoietin production in renal carcinoma cells. Biochem Biophys Res Commun 154:773–780

Yasuda H, Kishiro K, Izumi N, Nakanishi M (1985) Biphasic liberation of arachidonic and stearic acid during cerebral ischemia. J Neurochem 45:168–172

CHAPTER 4

The Mechanism of Action of Erythropoietin: Erythroid Cell Response

J.L. Spivak

A. Introduction

Erythropoiesis is regulated by erythropoietin (Ep), a glycoprotein hormone produced in the kidneys and to a lesser extent in the liver, which promotes the proliferation and differentiation of committed erythroid progenitor cells. Ep is not the only growth factor which interacts with erythroid progenitor cells, but it is the most important, and a lack of it is associated clinically with severe anemia, while in vitro, erythroid progenitor cells cannot survive without it. Ep is unique amongst hematopoietic growth factors for several reasons. It was the first one to be identified (Reissmann 1956) and the only one which fits the definition of a hormone. In contrast to the other hematopoietic growth factors, Ep was not initially recognized as a colony stimulating factor and has no influence on the behavior of the mature progeny of its target cells. With perhaps the exception of macrophage colony stimulating factor (CSF-1), Ep is more restricted in its progenitor cell nteractions than any other hematopoietic growth factor. Interestingly, Ep also shares in common with CSF-1 and granulocyte colony stimulating factor (G-CSF) the expression of its receptors by cells of placental origin (Muller et al. 1983; Rettenmier et al. 1986; Koury et al. 1988; Uzumaki et al. 1989). Although the reason for placental expression is unknown, it is noteworthy that the CSF-1 receptor is the product of the c-*fms* protooncogene (Sherr et al. 1985).

Although all of the major hematopoietic growth factors have been purified and their genes cloned, none has attracted more attention from biochemists and cell biologists than Ep. Several years ago, shortly after the gene for the human form was cloned, a review of the literature concerning the mechanism of action of Ep was published (Spivak 1986). Although such a review might have been deemed premature given that adequate quantities of pure Ep had only just become available, it served a useful purpose by summarizing the literature for scientists newly attracted to the study of this fascinating glycoprotein. A second review of the same subject only 5 years later should also not be judged as untimely considering the remarkable advances that have occurred since, including the cloning of the mouse Ep receptor (D'Andrea et al. 1989) followed by the cloning of the human Ep receptor (Jones et al. 1990; Winkelman et al. 1990). However, it must be acknowledged that there is still much to be learned about the physiology of Ep.

I. The Erythropoietin Gene

The gene for human Ep is present as a single copy on chromosome 7 in the region q11-q22 (POWELL et al. 1986; LAW et al. 1986; WATKINS et al. 1986), and restriction fragment length polymorphisms, inherited in a Mendelian fashion, have been identified at a frequency of approximately 20% in Caucasians and Orientals using the enzymes *XBa*I or *Hin*dIII and *Hin*fl, respectively (SEMENZA et al. 1987; LIN 1987). The human Ep gene is composed of 5 exons (582 base pairs) and 4 introns (1562 base pairs) and encodes a protein of 193 amino acids (JACOBS et al. 1985; LIN et al. 1985). The first 27 amino acids represent a hydrophobic leader sequence, while the remaining 166 constitute the mature protein before posttranslational processing. Computer-assisted homology studies have failed to reveal significant similarities between human Ep and any other protein (JACOBS et al. 1985; LIN et al. 1985).

As might be expected of a protein which is fully interactive amongst various mammalian species, the gene for erythropoietin (Ep) is highly conserved, more so than interleukin-2 (IL-2), granulocyte-macrophage colony stimulating factor (GM-CSF), or the interferons (SHOEMAKER and MITSOCK 1986). When the cloned human, simian, and mouse Ep genes were compared, a high degree of homology was observed: over 90% between the human and simian genes (MCDONALD et al. 1986) and approximately 80% for the human and murine genes (SHOEMAKER and MITSOCK 1986; MCDONALD et al. 1986). The most extensive homology was observed for the five exons, the first intron, the intron-exon boundaries, and the transcriptional control region (SHOEMAKER and MITSOCK 1986; MCDONALD et al. 1986). Interestingly, within the putative promoter site of the human gene, there are no sequences equivalent to the canonical TATA or CAAT boxes, which is true of other tissue-specific genes, nor was promoter function observed when the nominal murine promoter region, which does contain a CAAT-like element and shares a GATAACA sequence in common with the human gene, was inserted into a mammalian cell line (SHOEMAKER and MITSOCK 1986). It is of interest that both GM-CSF (MIYATAKE et al. 1985) and G-CSF (NAGATA et al. 1986a) contain TATA sequences but lack an upstream CAAT sequence, while IL-3 (YANG et al. 1986), GM-CSF, and G-CSF share in common noncoding 3′-ATTTA sequences which are not present in Ep and which may influence the degradation of mRNA for transiently expressed genes (SHAW and KAMEN 1986). Based on such observations, it was concluded that the proposed Ep promoter was more like that of a housekeeping gene than an inducible one (SHOEMAKER and MITSOCK 1986). This would be in keeping with the fact that Ep is constitutively produced, since it is never absent from plasma (SPIVAK and HOGANS 1987), even when there is extreme erythrocytosis (MOCCIA et al. 1980). Additionally, BERU et al. (1990) have identified several nuclear factors, one a 47K protein, the other a ribonucleoprotein, which bind to the Ep gene promoter in the -61 to -45 region relative to the transcription start site. The ribonucleoprotein was downregulated following cobalt chloride exposure, suggesting that it may act as a negative regulator of Ep gene expression. Recent studies using the Ep-producing hepatoma cell line, Hep3b (GOLDBERG et al. 1988), have implicated a heme protein as the intracellular oxygen sensor mediating Ep production and also documented that hypoxia influences Ep mRNA expression both transcriptionally and posttranscriptionally (GOLDBERG et al. 1991).

Recent studies of human Ep gene expression in transgenic mice have indicated that there are different sites for the induction of expression in the liver and kidneys, with the renal inducible element located greater than 6 kilobases (kb) 5′ or 0.7 kb 3′ to the gene, while the hepatic inducible element is present in a 4 kb region from 0.4 kb 5′ to 0.7 kb 3′ to the gene (SEMENZA et al. 1990). A negative regulatory element was identified between 0.4 and 6 kb 5′ to the gene. Multiple transcription initiation sites were also noted which demonstrated differential regulation, with downstream start sites being primarily utilized in the liver during tissue hypoxia, while upstream start sites appeared to be employed in the kidneys as well as during hypoxia.

II. The Erythropoietin Molecule

Based on its amino acid composition, the molecular weight of Ep is 18398 (JACOBS et al. 1985; LIN et al. 1985). Estimates of the molecular weight of the fully glycosylated protein based on gel filtration under denaturing conditions and sodium dodecyl sulfate (SDS)-polyacrylamide gel electrophoresis have ranged from 27000 (O'SULLIVAN et al. 1970) to 39000 (MIYAKE et al. 1977). Most recently, careful studies of the protein by sedimentation equilibrium have yielded a molecular weight of 30400 (DAVIS et al. 1987). As demonstrated by its hydropathic plot (Fig. 1), Ep is a hydrophobic protein

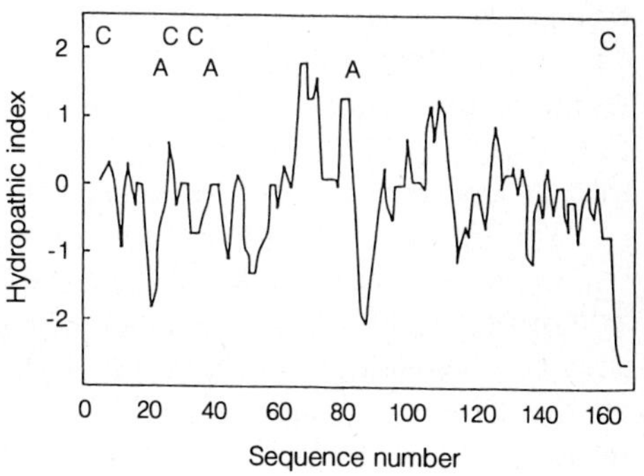

Fig. 1. Hydropathic analysis of human erythropoietin from its amino acid sequence *C*, cysteine residues; *A*, glycosylation sites (from SYTKOWSKI and DONAHUE 1987)

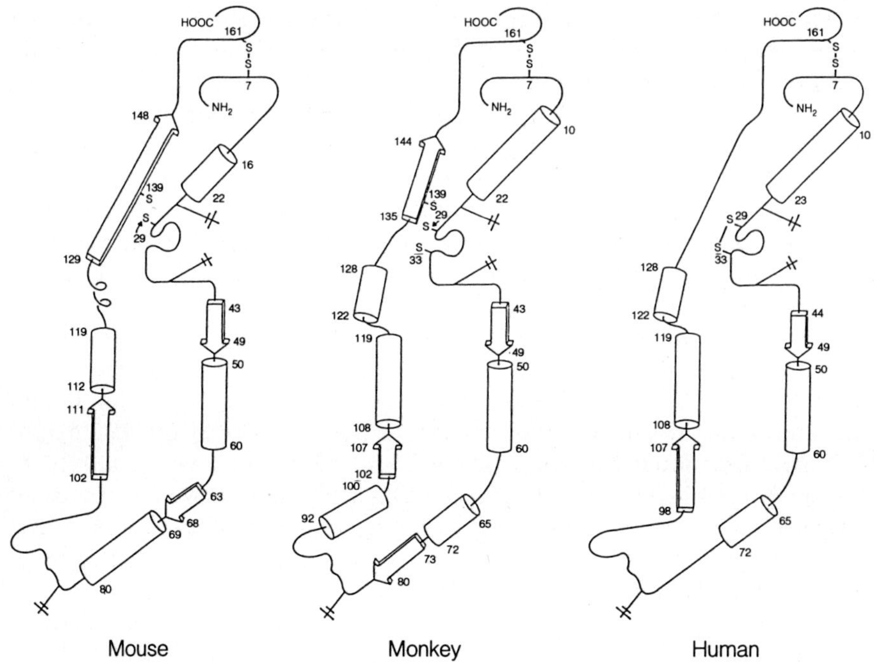

Fig. 2. Predicted secondary structures of mouse, monkey, and human erythropoietins based on their primary amino acid sequences. α-Helices are indicated by a *cylinder*, β-strands by an *arrow*, and β-turns by a *turn* in the amion acid backbone (from Shoemaker and Mitsock 1986)

(Sytkowski and Donahue 1987). The predicted secondary structures of mouse, primate, and human Eps based on their amino acid sequences are shown in Fig. 2 (McDonald et al. 1986). With regard to the amino acid composition, recent studies of its carboxy-terminus by peptide mapping and fast atom bombardment mass spectrometry have revealed that arginine-166 is absent from the mature, functionally active form of the hormone (Recny et al. 1987). The significance of this observation with respect to the biological activity of Ep is unknown, since an authentic Ep containing arginine-166 has not been examined. The absence of arginine-166 is common to both recombinant human Ep and human urine Ep, making it likely that this proteolytic modification occurs as part of posttranslational processing rather than as a nonspecific extracellular event (Recny et al. 1987).

The Ep molecule contains two internal disulfide bonds, and they or their conformational equivalent, since one of the four cysteine residues is absent in murine Ep (McDonald et al. 1986), appear to be necessary for biological activity. Alkylation of the sulfhydryl residues of these cysteines (Wang et al. 1985) or replacement of the cysteines by site-directed mutagenesis inactivated the hormone (Lin 1987). Under normal circumstances, however, the disulfide bonds are not exposed since Ep was not inactivated in vitro by reducing agents (ESPADA et al. 1973). Internal disulfide linkages are also a feature of GM-CSF (MIYATAKE et al. 1985), G-CSF (NAGATA et al. 1986a), and IL-3 (YANG et al. 1986). Although iodination of more than one tyrosine residue, occupation of lysine residues, or alteration of their charge inactivated Ep (GOLDWASSER 1981; SATAKE et al. 1990), this may be mainly a consequence of steric hindrance, since iodination of tyrosine-15 alone did not result in a loss of biologic activity, and site-directed mutagenesis of tyrosine-46, 145, or 156 did not affect biologic activity or failed to abolish it completely (LIN 1987; FELDMAN and CHUNG 1989).

Studies employing monoclonal antibodies as well as differences in the amino-terminal amino acid sequences of human and simian Eps suggest that the amino-terminus is also not involved in the functional behavior of the hormone (MCDONALD et al. 1986; SYTKOWSKI and DONAHUE 1987). Monoclonal antibodies produced against synthetic peptides corresponding to amino acid residues 99–118 and 111–129 of Ep neutralized its activity in vitro (SYTKOWSKI and DONAHUE 1987), suggesting that these hydrophilic regions may have a functional role. However, it must be noted that one of the hypervariable regions in murine Ep is present between residues 118–135 (MCDONALD et al. 1986), making it less likely that this area contains a biologically important domain.

Ep is a heavily glycosylated protein, containing one *O*- and three *N*-linked sites for oligosaccharide side chains. Carbohydrate residues make up 39% of the molecule by weight, and they include (in mole/mole of human urine Ep) fucose (2.9), mannose (9.2), galactose (12.9), *N*-acetylglucosamine (16.3), *N*-acetylgalactosamine (0.9), and *N*-acetylneuraminic acid (10.4) (SASAKI et al. 1987; TAKEUCHI et al. 1988). The carbohydrate composition of recombinant Ep is similar. The carbohydrate structure of Ep is complex and consists of bi-, tri-, and tetraantenary saccharides, some of which contain one to three *N*-acetyllactosaminyl repeats (SASAKI et al. 1987; TAKEUCHI et al. 1988); the degree of sialation as well as the degree of glycosylation also differ amongst the *N*-linked glycosylation sites (SASAKI et al. 1988). The carbohydrate residues of Ep appear to have a role in its biologic activity since cleavage of the oligosaccharide side chains with an endoglycosidase or alterations in glycosylation induced by site-directed mutagenesis diminished its in vitro biologic activity (DORDAL et al. 1985; DUBE et al. 1988), particularly when the core carbohydrate residues were removed (TAKEUCHI et al. 1990). The extent of glycosylation appears less important than the presence of *N*-linked sugars as incompletely glycosylated recombinant Ep produced by insect cells retained full biological activity (WOJCHOWSKI et al. 1987).

The carbohydrate structure is also important in maintaining Ep in the circulation; chemical or enzymatic removal of the terminal sialic acid residues exposes galactosyl residues which are recognized by hepatic galactosyl receptors (GOLDWASSER et al. 1974; SPIVAK and HOGANS 1989; FUKUDA et al. 1989). Asialoerythropoietin is cleared from the plasma 20-fold faster than the native hormone and accumulates primarily in the liver, where it is rapidly degraded (Spivak and Hogans 1989). Desigalation does not, however, impair biologic activity in vitro and may actually enhance it (Goldwasser et al. 1974) by reducing steric or charge hindrance.

The complex carbohydrate structure may serve several other purposes as well. Glycosylation of both *N*- and *O*- linked sites appears to be required for the processing and transport of the Ep molecule from its cell of origin (Dube et al. 1988) and may be involved in its transport across the blood-bone marrow endothelial cell barrier (Tavassoli 1979). Endothelial cells have been found to express receptors which recognize the galactosyl residues of transferrin (Regoeczi et al. 1980), and asialoerythropoietin reaches the bone marrow more quickly than its fully sialated derivative (Spivak and Hogans 1989). In this regard, it is of interest that oxidation of the exposed galactosyl residues of desialated Ep restores its plasma clearance to normal, suggesting that determinants other than carbohydrates are involved (Spivak and Hogans 1989). A recent report suggests that endothelial cells may express receptors for Ep (Anagnostou et al. 1990), but their affinity was low.

Like Ep, the CSFs are heavily glycosylated. GM-CSF has one *O*- and two *N*-linked sites for glycosylation (Donahue et al. 1986), IL-3 two *N*-linked sites (Yang et al. 1986), G-CSF one *O*-linked site (Nagata et al. 1986b), and M-CSF two *N*-linked sites (Kawasaki et al. 1985). Unlike Ep, however, there is substantial heterogeneity with respect to the extent of glycosylation of some of these proteins (Donahue et al. 1986) and, for GM-CSF at least, heterogeneity with respect to the degree of sialation (Nicola et al. 1979), which may be a feature of the site of its production. Also, in contrast to Ep, the biological activity of GM-CSF may be influenced by the extent of its glycosylation (Donahue et al. 1986). Modification of its glycosylation alters its plasma clearance kinetics and renal accumulation (Donahue et al. 1986).

When human urine Ep was first purified, two forms of equal potency, designated α and β, were identified on the basis of hydroxylapatite chromatography (Miyake et al. 1977). These were found to differ with respect to their carbohydrate content (Dordal et al. 1985). Recombinant human Ep produced in Chinese hamster ovary cells is identical to human urine Ep with respect to amino acid composition and sequence, carbohydrate composition and oligosaccharide structure, protein conformation, pharmacokinetics, biological activity, and specific activity. Based on carbohydrate content, α and β isoforms of the recombinant hormone have not been identified, and they may actually reflect in vivo processing of the urinary Ep or, perhaps, a genetic polymorphism considering the source of the crude starting material (Miyake et al. 1977). Given the identical physico-chemical and biological characteristics of native human and recombinant Ep and the wider availability of the recombinant protein, the latter is now generally employed for physiology studies.

III. Erythropoietin-Responsive Cells

Normally, maturation of hematopoietic progenitor cells proceeds serially from primitive, pluripotent progenitor cells to committed, lineage-restricted progenitors destined for terminal differentiation. The most primitive progenitors have the capacity for self-renewal as well as for differentiation to multipotent progenitor cells. The latter are restricted in their ability for self-renewal but can differentiate along multiple, lineage-specific pathways. As maturation advances, differentiation becomes progressively restricted to one particular pathway. The progeny of the most restricted hematopoietic progenitor cells gives rise to the morphologically recognizable, terminally dividing hematopoietic cells which constitute the majority of cells within the marrow cavity.

At each level of commitment, the proliferation and differentiation of hematopoietic progenitor cells are regulated by particular glycoproteins whose target cell specificity may be broad as in the case of IL-3 or restricted as in the case of CSF-1 or Ep. It is generally held, based on data derived from in vivo and in vitro clonal assays, that the process of stem cell commitment and differentiation is a stochastic process (Till et al. 1964; Nakahata et al. 1982a). According to this theory, glycoprotein regulatory factors serve to facilitate proliferation and commitment but do not direct it (Suda et al. 1983). Given the complex cellular composition of the bone marrow as well as its morphological and biochemical diversity, it is likely that while commitment may be a random process, it is facilitated or inhibited by local extracellular matrix and cell-cell interactions (Dexter et al. 1981; Eastment and Ruscetti 1985).

Early studies of Ep focused on its ability to stimulate globin synthesis and iron incorporation into heme (Krantz and Jacobson 1970), biochemical processes which we now recognize as occurring relatively late during erythroid maturation. However, given the crude nature of early Ep preparations and the diversity of the target cell populations within the bone marrow, these were at least erythroid cell specific, while other biochemical processes such as total protein or RNA synthesis were potentially nonspecific with respect to the cell of origin.

The development of in vivo and in vitro clonal assays for hematopoietic progenitor cells provided methods for analyzing target cell specificity and defining the site of action of the various hematopoietic growth factors. With respect to Ep, its target cell activity appears largely restricted to committed erythroid progenitor cells. For example, neither hypoxia nor hypertransfusion, both of which are known to alter the synthesis and plasma concentration of Ep, affect the proliferation of pluripotent hematopoietic stem cells (CFU-S) (Bruce and McDulloch 1964; Schooley 1966). Attempts to influence spleen colony formation by CFU-S through exposure to Ep in vitro (Van Zant and Goldwasser 1977) have not been reproducible (Schooley 1966; Krantz and Fried 1968; Spivak et al. 1989). Furthermore, using both in vitro and in vivo clonal assays, no correlation was observed between the number of CFU-S and the number of erythroid colony forming cells (CFU-E) in a spleen colony, suggesting that the two types of progenitor cells are separated by a number of cell divisions and do not share a direct precursor-progeny relationship (GREGORY et al. 1973). CFU-S and Ep-dependent erythroid progenitor cells also have different physical characteristics, as identified by their behavior during sedimentation at unit gravity (STEPHENSON and AXELRAD 1971). In addition, it is possible to inhibit the proliferation of pluripotent stem cells without impairing expansion of the erythroid progenitor cell pool by Ep (REISSMAN and SAMORAPOOMPICHIT 1970). Perhaps the most compelling evidence that Ep is restricted with respect to its target cell activity comes from clinical observations as well as attempts to manipulate its gene.

In patients with cyanotic congenital heart disease as well as in those with tissue hypoxia from other causes, erythrocytosis due to increased Ep production is not associated with leukocytosis or thrombocytosis. Similarly, patients receiving recombinant human Ep in pharmacologic doses for correction of anemia do not develop elevations of their leukocyte or platelet counts (ESCHBACH et al. 1987). Finally, transgenic mice bearing multiple copies of the Ep gene develop erythrocytosis but not leukocytosis or thrombocytosis (SEMENZA et al. 1989). Enhanced in vitro colony formation by CFU-GEMM, CFU-GM, and CFU-Meg has been demonstrated with bone marrow cells from anemic patients with either rheumatoid arthritis (MEANS et al. 1987) or end-stage renal disease (STONE et al. 1988; GANSER et al. 1989) who were treated with recombinant human Ep. However, such in vitro effects were not correlated with in vivo changes in leukocyte or platelet counts and could in part reflect a generalized improvement in marrow function during the correction of the anemia. Evidence has been presented, however, which suggests that augmentation of primitive progenitor cell proliferation in vitro by IL-3 is enhanced by Ep, which by itself had no effect on these progenitor cells (MIGLIACCIO et al. 1988). In this regard, the recent observation that in vitro high concentrations of Ep suppress granulocyte production is of interest (CHRISTENSEN et al. 1989). In vivo, however, no such stem cell competition has been observed in humans in numerous clinical trials and in animal studies (KOENIG et al. 1990).

The possible interaction of Ep with megakaryocyte progenitor cells has been widely examined with both positive and negative results. For example, in hypoxic mice, Ep production and erythropoiesis increased, but there was no augmentation in thrombopoiesis, while hypertransfusion, which suppresses erythropoiesis, failed to inhibit thrombopoiesis (EVATT et al. 1976). In in vitro culture assays, Ep did potentiate the proliferation of murine megakaryocyte colonies, but a high concentration of the hormone was required, and the number of colonies was small compared with that obtained with spleen-cell-conditioned medium (SAKAGUCHI et al. 1987a). Expression of low-affinity Ep receptors on megakaryocytes has been demonstrated by some investigators (FRASER et al. 1989) but not others (AKAHANE et al. 1989), and increases in rat platelet counts have been observed following administration of recombinant human Ep (BERRIDGE et al. 1988). However, in these experiments, the platelet count rose after the reticulocyte count (possibly reflecting relative iron deficiency), but the increase was not sustained, a transient increase in the leukocyte count occurred, and the appropriate controls receiving the vehicle but not Ep were not employed. In other studies, extremely high concentrations of Ep did not significantly increase platelet number (McDONALD et al. 1987). Furthermore, recombinant human Ep does not enhance human megakaryocyte colony formation in vitro (BRUNO et al. 1988) and does not increase the platelet count in humans when administered in vivo (ESCHBACH et al. 1987). In spite of the substantial homology amongst mammalian Eps, in vivo results obtained across species lines must be interpreted with caution.

It would, however, not be surprising if Ep influenced megakaryocyte colony formation since bipotent erythroid-megakaryocyte progenitor cells have been identified employing in vitro clonal assays (McLEOD et al. 1980), and one could envision a nonspecific enhancement of megakaryocytopoiesis through receptor down-regulation by Ep. In addition, bipotent erythroid-eosinophil and erythroid-mast cell progenitors have also been described (NAKAHATA et al. 1982b; WENDLING et al. 1985; NAKAZAWA et al. 1989). It is of interest in this regard that an important DNA binding protein (GATA-1, previously known as GF-1, NF-ε1, Ery*f*-1) (MARTIN et al. 1988; WALL et al. 1988; EVANS et al. 1988; TSAI et al. 1989) which is erythroid-specific is also expressed in megakaryocytes and mast cells (MARTIN et al. 1990; ROMEO et al. 1990). There is no evidence, however, that Ep causes an increase in eosinophil or mast cell production either in vitro or in vivo. The inherent difficulty in making inferences concerning clinical effects from in vitro observations is well illustrated by the research in this area.

If controversy exists concerning the interaction of Ep with nonerythroid cells, this is not the situation with erythroid progenitor cells. These cells can be cultivated in vitro in a variety of viscous media including agar (HORLAND et al. 1977), fibrin (STEPHENSON et al. 1971), and methylcellulose (ISCOVE et al. 1974) as well as in liquid culture (KRANTZ and JACOBSON 1970). Each type of culture system offers advantages lacking in others, and consequently, they can be employed in a complementary fashion. The assays using viscous media provide an opportunity to evaluate progenitor cell behavior on a clonal basis while liquid culture systems lend themselves well to either short- (GLASS et al. 1975) or long-term (DEXTER et al. 1981; EASTMENT and RUSCETTI 1985; ELIASON et al. 1979) studies. In addition, erythroid progenitors can be assayed in vivo with the spleen colony technique (GREGORY et al. 1975), in diffusion chambers (STEINBERG et al. 1976), or by incorporation of radioactive iron (KRANTZ and JACOBSON 1970). Each of these systems also has its faults and must be employed critically. A major problem is the presence of undefined, complex, or impure ingredients in the culture medium which can produce effects that may be trivial rather than physiologically significant. Serum is a frequent cause of experimental and interlaboratory variability, and results obtained when culture conditions are suboptimal will certainly not have the same relevance as when optimal culture conditions are achieved. In vitro systems, of course, cannot faithfully mimic the in vivo environment. For example, normal human erythroid progenitor cells cultured in vitro yield progeny which exhibit morphologic abnormalities similar to those seen clinically in certain dyserythropoietic states, indicating that the in vitro environment is not totally hospitable (PARMLEY et al. 1978). Finally, given the complexity of the cell populations in hematopoietic organs and the over-lapping effects of many of the hematopoietic growth factors and interleukins as well as the nonspecific contributions of agents such as endotoxin, it is apparent that caution must always be employed when interpreting the results of in vitro or in vivo assays of hematopoietic progenitor cells.

Amongst erythroid progenitor cells, as with hematopoietic progenitor cells in general, there exists a hierarchy based on age, and the various classes of erythroid progenitor cells within this hierarchy can be distinguished by physical properties using sedimentation behavior (HEATH et al. 1976; MISITI and SPIVAK 1979b; OGAWA et al. 1977; GREGORY and EAVES 1978), by sensitivity to other hematopoietic growth factors as well as to Ep (AYE 1977; ISCOVE 1978a,b), by cell cycle status (GREGORY and EAVES 1978; ISCOVE 1977), and by the kinetics and morphology of the colonies they form in vitro (STEPHENSON et al. 1971; OGAWA et al. 1977; GREGORY and EAVES 1977, 1978; AXELRAD et al. 1974; ISCOVE and SIEBER 1975) and in vivo (GREGORY et al. 1975; GERARD et al. 1978; GREENBERG and ROBINSON 1978). Based on these characteristics, at least five classes of erythroid progenitor cells capable of forming colonies in vitro can be identified: the macroscopic burst-forming unit (BFU-E) (HUMPHRIES et al. 1979), the early (microscopic) erythroid burst-forming unit (AXELRAD et al. 1974), the late erythroid burst-forming unit (OGAWA et al. 1977; GREGORY 1976), the early erythroid colony-forming unit (CFU-E) (STEPHENSON et al. 1971), and the late erythroid cluster-forming unit (MISITI and SPIVAK 1979b); the latter may correspond to the proerythroblast which is also Ep-sensitive (GLASS et al. 1975).

The macroscopic BFU-E is the earliest "erythroid" progenitor cell identified in vitro but is actually a multipotent progenitor cell of very high proliferative but limited self-renewal capacity which is closely related to the pluripotent hematopoietic stem cell (CFU-S) and for which erythroid differentiation is but one potential (HUMPHRIES et al. 1979). Only the other four classes of will concern us here, since these cells are restricted in their differentiation to the erythroid pathway and are directly influenced by Ep.

IV. The Erythroid Burst-Forming Unit

As indicated above, the BFU-E, so designated because of the morphology of the colonies it produces in vitro, can be divided into early and late forms.

The early one is developmentally related to the CFU-S but not as closely as the macroscopic burst-forming unit (HUMPHRIES et al. 1979; GREGORY 1976). Early BFU-E are found in the circulation (HARA and OGAWA 1976; CLARKE and HOUSMAN 1977) as well as the marrow and at least in vitro demonstrate a requirement for growth factors such as interleukin-3 (IL-3) (ISCOVE 1978a,b; GOLDWASSER et al. 1983; ISCOVE et al. 1982) or granulocyte-macrophage colony stimulating factor (GM-CSF) (METCALF et al. 1980; DONAHUE et al. 1985), as well as Ep (ISCOVE 1978). Recently, IL-9 has been shown to support BFU-E proliferation (DONAHUE and YANG 1990). In this regard, fetal liver BFU-E appear to differ from adult periheral blood BFU-E since the former require only Ep for colony formation in vitro, while the latter require IL-3 or GM-CSF as well as Ep (EMERSON et al. 1989; VALTIERI et al. 1989).

Ep sensitivity in vitro appears to be acquired as BFU-E mature and can be employed to define their state of maturation (STEFF et al. 1986). For example, peripheral blood BFU-E appear to be the most primitive since they can proliferate the longest in vitro in the absence of Ep (LIPTON et al. 1981). The extent to which Ep might be required in vivo, however, is another issue. The conclusion that early BFU-E are Ep-independent was based on data derived using hypertransfused mice, in which it was assumed that Ep production was almost completely suppressed. However, with more sensitive assay techniques, it is now clear that Ep production persists in this situation (MOCCIA et al. 1980). Consequently, the actual in vivo behavior of BFU-E in the absence of Ep is unknown. What is clear is that the majority of BFU-E are not in cell cycle (ISCOVE 1977), and neither hypoxia nor hypertransfusion have more than a transient effect on their proliferation (PESCHLE et al. 1979, 1980), but when there is a sustained demand for erythrocytes, BFU-E proliferation increases (ISCOVE 1977).

Kinetic studies indicate that the early BFU-E pool is maintained by multipotent or pluripotent stem cells (GREGORY et al. 1975) and that early BFU-E are responsible for replenishing the late or mature BFU-E pool (ISCOVE 1977; GREGORY 1976; UMEMURA et al. 1989). It is these latter cells which acquire sufficient sensitivity to Ep to function as those responsible for replenishing or expanding the population of erythroid progenitors (CFU-E) which terminally differentiate (GREGORY 1976; ISCOVE 1978a,b; UDUPA and REISSMAN 1979). The late BFU-E appears to represent a crucial transition phase in erythroid differentiation, since it is at this stage that endotoxin interrupts erythropoiesis (UDUPA and REISSMAN 1977), clonal suppression arises in polycythemia vera (ADAMSON et al. 1980), and infection with certain viruses occurs (KOST et al. 1979).

V. The Colony-Forming Unit Erythroid

CFU-E represent committed erythroid progenitor cells which differentiate into recognizable erythroid cells (STEPHENSON et al. 1971). CFU-E are the most Ep-dependent of the various classes of erythroid progenitor cells, and the majority are in cell cycle (Gregory and Eaves 1978; Iscove 1977). In vitro, these cells do not survive long in the absence of Ep (Iscove 1978a,b). The proliferative capacity of CFU-E is very limited, and it is capable of forming colonies with usually no more than 50 cells. The clonality of CFU-E has been demonstrated by time-lapse photography (Cormack 1976) and karyotypic (Strome et al. 1978) and isoenzyme analysis (Prchal et al. 1976). Although CFU-E can form colonies under serum-free conditions in the presence of Ep (Iscove et al. 1980) and appears not to respond to physiologic concentrations of IL-3 (Goldwasser et al. 1983), it is responsive to other growth factors present in serum (Dexter et al. 1981; Oddos et al. 1987) and spleen cell conditioned medium (Fagg 1981; Fagg and Roitsch 1986). Of particular importance in this regard is insulin-like growth factor I (Sawada et al. 1989).

The CFU-E appears to be the basic erythroid forming unit into which early erythroid progenitors mature, and it exists at the interface between the progenitor cell pool and the morphologically recognizable differentiating erythroid cell pool. This is well demonstrated in cases of iron deficiency, in which there is a reduction in the number of differentiating erythroid cells while the number of CFU-E is actually increased (Kimura et al. 1986).

The final erythroid progenitor cell is the late erythroid colony or cluster forming unit, a cell first identified following isokinetic gradient centrifugation of mouse marrow (Misiti and Spivak 1979b) and subsequently noted in humans as well. It is more numerous in the marrow and migrates differently during sedimentation than the classic CFU-E (Misiti and Spivak 1979), is exquisitely sensitive to Ep, and requires only 24 h for terminal differentiation and nuclear extrusion in vitro (Ouellette and Monette 1980; Monette et al. 1981). In contrast to the CFU-E, the colonies it forms usually only have 4 cells. Presumably, these cells represent erythroid progenitors which have passed beyond the CFU-E maturation stage and are committed to terminal differentiation at the time of harvest.

B. Model Systems for Studying the Interaction of Erythropoietin with Erythroid Progenitor Cells

Erythropoiesis provides an ideal system for studying cell differentiation. Marrow is easy to sample and requires virtually no disaggregation to obtain single cell preparations. Unique morphological and biochemical changes facilitate the identification of the various phases of erythroid cell differentiation, and the differentiation process is characterized by the synthesis of certain erythroid-specific proteins, most notably hemoglobin. The major problems in studying erythropoiesis from a biochemical perspective are the heterogeneity of the bone marrow with respect to its cell composition, the intrinsic heterogeneity of erythroid cells with respect to their differentiation state, the number of cells that can be obtained for study from a single donor, and the restricted ability of erythroid cells to propagate in vitro. While cell-to-cell and short-range humoral interactions are intimately involved in erythropoiesis in vivo and the technology to recapitulate these interactions in vitro has been developed (DEXTER et al. 1977, 1981; EASTMENT and RUSCETTI 1985; ELIASON et al. 1979; COREY et al. 1990; MAYANI et al. 1990) in vitro dissection of the nature of the specific interactions of Ep and other growth factors with erythroid cells requires that both the growth factors and the target cells be as pure as possible. The development of in vitro clonal assays for erythroid progenitor cells greatly facilitated the study of erythropoiesis since a specific end point, erythroid colonies, could be employed. However, this did not solve the problem of interacting cell populations, nor are erythroid colony-forming cells present in large numbers in normal marrow.

To obtain cell populations enriched for erythroid progenitor cells, a variety of techniques have been employed. They include suppression of the proliferation of mature erythroid precursors by hypertransfusion (GURNEY et al. 1962), enhancement of erythropoiesis by induction of hemolysis (SPIVAK et al. 1972), immune lysis of unwanted mature erythroid cells (BORSOOK et al. 1969; FIBACH et al. 1989), physical separation of erythroid cells from other marrow cells by continuous (BORSOOK et al. 1969; SHORTMAN and SELIGMAN 1969) and discontinuous (ZUCALL et al. 1974; CLISSOLD 1974) gradient centrifugation, flow cytometry (BEVERLEY et al. 1980), immunological panning (EMERSON et al. 1985), centrifugal elutriation (NIJHOF and WIERENGA 1983), velocity sedimentation at unit gravity (GLASS et al. 1975; HEATH et al. 1976; MCCOOL et al. 1970; DENTON and ARNSTEIN 1973), and isokinetic gradient sedimentation (MISITI and SPIVAK 1979b). None of these techniques alone will provide a pure population of erythroid cells, but when used in conjunction with other techniques which enhance specificity such as erythroid colony formation, they become powerful tools for obtaining erythroid progenitor cells for study (SAWADA et al. 1987).

The use of cell lines derived from spontaneous or virally transformed cells provides an alternative to the use of freshly explanted hematopoietic cells. Human cell lines derived from patients with myeloproliferative disorders which express erythroid features include K562 (LOZZIO and LOZZIO 1975), HEL (MARTIN and PAPAYANNOPOULOU 1982), JK-1 (HITOMI et al. 1988) and OCIM1 (BROUDY et al. 1988). Although these cells express erythroid features, they are not usually Ep-responsive, and their expression of the erythroid phenotype is incomplete. For example, when K562 cells are induced chemically with hemin to synthesize hemoglobin, they do not initiate the other components of the differentiation process normally associated with this (DEAN et al. 1981).

Like the human erythroid cell lines, virally transformed murine erythroleukemia cell lines are usually insensitive to Ep and undergo terminal differentiation only after exposure to certain classes of chemical agents (FRIEND et al. 1971). When such cells are Ep-responsive, it is usually only to a limited degree (PREISLER and GILADI 1974; SYTKOWSKI et al. 1980). An exception to this is the HCD-57 line developed by HANKINS et al. (1987) from mouse spleen cells infected with a molecularly-cloned, replication-competent, Friend virus isolate free from spleen focus-forming activity. HCD-57 cells proliferate vigorously in the presence of Ep but arrest in a G_0-G_1 state in its absence (SPIVAK et al. 1990, 1991). Although virally transformed, HCD-57 cells do provide a useful model for studying the mechanism of action of Ep and identifying the potential biochemical pathways which might be operative in normal erythroid cells (CARROLL et al. 1990a,b). Importantly, such cell lines provide a means of obtaining adequate tissue for biochemical studies which is not currently possible using normal cells. IL-3-dependent cell lines which express Ep receptors such as DA-1 (BRANCH et al. 1987; TSUDA et al. 1989), 32D (SHIMADA et al. 1990), and ELM-1 (SHIOZAKI et al. 1990) have also been employed to study the mechanism of action of Ep. Additionally, permanent transfection of the Ep receptor into IL-3-dependent cells has also been used productively to study the behavior of the Ep receptor (LI et al. 1990).

With regard to obtaining adequate quantities of erythroid progenitor cells for study in species other than man, it is possible to exploit ontogeny or specialized tissue behavior. For example, during embryogenesis, the liver becomes a major site of erythropoiesis, and in mice at 14.5 days of gestation, over 70% of the liver cell population is erythroid (PAUL et al. 1969; TARBUTT and COLE 1970). Fetal liver erythropoiesis has been well characterized not only in rodents (RIFKIND et al. 1969; PAUL et al. 1973) but also in humans (MIGLIACCIO et al. 1986; ROWLEY et al. 1978), and fetal liver is thus a useful source of erythroid tissue. Furthermore, because of limited intramedullary space, the spleen becomes a major site of erythropoiesis in adult rodents following the induction of anemia, and splenic erythropoiesis in this situation has also been well characterized (SPIVAK et al. 1972). Since the spleen is easily accessible, it provides an attractive source of erythroid cells. Having chosen a tissue rich in erythroid precursors, it is next necessary to separate them from noneryhtroid cells. Of all the techiques employed for this purpose, three have proved particularly useful: centrifugal elutriation combined with density gradient centrifugation (EMERSON et al. 1985), infection with the Friend virus complex (HANKINS et al. 1978; SAWYER et al. 1987a), and immunologic panning (EMERSON et al. 1985).

Induction of erythropoiesis in mice by bleeding coupled with continuous exposure to thiamphenicol (which arrests erythropoiesis) produces a 100-fold enrichment for CFU-E in the spleens of these mice as compared with the bone marrow; other progenitor cells are also proportionately increased in number (NIJHOF and WIERENGA 1983). The CFU-E can be recovered by sequential centrifugal elutriation and Percoll density gradient centrifugation with a purity of over 80% by seeding efficiency and a yield of around 10^6 cells per spleen (NIJHOF and WIERENGA 1983). The in vitro kinetics of colony formation by these cells suggests a mixed population with respect to proliferative capacity, with many of the cells being unable to divide more than one or two times. The extent to which thiamphenicol toxicity persists is unknown, but this system provides a means of obtaining highly purified late stage erythroid progenitor cells, although a large number of animals must be employed to obtain an adequate number of cells for biochemical studies.

The Friend virus complex has proved very useful in studying erythropoiesis. Two replication-defective spleen focus forming virus (SFFV) strains have been identified, one of which when complexed with a replication-competent murine leukemia virus (MuLV) produces anemia in mice; the other produces polycythemia (MacDonald et al. 1980). While the genetic composition of the host influences its response to these viruses (Shibuya et al. 1982), the viruses themselves appear to affect the Ep sensitivity of their target cells at least in vitro (Hankins 1983). Thus, cells infected with either the polycythemia-inducing strain (FVP) or the anemia-inducing strain (FVA) require Ep for terminal differentiation in vitro but differ in their absolute requirements (Hankins 1983). Recognition that mouse marrow cells could be infected with FVA in vitro (Hankins et al. 1978) led to a model system to study erythroid differentiation since such cells proliferate but fail to differentiate in the absence of Ep. The target cell for the virus appears to be the late or mature BFU-E (Kost et al. 1979; Behringer and Dewey 1985).

A drawback of this in vitro model was the need to isolate manually the FVA-infected erythroid colonies to obtain cells for biochemical studies (Koury et al. 1982). However, when mice are injected with FVA by the intravenous route, the spleen becomes a major site of erythropoiesis within 13–18 days. The erythropoietin-dependent splenic erythroblasts can be separated from the other spleen cells by sedimentation at unit gravity, yielding approximately 10^8 erythroid cells per spleen (Sawyer et al. 1987a). It is important to remember that due to the genetic influence of the host animal on the expression of the viral genome (Mak et al. 1979), mouse strains will vary in their response to infection with the Friend virus (Shibuya and Mak 1982).

Immunologic panning using a panel of monoclonal antibodies has been successfully employed to obtain highly purified erythroid progenitor cell populations from human fetal liver (Emerson et al. 1985) and human peripheral blood (Sawada et al. 1987) and marrow (Sieff et al. 1986). With this technique, disaggregated liver or marrow cells are first subjected to density gradient centrifugation in Ficoll-Hypaque, followed by adherence depletion. The cells are then exposed to a panel of monoclonal antibodies specific for various classes of nonerythroid marrow cells and subjected to adherence depletion in dishes coated with antibodies to IgG. With this type of negative selection technique, it has been possible to obtain a 150-fold enrichment of erythroid colony-forming cells with an 85% recovery rate (Sawada et al. 1987). These cells are biologically active and can be obtained in sufficient numbers for studying ligand-receptor interactions. This technique is the most useful one currently available for isolating human erythroid progenitor cells.

I. The Erythropoietin Receptor

Defining the receptor-ligand interaction involving Ep and its target cells is central to understanding the mechanism of action of Ep, and perhaps in no other area of Ep research has there been so much activity over the past several years. The concept that Ep interacts with erythroid progenitor cells through surface receptors was supported initially by studies of marrow cells treated with trypsin and cycloheximide (Chang et al. 1974). Marrow cells treated in this fashion lost the ability to respond to Ep, while marrow cells treated with either trypsin or cycloheximide alone did not, suggesting that Ep-responsive cells had a trypsin-sensitive Ep receptor which was regenerated by de novo protein synthesis. Morphological evidence for such a ligand-surface receptor interaction was provided by the demonstration of erythroid colony formation on agarose beads bearing covalently bound phytohemagglutinin-Ep complexes (Roodman et al, 1981b).

Initial attempts to study the interaction of pure human urine Ep with erythroid cells were frustrated by the inactivation of Ep following iodination by a variety of techniques (Goldwasser 1981). Using a fluorescent adduct of Ep, it was possible to demonstrate labeling of approximately 1.5% of cells in unstimulated rat bone marrow, a frequency which rose to 4.5% following induction of anemia (Weiss et al. 1985). More recently, using biotinylated Ep, Ep receptors were identified on 5%–10% of normal mouse bone marrow cells (Wognum et al. 1990).

Introduction of radioactive tritium into the sialic acid residues of oxidized Ep by sodium borohydride reduction provided the first quantitative approach to the study of its interaction with its receptor (Krantz and Goldwasser 1984). With this technique, Ep was observed to bind with a K_d of 5.2 nM to specific high affinity receptors on FVA-infected splenic erythroblasts, which were present at 660 copies per cell. Due to the low specific activity of the Ep preparation, it was necessary to use high cell concentrations for these studies, and as described below, subsequent studies of receptor affinity and copy number using biologically active iodinated recombinant Ep have led to a revision of these data (Sawyer et al. 1987b).

The development of recombinant human Ep provided an opportunity to study Ep receptors under more appropriate conditions. To date, 31 reports of the ligand-receptor interaction involving target cells from normal, embryonic, and adult rodent and human tissues as well as transformed cells have been published (Table 1; see also D'Andrea and Zon 1990).

The accumulated data confirm that Ep interacts in a specific, temperature-dependent, saturable, and reversible fashion with pronase-sensitive receptors on the surface of its target cells. Studies with metabolically labeled, biologically active, recombinant human Ep have supported results obtained

Table 1. Characteristics of the erythropoietin receptor

Cell type	K_d (nm)	Copy number	Molecular weight	Reference
FVA-infected mouse splenic erythroblasts	0.09	300	100 000 and 85 000	SAWYER et al. 1987
	0.57	650		
MEL (745)	1.3	760	–	SAWYER et al. 1987
MEL (745)	0.49	500	–	MAYEUX et al. 1987
MEL (SKT6)	0.15	470	63 000, 94 000 and 119 000	TODOKORO et al. 1987
MEL (TSA8)	0.25	90	–	FUKAMACHI et al. 1987
(induced)	0.55	400		
Rat fetal liver erythroblasts	0.16	500	255 000 (78 000 and 94 000 reduced)	MAYEUX et al. 1987
Mouse fetal liver erythroblasts	0.41	920	110 000 and 95 000	FUKAMACHI et al. 1987
	3.13	300		SASAKI et al. 1987
	0.14	400		
Human fetal liver cells	4.1	–	86 000 and 41 000	PEKONEN et al. 1987
Human marrow cells	15.0	500	–	ROSENLOF et al. 1987
	33.0	280		FRASER et al. 1987
Mouse splenic erythroblasts	0.07	150	106 000	LANDSCHULZ et al. 1987
	0.81	220	91 000	
Mouse splenic erythroblasts	0.75	200	–	MUFSON and GESNER 1987
Mouse splenic erythroblasts	0.70	450	–	FRASER et al. 1988
Human peripheral blood	0.10	210	–	SAWADA et al. 1988
Erythroid progenitor cells	0.57	840	100 000 and 85 000	SAWYER et al. 1989
Hamster yolk sac	0.01–0.37	30–700	–	BOUSSIOS and BERTLE 1987, 1989
K562	0.27	5	–	FRASER et al. 1988
JK-1 human erythroleukemia	0.06	110	250 000 (110 000 and 90 000 reduced)	HITOMI et al. 1988
	0.40	130		
MEL (Rauscher)	0.44	1700	105 000 and 95 000	BROUDY et al. 1988
				WEISS et al. 1988
MEL (GM 979)	0.66	1600	–	BROUDY et al. 1988
DA-1	0.54	130	–	SAKAGUCHI et al. 1987

Table 1 (continued)

Cell type	K_d (nm)	Copy number	Molecular weight	Reference
DA-1	1.16	50	–	Tsao et al. 1988
DA-1	0.53	500	–	Broudy et al. 1990
B6Suta	0.38	310	–	Broudy et al. 1990
IC-2	0.84	20	–	Tsao et al. 1988
FDC-P2	1.39	20	–	Tsao et al. 1988
Human erythroleukemia				
(OCIM1)	0.11	2600	–	Broudy et al. 1988
(HEL)	0.29	30	–	Fraser et al. 1988
TF-1	0.40	1630	105 000 and 90 000	Kitamura et al. 1989
MEL (745)	0.21	113	250 000 (110 000 and 90 000 reduced)	Sasaki et al. 1987
(induced)	0.26	177		
TSA8	0.14	90	–	Sasaki et al. 1987
(induced)	0.25	350		
Rat bone marrow cells				
Normal	0.18	38	165 000 (75 000 reduced)	Akahane et al. 1989
Anemic	0.18	52		
Murine fetal liver cells	0.41	650	224 000 (102 000 and (85 000 reduced)	McCaffery et al. 1989
Bone marrow cells	0.67	80		
Murine FVA-infected erythroblasts	1.18	575		
MEL	0.06 0.60	500–1000	110 000 and 90 000	Hitomi et al. 1989
MEL (B8)	1.20	350–650	109 000 and 94 000	Tojo et al. 1988
(induced)	1.20	1300		
MEL (T3C1-2-0, K-1) (GM86, 707)	0.27–0.78	110–930	63 000	Todokoro et al. 1988
Human leukemia cells KU 812	0.25	205	–	Nakazawa et al. 1990
Murine fetal liver cell line J2E	0.27	1035	–	Klinken et al. 1988

FVA, friend virus anemia-inducing strain; MEL, murine erythroleukemia cells.

concentration (GOLDWASSER et al. 1983). Given the small extent of down-regulation by Ep of its own receptor, it is unlikely that IL-3 has a significant physiologic effect on late erythroid progenitors (CFU-E).

Although no other growth factor appears to interact with the Ep receptor, it has recently been demonstrated that the GP55 membrane glycoprotein of SFFV binds to the Ep receptor, an interaction which appears to take place largely in the endoplasmic reticulum, prolongs receptor half-life, and provides a means of abrogating Ep dependence (LI et al. 1990; RUSCETTI et al. 1990; YOSHIMURA et al. 1990).

There are conflicting data concerning the biochemical characteristics of the Ep receptor. Chemical cross-linking studies in different types of erythroid cells have identified a number of proteins which bind Ep in a specific fashion (Table 1). Studies of FVA-infected splenic erythroblasts revealed two proteins with molecular weights of 100 and 85 kDa under reducing and nonreducing conditions which bound Ep equally (SAWYER et al. 1987c, 1989; TOJO et al. 1987; MAYEUX et al. 1990) and exist in a ratio of 0.5; similar results have been obtained with human erythroid progenitor cells, FVP and MEL cells, and rodent placenta (SIEFF et al. 1986). There appears to be no correlation between these proteins and high- or low-affinity binding sites for Ep, since erythroleukemia cells which had only low-affinity ones binding expressed both proteins (BROUDY et al. 1988; SASAKI et al. 1987b; UMEMURA et al. 1989). In several studies, the molecular weights of the Ep-binding proteins varied under reducing and nonreducing conditions (HITOMI et al. 1988; MAYEUX et al. 1987b; SASAKI et al. 1987; MCCAFFERY et al. 1989), in contrast to the situation in FVA-infected cells or mouse fetal liver cells or certain erythroleukemia cell lines, suggesting that the Ep receptor was a disulfide-linked heterodimer. However, the possibility that the larger molecular weight Ep-receptor complex observed under non-reducing conditions was merely a product of nonspecific aggregation or incomplete solubilization of cross-linked membranes was not rigorously excluded in these studies (SAWYER et al. 1989; SAWYER 1989). Smaller molecular weight complexes may reflect the effects of proteolysis during in vitro manipulation. Recent data suggest that the 100 and the 85 kDa proteins are derived from the same gene, and the smaller protein may represent the consequence of proteolysis (SAWYER 1989).

The most important advance to date in Ep receptor research has been the cloning of the receptor from murine erythroleukemia cells (MEL) exhibiting only a single low-affinity receptor (K_d = 0.21 nM) by an expression strategy using transfected COS cells (D'ANDREA et al. 1989). The surprising result of this approach was the identification of 1.8-kilobase cDNA which when transfected into COS cells yielded both high (K_d = 0.03 nM) and low (K_d = 0.21 nM) -affinity receptors. There was no competition by other growth factors, and endocytosis of receptor-ligand complexes occurred at 37°C. Furthermore, receptor mRNA expression was only observed in erythroid cells, and cross-linking studies revealed two binding

to the 100-kDa and 85-kDa Ep binding proteins identified by cross-linking studies is also unclear.

C. Interaction of Other Growth and Developmental Factors with Erythroid Progenitor Cells

Ep is obligatory for erythroid cell proliferation and differentiation, but it is not the only growth or developmental factor which interacts with erythroid progenitor cells. Both IL-3 and GM-CSF support the proliferation of BFU-E (Metcalf and Johnson 1979; Emerson et al. 1988; Migliaccio et al. 1988) but do not support the terminal differentiation of erythroid cells (Iscove 1977; Goldwasser et al. 1983), although there are conflicting data concerning this (Goodman et al. 1985; Suda et al. 1986; Migliaccio et al. 1987). IL-3 may, in fact, inhibit terminal differentiation of erythroid precursors (Goldwasser et al. 1983). Controversy also exists as to whether EPA, a lymphokine obtained from a T-lymphoblast cell line (Westbrook et al. 1984), enhances erythroid colony formation in vitro (Westbrook et al. 1984) or has no effect as all (Sieff et al. 1985). There is evidence that EPA enhances erythropoiesis in vivo, but the mechanism for this is unknown (Niskanen et al. 1988a). Human lymphocytes also express a membrane-bound, 28-kDa glycoprotein thought to be distinct from EPA and BPA produced by T cells, which selectively enhances colony formation by BFU-E (Feldman et al. 1987, 1989).

Mouse spleen cell conditioned medium contains an interesting 20-kDa protein designated "erythropoietin-like activity" (EpLA) which promotes erythroid colony formation by CFU-E in vitro and has a minimal effect on ^{59}Fe incorporation in vivo (Fagg 1981; Fagg and Roitsch 1986). EpLA appears to act on a subset of CFU-E but is neither as potent as Ep nor does it appear to compete with it. Neither the chemical composition of EpLA nor its cell of origin have been defined, and it is not known whether this material is related to a soluble erythropoietic growth factor identified in medium from long-term mouse bone marrow cultures (Oddos et al. 1987).

Perhaps the most interesting protein identified to date which interacts with erythroid cells is an "erythroid differentiating factor" (EDF) isolated from a human leukemia cell line (Eto et al. 1987) which induces murine erythroleukemia cells and K562 cells to differentiate and enhances the effect of Ep on colony formation by human CFU-E (Yu et al, 1987). EDF appears to be identical with follicle stimulating hormone (FSH)-releasing protein, a homodimer of the chains of the protein inhibin (Murata et al. 1988). Inhibin antagonizes low concentrations of Ep in vitro and blocks the effect of EDF (Yu et al. 1987). The physiologic significance of these proteins is unknown. In some studies, it appears that they do not interact directly with erythroid progenitor cells (Broxmeyer et al. 1988), but in others, specific, saturable receptors have been identified on erythroid cells (Hino et al.

1989). Further elucidation of their biology could enhance our understanding of the mechanisms by which Ep interacts with its target cells.

Erythrotropin II, isolated from fetal calf intestine, is another as yet uncharacterized peptide which enhances the effect of Ep on thymidine incorporation by fetal liver cells (CONGOTE 1983). Recently, an 8-kDa peptide was isolated from the serum of an anephric patient which stimulated thymidine corporation by fetal liver cells and also colony formation by CFU-E (BROX and CONGOTE 1989). It seems to be similar to the erythrotropins and perhaps insulin-like growth factors, but it has not yet been chemically analyzed.

In addition to the factors described above, a variety of hormones such as glucocorticoids, growth hormone, insulin, insulin-like growth factors (IGF-I and -II), platelet-derived growth factor, thyroid hormones, androgens, estrogens, progesterone, and prolactin as well as agents such as prostaglandins and hemin have been observed to modulate the behavior of Ep-responsive cells either in vivo or in vitro. The interpretation of many of these studies is difficult because of the lack of specificity imposed by the experimental protocols. For example, target cell specificity or mechanism of action is difficult if not impossible to define in whole animal experiments, and similar considerations apply to in vitro studies when unseparated bone marrow cells are employed. Further, as mentioned previously, if culture conditions are not optimal then the observed effects of the agent under scrutiny may have no physiologic relevance. The choice of experimental host with respect to species, gender, and developmental or physiologic state as well as the particular tissue studied will also influence the results obtained. Indeed, the fastidious growth requirements of hematopoietic progenitor cells coupled with the competitive atmosphere of the scientific environment have conspired in the generation of experimental data which are often ambiguous with respect to their interpretation if not their significance.

The interaction of glucocorticoids with erythroid cells provides an excellent example of how the choice of experimental model influences the results obtained. Glucocorticoids at physiological concentrations enhance to a small extent colony formation by adult human BFU-E and CFU-E (URABE et al. 1979; KING et al. 1987; GOLDE et al. 1976) but inhibit the proliferation of CFU-E from adult mice when a range of concentrations is evaluated (URABE et al. 1979). Since both the inhibitory (LEUNG and GIDARI 1981) and stimulatory effects (BILLAT et al. 1982) of the glucocorticoids were reversed by 17α-methyltestosterone, it was concluded that the glucocorticoids were acting through a classic steroid receptor. In fetal liver, both enhancement (LEUNG and GIDARI 1981) and inhibition of erythroid colony formation (GIDARI and LEVERE 1979) have been observed with glucocorticoids. Glucocorticoid receptors have been identified in fetal rat liver cells (MAYEUX et al. 1983) and appear to decline in number with progenitor cell maturation and also as a function of gestational age (BILLAT et al. 1981). There appears to be an inverse correlation between the effect of glucocorticoids on colony formation by fetal liver erythroid progenitor cells and the concentration of Ep (BILLAT et al. 1982). Thus, glucocorticoids are inhibitory when the concentration of Ep is low. Increasing the glucocorticoid concentration also causes inhibition of colony formation, while at saturating concentrations of Ep, physiological concentrations of glucocorticoids have no effect on fetal liver erythroid colony formation. Since there is a reciprocal fluctuation of Ep and glucocorticoid levels in utero during gestation, it has been postulated that these changes may regulate hepatic erythropoiesis (BILLAT et al. 1982).

The antiproliferative effect of glucocorticoids appears to be due to inhibition of DNA synthesis (GIDARI 1981), but it is unclear to what extent glucocorticoids are acting through accessory cells as opposed to acting directly on erythroid progenitor cells. Discrepancies between different laboratories with respect to the inhibitory or stimulatory effects of glucocorticoids may, therefore, merely reflect the stage of development of the progenitor cells studied, the gestational age of the host, and the concentration of Ep employed in the particular study. From a mechanistic perspective, however, glucocorticoids do not appear to have a direct physiological role in the regulation of erythropoiesis postpartum.

Androgenic steroids can have a profound effect on erythropoiesis clinically (reviewed in SHAHIDI 1973) and consequently have been widely examined experimental both in vivo and in vitro. It is generally accepted that androgenic steroids enhance erythropoiesis either by increasing Ep production (ALEXANIAN et al. 1967; NECHELES and RAI 1969) or by influencing the behavior of erythroid progenitor cells. Once again, a variety of experimental models have been employed, and not unexpectedly, conflicting results have been obtained according to the model employed and the end-point measured. As with glucocorticoids, species differences as well as developmental stage may influence the results. Additionally, the ability of certain of these steriods to enhance heme synthesis, presumably through induction of α-aminolevulinic acid (ALA) synthetase (NECHELES and RAI 1969; MIZOGUCHI and LEVERE 1971), may have no physiologic relevance with respect to the regulation of erythropoiesis. It is apparent that androgenic steroids act on a variety of classes of hematopoietic progenitor cells, and consequently some of their effects on erythropoiesis may be indirect.

Several studies have indicated that both marrow (VALLADARES and MINGUELL 1975) and spleen cells, following the induction of erythropoiesis in that organ (HADJIAN et al. 1976), contain receptors for testosterone, but there is no available evidence that erythroid cells can metabolize testosterone to its active metabolites. Careful structure-function studies suggest, as least for rat marrow cells, that the most erythropoietically-active steroids are the 5′-H-androstanes, although important exceptions to this exist (SINGER et al. 1975). Limited studies with the Tfm mutant mouse which lacks cytosolic androgen receptors indicate that these are not essential for a normal response to Ep (BYRON 1977).

In the rabbit, both testosterone and its 5β-metabolite enhanced Ep-induced erythroid colony formation, while the 5α-H-epimers did not (MODDER et al. 1978). More importantly, these steroids appear to interact with different classes of target cells, and within the erythroid progenitor cell pool, at various stages of maturity. Thus, in vivo injection of testosterone in ex-hypoxic polycythemic mice enhances the size of the BFU-E pool but not the CFU-E pool (PESCHLE et al. 1977a). In polycythemic mice receiving carmustine (BCNU), however, regeneration of the Ep-responsive cell pool was accelerated by Ep but not by testosterone, although the latter hormone enhanced the recovery of CFU-GM (REISSMANN et al. 1974). These contradictory data can be resolved by the observation that erythroid progenitor cells are heterogenous with respect to their responsiveness to androgens (GROSS and GOLDWASSER 1976). Thus, the 5β-androstane, etiocholanolone, appears to interact with erythroid progenitor cells which are not in cell cycle, while a fluorinated 5α-androstane, fluoxymetholone, acts only on cell cycle active progenitors and has no effect in the presence of saturating concentrations of Ep (SINGER and ADAMSON 1975, 1976). The target cells for these different types of steroids are physically separable, and the effects of the steroids are additive when they are employed together. These data support the contention that androgenic steroids can modulate erythropoiesis by increasing the size of the Ep-responsive cell population by triggering cells into active cycle and by recruiting cells from more primitive progenitor cell pools as well as by increasing the concentration of Ep in the circulation.

In contrast to androgens, estrogens appear to have no direct effect on erythroid colony formation in vitro (SINGER et al. 1975), while in vivo in mice, suppression of marrow erythropoiesis follows estrogen administration (PESCHLE et al. 1977b), and in guinea pigs such suppression was associated with an increase in splenic erythropoiesis (SANDBERG and BJORKHOLM 1974). Other hormones which have been examined for their effect on erythropoiesis include progesterone (SINGER et al. 1975) and parathormone (DUNN and TRENT 1981), which have no effect, prolactin, which is inhibitory to erythroid colony formation at high concentrations (GOLDE and BERSCH 1977), and growth hormone (GOLDE and BERSCH 1977), thyroid hormones (GOLDE et al. 1977; DAINIAK et al. 1978; POPOVIC et al. 1977), insulin (KURTZ et al. 1983; PERRINE et al. 1986; DAINIAK and KRECZKO 1985), IGF-I (KURTZ et al. 1982; AKAHANE et al. 1987; SAWADA et al. 1989; CLAUSTRES et al. 1987; CONGOTE 1987; SONODA et al. 1988), IGF-II (DAINIAK and KRECZKO 1985), and PDGF (DAINIAH and DRECZKO 1985; DAINIAK et al. 1983; DELWICHE et al. 1985), all of which enhance erythroid colony formation in vitro. The effect of growth hormone and prolactin on erythroid colony formation is of particular interest in view of the fact that the growth hormone, prolactin, and Ep receptors belong to a common family (BAZAN 1989). However, this does not exclude indirect effects through accessory cells, and a recent study indicates that growth hormone may interact with erythroid cells by stimulating monocytes to release IGF-I (MERCHAV et al. 1988).

The fact that high concentrations of insulin were required to stimulate erythroid colony formation, together with the positive trophic effect of growth hormone, suggested that insulin-like growth factors might influence erythropoiesis. This contention was substantiated by the observation that IGF-I promoted colony formation by CFU-E in the absence of Ep with both fetal liver and adult human or murine marrow cells under serum-free conditions (KURTZ et al. 1982; AKAHANE et al. 1987). Recent studies with purified human erythroid progenitor cells indicate that insulin or IGF-I are obligatory growth factors and that IGF-I acts directly with erythroid progenitor cells (SAWADA et al. 1989). Additionally, in serum-free medium, IGF-I and Ep were sufficient to promote erythroid colony formation (SAWADA et al. 1989).

Thyroid hormones enhance Ep-induced erythroid colony formation in vitro with canine (POPOVIC et al. 1977), murine (GOLDE et al. 1977), and human marrow cells (GOLDE et al. 1977; DAINIAK et al. 1978). In animal studies, both D and L isomers were active, while in humans, only the L isomer was biologically active, and T_3 was more potent than T_4 (DAINIAK et al. 1978). Thyroid hormones augmented colony formation by BFU-E as well as CFU-E (DAINIAK et al. 1978), and their effects were inhibited by propranolol which by itself had no influence on erythroid colony formation. In canine studies, the thyroid hormone effect appeared to be mediated by a receptor with two specificities (POPOVIC et al. 1977), and it is of interest that in the setting of clinical hypothyroidism, two-receptor responsiveness was lost in vitro while α adrenergic responsiveness was acquired (POPOVIC et al. 1979). In addition, BFU-E were more sensitive to thyroid hormones than CFU-E (DAINIAK et al. 1978), and amongst CFU-E, there was heterogeneity with respect to thyroid hormone responsiveness (POPOVIC et al. 1977). The thyroid hormone-responsive population had a sedimentation profile similar to that of CFU-E not in active cell cycle (POPOVIC et al. 1977). Thus, thyroid hormones, like certain androgenic steroids, are capable of modulating the effects of Ep and appear to act on distinct subpopulations of Ep-responsive cells which are not in cell cycle or which are less mature than the CFU-E. The mechanisms for this are unclear, i.e., it is not known whether thyroid hormones act at the level of the nucleus, at the level of the plasma membrane, or both. Erythrocytes have cytosolic thyroid binding proteins (YOSHIDA and DAVIS 1977), and L-T_3 is actively transported across the red cell membrane (OSTY et al. 1988), so it is conceivable that these hormones may influence cell behavior at the level of the nucleus. However, the observed alteration of adrenergic receptors in the hypothyroid state supports an effect directly or indirectly at the level of the plasma membrane, if these agents are acting directly on erythroid cells. Current evidence, however, suggests that thyroid hormones may exert some of their effects through accessory cells (DAINIAK et al. 1986).

Other agents which influence erythropoiesis in vitro include prostaglandins (ROSSI et al. 1980; MAYEUX et al. 1986b; CHAN et al. 1980), hemin (PORTER et al. 1979; MAYEUX et al. 1986a; MONETTE and HOLDEN 1982; BONANOU-TZEDAKI et al. 1981), and atrial naturetic factor (NISKANEN et al. 1989b). With respect to prostaglandins, in vitro studies indicate species differences as well as variations in the response of early and late erythroid progenitor cells (ROSSI et al. 1980). PGE_1 inhibits colony formation by murine BFU-E but not CFU-E and stimulates colony formation by human BFU-E and CFU-E (ROSSI et al. 1980). In part, many of the changes observed reflect the interaction of the prostaglandins with accessory cells (ROSSI et al. 1980) rather than directly with erythroid progenitor cells, and it is unlikely that prostaglandins influence erythropoiesis under normal circumstances. Hemin has been observed to enhance erythroid colony formation by murine (PORTER et al. 1979; MONETTE and HOLDEN 1982) and fetal liver cells (MAYEUX et al. 1986a) and DNA and heme synthesis in erythroid colony-forming cells in vitro (MAYEUX et al. 1986), while in more mature cells, differentiation was accelerated (BONANOU-TZEDAKI et al. 1981). The physiological significance of these observations for the normal situation is unclear since in vivo an efficient mechanism exists for removal of free heme from the circulation.

D. The Erythroid Differentiation Program

Erythrocytes initially develop as nucleated cells, shedding their nucleus at the termination of the differentiation process. The transformation of the erythrocyte from a stationary, extravascular, nucleated cell to a non-nucleated one capable of oxygen transport while surviving in the circulation for a period of 120 days involves marked changes in the composition, structure, and function of its membrane, cytoskeleton, and cytosol which confer upon the cell the necessary elasticity, strength, and metabolic repertoire required for this purpose. The erythroid differentiation program has been studied in a number of model systems involving various species and other means of enhancing erythropoiesis, and while the details vary, each experimental model of erythroid differentiation has many features in common with the others.

Early erythroid progenitor cells synthesize major membrane or cytoskeletal proteins such as α- and β-spectrin and ankrin (reviewed in LAZARIDES 1987) and proteins such as the transferrin receptor (SAWYER and KRANTZ 1986), the fibronectin receptor (PATEL and LODISH 1986), certain lectin-binding proteins whose physiological function is unknown (GEIDUSCHEK and SINGER 1979), the Tn (VAINCHENKER et al. 1982) and Rh blood groups (REARDEN, MASOUREDIS 1977), and HLA-DR antigens (ROBINSON et al. 1981), and the Ep receptor. Some, such as the receptors for transferrin, Ep, fibronectin, lectins, and the HLA-DR antigens, are lost from the cell at successive stages of maturation, while others either remain unchanged or decrease in concentration (HINSSEN et al. 1987); at the same time, there is de novo synthesis of still other proteins (KOURY et al. 1986).

Mechanisms for protein loss following cessation of protein synthesis include shedding (PAN and JOHNSTONE 1983) and membrane remodeling following nuclear extrusion (GEIDUSCHEK and SINGER 1979) or passage from the bone marrow or through the spleen (PATEL and LODISH 1986) as well as proteolytic degradation.

Exposure of erythroid progenitor cells to Ep results in an increase in protein synthesis, but only a small percentage of this represents new gene expression. For example, the synthesis of bands 3 and 4.1 is only observed after exposure to Ep (KOURY et al. 1986, 1987a; TONG and GOLDWASSER 1981; NIJHOF and WIERENGA 1988), and these proteins permit an increase in the accumulation from the cytosol pool of membrane-associated spectrin due to their stabilizing influence. In their absence, cytosol spectrin chains, in contrast to membrane-bound spectrin (KOURY et al. 1986; HANSPAL and PALEK 1987), turnover rapidly. In addition, a recent study indicates that Ep enhances the production of spectrin, balancing it with α-spectrin (HANSPAL and KALRAIYA 1989). The induction of heme and globin synthesis are major features of erythroid cell differentiation, and recent studies suggest that globin mRNA expression precedes the induction of heme synthesis in murine CFU-E (BISHOP et al. 1987). Of course, activation of either of these biosynthetic pathways is temporally remote from the initiation of the erythroid differentiation program (KOURY et al. 1982; BERU and GOLDWASSER 1985; IBRAHIM et al. 1982) and is presumably dependent on the synthesis or activation of particular proteins which regulate transcription (BONDURANT and KOURY 1988). In this regard, it is of interest to note that chromosomal protein content varies during erythroid cell differentiation, being greatest in early erythroid cells (SPIVAK 1975). An increase in nonhistone protein synthesis is an early effect of Ep in its target cells (SPIVAK 1976). Histone synthesis also increases but is delayed relative to nonhistone protein synthesis (SPIVAK 1976). The role of these proteins with regard to transcriptional activation is unknown.

An important feature of erythropoiesis is the ability of erythroid differentiation to proceed in the absence of Ep once a critical stage in development has been reached (GLASS et al. 1975). While this concept is, for obvious reasons, based on observations of the in vitro behavior of erythroid cells, it appears physiologically valid because erythroid cells do not appear to retain Ep receptors as they mature (FRASER et al. 1988c), in contrast to myeloid cells which do retain receptors for colony stimulating factors (CLARK and KAMEN 1987). Although the issue is not completely settled, it appears that Ep does not interact with erythroid cells beyond the basophilic normoblast stage (GLASS et al. 1975).

I. Gene Expression During Erythroid Cell Differentiation

The earliest recognizable erythroid progenitors are characterized morphologically by an abundance of both ribosomes and mitochondria (ORLIC et al.

1968), and from the inception of Ep research, the effect of the hormone on RNA metabolism and, in essence, on erythroid-specific gene expression has been a subject of major interest. The initial cytochemical studies of erythropoiesis indicated that RNA synthesis was most active in early erythroid precursors (GRASSO et al. 1963), and indeed, one of the first observed effects of Ep was an increase in uridine incorporation into erythroblast nuclei, which occurred within 1 h after administration of the hormone in vivo (ORLIC et al. 1968). In vitro, a rise in uridine incorporation into RNA was observed within 15 min after exposure to Ep (GROSS and GOLDWASSER 1969), and a variety of species of newly synthesized RNA were identified which appeared to vary according to the cell population under scrutiny (GROSS and GOLDWASSER 1969; MANIATIS et al. 1973). Although it was at first supposed that Ep directly stimulated the synthesis of globin mRNA, it is now clear that this is not an early event but one that is dependent on initiation of the erythroid differentiation program in general (BONDURANT et al. 1985; NIJHOF et al. 1987).

The importance of transcriptional activation in erythroid cell differentiation was underscored by the demonstration that concentrations of actinomycin D which were too low to inhibit myelopoiesis, lymphopoiesis, or megakaryocytopoiesis could completely abolish erythropoiesis when administered in vivo (REISSMANN and ITO 1966; KEIGHLEY and LOWY 1966). Actinomycin-D-induced inhibition of erythroid differentiation also appeared to be specific for a particular stage of maturation, since proerythroblasts were less affected by the drug than their immediate progenitors (HITOMI et al. 1989). Studies of RNA synthesis in the erythropoietic mouse spleen clearly demonstrated that activation of ribosomal RNA synthesis was an early and important event in erythroid differentiation (SPIVAK et al. 1972), a feature in keeping with the known importance of ribosomes in cell proliferation in general (TUSHINSKI and WARNER 1982) and the morphological characteristics of primitive erythroblasts (ORLIC et al. 1968).

Although many studies of erythropoietin-induced RNA synthesis failed to take into consideration changes in nucleotide transport and pool size, other studies have substantiated that the enhancement of RNA synthesis by Ep in its target cells does, indeed, involve the activation of transcription (PIANTADOSI et al. 1976). For example, within 30 min after administration of Ep to ex-hypoxic polycythemic mice, there was a transient increase in splenic nuclear RNA polymerase II activity, which was followed by an increase in RNA polymerase I activity and a secondary increase in RNA polymerase II activity (PIANTADOSI et al. 1976). These changes correlated well with the morphological alterations in differentiating splenic erythroblasts and provided an enzymatic basis for the synthesis of the wide spectrum of RNA molecules observed by various investigators following exposure of erythroid cells to Ep. Since a number of laboratories have indicated that Ep can stimulate RNA synthesis in the absence of protein synthesis (MANIATIS et al. 1973; GROSS and GOLDWASSER 1972), it is unlikely that the initial activation of transcription by the hormone is due to either an increase in the number of polymerase molecules or a change in chromosomal protein synthesis.

Changes in the synthesis of chromosomal proteins may be involved in regulating gene expression during erythroid cell differentiation (BONDURANT and KOURY 1988; SPIVAK 1975, 1976), but such changes have not been observed earlier than 3 h following administration of the hormone (SPIVAK 1976) and thus are probably not involved in the initial activation of transcription by Ep. Limited studies of the modification of chromosomal proteins by acetylation or methylation also indicate that these are late events and cannot be invoked as an explanation for transcriptional activation (SPIVAK and PECK 1979; THREADGILL and ARNSTEIN 1985). Transacting factors, both erythroid specific and nonspecific, which bind to DNA promoter and enhancer elements in globin genes have also been described in erythroid cells (WALL et al. 1988; BARNHART et al. 1989). Recently, one such erythroid restricted and highly conserved DNA-binding protein was cloned and identified as a member of the zinc-finger family (TSAI et al. 1989). As mentioned previously, the role of such proteins in the determination of the erythroid differentiation program and the mechanism of action of Ep remains to be clarified. A proposed but unsubstantiated mechanism for activation of transcription in Ep-responsive cells is that Ep generates a cytoplasmic factor which is responsible for such activation (CHANG and GOLDWASSER 1973).

DNA synthesis is also not a prerequisite for activation of transcription by Ep (DJALDETTI et al. 1972; DATTA and DUKES 1975; BEDARK and GOLDWASSER 1976; SPIVAK et al. 1991), and an increase in DNA polymerase activity is not an early event following exposure to Ep (ROODMAN et al. 1975).

Since androgenic steroids enhance erythropoiesis, it is instructive to examine their effects on transcription in erythroid cells. In fetal liver cells, induction of heme synthesis by testosterone required RNA synthesis (CONGOTE et al. 1974), and the hormone appeared to stimulate the synthesis of RNA with the characteristics of globin mRNA (FERNANDO et al. 1975) but only in cells of a certain gestational age (CONGOTE et al. 1974). By contrast, Ep stimulated a variety of species of RNA in fetal liver cells (GROSS and GOLDWASSER 1969; MANIATIS et al. 1973; NICOL et al. 1972). In adult rat marrow cells, testosterone enhanced the activity of RNA polymerase I and the synthesis of ribosomal RNA mainly in late erythroblasts, while Ep stimulated RNA polymerase II activity and the synthesis of a variety of RNA species including a putative 9*S* globin mRNA (PERRETTA et al. 1980). These differences between testosterone and Ep (PIANTADOSI et al. 1976) are in keeping with their known biologic influence on erythropoiesis in general.

The expression of genes unique to erythroid cells other than the globin gene has been investigated by a number of laboratories (OBINATA and IKAWA 1980; MISHINA et al. 1984, 1988; AFFARA et al. 1983). Nonglobin gene expression in erythroid cells appears to involve three categories of genes:

those unique to erythroid cells, those shared with a restricted group of cell types, and those shared in common with many other cells (Affara et al. 1983). The latter category includes both housekeeping genes whose expression is common to many tissues, although their temporal patterns of expression may be unique to a particular tissue, and those protooncogenes which are involved in the control of cell proliferation and differentiation.

In general, as erythroid differentiation proceeds, there appears to be a decrease in the varieties of nonglobin mRNA synthesized, but this is a coordinated and selective process rather than a random one (Mishina et al. 1984), and it has been suggested that specific genes are expressed at certain stages during erythroid maturation (Mishina et al. 1988; Boyer et al. 1987). This contention is supported with regard to protooncogene expression during erythroid differentiation. Induction of murine erythroleukemia cells by dimethyl sulfoxide (DMSO) is associated with sequential changes in the expression of a number of protooncogenes. The expression of c-*myc*, which is constitutive throughout the cell cycle in these cells, terminates several hours after DMSO exposure and is then reinitiated approximately 10 h later, only to decline again in association with terminal differentiation (Lachman and Skoultchi 1984). The reaccumulation of c-*myc* after exposure to an inducing agent appears to occur during the G_1 phase of the cell cycle (Lachman et al. 1985). Sequential changes in expression are observed for other protooncogenes as well. There is a brief expression of c-*fos*, which is not constitutively expressed in murine erythroleukemia cells (Todokoro and Ikawa 1986), and c-*myb*, which is constitutively expressed, follows a time course with respect to increased expression that is similar but less prolonged than in c-*myc*, while expression of c-K-*ras* follows that of the other protooncogenes (Todokoro and Ikawa 1986; Ramsay et al. 1986; Kirsch et al. 1986). In nontransformed human BFU-E, c-*myc* expression appears constitutive and declines with terminal differentiation (Umemura et al. 1986), and c-*fos* expression is coordinated with c-*myc* (Umemura et al. 1988; Badiavas et al. 1989). In the erythropoietic mouse spleen, c-*myc* and c-K-*ras* expression resembled that of induced murine erythroleukemia cells (Bering et al. 1984), while in another study differentiating erythroblasts strongly expressed c-*fos* in contrast to other marrow cells (Caubet et al. 1989). Transfection studies suggest that regulation of c-*myc* expression is important for the entry of cells into terminal differentiation. For example, the rate at which c-*myc* is reexpressed following exposure of murine erythroleukemia cells to an inducing agent correlates directly with the rate of initiation of terminal differentiation (Lachman et al. 1986), while inhibition of the initial decline in c-*myc* expression prevents terminal differentiation (Prochownik and Kukowska 1986; Dmitrovsky et al. 1986). Other studies have indicated that down-regulation of c-*myb* expression is essential for the induction of erythroid differentiation (Todokoro et al. 1988b).

We have employed an Ep-dependent murine erythroleukemia cell line, HCD-57, to study changes in protooncogene expression following exposure to Ep (Spivak et al. 1990). Expression of c-*myc*, c-*fos*, and c-*myb* was constitutive in HCD-57 cells in log phase growth and also in those in the G_0-G_1 phase of the cell cycle. Following exposure of HCD-57 cells synchronized in G_0/G_1 to Ep, only the expression of c-*myc* was enhanced (Spivak et al. 1990), and subsequent nuclear run-on studies have suggested that the increase in c-*myc* mRNA was not due to an increase in gene transcription.

E. Signal Transduction in Erythroid Progenitor Cells

The plasma membrane provides a protective barrier between cells and their environment as well as a means for communicating with that environment through highly specialized receptors which span the lipid bilayer. These receptors selectively recognize and bind with specific high affinity polypeptide ligands and as a consequence generate transmembrane signals which activate particular intracellular biochemical pathways. In mammalian cells, three basic mechanisms for transmembrane signaling associated with receptor-ligand binding have been recognized (for a concise review, see Hollenberg 1986): (a) activation of intrinsic kinase activity within the cytoplasmic domain of the membrane receptor, (b) activation of the catalytic subunit of an associated plasma membrane protein which in turn interacts with adenylate cyclase or possibly a phosphodiesterase, and (c) alterations in transmembrane ion transport. These are not, of course, mutually exclusive. Since the Ep receptor has not been completely characterized, the mechanism of transmembrane signaling evoked by Ep is unknown, although it does not appear from its structure that the receptor possesses tyrosine kinase activity (D'Andrea et al. 1989). A number of attempts have been made by indirect means to uncover the mechanism through which the hormone promotes the proliferation and differentiation of its target cells. Activation of receptor-intrinsic tyrosine kinase activity is a feature of a number of hormones and growth factors including EGF, insulin, IGF-1, M-CSF, and PDGF (Yarden and Ullrich 1988), and unregulated tyrosine kinase activity is a feature of a number of oncogenes such as v-*fms* and v-*abl* which can induce factor-independent proliferation of hematopoietic cells by a nonautocrine mechanism (Wheeler et al. 1987; Cook et al. 1985; Pierce et al. 1985; Waneck et al. 1986). It is of considerable interest that the oncogenes *erb* B (Graf and Beug 1983), *src* (Anderson et al. 1985), H-*ras*, and K-*ras* (Hankins and Scolnick 1981), all of which have tyrosine kinase activity, can transform erythroblasts that remain Ep-dependent with respect to differentiation. In this regard, introduction of v-*abl* into H-*ras*-containing erythroblasts abrogates this Ep-dependence, suggesting that v-*abl* is capable of influencing both proliferation and differentiation while H-*ras* influences proliferation alone (Waneck et al. 1986). It has also been demonstrated that tyrosine phosphorylation can be stimulated by IL-2, IL-3, IL-4, and GM-CSF through their respective surface receptors, even though these receptors themselves lack intrinsic tyrosine kinase activity (Morla et al. 1988; Mills et al. 1990; Itoh et al. 1990; Siegel et al. 1990; Idzerda et al. 1990; Sorensen et al. 1989; Kanakura et al. 1990). DMSO can also increase tyrosine phosphorylation in the membranes of murine erythroleukemia cells, but the concentrations of DMSO employed were much higher than those required for differentiation (Earp et al. 1983).

Thus, biological precedence exists for tyrosine kinase activation as a possible mechanism by which Ep might induce the proliferation or differentiation of its target cells. Few data are available with respect to Ep on this issue, but it is noteworthy that both insulin (Kurtz et al. 1983; Perrine et al. 1986; Dainiak and Kreczko 1985) and IGF-1 (Kurtz et al. 1982; Akahane et al. 1987; Claustres et al. 1987; Congote 1987; Sonoda et al. 1988) promote the proliferation of erythroid progenitor cells in vitro, and they appear to be able to act directly on erythroid cells (Sawada et al. 1989). Recently, Im et al. (1990) presented data employing partially purified solubilized Ep receptors that Ep stimulates tyrosine phosphorylation of its receptor. The residues phosphorylated were not identified. Evidence has also been given that Ep rapidly promotes the dephosphorylation of a 43 000 MW protein in isolated membranes of either murine erythroblasts or Rauscher erythroleukemia cells (Choi et al. 1987). However, the same events were not studied in intact cells, and their physiological significance is unclear, particularly since it has been shown that phosphorylation of the transferrin receptor is not required for endocytosis or recycling (Zerial et al. 1987).

Phosphorylation of the c-*raf* protein, a cytosolic serine/threonine kinase involved in signal transduction, is an early event following receptor-ligand interaction in IL-2-, IL-3- and GM-CSF-dependent cells (Carroll et al. 1990, Siegel et al. 1990) and is involved in signal transduction in non-hematopoietic cells (Morrison et al. 1988; Kovacina et al. 1990). To determine whether or not phosphorylation of the c-*raf* protein was involved in Ep-mediated signal transduction, we studied the phosphorylation of the c-*raf* protein following exposure of HCD-57 cells to Ep (Carroll et al. 1991). Within 1 min after exposure to Ep, c-*raf* protein was phosphorylated on both serine and tyrosine in a dose-dependent fashion, and there was activation of intrinsic c-*raf* kinase activity. Since similar observations have been made for IL-3 and GM-CSF, it appears that c-*raf* protein phosphorylation may serve as a common mechanism for signal transduction in hematopoietic cells. The target of the *raf* kinase and the relationship between its phosphorylation and receptor-ligand binding remain to be determined, but it is noteworthy that v-*raf* has been implicated in stimulating erythroid differentiation in retroviral infection studies (Klinken et al. 1988).

Receptor-initiated activation or inhibition of adenylate cyclase through intermediary guanine-nucleotide-binding regulatory proteins is an important mechanism for transmembrane signaling common to a number of polypeptide hormones (Casey and Gilman 1988). Many investigators have attempted to implicate this system in the mechanism of action of Ep, but, to date, the data are not conclusive. In some in vitro systems, cAMP enhanced heme synthesis in vitro in a subpopulation of erythroid cells (BROWN and ADAMSON 1977a), while in others it did not (GRABER et al. 1972), and the effective concentration of cAMP was pharmacologic, not physiologic. Neither cAMP nor adrenergic agonists supported or enhanced the proliferation of rabbit erythroblasts in vitro in the absence or presence of Ep (BONANOU-TZEDAKI et al. 1987), although the same laboratory reported that Ep enhanced GTP-dependent adenylate cyclase activity in these cells (BONANOU-TZEDAKI et al. 1986). An increase in cAMP has also been observed in unfractionated rabbit marrow cells incubated with crude Ep (CHIUINI et al. 1979) but not in an Ep-dependent cell line (TSUDA 1989). On the other hand, fetal liver cells which are very sensitive to Ep failed to increase their cAMP level when exposed to that hormone, whereas epinephrine generated a substantial increase in cAMP in the same cells (GRABER et al. 1974).

Adrenergic agents which enhance erythroid colony formation in vitro did so only in the presence of Ep (BROWN and ADAMSON 1977b; PRZALA et al. 1979) and appeared to act only on a subpopulation of erythroid cells (BROWN and ADAMSON 1977). Since these agents were active even in the presence of saturating concentrations of Ep, it is unlikely that the hormone was modulating adenylate cyclase activity. It is, of course, unclear from the design of many of these studies whether the adrenergic agents were acting directly on erythroid progenitor cells as opposed to accessory cells. It is also worth noting that agents which elevate cAMP in murine erythroleukemia cells block their differentiation (SHERMAN et al. 1988), and in an Ep-dependent cell line a similar effect was observed (TSUDA 1989). The alternative possibility that cGMP is involved in the mechanism of action of Ep (RODGERS et al. 1976) has not been substantiated (GRABER et al. 1977).

Cholera toxin has been reported to enhance erythroid colony formation by CFU-E (BROWN and ADAMSON 1977b). Since maturing hematopoietic cells, in contrast to their primitive progenitor cells, contain the membrane sialoganglioside GM1, which binds cholera toxin (LANOTTE et al. 1986), it is possible but not proven that the cholera toxin affected the erythroid progenitors directly through the adenylate cyclase pathway. Two recent preliminary studies have implicated G-binding proteins but did not confirm a role for cholera toxin (MILLER and FOSTER 1989; HILTON and TAN 1989).

A more recently appreciated receptor-initiated system for signal transduction involves the phosphodiesterase-mediated hydrolysis of phosphatidylinositols, releasing diacylglycerol, which activates protein kinase C, and inositol trisphosphate, which mobilizes calcium from the endoplasmic reticulum (BERRIDGE and IRVINE 1984). While the mechanism for activation of the membrane-associated phosphodiesterase is not completely resolved, it may involve either a conformational change in the receptor which perturbs the plasma membrane (BERRIDGE and IRVINE 1984), allowing substrate and enzyme to interact, or a guanine-nucleotide binding protein distinct from those taking part in adenylate cyclase modulation (Casey and Gilman 1988). Whatever the activation mechanism, this dual pathway is involved in signal transduction in a variety of cells, and recently, tyrosine phosphorylation was implicated as part of the signal cascade (Gilmore and Martin 1983). This indicates that different methods of transmembrane signaling are not mutually exclusive and may act through the same final common pathways.

Tumor-promoting phorbol esters, which mimic the effect of diacylglycerol, activate protein kinase C in their target cells, while agents which mobilize calcium enhance the effects of the phorbol esters (Nishizuka 1984). With respect to hematopoietic cells, tumor-promoting phorbol esters enhance the in vitro proliferation of CFU-S- (Spivak et al. 1989), GFU-GM- (Stuart and Hamilton 1980), CFU-Meg- (Long et al. 1985), and IL-3-dependent cell lines (Hogans and Spivak 1988). Interestingly, while these agents promoted the proliferation of murine CFU-GM in vitro, they inhibited the proliferation of murine BFU-E; CFU-E were unaffected (Sieber et al. 1981). Since the phorbol esters activate protein kinase C in IL-3-dependent cells (Farrar et al. 1985) and promote their proliferation in serum-free medium (Hogans and Spivak 1988), it appears that these effects are not mediated through accessory cells. With regard to erythroid progenitor cells, it is unlikely that inhibition of colony formation by the phorbol esters represents a toxic effect since it was observed at a concentration as low as 10 n*M*, occurred with only 45 min of exposure, and was only seen if the phorbol esters were present during the first 3 days of culture (Sieber et al. 1981). These results suggest that the phorbol esters may have caused receptor inactivation or down-regulation. In human erythroleukemia cells, phorbol esters decreased the number of Ep-binding sites without affecting their affinity (Broudy et al. 1988), and these agents also inhibited the differentiation of murine erythroleukemia cells (Faletto et al, 1985), as did protein kinase C inhibitors (Jenis et al. 1989). Alternatively, Ep might activate a nuclear protein kinase C (Mason-Garcia et al. 1990) or act to translocate one to the nucleus. There is precedence for nuclear translocation of protein kinase C in hematopoietic cells (Fields et al. 1990). Thus, activation or inhibition of protein kinase C at certain stages of erythroid differentiation in both normal and transformed cells alters their differentiation program.

To date, however, there is no evidence that generation of inositol trisphosphate has an important role in the activation of proliferation or differentiation of hematopoietic progenitor cells. Thus, neither IL-3 nor M-CSF altered phosphatidylinositol metabolism in macrophages (Whetton et al. 1986), while in murine erythroleukemia cells, there was actually a decrease in phosphatidylinositol turnover following exposure to differentiation inducers (Faletto et al. 1985). Interestingly, this was associated with a decrease in c-*myc* expression, an event which is closely correlated with

In studies with human fetal liver cells (Linch et al. 1987), however, no changes were observed in free intracellular calcium following exposure to Ep, while in rabbit erythroblasts, a calcium ionophore did not enhance the effect of Ep, although EGTA, verapamil, or TMB-8, all of which interfere with calcium metabolism, antagonized Ep (Bonanou-Tzedaki et al. 1987). Furthermore, in another study employing flow cytometry, no change in free intracellular calcium was demonstrated following exposure of splenic erythroblasts to Ep (Imagawa et al. 1989). Finally, it was recently demonstrated that Ep, after prolonged incubation, reduces Ca^{2+}-ATPase activity in reticulocyte membranes (Lawrence et al. 1987). Since intact cells were not examined and late erythroblasts are not thought to be Ep-responsive, the physiologic relevance of these findings remains to be determined.

In summary, there is considerable evidence that alterations in intracellular calcium level may be involved in the mechanism of action of Ep, particularly with respect to differentiation, but definitive proof for this has not yet been obtained. In this regard, negative results may be a consequence of the particular state of differentiation of the erythroid progenitor cell under study.

The arachidonic acid pathway provides another possible mechanism for signal transduction in erythroid progenitor cells. This pathway is linked to phosphatidylinositol metabolism, and data have been reported indicating that murine fetal liver cells have lipoxygenase activity and that lipoxygenase antagonists inhibit in vitro erythroid colony formation by these cells (Beckman et al. 1987). The relevance of these observations to Ep-mediated signal transduction remains to be established.

F. Erythropoietin as a Competence or Progression Factor

Many growth factors act at a specific stage in the cell cycle of their target tissue. Those that stimulate resting cells to enter the cell cycle have been designated as competence factors, while those that act to permit cells to proceed through DNA synthesis are progression factors. Thus, for quiescent, confluent fibroblasts, PDGF is a competence factor, while EGF serves as a progression factor (Stiles et al. 1980). IL-3 can serve as both a competence and a progression factor for IL-3-dependent cells (London and McKearn 1987; Kelvin et al. 1986) while for these same cells, IL-4 and GM-CSF function mainly as progression factors (London and McKearn 1987). Additionally, the hematopoietic growth factors appear to confer the capacity not only for competence or progression but also serve as maintenance or survival factors. For example, it has been demonstrated for IL-3-dependent cells that the presence of IL-3 is critical for the maintenance of intracellular ATP levels and thus cell viability (Whetton and Dexter 1983;

WILLIAMS et al. 1990), while M-CSF is critical for the maintenance of protein synthesis in resting macrophages (TUSHINSKI and STANLEY 1983).

Any definition of the mechanism of action or function of Ep is complicated by the heterogeneity of its target cell population with respect to age, proliferative capacity, and requirement for Ep as well as other growth factors. For example, Ep is widely considered a mitogen, and indeed, an in vitro assay based on its ability to stimulate the incorporation of labeled thymidine into the DNA of splenic erythroblasts is widely employed in lieu of more cumbersome and less sensitive in vivo bioassays (KRYSTAL 1983). While the hormone appears to be a mitogen for early erythroid progenitor cells (BFU-E) (DESSYPRIS and KRANTZ 1984), it is noteworthy that when labelled thymidine incorporation was evaluated with purified populations of late splenic erythroblasts either from phenylhydrazine-treated (SPIVAK, unpublished observations) or FVA-infected mice (KOURY and BONDURANT 1988), it was immediately apparent that Ep had no effect on DNA synthesis in these cell populations, although Ep-mediated maintenance of protein synthesis and stimulation of RNA synthesis were evident (KOURY and BONDURANT 1988). Somewhat similar aspects were noted with mouse fetal liver cells (FREDRICKSON et al. 1977), but the extent of autonomous thymidine incorporation in the absence of Ep was less durable. These observations are not surprising if one considers that the bulk of late erythroid progenitors (CFU-E) are already in active cell cycle (ISCOVE 1977; HARA and OGAWA 1977), and this is true even if the ambient Ep level is reduced by hypertransfusion. In this situation, while the number of late erythroid progenitors diminishes, the fraction in cell cycle does not change markedly (ISCOVE 1977; HARA and OGAWA 1977). Presumably, the reduction in CFU-E following hypertransfusion reflects both a decrease in input from the BFU-E pool and egress from the CFU-E pool through either maturation or cell death (PESCHLE et al. 1977c).

Importantly, Ep, if not a mitogen in late erythroid progenitor cells in the sense of increasing DNA synthesis, does appear to maintain DNA synthesis, and in the absence of the hormone, there is rapid breakdown of DNA in these cells (KOURY and BONDURANT 1988, 1990; BISHOP et al. 1990). Similar observations have been made with IL-3-dependent cells (WILLIAMS et al. 1990). This may be analogous to the situation observed on the rat prostate in which androgen deprivation is associated with fragmentation of DNA into low molecular weight oligomers followed by complete digestion (KYPRIANOU and ISAACS 1988). Since Ca-dependent nuclease activity is involved in this process, it is conceivable that Ep could modulate this activity by altering intracellular calcium pools.

Studies of the ability of CFU-E to survive in vitro in the absence of Ep have revealed a heterogeneity in Ep effects (KENNEDY et al. 1980; ROODMAN et al. 1981). Ep does not appear to be merely required for progression since a delay of only a few hours in exposing erythroid cells to Ep results in substantial cell loss or damage as measured either by in vitro colony formation (Kennedy et al. 1980; Roodman et al. 1981) or thymidine incorporation into DNA (Koury and Bondurant 1988). Whether the critical role of Ep is to maintain the transport of nutrients such as glucose (Koury et al. 1987b) or amino acids (Vadgama et al. 1987) or the generation of ATP is unknown, but its function appears highly specific and time-dependent since cells reaching the basophilic normoblast stage no longer require the hormone for survival in vitro (Glass et al. 1975).

It is of interest that when late-stage murine erythroid progenitor cells are deprived of Ep, they are initially able to proceed through one to two cycles of DNA synthesis but then arrest in a G_0/G_1 state (Nijhof et al. 1984; Spivak et al. 1990). The accumulation of these cells in G_1 may account for the observation that reduction of Ep levels in vivo by hypertransfusion resulted in a delay in the formation of erythroid colonies by CFU-E in vitro, while injection of exogenous Ep abolished this delay (Udupa and Lipschitz 1986). There is no evidence that Ep shortens cell cycle progression significantly (Papayannopoulou et al. 1972; Spivak et al. 1990).

A number of studies have addressed the issue of at which phase in the cell cycle Ep acts (Bedard and Goldwasser 1976; Morse et al. 1970), but many investigators have not appreciated that the bulk of late erythroid progenitor cells are in active cell cycle nor taken the precaution of separating cells according to their cell cycle status. When this was done, it became apparent that Ep interacted with cells in all phases of the cell cycle, although those not in S phase were less sensitive to the hormone (Udupa and Reissmann 1978; Monette et al. 1980). In studies with Ep-dependent cell lines, Ep deprivation caused an arrest of cells in G_1 (Tsuda et al. 1989; Spivak et al. 1990), suggesting that the hormone has its principle effect during this phase of the cell cycle. Once exposed to the hormone, there is a lag phase of approximately 10h before DNA synthesis is initiated (Tsuda et al. 1989; Spivak et al. 1991). Using acridine orange staining and flow cytometry, we also determined that Ep deprivation causes Ep-dependent HCD-57 cells to enter a G_0 state (Spivak et al. 1990). In these cells, DNA fragmentation appears to be a constant process, but Ep deprivation accelerates it (Spivak et al. 1991).

Like late erythroid progenitor cells, BFU-E form a heterogenous population, but in contrast to CFU-E, the bulk of BFU-E are not in cell cycle (Iscove 1977). Although BFU-E are less sensitive to Ep (Gregory 1976), a number of in vivo (Iscove 1977; Gerard et al. 1978; Greenberg and Robinson 1978) and in vitro (Dessypris and Krantz 1984; Umemura et al. 1989) studies have firmly established that these cells are not only Ep-responsive but also that Ep appears to act as a mitogen. Classically, BFU-E require both a burst promoting factor such as IL-3 or GM-CSF and Ep, with the latter not being required during the initial rounds of cell division, at least in vitro (Metcalf et al. 1980). As mentioned previously, Ep is always present in vivo, and thus, the extent to which BFU-E are Ep-independent is unknown. Certainly, Ep can trigger BFU-E into DNA synthesis, and it seems likely that the hormone functions to release these cells from a G_0/G_1 state and facilitates their progression through S phase of the cell cycle (SPIVAK et al. 1991). A second, undefined function of Ep is to recruit BFU-E into the CFU-E pool as indicated by numerous kinetic studies performed in the presence of agents that inhibit hematopoietic stem cell proliferation (REISSMANN and SAMORAPOOMPICHIT 1969; REISSMANN and UDUPA 1972; WAGEMAKER and VISSER 1980). How this function differs from the triggering of CFU-E to form recognizable erythroblasts is unknown. In the latter situation, Ep's function may be permissive, that is, it may merely act as a survival factor or regulate nuclear involution; in the former, it appears instructive since normally Ep in the circulation is maintained at a low level. Only when an increase in red cell mass is required does the Ep level rise, and this is usually a transient event (ABBRECHT and LITTELL 1972). Certainly, Ep alone is not sufficient to cause CFU-E to differentiate into recognizable erythroblasts since in iron-deficiency anemia, in which the Ep level is elevated, CFU-E proliferation is enhanced, but erythroid differentiation is impaired (KIMURA et al. 1986).

G. Conclusion

From the foregoing, it is clear that while much has been learned about the physiology of Ep and erythroid progenitor cells, much remains to be learned. However, the opportunities for rapid progress are greater than ever, given the cloning of both the gene for Ep and its receptor, the development of techniques for obtaining purified populations of erythroid progenitor cells, the development of Ep-dependent cell lines, and the concomitant progress in general in the areas of signal transduction and oncogene biology. It is clear that Ep acts as both a mitogen and a survival factor, that its effects on erythroid progenitor cells vary according to their maturation stage, and that phosphorylation of the c-*raf* protein is an early event following the interaction of Ep with its receptor. Rather less clear are the events in primitive progenitor cells which establish the commitment to an erythroid-specific developmental program or those involved in signal transduction from the plasma membrane to the nucleus. However, given current scientific technology, it can be anticipated that not only will answers to these issues be forthcoming rapidly, but future reviews will be correspondingly more concise.

Acknowledgements. The excellent secretarial assistance of Mrs. Nancy Dietz is acknowledged with gratitude. Research supported in part by grant DK-16702 from the National Institute of Diabetes, Digestive, and Kidney Diseases.

References

Abbrecht PH, Littell JK (1972) Plasma erythropoietin in men and mice during acclimatization to different altitudes. J Appl Physiol 32:54–58

Adamson JW et al. (1980) Polycythemia vera: further in vitro studies of hematopoietic regulation. J Clin Invest 66:1363–1368

Affara N et al. (1983) Patterns of expression of erythroblast non-globin mRNAs. Nucl Acids Res 11:931–945

Akahane K et al. (1987) Pure erythropoietic colony and burst formations in serum-free culture and their enhancement by insulin-like growth factor I. Exp Hematol 15:797–802

Akahane K et al. (1989) Binding of iodinated erythroopietin to rat bone marrow cells under normal and anemic conditions. Exp Hematol 17:177–182

Alexanian R et al. (1967) Erythropoietin excretion in man following androgens. J Lab Clin Med 70:777–785

Anagnostou A et al. (1990) Erythropoietin has a mitogenic and positive chemotactic effect on endothelial cells. Proc Natl Acad Sci 87:5978–5982

Anderson SM et al. (1985) A murine recombinant retrovirus containing the src oncogene transforms erythroid precursor cells in vitro. Molec Cell Biol 5: 3369–3375

Atkins H, Broudy VC (1989) The structure of the erythropoietin receptor by ligand blotting. Blood 74:5a

Axelrad AA et al. (1974) Properties of cells that produce erythrocytic colonies in vitro. In: Robinson W (ed) Hemopoiesis in culture. US Government Printing Office, Washington DC, pp 226–234

Aye MT (1977) Erythroid colony formation in cultures of human marrow: effect of leukocyte conditioned medium. J Cell Physiol 91:69–78

Badiavas EV et al. (1989) An in vivo analysis of c-myc and c-fos expression during terminal erythroid differentiation in mouse spleen progenitors. Int J Cell Cloning 7:179–189

Bailey SC et al. (1990) Identification of the native erythropoietin receptor and higher molecular weight related proteins using anti-peptide antibodies. Blood 76:131a

Barnhart KM et al. (1989) Purification and characterization of an erythroid cell-specific factor that binds the murine α- and B-globin genes. Mol Cell Biol 9:2606–2614

Bartocci A et al. (1987) Macrophages specifically regulate the concentration of their own growth factor in the circulation. Proc Natl Acad Sci 84:6179–6183

Bazan JF (1989) A novel family of growth factor receptors. Biochem Biophys Res Commun 164:788–796

Beckman BS et al. (1987) The action of erythropoietin is mediated by lipoxygenase metabolites in murine fetal liver cells. Biochem Biophys Res Comm 147: 392–398

Bedard DL, Goldwasser E (1976) On the mechanism of erythropoietin-induced differentiation. XV. Induced transcription restricted by cytosine arabinoside. Exp Cell Res 102:376–384

Behringer RR, Dewey MJ (1985) Cellular site and mode of Fv-2 gene action. Cell 40:441–447

Bering HA et al. (1984) Proto-oncogene expression during erythroid proliferation. Clin Res 32:304a

Berridge MJ, Irvine RF (1984) Inositol trisphosphate, a novel second messenger in cellular signal transduction. Nature 312:315–321

Berridge MV et al. (1988) Effects of recombinant human erythropoietin on megakaryocytes and on platelet production in the rat. Blood 72:970–977

Beru N, Goldwasser E (1985) The regulation of heme biosynthesis during erythropoietin-induced erythroid differentiation. J Biol Chem 260:9251–9257

Beru N et al. (1990) Evidence suggesting negative regulation of the erythropoietin gene by ribonucleoprotein. J Biol Chem 265:14100–14104

Beverley PCL et al. (1980) Isolation of human haematopoietic progenitor cells using monoclonal antibodies. Nature 287:332–333

Billat C et al. (1981) Binding of glucocorticosteroids to hepatic erythropoietic cells of the rat fetus. J Endocrinol 89:307–315

Billat CL et al. (1982) In vitro and in vivo regulation of hepatic erythropoiesis by erythropoietin and glucocorticoids in the rat fetus. Exp Hematol 10:133–140

Bishop TR et al. (1987) Gene expression during CFU-E maturation differs from expression during Friend cell induction. Blood 70:148a

Bishop TR et al. (1990) Effects of erythropoietin on DNA stability and induction of B-globin gene transcription in murine CFU-E. Blood 76:84a

Bonanou-Tzedaki SA et al. (1981) Regulation of erythroid cell differentiation by haemin. Cell Diff 10:267–279

Bonanou-Tzedaki SA et al. (1986) Stimulation of the adenylate cyclase activity of rabbit bone marrow immature erythroblasts by erythropoietin and haemin. Eur J Biochem 155:363–370

Bonanou-Tzedaki SA et al. (1987) The role of cAMP and calcium in the stimulation of proliferation of immature erythroblasts by erythropoietin. Exp Cell Res 170:276–289

Bondurant MC et al. (1985) Control of globin gene transcription by erythropoietin in erythroblasts from Friend virus-infected mice. Mol Cell Biol 5:675–683

Bondurant MC, Koury MJ (1988) Three proteins in mouse erythroblasts bind to the 5′-CACACCC-3′ sequence of the B major globin gene promoter. Blood 72:80a

Borsook H et al. (1969) Studies on erythropoiesis: II. A method of segregating immature from mature adult rabbit erythroblasts. Blood 34:32–41

Boussios T, Bertles JF (1987) Receptors specific for erythropoietin on yolk-sac erythroid cells. In: Developmental control of globin gene expression. Alan R, New York, pp 35–41

Boussios T, Bertles JF (1989) Erythropoietin: receptor characteristics during the ontogeny of hamster yolk sac erythroid cells. J Biol Chem 264:16017–16021

Boyer SH et al. (1987) Patterns of differential gene expression during maturation of erythroid colony forming units. In: Developmental control of globin gene expression. Alan R, New York, pp 43–54

Branch DR et al. (1987) Identification of an erythropoietin-sensitive cell line. Blood 69:1782–1785

Broudy VC et al. (1988) Identification of the receptor for erythropoietin on human and murine erythroleukemia cells and modulation by phorbol ester and dimethyl sulfoxide. Proc Natl Acad Sci 85:6513–6517

Broudy VC et al. (1990) Dynamics of erythropoietin receptor expression on erythropoietin-responsive murine cell lines. Blood 75:1622–1626

Brown JE, Adamson JW (1977a) Studies of the influence of cyclic nucleotides on in vitro haemoglobin synthesis. Brit J Haematol 35:193–208

Brown JE, Adamson JW (1977b) Modulation of in vitro erythropoiesis. The influence of B-adrenergic agonists on erythroid colony formation. J Clin Invest 60:70–77

Brox AG, Congote LF (1989) Identification and characterization of an 8-kd peptide stimulating late erythropoiesis. Exp Hematol 17:769–773

Broxmeyer HE et al. (1988) Selective and indirect modulation of human multipotential and erythroid hematopoietic progenitor cell proliferation by recombinant human activin and inhibin. Proc Natl Acad Sci 85:9052–9056

Bruce WR, McCulloch EA (1964) The effect of erythropoietic stimulation on the hemopoietic colony-forming cells of mice. Blood 23:216–232

Bruno E et al. (1988) Effect of recombinant and purified hematopoietic growth factors on human megakaryocyte colony formation. Exp Hematol 16:371–377

Byron JW (1977) Analysis of receptor mechanisms involved in the hemopoietic effects of androgens: use of the Tfm mutant. Exp Hematol 5:429–435

Carroll MP et al. (1990) Interleukin-3 and granulocyte-macrophage colony-stimulating mediate rapid phosphorylation and activation of cytosolic c-raf. J Biol Chem 265:19812–19817

Carroll MP et al. (1991) Erythropoietin induces raf-1 activation and raf-1 is required for erythropoietin-mediated proliferation. J Biol Chem: 14964–1496

Casey PJ, Gilman AG (1988) G protein involvement in receptor-effector coupling. J Biol Chem 263:2577–2580
Caubet JF et al. (1989) Expression of the c-fos protooncogene by human and murine erythroblasts. Blood 74:947–951
Chan HSL et al. (1980) Modulation of human hematopoiesis by prostaglandins and lithium. J Lab Clin Med 95:125–132
Chang SCS et al. (1974) Evidence for an erythropoietin receptor protein on rat bone marrow cells. Biochem Biophys Res Comm 57:399–405
Chang CS, Goldwasser E (1973) On the mechanism of erythropoietin-induced differentiation: XII. A cytoplasmic protein mediating induced nuclear RNA synthesis. Develop Biol 34:246–254
Cheung WY (1980) Calmodulin plays a pivotal role in cellular regulation. Science 207:19–27
Chiuini F et al. (1979) Early increase of cyclic adenosine monophosphate level induced by erythropoietin on rabbit bone marrow cell suspensions. Acta Haematol 61:251–257
Choi HS et al. (1987) Erythropoietin rapidly alters phosphorylation of pp43, an erythroid membrane protein. J Biol Chem 262:2933–2936
Christensen RD et al. (1989) Down-modulation of neutrophil production by erythropoietin in human hematopoietic clones. Blood 74:817–822
Clark SC, Kamen R (1987) The human hematopoietic colony-stimulating factors. Science 236:1229–1237
Clarke BJ, Housman D (1977) Characterization of an erythroid precursor cell of high proliferative capacity in normal human peripheral blood. Proc Natl Acad Sci 74:1105–1109
Claustres M et al. (1987) Insulin-like growth factor I stimulates human erythroid colony formation in vitro. J Clin Endocrinol Metab 65:78–82
Clissold PM (1974) Differentiation studies on separated rabbit early erythroid cells. Exp Cell Res 89:389–398
Congote LF (1983) Isolation of two biologically active peptides, erythrotropin I and erythrotropin II from fetal calf intestine. Biochem Biophys Res Comm 115: 477–483
Congote LF (1987) Effects of insulin-like growth factor I, platelet-derived growth factor, fibroblast growth factor, and transforming growth factor-beta on thymidine incorporation into fetal liver cells. Exp Hematol 15:936–941
Congote LF et al. (1974) Hormone control of heme synthesis in cultures of human fetal liver cells. Biochemistry 13:4255–4263
Cook WD et al. (1985) Malignant transformation of a growth factor-dependent myeloid cell line by Abelson virus without evidence of an autocrine mechanism. Cell 41:677–683
Corey CA et al. (1990) Erythropoiesis in murine long-term marrow cultures following transfer of the erythropoietin cDNA into marrow stromal cells. Exp Hematol 18:201–204
Cormack D (1976) Time-lapse characterization of erythrocytic colony-forming cells in plasma cultures. Exp Hemat 4:319–327
Cosman D et al. (1990) A new cytokine receptor superfamily. Trends Biochem Sci 15:265–269
Dainiak N, Kreczko S (1985) Interactions of insulin, insulinlike growth factor II, and platelet-derived growth factor in erythropoietic culture. J Clin Invest 76: 1237–1242
Dainiak N et al. (1978) Potentiation of human erythropoiesis in vitro by thyroid hormone. Nature 272:260–262
Dainiak N et al. (1983) Platelet-derived growth factor promotes proliferation of erythropoietic progenitor cells in vitro. J Clin Invest 71:1206–1214
Dainiak N et al. (1986) L-triiodothyronine augments erythropoietic growth factor release from peripheral blood and bone marrow leukocytes. Blood 68: 1289–1297

D'Andrea A, Zon LI (1990) Erythropoietin receptor: subunit structure and activation. J Clin Invest 86:681–687

D'Andrea AD et al. (1989) Expression cloning of the murine erythropoietin receptor. Cell 57:277–285

D'Andrea et al. (1990) The cytoplasmic region of the erythropoietin receptor contains non-overlapping positive and negative growth regulatory domains. Blood 76:89a

Datta MC, Dukes PP (1975) Erythropoietin action in rat marrow cell cultures in complete absence of DNA synthesis: 1. Early effect on RNA synthesis. Biochem Biophys Res Comm 66:293–302

Davis JM et al. (1987) Characterization of recombinant human erythropoietin produced in Chinese hamster ovary cells. Biochemistry 26:2633–2638

Dean A et al. (1981) Induction of hemoglobin accumulation in human K562 cells by hemin is reversible. Science 212:459–461

Delwiche F et al. (1985) Platelet-derived growth factor enhances in vitro erythropoiesis via stimulation of mesenchymal cells. J Clin Invest 76:137–142

Denton MJ, Arnstein HRV (1973) Characterization of developing adult mammalian erythroid cells separated by velocity sedimentation. Brit J Haematol 24:7–17

Dessypris EN, Krantz SB (1984) Effect of pure erythropoietin on DNA-synthesis by human marrow day 15 erythroid burst forming units in short-term liquid culture. Brit J Haematol 56:295–306

Dexter TM, Allen TP, Lajtha LG (1977) Conditions controlling the proliferation of haemopoietic stem cells in vitro. J Cell Physiol 91:335–344

Dexter TM et al. (1981) Molecular and cell biologic aspects of erythropoiesis in long-term bone marrow cultures. Blood 58:699–707

Djaldetti M et al. (1972) Erythropoietin effects on fetal mouse erythroid cells. J Biol Chem 247:731–735

Dmitrovsky E et al. (1986) Expression of a transfected human c-myc oncogene inhibits differentiation of a mouse erythroleukaemia cell line. Nature 322: 748–750

Docherty AJP et al. (1985) Sequence of human tissue inhibitor of metalloproteinases and its identity to erythroid-potentiating activity. Nature 318:66–69

Donahue RE et al. (1985) Demonstration of burst-promoting activity of recombinant human GM-CSF on circulating erythroid progenitors using an assay involving the delayed addition of erythropoietin. Blood 66:1479–1481

Donahue RE et al. (1986) Effects of N-linked carbohydrate on the in vivo properties of human GM-CSF. Cold Spring Harbor Symp Quant Biol 51:685–692

Donahue RE et al. (1990) Human P40 T-cell growth factor (Interleukin 9) supports erythroid colony formation. Blood 75:2271–2275

Dordal MS et al. (1985) The role of carbohydrate in erythropoietin action. Endocrinology 116:2293–2299

Dube S et al. (1988) Glycosylation at specific sites of erythropoietin is essential for biosynthesis, secretion, and biological function. J Biol Chem 263:17516–17521

Dukovich M et al. (1987) A second human interleukin-2 binding protein that may be a component of high-affinity interleukin-2 receptors. Nature 327:518–521

Dunn CDR, Trent D (1981) The effect of parathyroid hormone on erythropoiesis in serum-free cultures of fetal mouse liver cells. Proc Soc Exp Biol Med 166: 556–561

Earp HS et al. (1983) DMSO increases tyrosine residue phosphorylation in membranes from murine erythroleukemia cells. Biochem Biophys Res Comm 112: 413–418

Eastment CE, Ruscetti FW (1985) Regulation of erythropoiesis in long-term hamster marrow cultures: a role of bone marrow-adherent cells. Blood 65:736–743

Eliason JF et al. (1979) Erythropoietin-stimulated erythropoiesis in long-term bone marrow culture. Nature 281:382–384

Emerson SG et al. (1985) Purification of fetal hematopoietic progenitors and demonstration of recombinant multipotential colony-stimulating activity. J Clin Invest 76:1286–1290

Emerson SG et al. (1988) Human recombinant granulocyte-macrophage colony stimulating factor and interleukin 3 have overlapping but distinct hematopoietic activities. J Clin Invest 82:1282–1287

Emerson SG et al. (1989) Developmental regulation of erythropoiesis by hematopoietic growth factors: analysis on populations of BFU-E from bone marrow, peripheral blood, and fetal liver. Blood 74:49–55

Enver T et al. (1988) Erythropoietin changes the globin program of an interleukin 3-dependent multipotential cell line. Proc Natl Acad Sci 85:9091–9095

Eschbach JW et al. (1987) Correction of the anemia of end-stage renal disease with recombinant human erythropoietin: results of a combined phase I and II clinical trial. N Engl J Med 316:73–78

Espada J et al. (1973) Effect of chemical and enzymatic agents on the biological activity of erythropoietin. Acta Physiol Latinoam 23:193–201

Eto Y et al. (1987) Purification and characterization of erythroid differentiation factor (EDF) isolated from human leukemia cell line THP-1. Biochem Biophys Res Comm 142:1095–1103

Evans T et al. (1988) An erythrocyte-specific DNA-binding factor recognizes a regulatory sequence common to all chicken globin genes. Proc Natl Acad Sci 85:5976–5980

Evatt BL et al. (1976) Relationships between thrombopoiesis and erythropoiesis: with studies of the effects of preparations of thrombopoietin and erythropoietin. Blood 48:547–557

Fagg B (1981) Is erythropoietin the only factor which regulates late erythroid differentiation? Nature 289:184–186

Fagg B, Roitsch CA (1986) Characterization of erythropoietin-like activity from mouse spleen cells. J Cell Physiol 126:1–9

Faletto DL, Macara IG (1985) The role of Ca^{2+} in dimethyl sulfoxide-induced differentiation of Friend erythroleukemia cells. J Biol Chem 260:4884–4889

Faletto DL et al. (1985) An early decrease in phosphatidylinositol turnover occurs on induction of Friend cell differentiation and precedes the decrease in c-myc expression. Cell 43:315–325

Farrar WL et al. (1985) Altered cytosol/membrane enzyme redistribution on interleukin-3 activation of protein kinase C. Nature 315:235–237

Feldman L, Chung T (1989) Identification of a structural role for tyrosine-145 in human erythropoietin. Blood 74:194a

Feldman L et al. (1987) Purification of a membrane-derived human erythroid growth factor. Proc Natl Acad Sci 84:6775–6779

Feldman L et al. (1989) B-lymphocyte-derived erythroid burst-promoting activity is distinct from other known lymphokines. Blood 73:1814–1820

Fernando L et al. (1975) Testosterone stimulation of a rapidly labeled, low-molecular-weight RNA fraction in human hepatic erythroid cells in culture. Proc Natl Acad Sci 72:523–527

Fibach E et al. (1989) Proliferation and maturation of human erythroid progenitors in liquid culture. Blood 73:100–103

Fields AP et al. (1989) Interleukin-3 and bryostatin 1 mediate rapid nuclear envelope protein phosphorylation in growth factor-dependent FDC-P1 hematopoietic cells. J Biol Chem 264:21896–21901

Fraser JK et al. (1988a) Down-modulation of high-affinity receptors for erythropoietin on murine erythroblasts by interleukin 3. Exp Hematol 16:769–773

Fraser JK et al. (1988b) Expression and modulation of specific, high affinity binding sites for erythropoietin on the human erythroleukemic cell line K562. Blood 71:104–109

Fraser JK et al. (1988c) Expression of high affinity receptors for erythropoietin on human bone marrow cells and on the human erythroleukemic cell line, HEL. Exp Hematol 16:836–842

Fraser JK et al. (1989) Expression of specific high-affinity binding sites for erythropoietin on rat and mouse megakaryocytes. Exp Hematol 17:10–16

Fredrickson TN et al. (1977) The interaction of erythropoietin with fetal liver cells: I. Measurement of proliferation by tritiated thymidine incorporation. Exp Hematol 5:254–265

Friend C et al. (1971) Hemoglobin synthesis in murine virus-induced leukemic cells in vitro: stimulation of erythroid differentiation by dimethylsulfoxide. Proc Natl Acad Sci 68:378–382

Fukamachi H et al. (1987a) Binding of erythropoietin to CFU-E derived from fetal mouse liver cells. Exp Hematol 15:833–837

Fukamachi H et al. (1987b) Internalization of radioiodinated erythropoietin and the ligand-induced modulation of its receptor in murine erythroleukemia cells. Int J Cell Cloning 5:209–219

Fukuda MN et al. (1989) Survival of recombinant erythropoietin in the circulation: the role of carbohydrates. Blood 73:84–89

Fukunaga R et al. (1990a) Expression cloning of a receptor for murine granulocyte colony-stimulating factor. Cell 62:341–350

Fukunaga R et al. (1990b) Purification and characterization of the receptor for murine granulocyte colony-stimulating factor. J Biol Chem 265:14008–14015

Gallicchio VS et al. (1982) Effects of ouabain and valinomycin on in vitro erythroid colony formation (CFU-e and BFU-e). Exp Cell Biol 50:295–299

Ganser A et al. (1989) In vivo effects of recombinant human erythropoietin on circulating human hemopoietic progenitor cells. Exp Hematol 17:433–435

Geiduschek JB, Singer SJ (1979) Molecular changes in the membranes of mouse erythroid cells accompanying differentiation. Cell 16:149–163

Gerard E et al. (1978) The proliferative potential of plasma clot erythroid colony-forming cells in diffusion chambers. Blood Cells 4:105–128

Gidari AS (1981) Mechanism of glucocorticoid-mediated inhibition of murine erythroid colony formation in vitro. J Cell Physiol 109:419–427

Gidari AS, Levere RD (1979) Glucocorticoid-mediated inhibition of erythroid colony formation by mouse bone marrow cells. J Lab Clin Med 93:872–878

Gilmore T, Martin GS (1983) Phorbol ester and diacylglycerol induce protein phosphorylation at tyrosine. Nature 306:487–490

Glass J et al. (1975) Use of cell separation and short-term culture techniques to study erythroid cell development. Blood 46:705–711

Goldberg MA et al. (1988) Regulation of the erythropoietin gene: evidence that the oxygen sensor is a heme protein. Science 242:1412–1415

Goldberg MA et al. (1991) Erythropoietin mRNA levels are governed by both the rate of gene transcription and posttranscriptional events. Blood 77:271–277

Golde DW, Bersch N (1977) Growth hormone: species-specific stimulation of erythropoiesis in vitro. Science 196:1112–1113

Golde DW et al. (1976) Potentiation of erythropoiesis in vitro by dexamethasone. J Clin Invest 57:57–62

Golde DW et al. (1977) Thyroid hormones stimulate erythropoiesis in vitro. Brit J Haematol 37:173–177

Goldwasser E (1981) Erythropoietin and red cell differentiation. In: Cunningham D et al. (ed) Control of cellular division and development: Part A. Alan R Liss, New York, pp 487–494

Goldwasser E et al. (1974) On the mechanism of erythropoietin-induced differentiation: XII. The role of sialic acid in erythropoietin action. J Biol Chem 249: 4202–4206

Goldwasser E et al. (1983) The effect of interleukin-3 on hemopoietic precursor cells. In: Normal and Neoplastic Hematopoiesis, Alan R Liss, New York, pp 301–309

Goodman JW et al. (1985) Interleukin 3 promotes erythroid burst formation in "serum-free" cultures without detectable erythropoietin. Proc Natl Acad Sci 82:3291–3295

Iscove NN et al. (1982) Molecules stimulating early red cell, granulocyte, macrophage and megakaryocyte precursors in culture: similarity in size, hydrophobicity and charge. J Cell Physiol (Suppl 1) 1:65–78

Itoh N et al. (1990) Cloning of an interleukin-3 receptor gene: a member of a distinct receptor gene family. Science 249:324–327

Ives HE, Daniel TO (1987) Interrelationship between growth factor-induced pH changes and intracellular Ca^{2+}. Proc Natl Acad Sci 84:1950–1954

Jacobs K et al. (1985) Isolation and characterization of genomic and cDNA clones of human erythropoietin. Nature 313:806–809

Jenis DM et al. (1989) Effects of inhibitors and activators or protein kinase C on late erythroid progenitor (CFU-e) colony formation in vitro. Int J Cell Cloning 7:190–202

Jones SS et al. (1990) Human erythropoietin receptor: cloning, expression, and biologic characterization. Blood 76:31–35

Kanakura Y et al. (1990) Signal transduction of the human granulocyte-macrophage colony-stimulating factor and interleukin-3 receptors involves tyrosine phosphorylation of a common set of cytoplasmic proteins. Blood 76:706–715

Kawasaki ES et al. (1985) Molecular cloning of a complementary DNA encoding human macrophage-specific colony-stimulating factor (CSF-1). Science 230: 291–296

Keighley G, Lowy PH (1966) Actinomycin and erythropoiesis and the production of erythropoietin in mice. Blood 27:637–645

Kelvin DJ et al. (1986) Interleukin 3 and cell cycle progression. J Cell Physiol 127:403–409

Kennedy WL et al. (1980) Regulation of red blood cell production by erythropoietin: normal mouse marrow in vitro. Exp Hematol 8:1114–1122

Kimura H et al. (1986) Hematopoiesis in the rat: quantitation of hematopoietic progenitors and the response to iron deficiency anemia. J Cell Physiol 126: 298–306

King DJ et al. (1987) Modulation of human erythropoiesis by hydrocortisone in vitro. Eur J Haematol 38:137–140

Kirsch IR et al. (1986) Regulated expression of the c-myb and c-myc oncogenes during erythroid differentiation. J Cell Biochem 32:22–21

Kitamura T et al. (1989) Identification and analysis of human erythropoietin receptors on a factor-dependent cell line, TF-1. Blood 73:375–380

Klinken SP et al. (1988) In vitro-derived leukemic erythroid cell lines induced by a raf- and myc-containing retrovirus differentiate in response to erythropoietin. Proc Natl Acad Sci 85:8506–8510

Koenig JM, Christensen RD (1990) Effect of erythropoietin on granulocytopoiesis: in vitro and in vivo studies in weanling rats. Pediat Res 27:583–587

Kost TA et al. (1979) Target cells for Friend virus-induced erythroid bursts in vitro. Cell 18:145–152

Koury MJ, Bondurant MC (1988) Maintenance by erythropoietin of viability and maturation of murine erythroid precursor cells. J Cell Physiol 137:65–74

Koury MJ, Bondurant MC (1990) Erythropoietin retards DNA breakdown and prevents programmed death in erythroid progenitor cells. Science 248:378–381

Koury MJ et al. (1982) Specific differentiation events induced by erythropoietin in cells infected in vitro with the anemia strain of Friend virus. Proc Natl Acad Sci 79:635–639

Koury MJ et al. (1986) The role of erythropoietin in the production of principal erythrocyte proteins other than hemoglobin during terminal erythroid differentiation. J Cell Physiol 126:259–265

Koury MJ et al. (1987a) Changes in erythroid membrane proteins during erythropoietin-mediated terminal differentiation. J Cell Physiol 133:438–448

Koury MJ et al. (1987b) Erythropoietin control of terminal erythroid differentiation: maintenance of cell viability, production of hemoglobin, and development of the erythrocyte membrane. Blood Cells 13:217–226

Koury MJ et al. (1988) Erythropoietin messenger RNA levels in developing mice and transfer of ^{125}I-erythropoietin by the placenta. J Clin Invest 82:154–159
Kovacina KS et al. (1990) Insulin activates the kinase activity of the raf-1 proto-oncogene by increasing its serine phosphorylation. J Biol Chem 265: 12115–12118
Krantz SB, Fried W (1968) In vitro behavior of stem cells. J Lab Clin Med 72: 157–164
Krantz SB, Goldwasser E (1984) Specific binding of erythropoietin to spleen cells infected with the anemia strain of Friend virus. Proc Natl Acad Sci 81: 7574–7578
Krantz SB, Jacobson LO (1970) Erythropoietin and the regulation of erythropoiesis. University Press, Chicago
Krystal G (1983) A simple microassay for erythropoietin based on ^{3}H-thymidine incorporation into spleen cells from phenylhydrazine treated mice. Exp Hematol 11:649–660
Kurtz A et al. (1982) A new candidate for the regulation of erythropoiesis. Insulin-like growth factor I. FEBS Lett 149:105–108
Kurtz A et al. (1983) Insulin stimulates erythroid colony formation independently of erythropoietin. Brit J Haematol 53:311–316
Kyprianou N, Isaacs JT (1988) Activation of programmed cell death in the rat ventral prostate after castration. Endocrinology 122:552–562
Lachman HM, Skoultchi AI (1984) Expression of c-myc changes during differentiation of mouse erythroleukaemia cells. Nature 310:592–594
Lachman HM et al. (1985) C-myc mRNA levels in the cell cycle change in mouse erythroleukemia cells following inducer treatment. Proc Natl Acad Sci 82: 5323–5327
Lachman HM et al. (1986) Transfection of mouse erythroleukemia cells with myc sequences changes the rate of induced commitment to differentiate. Proc Natl Acad Sci 83:6480–6484
Landschulz K et al. (1989) Erythropoietin receptors on murine erythroid colony-forming units: natural history. Blood 73:1476–1486
Lannigan DA, Knauf PA (1985) Decreased intracellular Na^{+} concentration is an early event in murine erythroleukemic cell differentiation. J Biol Chem 260: 7322–7324
Lanotte M et al. (1986) Selective inhibition of the proliferation of various murine hemopoietic progenitor cells by cholera toxin. Exp Hematol 14:724–731
Law ML et al. (1986) Chromosomal assignment of the human erythropoietin gene and its DNA polymorphism. Proc Natl Acad Sci 83:6920–6924
Lawrence WD et al. (1987) Action of erythropoietin in vitro on rabbit reticulocyte membrane Ca^{2+}-ATPase activity. J Clin Invest 80:586–589
Lazarides E (1987) From genes to structural morphogenesis: the genesis and epigenesis of a red blood cell. Cell 51:345–356
Leung P, Gidari AS (1981) Glucocorticoids inhibit erythroid colony formation by murine fetal liver erythroid progenitor cells in vitro. Endocrinology 108: 1787–1794
Levenson R et al. (1983) Ionic regulation of MEL cell commitment. J Cell Biochem 21:1–8
Li JP et al. (1990) Activation of cell growth by binding of Friend spleen focus-forming virus gp^{55} glycoprotein to the erythropoietin receptor. Nature 343: 762–764
Lin FK (1987) The molecular biology of erythropoietin. In: Rich IN (ed) Molecular and cellular aspects of erythropoietin and erythropoiesis, series H. Springer, Berlin Heidelberg, New York pp 23–36 (Cell biology, vol VIII)
Lin FK et al. (1985) Cloning and expression of the human erythropoietin gene. Proc Natl Acad Sci 82:7580–7584
Linch DC et al. (1987) The effects of erythropoietin on primitive human erythroid cells. Blood 70:177a

Modder B et al. (1978) The in vitro and in vivo effects of testosterone and steroid metabolites on erythroid colony forming cells (CFU-E). J Pharmacol Exp Therap 207:1004–1012
Monette FC, Holden SA (1982) Hemin enhances the in vitro growth of primitive erythroid progenitor cells. Blood 60:527–530
Monette FC et al. (1980) Cell-cycle properties and proliferation kinetics of late erythroid progenitors in murine bone marrow. Exp Hematol 8:484–493
Monette FC et al. (1981) Characterization of murine erythroid progenitors with high erythropoietin sensitivity in vitro. Exp Hematol 9:249–256
Morla AO et al. (1988) Hematopoietic growth factors activate the tyrosine phosphorylation of distinct sets of proteins in interleukin-3-dependent murine cell lines. Mol Cell Biol 8:2214–2218
Morrison DK et al. (1988) Signal transduction from membrane to cytoplasm: growth factors and membrane-bound oncogene products increase raf-1 phosphorylation and associated protein kinase activity. Proc Natl Acad Sci 85:8855–8859
Morse BS et al. (1970) Relationship of erythropoietin effectiveness to the generative cycle of erythroid precursor cell. Blood 35:761–774
Mufson RA, Gesner TG (1987) Binding and internalization of recombinant human erythropoietin in murine erythroid precursor cells. Blood 69:1485–1490
Muller R et al. (1983) Transcription of c-onc genes c-ras^{Ki} and c-fms during mouse development. Mol Cell Biol 3:1062–1069
Murata M et al. (1988) Erythroid differentiation factor is encoded by the same mRNA as that of the inhibin B_A chain. Proc Natl Acad Sci 85:2434–2438
Nagata S et al. (1986a) The chromosomal gene structure and two mRNAs for human granulocyte colony-stimulating factor. EMBO J 5:575–581
Nagata S et al. (1986b) Molecular cloning and expression of cDNA for human granulocyte colony-stimulating factor. Nature 319:415–418
Nakahata T et al. (1982a) A stochastic model of self-renewal and commitment to differentiation of the primitive hemopoietic stem cells in culture. J Cell Physiol 113:455–458
Nakahata T et al. (1982b) Clonal origin of human erythro-eosinophilic colonies in culture. Blood 59:857–864
Nakazawa M et al. (1989) KU 812: a pluripotent human cell line with spontaneous erythroid terminal maturation. Blood 73:2003–2013
Necheles TF, Rai US (1969) Studies on the control of hemoglobin synthesis: the in vitro stimulating effect of a 5B-H steroid metabolite on heme formation in human bone marrow cells. Blood 34:380–384
Nicol AG et al. (1972) Characteristics of erythropoietin-induced RNA from foetal mouse liver erythropoietic cell cultures and the effects of 5-fluorodeoxyuridine. Biochim Biophys Acta 277:342–353
Nicola NA et al. (1979) Similar molecular properties of granulocyte-macrophage colony-stimulating factors produced by different mouse organs in vitro and in vivo. J Biol Chem 254:5290–5299
Nijhof W, Wierenga PK (1983) Isolation and characterization of the erythroid progenitor cell: CFU-E. J Cell Biol 96:386–392
Nijhof W, Wierenga PK (1988) Biogenesis of the red cell membrane and cytoskeletal proteins during erythropoiesis in vitro. Exp Cell Res 177:329–337
Nijhof W et al. (1984) Cell kinetic behaviour of a synchronized population of erythroid precursor cells in vitro. Cell Tissue Kinet 17:629–639
Nijhof W et al. (1987) Induction of globin mRNA transcription by erythropoietin in differentiating erythroid precursor cells. Exp Hematol 15:779–784
Nishizuka Y (1984) The role of protein kinase C in cell surface signal transduction and tumour promotion. Nature 308:693–698
Niskanen E et al. (1988a) In vivo effect of human erythroid-potentiating activity on hematopoiesis in mice. Blood 72:806–810
Niskanen E et al. (1988b) Physiological concentrations of atrial natriuretic factor stimulate human erythroid progenitors in vitro. Biochem Biophys Res Commun 156:15–21

Obinata M, Ikawa Y (1980) Change in message sequences during erythrodifferentiation. Nucl Acids Res 8:4271–4282

Oddos T et al. (1987) Erythropoiesis in murine long-term bone-marrow cell cultures: dependence on erythropoietin and endogenous production of an erythropoietic stimulating activity. J Cell Physiol 133:72–78

Ogawa M et al. (1977) Human marrow erythropoiesis in culture: II. Heterogeneity in the morphology, time course of colony formation, and sedimentation velocities of the colony-forming cells. Am J Hematol 3:29–36

Orlic D et al. (1968) Ultrastructural and autoradiographic studies of erythropoietin-induced red cell production. Ann NY Acad Sci 149:198–216

Osty J et al. (1988) Characterization of triiodothyronine transport and accumulation in rat erythrocytes. Endocrinology 123:2303–2311

O'Sullivan MB et al. (1970) Some molecular characteristics of human urinary erythropoietin determined by gel filtration and density-gradient ultracentrifugation. J Lab Clin Med 75:771–779

Ouellette PL, Monette FC (1980) Erythroid progenitors forming clusters in vitro demonstrate high erythropoietin sensitivity. J Cell Physiol 105:181–184

Pan BT, Johnstone RM (1983) Fate of the transferrin receptor during maturation of sheep reticulocytes in vitro: selective externalization of the receptor. Cell 33:967–977

Papayannopoulou T et al. (1972) On the in vivo action of erythropoietin: a quantitative analysis. J Clin Invest 51:1179–1185

Parmley RT et al. (1978) Human marrow erythropoiesis in culture: III. Ultrastructural and cytochemical studies of cellular interactions. Exp Hemat 6:78–90

Patel VP, Lodish HF (1986) The fibronectin receptor on mammalian erythroid precursor cells: characterization and developmental regulation. J Cell Biol 102:449–456

Paul J et al. (1969) Erythropoietic cell population changes during the hepatic phase of erythropoiesis in the foetal mouse. Cell Tissue Kinet 2:283–294

Paul J et al. (1973) Effects of erythropoietin on cell populations and macromolecular syntheses in foetal mouse erythroid cells. J Embryol Exp Morph 29:453–472

Pekonen F et al. (1987) Erythropoietin binding sites in human foetal tissues. Acta Endocrinol 116:561–567

Perretta M et al. (1980) Hormonal control of RNA polymerases in rat bone marrow nuclei. The action of erythropoietin and testosterone. Arch Biol Med Exp 13:247–257

Perrine SP et al. (1986) Insulin stimulates cord blood erythroid progenitor growth: evidence for an aetiological role in neonatal polycythaemia. Brit J Haematol 64:503–511

Peschle C et al. (1977a) Enhanced erythroid burst formation in mice after testosterone treatment. Life Sci 21:773–778

Peschle C et al. (1977b) Erythroid colony formation and erythropoietin activity in mice treated with estradiol benzoate. Life Sci 21:1303–1310

Peschle C et al. (1977c) Kinetics of erythroid and myeloid stem cells in post-hypoxia polycythaemia. Brit J Haematol 37:345–352

Peschle C et al. (1979) Early fluctuations of BFU-E pool size after transfusion or erythropoietin treatment. Exp Hemat 7:87–93

Peschle C et al. (1980) Fluctuations of BFU_e and CFU_e cycling after erythroid perturbations: correlation with variations of pool size. Exp Hemat 8:96–102

Piantadosi CA et al. (1976) Sequential activation of splenic nuclear RNA polymerases by erythropoietin. J Clin Invest 57:20–26

Pierce JH et al. (1985) Neoplastic transformation of mast cells by Abelson-MuLV: abrogation of IL-3 dependence by a nonautocrine mechanism. Cell 41:685–693

Popovic WJ et al. (1977) The influence of thyroid hormones on in vitro erythropoiesis. J Clin Invest 60:907–913

Popovic WJ et al. (1979) Modulation of in vitro erythropoiesis. Studies with euthyroid and hypothyroid dogs. J Clin Invest 64:56–61

Porter PN et al. (1979) Enhancement of erythroid colony growth in culture by hemin. Exp Hemat 7:11–16
Powell JS et al. (1986) Human erythropoietin gene: high level expression in stably transfected mammalian cells and chromosome localization. Proc Natl Acad Sci 83:6465–6469
Prchal JF et al. (1976) Human erythroid colony formation in vitro: evidence for clonal origin. J Cell Physiol 89:489–492
Preisler HD, Giladi M (1974) Erythropoietin responsiveness of differentiating Friend leukaemia cells. Nature 251:645–646
Prochownik EV, Kukowska J (1986) Deregulated expression of c-myc by murine erythroleukaemia cells prevents differentiation. Nature 322:848–850
Przala F et al. (1979) Influence of albuterol on erythropoietin production and erythroid progenitor cell activation. Am J Physiol 236:H422–H426
Ramsay RG et al. (1986) Changes in gene expression associated with induced differentiation of erythroleukemia: protooncogenes, globin genes, and cell division. Proc Natl Acad Sci 83:6849–6853
Rearden A, Masouredis SP (1977) Blood group D antigen content of nucleated red cell precursors. Blood 50:981–986
Recny MA et al. (1987) Structural characterization of natural human urinary and recombinant DNA-derived erythropoietin. J Biol Chem 262:17156–17163
Regoeczi E et al. (1980) Galactose-specific elimination of human asialotransferrin by the bone marrow in the rabbit. Arch Biochem Biophys 205:76–84
Reissmann KR (1956) Studies on the mechanism of erythropoietic stimulation in parabiotic rats during hypoxia. Blood 5:372–380
Reissmann KR, Ito K (1966) Selective eradication of erythropoiesis by actinomycin D as the result of interference with hormonally controlled effector pathway of cell differentiation. Blood 28:201–212
Reissmann KR, Samorapoompichit S (1969) Effect of erythropoietin on regeneration of hematopoietic stem cells after 5-fluorouracil administration. J Lab Clin Med 73:544–550
Reissmann KR, Samorapoompichit S (1970) Effect of erythropoietin on proliferation of erythroid stem cells in the absence of transplantable colony-forming units. Blood 36:287–296
Reissmann KR, Udupa KB (1972) Effect of erythropoietin on proliferation of erythropoietin-responsive cells. Cell Tissue Kinet 5:481–489
Reissmann KR et al. (1974) Effects of erythropoietin and androgens on erythroid stem cells after their selective suppression by BCNU. Blood 44:649–657
Rettenmier CW et al. (1986) Expression of the human c-fms proto-oncogene product (colony-stimulating factor-1 receptor) on peripheral blood mononuclear cells and choriocarcinoma cell lines. J Clin Invest 77:1740–1746
Rifkind RA et al. (1969) An ultrastructural study of early morphogenetic events during the establishment of fetal hepatic erythropoiesis. J Cell Biol 40:343–365
Robinson J et al. (1981) Expression of cell-surface HLA-DR, HLA-ABC and glycophorin during erythroid differentiation. Nature 289:68–71
Rodgers GM et al. (1976) Elevated cyclic GMP concentrations in rabbit bone marrow culture and mouse spleen following erythropoietic stimulation. Biochem Biophys Res Comm 70:287–294
Romeo PH et al. (1990) Megakaryocytic and erythrocytic lineages share specific transcription factors. Nature 344:447–449
Roodman GD et al. (1975) DNA polymerase activities during erythropoiesis. Exp Cell Res 91:269–278
Roodman GD et al. (1981a) Effects of shortened erythropoietin exposure on sheep marrow cultures. Brit J Haematol 47:195–201
Roodman GD et al. (1981b) Stimulation of erythroid colony formation in vitro by erythropoietin immobilized on agarose-bound lectins. J Lab Clin Med 98: 684–690

Rosenlof K et al. (1987) Receptors for recombinant erythropoietin in human bone marrow cells. Scand J Clin Lab Invest 47:823–827

Rossi GB et al. (1980) In vitro interactions of PGE and cAMP with murine and human erythroid precursors. Blood 56:74–79

Rowley PT et al. (1978) Erythroid colony formation from human fetal liver. Proc Natl Acad Sci 75:984–988

Rowley PT et al. (1981) Erythropoiesis in vitro: enhancement by neuraminidase. Blood 57:483–490

Rozengurt E (1986) Early signals in the mitogenic response. Science 234:161–166

Ruscetti SK et al. (1990) Friend spleen focus-forming virus induces factor independence in an erythropoietin-dependent erythroleukemia cell line. J Virol 63:1057–1062

Sakaguchi M et al. (1987a) Human erythropoietin stimulates murine megakaryopoiesis in serum-free culture. Exp Hematol 15:1028–1034

Sakaguchi M et al. (1987b) The expression of functional erythropoietin receptors on an interleukin-3 dependent cell line. Biochem Biophys Res Comm 146:7–12

Sandberg G, Bjorkholm (1974) Differing effects of estradiol on erythroid cells in the bone marrow and spleen of guinea pigs. Exp Hematol 2:317–327

Sasaki H et al. (1987) Carbohydrate structure of erythropoietin expression in Chinese hamster ovary cells by a human erythropoietin cDNA. J Biol Chem 262:12059–12076

Sasaki H et al. (1988) Site-specific glycosylation of human recombinant erythropoietin: analysis of glycopeptides or peptides at each glycosylation site by fast atom bombardment mass spectrometry. Biochemistry 27:8618–8626

Sasaki R et al. (1987) Characterization of erythropoietin receptor of murine erythroid cells. Eur J Biochem 168:43–48

Satake et al. (1990) Chemical modification of erythropoietin: an increase in in vitro activity by guanidination. Biochim Biophys Acta 1038:125–129

Sawada K et al. (1987) Purification of human erythroid colony-forming units and demonstration of specific binding of erythropoietin. J Clin Invest 80:357–366

Sawada K et al. (1988) Quantitation of specific binding of erythropoietin to human erythroid colony-forming cells. J Cell Physiol 137:337–345

Sawada K et al. (1989) Human colony-forming units-erythroid do not require accessory cells, but do require direct interaction with insulin-like growth factor I and/or insulin for erythroid development. J Clin Invest 83:1701–1709

Sawada K et al. (1990) Purification of human blood burst-forming units-erythroid and demonstration of the evolution of erythropoietin receptors. J Cell Physiol 142:219–230

Sawyer ST (1989) The two proteins of the erythropoietin receptor are structurally similar. J Biol Chem 264:13343–13347

Sawyer ST, Hankins WD (1988) Erythropoietin receptor metabolism in erythropoietin-dependent cell lines. Blood 72:132a

Sawyer ST, Krantz SB (1984) Erythropoietin stimulates $^{45}Ca^{2+}$ uptake in Friend virus-infected erythroid cells. J Biol Chem 259:2769–2774

Sawyer ST, Krantz SB (1986) Transferrin receptor number, synthesis, and endocytosis during erythropoietin-induced maturation of Friend virus-infected erythroid cells. J Biol Chem 261:9187–9195

Sawyer ST, Sawada KI (1989) Conversion of low affinity binding sites for erythropoietin into higher affinity binding sites by chymopapain digestion of the cell surface in mouse and human erythroid cells. Blood 74:152a

Sawyer ST et al. (1987a) Large-scale procurement of erythropoietin-responsive erythroid cells: assay for biological activity of erythropoietin. Meth Enzymol 147:340–352

Sawyer ST et al. (1987b) Binding and receptor-mediated endocytosis of erythropoietin in Friend virus-infected erythroid cells. J Biol Chem 262:5554–5562

Sawyer ST et al. (1987c) Identification of the receptor for erythropoietin by cross-linking to Friend virus-infected erythroid cells. Proc Natl Acad Sci 84:3690–3694

Sawyer ST et al. (1989) Receptors for erythropoietin in mouse and human erythroid cells and placenta. Blood 74:103–109
Schooley JL (1966) The effect of erythropoietin on the growth and development of spleen colony-forming cells. J Cell Physiol 68:249–262
Semenza GL et al. (1987) An Xba I polymorphism 3′ to the human erythropoietin (EPO) gene. Nucleic Acids Rec 15:6768
Semenza GL et al. (1989) Polycythemia in transgenic mice expressing the human erythropoietin gene. Proc Natl Acad Sci 86:2301–2305
Semenza GL et al. (1990) Human erythropoietin gene expression in transgenic mice: multiple transcription initiation sites and cis-acting regulatory elements. Mol Cell Biol 10:930–938
Shahidi NT (1973) Androgens and erythropoiesis. N Engl J Med 289:72–80
Shaw G, Kamen R (1986) A conserved AU sequence from the 3′untranslated region of GM-CSF mRNA mediates selective mRNA degradation. Cell 46:659–667
Sherman ML et al. (1988) Modulation of cyclic AMP levels and differentiation by adenosine analogs in mouse erythroleukemia cells. J Cell Physiol 134:429–436
Sherr CJ et al. (1985) The c-fms proto-oncogene product is related to the receptor for the mononuclear phagocyte growth factor, CSF-1. Cell 41:665–667
Shibuya T, Mak TW (1982) A host gene controlling early anaemia or polycythaemia induced by Friend erythroleukaemia virus. Nature 296:577–579
Shibuya T et al. (1982) Erythroleukemia induction by Friend leukemia virus. A host gene locus controlling early anemia or polycythemia and the rate of proliferation of late erythroid cells. J Exp Med 156:398–414
Shimada Y et al. (1990) Cell cycle control in lineage-restricted subclones of the IL-3-dependent cell line 32D. Exp Hematol 18:621a
Shiozaki M et al. (1990) Proliferation and differentiation of erythroleukemia cell line (ELM-I-1) in response to erythropoietin and interleukin 3. Leuk Res 14: 287–291
Shoemaker CB, Mitsock LD (1986) Murine erythropoietin gene: cloning, expression, and gene homology. Mol Cell Biol 6:849–858
Shortman K, Seligman K (1969) The separation of different cell classes from lymphoid organs: III. The purification of erythroid cells by pH-induced density changes. J Cell Biol 42:783–793
Sieber F (1976) Erythroid colony growth in culture: effects of desialated erythropoietin, neuraminidase, dimethyl sulfoxide, and amphotericin B. In: Muller-Berat N (ed) Progress in differentiation research. North-Holland, Amsterdam, pp 521–528
Sieber F et al. (1981) Tumor-promoting phorbol esters stimulate myelopoiesis and suppress erythropoiesis in cultures of mouse bone marrow cells. Proc Natl Acad Sci 78:4402–4406
Sieff CA et al. (1985) Human recombinant granulocyte-macrophage colony-stimulating factor: a multilineage hematopoietin. Science 230:1171–1173
Sieff CA et al. (1986) Dependence of highly enriched human bone marrow progenitors on hemopoietic growth factors and their response to recombinant erythropoietin. J Clin Invest 77:74–81
Siegel JN et al. (1990) T cell antigen receptor engagement stimulates c-raf phosphorylation and induces c-raf-associated kinase activity via a protein kinase C-dependent pathway. J Biol Chem 265:18472–18480
Singer JW, Adamson JW (1975) Steroids and hematopoiesis: II. The effect of steroids on in vitro erythroid colony growth: evidence for different target cells for different classes of steroids. J Cell Physiol 88:135–144
Singer JW, Adamson JW (1976) Steroids and hematopoiesis: III. The response of granulocytic and erythroid colony-forming cells to steroids of different classes. Blood 48:855–863
Singer JW et al. (1975) Steroids and hematopoiesis: I. The effect of steroids on in vitro erythroid colony growth: structure/activity relationships. J Cell Physiol 88:127–134
Somlyo AP (1984) Cellular site of calcium regulation. Nature 309:516–517

Sonoda Y et al. (1988) Erythroid burst-promoting activity of purified recombinant human GM-CSF and interleukin-3: studies with anti-GM-CSF and anti-IL-3 sera and studies in serum-free cultures. Blood 72:1381–1386

Sorensen PHB et al. (1989) Interleukin-3, GM-CSF, and TPA induce distinct phosphorylation events in an interleukin 3-dependent multipotential cell line. Blood 73:406–418

Spivak JL (1975) Chromosomal protein synthesis during erythropoiesis in the mouse spleen. Exp Cell Res 91:253–262

Spivak JL (1976) Effect of erythropoietin on chromosomal protein synthesis. Blood 47:581–592

Spivak JL (1986) The mechanism of action of erythropoietin. Int J Cell Cloning 4:139–166

Spivak JL, Hogans BB (1987) Clinical evaluation of a radioimmunoassay for serum erythropoietin using reagents derived from recombinant erythropoietin. Blood 70:143a

Spivak JL, Hogans BB (1989) The in vivo metabolism of recombinant human erythropoietin in the rat. Blood 73:90–99

Spivak JL, Peck L (1979) Chemical modification of nuclear proteins by erythropoietin. Am J Hematol 7:45–51

Spivak JL et al. (1972) Studies on splenic erythropoiesis in the mouse: I. Ribosomal ribonucleic acid metabolism. J Lab Clin Med 79:526–540

Spivak JL et al. (1980) Suppression and potentiation of mouse hematopoietic progenitor cell proliferation by ouabain. Blood 56:315–317

Spivak JL et al. (1989) Tumor promoting phorbol esters support the in vitro proliferation of murine pluripotent hematopoietic stem cells. J Clin Invest 83: 100–107

Spivak JL et al. (1990) Cell cycle-specific effects of erythropoietin. Blood 76:121a

Spivak JL et al. (1991) Erythropoietin is both a mitogen and a survival factor. Blood 77:1228–1233

Steinberg HN et al. (1976) Assessment of erythrocytic and granulocytic colony formation in an in vivo plasma clot diffusion chamber culture system. Blood 47:1041–1051

Stephenson JR, Axelrad AA (1971) Separation of erythropoietin-sensitive cells from hemopoietic spleen colony-forming stem cells of mouse fetal liver by unit gravity sedimentation. Blood 37:417–427

Stephenson JR et al. (1971) Induction of colonies of hemoglobin-synthesizing cells by erythropoietin in vitro. Proc Natl Acad Sci 68:1542–1546

Stiles CD et al. (1980) Regulation of the Balb/c-3T3 cell cycle-effects of growth factors. J Supramolec Struct 13:489–499

Stone WJ et al. (1988) Treatment of the anemia of predialysis patients with recombinant human erythropoietin: a randomized, placebo-controlled trial. Am J Med Sci 296:171–179

Strome JE et al. (1978) Evidence for the clonal nature of erythropoietic bursts: application of an in situ method for demonstrating centromeric heterochromatin in plasma cultures. Exp Hemat 6:461–467

Stuart RK, Hamilton JA (1980) Tumor-promoting phorbol esters stimulate hematopoietic colony formation in vitro. Science 208:402–404

Suda T et al. (1983) Proliferative kinetics and differentiation of murine blast cell colonies in culture: evidence for variable G_0 periods and constant doubling rates of early pluripotent hemopoietic progenitors. J Cell Physiol 117:308–318

Suda J et al. (1986) Purified interleukin-3 and erythropoietin support the terminal differentiation of hemopoietic progenitors in serum-free culture. Blood 67: 1002–1006

Sytkowski AJ, Donahue KA (1987) Immunochemical studies of human erythropoietin using site-specific anti-peptide antibodies. J Biol Chem 262:1161–1165

Sytkowski AJ et al. (1980) Erythroid differentiation of clonal Rauscher erythroleukemia cells in response to erythropoietin or dimethyl sulfoxide. Science 210:74–76

Taga T et al. (1989) Interleukin-6 triggers the association of its receptor with a possible signal transducer, gp130. Cell 58:573–581

Takeuchi M et al. (1988) Comparative study of the asparagine-linked sugar chains of human erythropoietins purified from urine and the culture medium of recombinant Chinese hamster ovary cells. J Biol Chem 263:3657–3663

Takeuchi M et al. (1990) Role of sugar chains in the in vitro biological activity of human erythropoietin produced in recombinant Chinese hamster ovary cells. J Biol Chem 265:12127–12130

Tarbutt RG, Cole RJ (1970) Cell population kinetics of erythroid tissue in the liver of foetal mice. J Embryol Exp Morph 24:429–446

Tavassoli M (1979) The marrow-blood barrier. Brit J Haematol 41:297–302

Tenaglia AN et al. (1985) Amphotericin-B and monensin potentiation of murine erythropoiesis in vitro: a possible role for sodium ions. Exp Hematol 13: 512–519

Thompson ST et al. (1988) A search for the second messenger of erythropoietin. FASEB J 2:813a

Threadgill GJ, Arnstein HRV (1985) Changes in histone acetylation during the development of rabbit bone marrow erythroid cells. Biochim Biophys Acta 847:228–234

Till JE et al. (1964) A stochastic model of stem cell proliferation, based on the growth of spleen colony-forming cell. Proc Natl Acad Sci 51:29–36

Todokoro K, Ikawa Y (1986) Sequential expression of proto-oncogenes during a mouse erythroleukemia cell differentiation. Biochem Biophys Res Comm 135:1112–1118

Todokoro K et al. (1987) Specific binding of erythropoietin to its receptor on responsive mouse erythroleukemia cells. Proc Natl Acad Sci 84:4126–4130

Todokoro K et al. (1988a) Characterization of erythropoietin receptor on erythropoietin-unresponsive mouse erythroleukemia cells. Biochim Biophys Acta 943:326–330

Todokoro K et al. (1988b) Down-regulation of c-myb gene expression is a prerequisite for erythropoietin-induced erythroid differentiation. Proc Natl Acad Sci 85:8900–8904

Tojo A et al. (1987) Identification of erythropoietin receptors on fetal liver erythroid cells. Biochem Biophys Res Comm 148:443–448

Tojo A et al. (1988) Induction of the receptor for erythropoietin in murine erythroleukemia cells after dimethyl sulfoxide treatment. Canc Res 48: 1818–1822

Tong BD, Goldwasser E (1981) The formation of erythrocyte membrane proteins during erythropoietin-induced differentiation. J Biol Chem 256:12666–12672

Tsai SF et al. (1989) Cloning of cDNA for the major DNA-binding protein of the erythroid lineage through expression in mammalian cells. Nature 339:446–451

Tsao CJ et al. (1988) Expression of the functional erythropoietin receptors on interleukin 3-dependent murine cell lines. J Immunol 140:89–93

Tsuda H (1989) Mode of action of erythropoietin (Epo) in an Epo-dependent murine cell line: I. Involvement of adenosine 3′,5′-cyclic monophosphate not as a second messenger but as a regulator of cell growth. Exp Hematol 17:211–217

Tsuda H et al. (1989) Mode of action of erythropoietin (Epo) in an Epodependent murine cell line: II. Cell cycle dependency of Epo action. Exp Hematol 17: 218–222

Tsudo M et al. (1986) Demonstration of a non-tac peptide that binds interleukin 2: a potential participant in a multichain interleukin 2 receptor complex. Proc Natl Acad Sci 83:9694–9698

Tushinski RJ, Stanley ER (1983) The regulation of macrophage protein turnover by a colony stimulating factor (CSF-1). J Cell Physiol 116:67–75

Udupa KB, Lipschitz DA (1986) Studies on the kinetics of the erythroid colony-forming cell. Exp Hematol 14:343–350

Udupa KB, Reissmann KR (1977) In vivo and in vitro effect of bacterial endotoxin on erythroid precursors (CFU-e and ERC) in the bone marrow of mice. J Lab Clin Med 89:278–284

Udupa KB, Reissmann KR (1978) Cell kinetics of erythroid colony-forming cells (CFU-E) studied by hydroxyurea injections and sedimentation velocity profile. Exp Hematol 6:398–404

Udupa KB, Reissmann KR (1979) In vivo erythropoietin requirements of regenerating erythroid progenitors (BFU-e, CFU-e) in bone marrow of mice. Blood 53:1164–1171

Umemura T et al. (1986) Expression of c-myc oncogene during differentiation of human burst-forming unit, erythroid (BFU-E). Biochem Biophys Res Comm 135:521–526

Umemura T et al. (1988) Hematopoietic growth factors (BPA and EPO) induce the expressions of c-myc and c-fos proto-oncogenes in normal human erythroid progenitors. Leuk Res 12:187–194

Umemura T et al. (1989) The mechanism of expansion of late erythroid progenitors during erythroid regeneration: target cells and effects of erythropoietin and interleukin-3. Blood 73:1993–1998

Urabe A et al. (1979) Dexamethasone and erythroid colony formation: contrasting effects in mouse and human bone marrow cells in culture. Brit J Haematol 43:479–480

Uzumaki M et al. (1989) Identification and characterization of receptors for granulocyte colony-stimulating factor on human placenta and trophoblastic cells. Proc Natl Acad Sci 86:9323–9326

Vadgama JV et al. (1987) Characterization of amino acid transport during erythroid cell differentiation. J Biol Chem 262:13273–13284

Vainchenker W et al. (1982) Clonal expression of the Tn antigen in erythroid and granulocyte colonies and its application to determination of the clonality of the human megakaryocyte colony assay. J Clin Invest 69:1081–1091

Vairo G, Hamilton JA (1988) Activation and proliferation signals in murine macrophages: stimulation of Na^+, K^+-ATPase activity by hemopoietic growth factors and other agents. J Cell Physiol 134:13–24

Valladares L, Minguell J (1975) Characterization of a nuclear receptor for testosterone in rat bone marrow. Steroids 25:13–21

Valtieri M et al. (1989) Erythropoietin alone induces erythroid burst formation by human embryonic but not adult BFU-E in unicellular serum-free culture. Blood 74:460–470

Van Zant G, Goldwasser E (1977) The effects of erythropoietin in vitro on spleen colony-forming cells. J Cell Physiol 90:241–252

Van Zant G, Goldwasser E (1979) Suppression of erythroid differentiation by colony-stimulating factor. In: Baum ST, Ledney SE (eds) Experimental hematology today. Springer, Berlin Heidelberg New York, pp 63–70

Wagemaker G, Visser TP (1980) Erythropoietin-independent regeneration of erythroid progenitor cells following multiple injections of hydroxyurea. Cell Tissue Kinet 13:505–517

Wall L et al. (1988) The human B-globin gene 3′ enhancer contains multiple binding sites for an erythroid-specific protein. Genes Dev 2:1089–1100

Waneck GL et al. (1986) Abelson virus drives the differentiation of Harvey virus-infected erythroid cells. Cell 44:337–344

Wang FF et al. (1985) Some chemical properties of human erythropoietin. Endocrinology 116:2286–2292

Watkins PC et al. (1986) Regional assignment of the erythropoietin gene to human chromosome region 7pter....q22. Cytogenet Cell Genet 42:214–218

Weiss TL et al. (1985) The frequency of bone marrow cells that bind erythropoietin. J Cell Biochem 27:57–65

Weiss TL et al. (1989) Erythropoietin binding and induced differentiation of Rauscher erythroleukemia cell line red 5-1.5. J Biol Chem 264:1804–1810

Wendling F et al. (1985) A self-renewing, bipotential erythroid/mast cell progenitor in continuous cultures of normal murine bone marrow. J Cell Physiol 125:10–18

Westbrook CA et al. (1984) Purification and characterization of human T-lymphocyte-derived erythroid-potentiating activity. J Biol Chem 259:9992–9996

Wheeler EF et al. (1987) The v-fms oncogene induces factor-independent growth and transformation of the interleukin-3-dependent myeloid cell line FDC-P1. Mol Cell Biol 7:1673–1680

Whetton AD et al. (1986) The haemopoietic growth factors interleukin 3 and colony stimulating factor-1 stimulate proliferation but do not induce inositol lipid breakdown in murine bone-marrow-derived macrophages. EMBO J 5: 3281–3286

Whetton AD, Dexter TM (1983) Effect of haematopoietic cell growth factor on intracellular ATP levels. Nature 303:629–631

Williams GT et al. (1990) Haemopoietic colony stimulating factors promote cell survival by suppressing apoptosis. Nature 343:76–79

Winkelmann JC et al. (1990) The gene for the human erythropoietin receptor: analysis of the coding sequence and assignment to chromosome 19p. Blood 76:24–30

Wognum AW et al. (1990) Detection and isolation of the erythropoietin receptor using biotinylated erythropoietin. Blood 76:697–705

Wojchowski D et al. (1987) Active human erythropoietin expressed in insect cells using a baculovirus vector: oxole for N-linked oligosaccharide. Biochim Biophys Acta 910:224–232

Wolf M et al. (1985) A model for intracellular translocation of protein kinase C involving synergism between Ca^{2+} and phorbol esters. Nature 317:546–549

Yang YC et al. (1986) Human IL-3 (multi-CSF): identification by expression cloning of a novel hematopoietic growth factor related to murine IL-3. Cell 47:3–10

Yarden Y, Ullrich A (1988) Molecular analysis of signal transduction by growth factors. Biochemistry 27:3113–3119

Yelamarty RV et al. (1990) Three-dimensional intracellular calcium gradients in single human burst-forming units-erythroid-derived erythroblasts induced by erythropoietin. J Clin Invest 85:1799–1809

Yoshida K, Davis PJ (1977) Binding of thyroid hormone by erythrocyte cytoplasmic proteins. Biochem Biophys Res Comm 78:697–705

Yoshimura A et al. (1990) Friend spleen focus-forming virus glycoprotein gp55 interacts with the erythropoietin receptor in the endoplasmic reticulum and affects receptor metabolism. Proc Natl Acad Sci 87:4139–4143

Youssoufian H et al. (1990) Structure and transcription of the mouse erythropoietin receptor gene. Mol Cell Biol 10:3675–3682

Yu J et al. (1987) Importance of FSH-releasing protein and inhibin in erythrodifferentiation. Nature 330:765–767

Zerial M et al. (1987) Phosphorylation of the human transferrin receptor by protein kinase C is not required for endocytosis and recycling in mouse 3T3 cells. EMBO J 6:2661–2667

Zon LI et al. (1990) Regulation of the erythropoietin receptor promoter by the cell-specific transcription factor GF-1 (ERYF-1, NF-E1). Blood 76:174a

Zucali JR et al. (1974) Separation of erythropoietin-responsive cells (ERC) from rat bone marrow. Exp Hemat 2:250–258

CHAPTER 5

The Arachidonic Acid Cascade and Erythropoiesis

B.S. BECKMAN and M. MASON-GARCIA

A. Introduction

I. Background

Ever since the Nobel prize in physiology/medicine was awarded to Sune Bergstrom, Bengt Samuelsson, and John Vane in 1982 for their discoveries concerning prostaglandins and related biologically active compounds (OATES 1982), attention has focussed more intently on the potential roles of the eicosanoids in erythropoiesis. Included amongst these are prostaglandin E_2 (PGE_2), prostaglandin $F_{2\alpha}$ ($PGF_{2\alpha}$), prostaglandin D_2 (PGD_2), prostacyclin (PGI_2), thromboxane A_2 (TXA_2), and the leukotrienes. All are potent chemical transmitters of intra- and intercellular signals that mediate a diversity of physiologic and pathologic functions. They are formed from the oxygenation of arachidonic acid, a polyunsaturated fatty acid containing 20 carbon atoms, and are therefore more generally termed "eicosanoids," from the Greek word for 20.

Their biologic effects include the regulation of vascular tone and permeability of capillaries and venules, contraction and relaxation of muscle, stimulation or inhibition of platelet function, activation of leukocytes, regulation of renal blood flow and mineral metabolism, and possible control of growth and metastases of neoplastic cells. This diversity is matched by the variety of arachidonic acid metabolite structures. Individual cells are highly selective in their metabolism of arachidonic acid, forming metabolites that are specific for a given cell function. For example, TXA_2, formed subsequent to the activation of platelets, is a potent stimulus for platelet aggregation and vasoconstriction, whereas prostacyclin, produced by endothelial cells, is a potent inhibitor of platelet aggregation and a vasodilator. The leukotrienes and PGD_2 are produced by basophils and mast cells among others and participate in the allergic responses that result from immunologic activation of these cells. The discovery of TXA_2 has significantly affected the understanding of platelet aggregation and revealed a potential for platelets to produce vasoconstriction through release of TXA_2.

Arachidonic acid can be found as an integral part of phospholipids, triglycerides, and cholesterol esters. As a consequence of cellular stimulation or damage, arachidonic acid is released and rapidly oxidized to subsequent metabolites via cyclooxygenase or lipoxygenase. The rapid formation of these compounds under conditions of cellular stimulation or damage and their structural versatility involving many functional groups and intermediate lipid:water solubility allow them to interact with a diverse group of other ions and proteins to modulate cellular function. Calcium plays an essential role in arachidonic acid metabolism, particularly in the release of substrate from membranes by way of phospholipase A_2.

Because of the wide range of metabolic products of arachidonic acid and the variation from species to species, it is probable that these compounds evolved rather recently on the evolutionary time scale and have retained an adaptability to the specific requirements of each species (GERRARD 1985). Fundamental to an understanding of the relationship between cell function and the arachidonic acid cascade is a knowledge of phospholipids and of their organization into a lipid bilayer. Most phospholipids are characterized by a glycerol backbone with a polar phosphate attached on the third carbon and two nonpolar fatty acid chains attached to carbons 1 and 2. To the phosphate group on carbon 3 there is usually a further polar constituent, either choline, ethanolamine, inositol, or serine. The resulting structure is a molecule with a polar head group, which is most compatible with a water environment, and a hydrophobic tail, which prefers to exist in a lipid environment. One conformation in which groups of these molecules can exist together is a bilayer, with one layer of phospholipids associated tail to tail with another layer of phospholipids. In such a bilayer, the hydrocarbon of the acyl (derived from fatty acids) tails of these molecules associates in the middle to give a central lipid layer. The polar head ends face the outside water phases. This structure forms the basis for cell membranes. The central lipid domain back to back with fatty acid chains is relatively impermeable to most polar constituents including ions such as sodium, calcium, potassium, and magnesium, proteins, and carbohydrates. This enables the cell to maintain an intracellular microenvironment very different from the extracellular milieu. The integrity of the lipid bilayer is of fundamental importance to cells, and any influence which affects it must be responded to by the cell. In addition to phospholipids within the bilayer there are several other lipids and proteins. Bilayer membranes must have a certain stiffness and a certain fluidity. Individual cellular membranes may vary somewhat in the relative degree of fluidity. The fluidity of a membrane depends on the lipid constituents and on the associated proteins, with the nature of the acyl or fatty acid chains of the phospholipids being one important factor. The polar head group of the phospholipid has important interactions with components of the water phase. Phosphatidylcholine, which has no net charge over a wide range of pH, has less interaction with the cations, sodium, potassium, and calcium, etc. and positively charged groups on proteins than phosphatidylinositol, phosphatidylserine, phosphatidylethanolamine, and phosphatidic acid, all of which carry a net negative charge at physiologic

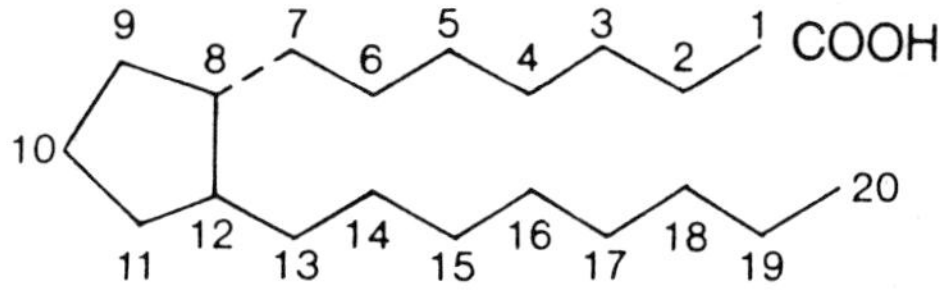

Fig. 1. The prostanoic acid structure

pH. Sphingomyelin, a sphingolipid which can function in a lipid bilayer similar to the above-mentioned phospholipids, has a slight net positive charge on the surface due to the presence of the free hydroxyl group of the 4-sphingosine, which lessens the acidity of the phosphate group by ion-dipole interaction. The phospholipids and sphingolipids are not uniformly distributed in cell membranes. Red blood cells and platelet plasma membranes are enriched in phosphatidylcholine and sphingomyelin on their outer face and in phosphatidyl ethanolamine, phosphatidyl serine and phosphatidylinositol on their inner face. Two other lipids which may contain arachidonic acid which could be released to make it available for prostaglandin are cholesterol esters and triglycerides.

II. Classification of Eicosanoids and Their Chemistry

1. Prostaglandins

All prostaglandins are derived from the basic prostanoic acid structure shown in Fig. 1. They have a cyclopentane ring, two aliphatic side chains, and a terminal carboxylic acid. In addition, all prostaglandins have a C-13:14 double bond and a 15-hydroxyl (or hydroperoxy) which are essential for their biological activity. The precise solution conformation is unknown, and indeed there is likely to be some flexibility in the exact position of the aliphatic side chains; however, the conformation of PGE_2 and other prostaglandins when crystallized has been determined (GERRARD 1985). During the synthesis of prostaglandins, the first stable intermediates formed by the prostaglandin synthase enzyme from arachidonic acid are the endoperoxides, PGG_2 and PGH_2.

Many nonsteroidal, antiinflammatory agents, including aspirin and indomethacin, exert their effects by inhibition of prostaglandin synthase (a component of cyclooxygenase). PGG_2 and PGH_2 are very unstable, with a half-life of about 5 min in water. Additional enzymes are involved in the metabolism of these endoperoxides to other prostaglandins. Specific isomerases convert PGH_2 to PGD_2 and PGE_2. A reductase converts PGH_2 to PGF_2. Prostacyclin synthase converts PGH_2 to PGI_2. PGI_2 is relatively stable in basic solutions but is unstable under neutral or acidic conditions, with a half-life of about 6 min in blood (pH 7.4). Its more stable end product, 6-keto-$PGF_{1\alpha}$, is the metabolite often detected in assays.

III. Erythropoiesis and Eicosanoids

The purpose of this review is to summarize the developments in this field since 1977, particularly focusing on the in vitro effects of both cyclooxygenase and lipoxygenase metabolites of arachidonic acid on erythropoiesis. For earlier work on the effects of prostaglandins on erythropoiesis, the reader is referred to reviews by FISHER and GROSS (1977) and by DUKES et al. (1975). For more detailed information of the arachidonic acid cascade, reviews by NEEDLEMAN et al. (1986) and by SAMUELSSON (1983) are recommended.

Early studies of the effects of prostaglandins on erythropoiesis centered around the effects of PGE_1, PGE_2, PGA_1, and PGA_2 in vivo. SCHOOLEY and MAHLMANN (1971a,b) were the first to demonstrate a stimulatory effect in plethoric mice. $PGF_{2\alpha}$ was ineffective, whereas PGE_1 and PGE_2 were effective and required the presence of erythropoietin. Both also enhanced the effects of hypoxia in mice. DUKES et al. (1973) demonstrated in ex-hypoxic polycythemic mice that PGA_1, PGA_2, PGE_1, and PGE_2 stimulated radioactive iron incorporation in newly formed red cells, but $PGF_{2\alpha}$ did not. PAULO et al. (1973) partially confirmed the work of Dukes when they reported a stimulatory effect of PGE_1 on radiolabelled iron incorporation in newly formed red cells of polycythemic mice and a stimulatory effect on erythropoietin (Ep) titers in the perfusates of isolated perfused dog kidneys previously exposed to hypoxia and infused with blood containing PGE_1. GROSS et al. (1976a,b) followed up this work with studies demonstrating that PGE_2, the primary renal prostaglandin, produced a significant dose-related increase in erythropoiesis in polycythemic mice and an increase in Ep in the isolated perfused dog kidney. The evidence, although indirect, supports the essential role of prostaglandins in the mechanism of Ep production by the kidney. Both DUKES et al. (1973) and FOLEY et al. (1978) found that the dehydrogenase-resistant prostaglandin analogues 15(s)-methy- and 16,16-dimethyl-PGE_2 were much more potent than the parent compound in terms of their ability to stimulate red blood cell production. NELSON et al. (1983) further reported that PGI_2 but not 6-keto-$PGF_{1\alpha}$ (its primary metabolite) also increased erythropoiesis in the ex-hypoxic polycythemic mouse assay.

B. Evidence for the Roles of Arachidonic Acid Metabolism in Erythropoiesis

I. Criteria for Implicating Eicosanoids

As a framework for studies of the role of arachidonic acid metabolites in erythropoiesis it is useful to consider specific criteria for implicating arachidonic acid metabolites in the physiologic response, in this case, Ep production or target cell proliferation and differentiation. P. NEEDLEMAN

(1987, personal communication) has suggested that the following criteria should apply:

1. Inhibition of the synthesis of the metabolite should abolish the response.
2. A specific agonist for the biological response should be capable of increasing arachidonic acid metabolite levels.
3. There should be a temporal and quantitative correlation between the production of the arachidonate metabolite and the biological response observed.
4. Addition of exogenous metabolite should mimic the biological response.
5. Exogenous administration of arachidonic acid should result in the synthesis of the metabolite and also elicit the biological response.

It is clear that arachidonic acid can enhance the production of erythropoietin by the kidney (Fig. 5). Inhibitors of the cyclooxygenase enzyme, sodium meclofenamate, indomethacin, and aspirin, can inhibit kidney production of erythropoietin (MUJOVIC and FISHER 1974; GROSS et al. 1976b; JELKMANN et al. 1979; SUSIC et al. 1979; GROSS and FISHER 1980; PAVLOVIC-KENTERA et al. 1980; RADTKE et al. 1980). Specific metabolites, such as the E prostaglandins, can mimic the response, although the level of ^{59}Fe incorporation in response to maximally effective doses of arachidonic acid was much lower than that elicited by PGE_2 (FOLEY et al. 1978). Subsequent studies (NELSON et al. 1983) demonstrated that an oxidation product of PGI_2, 6-keto-PGE_1, is a potent agonist for erythropoiesis in vivo. This metabolite, produced in a reaction catalyzed by NAD^+-dependent 9-

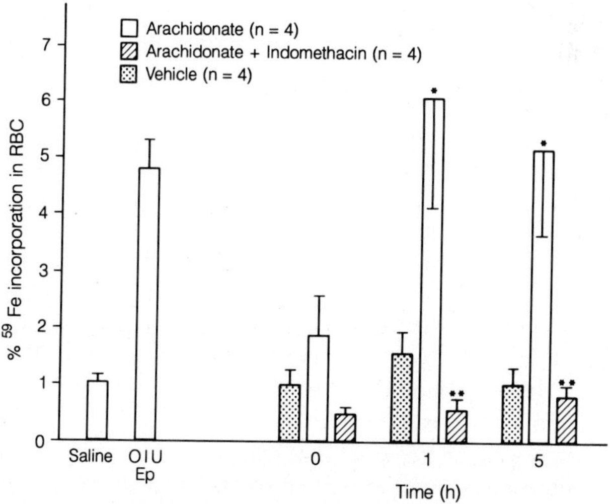

Fig. 5. Effect of arachidonate infusion (80 μg/min) on erythropoietin production in the posthypoxic, isolated perfused dog kidney. Each *bar* represents the mean ±SEM. *Significant difference ($P < 0.05$) between arachidonate-infused kidneys with and without pretreatment with indomethacin 01U, Ep concentration is 0.1 unit

hydroxyprostaglandin dehydrogenase, has not been identified as an endogenous effector of erythropoiesis as yet. Ep can enhance the production of PGE_2 and PGI_2 (FISHER and HAGIWARA 1984). Temporally and quantitatively the relationship between Ep and arachidonic acid metabolite production is also well supported. The mechanisms by which prostaglandins affect Ep release and/or synthesis remain unclear.

II. Target Cell Responses

Not so well documented are the roles of arachidonic acid metabolites in erythroid progenitor cell proliferation and differentiation. Although several laboratories have demonstrated effects of specific prostaglandins on erythroid colony forming units (CFU-E and BFU-E) in methylcellulose cultures in vitro, these effects depended on the presence of Ep in the culture and varied according to species and concentrations of metabolite studied. DUNN (1981) examined 10 prostaglandin derivatives for their ability to stimulate heme synthesis in serum-free cultures of fetal mouse liver cells in an attempt to define structural requirements of erythropoietic activity. Fetal liver is a rich source of erythroid progenitor cells at day 13–14 of gestation, at which time the stem cells reside in the liver on their migration from the yolk sac to the bone marrow (CHUI et al. 1971). Only PGE_2, $PGF_{2\alpha}$, and PGB_1 produced at least 50% stimulation of endogenous heme synthesis in the absence of serum or erythropoietin at concentrations of 10^{-16} to $10^{-5}\,M$. PGE_2 stimulated heme synthesis approximately 2.5 times at a concentration of $10^{-14}\,M$. This effect was evident at concentrations ranging from 10^{-14} to $10^{-10}\,M$. Inhibition of heme synthesis occurred at higher concentrations. When Ep was added to the cultures, the effects of PGE_2 were more variable, most often being inhibitory. Seven of the 10 prostaglandin derivatives tested were inhibitory at concentrations ranging between $5 \times 10^{-11}\,M$ ($PGF_{2\alpha}$) and $10^{-5}\,M$ (PGE_1, PGB_1). Both 15-epi-$PGF_{2\alpha}$ and PGB_2 were ineffective. Unit gravity cell sedimentation studies demonstrated that PGE_2 stimulated only the larger cells within the Ep responsive cell population. Very little characterization was done of the cell population involved. DATTA (1985) showed that PGE_2 ($1.5 \times 10^{-6}\,M$) in association with Ep stimulated the preferential synthesis of hemoglobin in PGE_2-treated, normal, adult, peripheral blood erythroid colonies. More recently, DATTA and his colleagues (1987) demonstrated that PGE_2 could play an active role in promoting the synthesis of hemoglobin F (HbF) in adults and in maintaining higher HbF synthesis following anemia or hypoxemia. DUKES et al. (1973), using [^{14}C]glucosamine uptake into rat bone marrow cells in vitro as the assay end-point, found PGE_2 to be the most potent of seven prostaglandins. However, PGA_2 was the most potent derivative when ^{59}Fe incorporation into heme was followed. Slight differences in the order of potency have been observed from laboratory to laboratory. While DUNN listed $PGE_2 > PGF_{2\alpha} > PGB_1$ as the order of potency, CHAN et al. (1980) employing erythroid burst formation and colony formation (BFU-E and CFU-E, respectively) demonstrated PGB_1 to be most potent, followed by $PGE_1 > PGF_{1\alpha} > PGA_1 > PGE_2 > PGF_{2\alpha} > PGB_2 > PGA_2$. A 20-min exposure was sufficient to elicit these effects when Ep was present. In DUNN's study, PGE_1, 15-epi-$PGF_{2\alpha}$, 6-keto-$PGF_{1\alpha}$, PGA_1, PGA_2, PGB_2, and prostacyclin had no effects. Undoubtedly, the assay systems used will influence the effects of added prostaglandins, i.e., adult bone marrow vs. fetal liver cells, amounts of fetal bovine serum, and endogenous levels of the prostanoids in serum, as well as availability of the substrate, arachidonic acid. High concentrations of fatty acid salts used in medium with a low albumin level will act in a "detergent" manner to cause lysis of erythroid cells. DUNN's structure-activity relationship (SAR) studies were the most extensive carried out to date for the cyclooxygenase products of arachidonic acid and suggest that the stimulatory properties of PGE_2 (on heme synthesis) are pharmacologically distinct from those of Ep. A prostaglandin antagonist, 15-epi-$PGF_{2\alpha}$, completely antagonized the PGE_2 effect without affecting the Ep response, implying that prostaglandins act by interaction with specific membrane receptors. BELEGU et al. (1983) found that murine bone marrow cells cultured in methylcellulose could form CFU-E-derived colonies in the presence of arachidonic acid (3×10^{-7} to 1×10^{-5} *M*) or PGE_2 or PGD_2 (Fig. 6, Fig. 7). Both of these prostaglandins have been shown to be produced in rat bone marrow (KOJIMA et al. 1980). ZIBOH et al. (1977) noted that rat bone marrow microsomes produce PGE_2 and PGF_2 as major metabolites. Sodium meclofenamate, a specific inhibitor of prostaglandin synthesis, significantly blocked the increase in CFU-E produced by arachidonic acid. ROSSI et al. (1980) reported species-specific

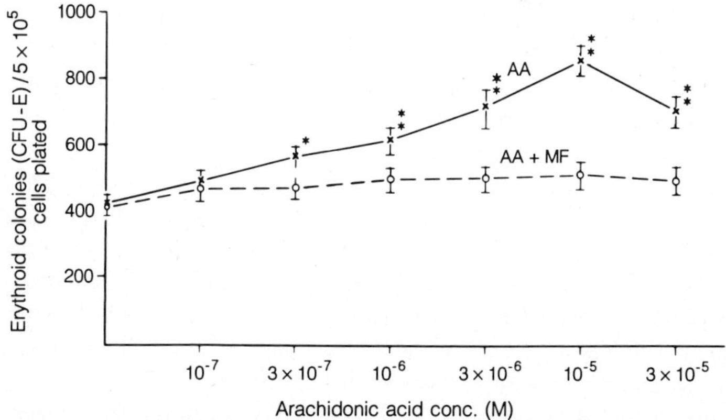

Fig. 6. Erythroid colony formation (CFU-E) in normal mouse bone marrow cultures (5×10^5 cells/plate) treated with several concentrations of arachidonic acid (*AA*) and meclofenamate (*MF*) (1×10^{-6} *M*). Each culture plate contained 0.2 U erythropoietin. *Bars* at each point represent SE of the mean of duplicate plates in 5 experiments. *Significantly different from erythropoietin alone ($P < 0.05$). **Significantly different from erythropoietin alone ($P < 0.001$)

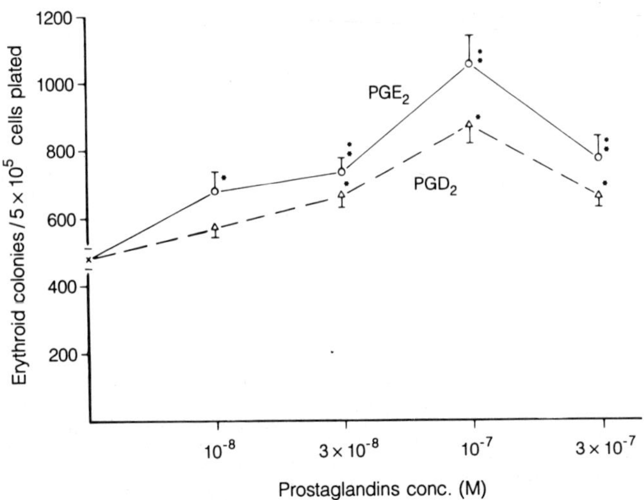

Fig. 7. Erythroid colony formation in normal mouse bone marrow cultures (n = 5) treated with several concentrations of prostaglandin E_2 (*PGE_2*) and prostaglandin D_2 (*PGD_2*). Each culture plate contained 0.2 U erythropoietin. *Significantly different from erythropoietin alone ($P < 0.05$). **Significantly different from erythropoietin alone ($P < 0.001$)

effects on CFU-E- and BFU-E-derived colonies in response to the addition of E prostaglandins (PGE_1 and PGE_2). The addition of PGE_1 to human marrow cultures exerted a significant enhancing effect on the clonogenic capacity of both CFU-E and BFU-E, which was abolished via removal of adherent cells. For murine hematopoietic precursors, PGE_1 inhibited BFU-E and colony forming unit–culture (CFU-C) (CFU-GM) colonies but had no effect on CFU-E. PGE_2 appears to be the most potent prostaglandin tested in all studies thus far, and its effect is likely to be distinct from that of Ep (Brown and Adamson 1977; Dunn 1981; Arce et al. 1981).

Feher and Gidali (1974) found that a 2.5-h preincubation of human bone marrow cells with PGE_2 (10^{-11} to 10^{-3} *M*) increased the fraction of spleen colony forming cells (CFU-S) killed by exposure to high concentrations of [^{3}H]thymidine to 30% from a control value of 5%. This suggests that the pluripotent hematopoietic stem cells of mice (CFU-S), which are normally in the resting (G_0) phase of the cell cycle, may be triggered by PGE_2 to commence DNA synthesis, indicating replication. The effects of PGE_1 and PGE_2 were also examined in vivo. Gidali and Feher (1977) found that the injection of 10^{-4} µg/g body weight caused a significant increase of the proportion of CFU-S in S-phase, without affecting their total number per animal.

III. Cell-Cell Interactions

Bone marrow stromal cells were shown either to enhance or to suppress erythroid colonies depending on the density of the marrow stromal cells in the culture underlayer (DeGowin and Gibson 1981; Werts et al. 1980). DeGowin et al. (1981) demonstrated that marrow stromal cells elaborate PGE which mediates both the enhancing and suppressing effects. Incremental doses of X-irradiation administered to replicating marrow stromal cells progressively decreased PGE levels and diminished enhancement of erythroid colonies. Dexter and colleagues (Dexter et al. 1977; Motomura and Dexter 1980) and Kurland and Moore (1977) have shown that PGE is suppressive to the formation of granulocyte-macrophage colonies (CFU-GM). Testa and Dexter (1977), also using long-term bone marrow cultures which allow the proliferation of multipotential stem cells (CFU-S), found that primitive BFU-E could be maintained for several weeks but failed to differentiate even with addition of Ep, as did CFU-E. This is similar to the result of Gibson et al. (1982) that confluent cultures of marrow stromal cells failed to support erythropoiesis. High cytotoxic doses of radiation (10000–20000 rad), however, released stimulatory concentrations of PGE. At doses of 100–800 rad, marrow stromal cell colony formation and PGE production were suppressed by a factor of 7.

Considerable evidence has accumulated indicating that either T lymphocytes (Nathan et al. 1978; Torok-Storb et al. 1981; Torok-Storb and Hansen 1982; Lipton et al. 1983) or monocyte-macrophages (Rossi et al. 1980; Rinehart et al. 1978; Kurland et al. 1980; Zuckerman 1981; Levitt et al. 1985), both populations (Mangan and Desforges 1980; Zuckerman 1980; Reid et al. 1981; Linch and Nathan 1984), or other cells (Linch et al. 1985) play roles in the regulation of BFU-E proliferation. Evidence by Lu et al. (1986) supports the specific enhancing effect of PGE_1 on colony formation by BFU-E expressing a high density distribution of major histocompatibility complex (MHC) class II antigens and that this effect requires the participation of a population of OKT8+ lymphocytes that do not need to express MHC class II antigens.

Kurland et al. (1978) have proposed, in a series of studies, a role for monocyte-macrophage-derived CSF and PGE in the positive and negative feedback control of myeloid stem cell proliferation, respective. The recognition that counterbalance mechanisms must exist to the positive feedback drive of this CSF (now identified as GM-CSF) caused these investigators to seek candidates for the negative feedback control. Limitation of CSF-dependent myelopoiesis may theoretically be mediated by activities inhibiting CSF production by mononuclear phagocytes, by direct inactivation of the CSF molecule, or by alteration in the responsiveness of the granulocyte-macrophage progenitor cells to CSF. E prostaglandins (PGE_1 and PGE_2) but not $PGF_{2\alpha}$ or PGF_1 profoundly inhibit CFU-GM (CFU-C) colony proliferation in vitro. In the presence of PGE, CFU-GM require an eight- or ninefold greater concentration of CSF in order to proliferate to the same extent as in the absence of PGE. Conversely, increasing the concentration of CSF counteracted the effectiveness of PGE-mediated inhibition, indicating that the control of production of both CSF and PGE may provide a dualistic modulation of committed stem cell proliferation. The physiologic relevance of PGE in myelopoiesis is suggested by the observation that the phagocytic mononuclear cells of human or murine origin actively synthesize and release PGE in vivo. In contrast, pure populations of lymphocytes and polymorphonuclear leukocytes do not possess detectable prostaglandin synthetase activity, and the level of PGE production by both normal and neoplastic monocyte-macrophages is dependent upon their state of stimulation. Thus, an important mechanism limiting inappropriate myelopoiesis is CSF-dependent macrophage PGE synthesis. The constitutive elaboration of CSF and PGE may account for the steady-state regulation of myelopoiesis. Recent studies have documented an in vivo inhibitory activity for PGE_2 on murine myelopoiesis; the total nucleated cellularity and the number of CFU-GM progenitor cells in both bone marrow and spleen were significantly suppressed in a mouse model by the intravenous administration of native PGE_2 as well as by a synthetic analogue, 16,16-dimethyl-PGE_2. A preferential inhibition of monocytopoiesis similar to the specificity demonstrated by PGE on monocyte production in vitro was also observed in the in vivo experiments. In addition, a reduction in the percentage of CFU-GM in the S-phase of the cell cycle and a decrease in the in vivo incorporation of [^{3}H] thymidine (TdR) was observed after the administration of PGE_2 to rebounding and steady-state mice.

IV. Specific Involvement of the Lipoxygenase Pathway

Although very few reports have appeared describing the effects of lipoxygenase metabolites in hematopoiesis or more specifically erythropoiesis (SNYDER and DESFORGES 1986; MILLER et al. 1986), there is suggestive evidence that they play a role because macrophages, which are central players in cell-cell interactions, can synthesize and secrete products of both the cyclooxygenase and lipoxygenase oxidative pathways (HUMES et al. 1977; ROUZER et al. 1980). When these cells are exposed to zymosan, the principal products of these pathways are PGE_2, PGI_2, and LTC_4. In addition to these enzymic pathways, resident mouse peritoneal macrophages contain a diversity of other lipoxygenases which give rise to 5-, 8-, 9-, 11-, 12-, and 15-HETEs (RIGAUD et al. 1979; RABINOVITCH et al. 1981; SCOTT et al. 1982). These HETEs can be further oxidized to their corresponding di-HETEs (MAAS et al. 1982).

Many studies have demonstrated that HPETEs and HETEs have regulatory effects on the enzymes of the arachidonic acid cascade. 12-HPETE, but not 12-HETE, inhibits platelet cyclooxygenase with a 50% inhibitory concentration of $3\,\mu M$ (SIEGEL et al. 1979). Lower concentrations of 12-

HPETE caused an increase in 12-lipoxygenase activity, presumably by acting as the hydroperoxy activator of lipoxygenases as described by HEMLER et al. (1978). Various other hydroperoxy compounds, including 15-hydroperoxy-PGE_1 and 15-HPETE have, in a similar manner, been shown by EGAN et al. (1981) to inactivate the cyclooxygenase associated with ram vesicular gland microsomes. EGAN and coworkers showed that an oxygen-centered radical was released from the hydroperoxy moiety of PGG_2 during its peroxidative reduction to PGH_2. This oxidant inactivates the cyclooxygenase as well as other enzymes of PG synthesis. Prostacyclin synthetase is particularly sensitive to this oxidative inactivation (HAM et al. 1981). In a similar manner, 15-HPETE is a potent inhibitor of both the 5- and 12-lipoxygenase from rabbit polymorphonuclear leukocytes and platelets (VANDERHOEK et al. 1982). In addition to the HPETE-mediated oxidative inactivation of cyclooxygenase and lipoxygenases, the corresponding HETEs are also inhibitors of these enzymes. 15-HETE has been shown to be a selective inhibitor of both the 5- and 15-lipoxygenase of rabbit polymorphonuclear leukocytes (VANDERHOEK et al. 1980) and also of the cyclooxygenase associated with ram vesicular gland microsomes (EGAN et al. 1981). Thus, both HPETEs and HETEs can regulate cyclooxygenase and lipoxygenases at the enzyme level. HUMES has concluded that lipoxygenase products such as 12- and 15-HETE must be considered potential intracellular regulators which can interact and regulate the synthesis of leukotrienes and prostaglandins. Certain inflammatory stimuli can stimulate prostaglandin synthesis exclusively without affecting lipoxygenase metabolism, whereas zymosan stimulates both oxidative pathways. Normal human bone marrow cells synthesize LTB_4, 5-HETE, 12-HETE, and 15-HETE, whereas bone marrow cells from patients with chronic myelocytic leukemia (CML) were found to produce significantly smaller amounts of both the double dioxygenation product 5*S*,12*S*-diHETE and the monohydroxy acid 12-HETE (965 ± 351 ng vs. 4390 ± 1801 ng indicating a 12-lipoxygenase deficiency; STENKE et al. 1987). The pattern of lipoxygenase products made in the bone marrow was similar to that for peripheral blood leukocytes after calcium ionophore stimulation. The levels of LTB_4 were also similar to those previously reported for peripheral blood granulocytes. This finding is consistent with an altered lipoxygenase activity in CML.

The finding that LTB_4 is produced by human bone marrow cells is of interest because of the work of CLAESSON et al. (1985) that LTB_4 stimulates human myelopoiesis in vitro, as determined by a CFU-GM assay. With CML the elevated LTB_4 levels may be responsible for excessive proliferation. Studies from other systems including glomerular epithelial cells (BAUD et al. 1985), epidermal keratinocytes (KRAGBALLE et al. 1985), and smooth muscle cells (PALMBERG et al. 1987) also support a role for leukotrienes in DNA synthesis (Table 1).

SNYDER and DESFORGES (1986) were the first to demonstrate that lipoxygenase metabolites of AA participate in the activation and of

Table 1. Evidence that leukotrienes initiate DNA synthesis

Metabolite	Target cell	Investigators
LTB_4	Granulocyte-macrophage progenitor cells	CLAESSON et al. 1985
LTC_4, LTD_4	Glomerular epithelial cells	BAUD et al. 1985
LTB_4, LTC_4, LTD_4	Epidermal keratinocytes	KRAGBALLE et al. 1985
LTB_4, LTC_4, LTD_4	Smooth muscle cells	PALMBERG et al. 1987

erythropoiesis as well as myelopoiesis. Their study was an indirect demonstration showing that the lipoxygenase-selective antagonists BW755C, 1-phenyl-3-pyrazolidone, butylated hydroxyanisole (BHA), and nordihydroguiaretic acid blocked all types of colony formation in a dose-dependent manner, whereas indomethacin, at concentrations which inhibited cyclooxygenase activity, had no significant effect. Although these findings are indirect, they suggest that certain lipoxygenase products may be important mediators of both CSF- and phorbol myristate acetate (PMA)-induced myelopoiesis and of burst promoting activity/erythropoietin (BPA/Ep)-induced erythropoiesis. The actual target cells involved could not be determined in these mixed cell populations of peripheral blood mononuclear cells and bone marrow cells from human sources, although the mononuclear cell preparations were well depleted of T cells and monocytes.

Since the lipoxygenase inhibitors were just as effective against PMA-induced monocytopoiesis as they were against CSF-induced myelopoiesis, the data suggest that lipoxygenase activation may be the final common intracellular pathway by which CSF, PMA, and BPA/Ep transmit their signals generated at the cell membrane.

Results from our laboratory support an important role for lipoxygenase metabolites in erythroid progenitor cell proliferation. Murine fetal liver cells (an enriched source of erythroid progenitor cells) respond to exogenous erythropoietin by proliferating and forming erythroid colonies (CFU-E) in semisolid media. Early erythroid progenitor cells (BFU-E) also form colonies in response to IL-3 or high concentrations of Ep. We found that inhibitors of the lipoxygenase pathway (BW755C, nordihydroguiaretic acid (NDGA), phenidone, and BHA) significantly inhibited both CFU-E- and BFU-E-derived colony formation, whereas the specific cyclooxygenase inhibitors, aspirin or sodium meclofenamate, did not (BECKMAN and NYSTUEN 1988). In addition, Ep stimulated the synthesis of 12-hydroxyeicosatetraenoic acid (12-HETE) and 15-HETE, as shown with high performance liquid chromatography and radioimmunoassay (BECKMAN et al. 1987). The addition of 12-HPETE but not 12-HETE or 15-HPETE/HETE could mimic the effect of Ep and stimulate erythroid colony formation (BECKMAN and SEFERYNSKA 1988). It is noteworthy that 5- and 12-lipoxygenase (LOX) products can activate guanylate cyclase, as this interaction could explain the

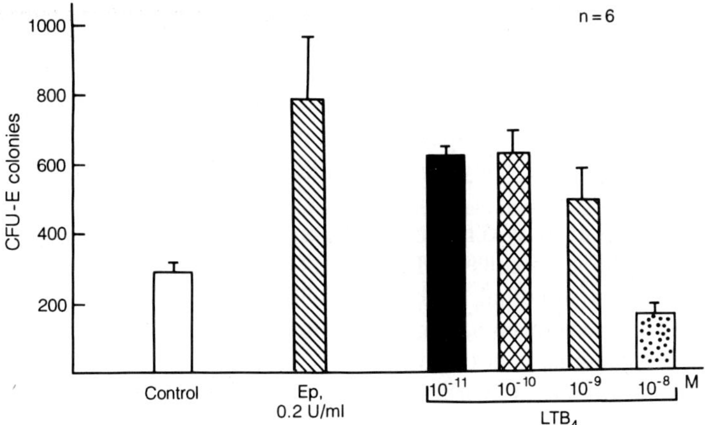

Fig. 8. Effect of the leukotriene *LTB*$_4$ on mouse fetal liver erythroid colony formation. At 10^{-11}, 10^{-10}, and 10^{-9} *M* LTB$_4$ significantly stimulated the formation of CFU-E-derived colonies in the absence of added erythropoietin ($n = 6$)

later increase in cGMP seen in response to Ep (White et al. 1980). As shown in Fig. 8, LTB$_4$ also significantly enhanced CFU-E colony formation in the absence of added Ep. Most recently, Beckman et al. (1990) have shown with specific radioimmunoassays that Ep induced a rapid rise in both LTB$_4$ and 12-HETE levels. Increases in both metabolites are detectable within 30 s and are significant by 2 min in the case of LTB$_4$ and 10 min in the case of 12-HETE. These elevations are sustained over 60 min for 12-HETE, but LTB$_4$ had returned to control levels by that time. It is therefore likely that lipoxygenase metabolites mediate cell proliferation in some way, perhaps by modulating intracellular calcium concentrations (Richter et al. 1987) or by activating protein kinase C. It is clear that intracellular calcium is involved at an early step in the mechanism of action of Ep (Miller et al. 1988; Mladenovic and Kay 1988), but the cascade of events between receptor activation and DNA synthesis await further study.

C. Future Directions for Research

In a progress report published in 1984, PGE$_2$ had been given to four patients with the anemia of end-stage renal disease (Ortega et al. 1984). There was a significant increase in peripheral blood BFU-E, which returned to baseline with cessation of therapy. A significant rise in serum Ep level was demonstrated in one patient. Side effects included local pain at the site of infusion and vomiting. Clinical trials of prostaglandins for end-stage renal disease became less important once the Ep gene was cloned in 1985 and became available through recombinant DNA technology (Jacobs et al. 1985). Sub-

Gross DM, Brookins J, Fink GD, Fisher JW (1976a) Effects of prostaglandins A_2, E_2 and F_2 on erythropoietin production. J Pharmacol Exp Ther 198:489–496

Gross DM, Mujovic VM, Jubiz W, Fisher JW (1976b) Enhanced erythropoietin and prostaglandin production in the dog following renal artery constriction. Proc Soc Exp Biol Med 151:498–501

Ham EE, Egan RW, Soderman DD, Gale PH, Kuehl FA Jr (1981) Peroxidase-dependent deactivation of prostacyclin synthetase. J Biol Chem 254:2191–2194

Hemler ME, Graff G, Lands WFM (1978) Accelerative autoactivation of prostaglandin biosynthesis by PGG_2. Biochem Biophys Res Commun 85: 1325–1331

Humes JL, Bonney RJ, Pelus L, Dahlgren ME, Sadowski SJ, Kuehl FA Jr, Davies P (1977) Macrophages synthesize and release prostaglandins in response to inflammatory stimuli. Nature 269:149–151

Jacobs K, Shoemaker C, Rudersdorf R, Neill SD, Kaufman RJ, Mufson M, Sukra J, Jones SS, Hewik R, Fritsch EF, Kaddkita M, Schimizu T, Miyake T (1985) Isolation and characterization of genomic and cDNA clones of human erythropoietin. Nature 313:806–810

Jelkmann W, Brookins J, Fisher JW (1979) Indomethacin blockade of albuterol-inducing erythropoietin production in isolated perfused dog kidney. Proc Soc Exp Biol Med 162:65–70

Keighley G, Cohen NS (1978) Stimulation of erythropoiesis in mice by adenosine 3′-5′-monophosphate and prostaglandin E_1. J Med 9:129–138

Kobayashi T, Levine L (1983) Arachidonic acid metabolism by erythrocytes. J Biol Chem 258:9116–9121

Kojima A, Shiraki M, Takahashi R, Orimo H, Morita I, Murota S-i (1980) Prostaglandin D_2 is the major prostaglandin of arachidonic acid metabolism in rat bone marrow homogenate. Prostaglandins 20:171–176

Kragballe K, Desjarlais L, Voorhees JJ (1985) Leukotrienes B_4, C_4 and D_4 stimulate DNA synthesis in cultured human epidermal keratinocytes. Br J Dermermatol 113:43–52

Kurland JI, Moore MAS (1977) Modulation of hemopoiesis by prostaglandins. Exp Hematol 5:357–373

Kurland JL, Bockman RS, Broxmeyer HE, Moore MAS (1978) Limitation of excessive myelopoiesis by the intrinsic modulation of macrophage derived prostaglandin E. Science 199:552

Kurland JI, Meyers PA, Moore MAS (1980) Synthesis and release of erythroid colony- and burst-potentiating activities by purified populations of murine peritoneal macrophages. J Exp Med 151:839–852

Levitt L, Kipps TJ, Engleman EG, Greenberg PL (1985) Human bone marrow and peripheral blood T lymphocyte depletion: efficacy and effects of both T cells and monocytes on growth of hematopoietic progenitors. Blood 65:663–679

Linch DC, Nathan DG (1984) T cell and monocyte derived burst-promoting activity directly act on erythroid progenitor cells. Nature 312:775–777

Linch DC, Lipton JM, Mathan DG (1985) Identification of three accessory cell populations in human bone marrow with erythroid burst-promoting properties. J Clin Invest 75:1278–1284

Lipton JM, Nadler LM, Canellos GP, Kudisch M, Reiss CS, Nathan DG (1983) Evidence for genetic restriction in the suppression of erythropoiesis by a unique subset of T-lymphocytes in man. J Clin Invest 72:694–706

Lu L, Broxmeyer HE (1985) Comparative influences of phytohemagglutinin-stimulated leukocyte conditioned medium, hemin, prostaglandin E_1 and low oxygen tension on colony formation by erythroid progenitor cells in normal human bone marrow. Exp Hematol 13:989–993

Lu L, Pelus LM, Broxmeyer HE (1984) Modulation of the expression of HLA-DR (IA) antigens and the proliferation of human erythroid (BFU-E) and multi-potential (CFU-GEMM) progenitor cells by prostaglandin E. Exp Hematol 12:741–748

Lu L, Pelus LM, Broxmeyer HE, Moore MAS, Wachter M, Walker D, Platzer E (1986) Enhancement of the proliferation of human marrow erythroid (BFU-E) progenitor cells by prostaglandin E requires the participation of OKT8-positive T lymphocytes and is associated with the density expression of major histocompatability complex class II antigens on BFU-E. Blood 68:126–133

Maas RL, Turk J, Oates TA, Brash AR (1982) Formation of a novel dihydroxy acid from arachidonic acid by lipoxygenase-catalyzed double oxygenation in rat mononuclear cells and human leukocytes. J Biol Chem 257:7056–7067

Mangan KF, Desforges JF (1980) The role of T lymphocytes and monocytes in the regulation of human erythropoietic peripheral blood burst forming units. Exp Hematol 8:717–727

Mayeux P, Billat C, Felix JM, Jacquot R (1986) Mode of action of erythropoietin and gluco-corticoids on the hepatic erythroid precursor cells: role of prostaglandins. Cell Differ 18:17–26

Miller AM, Russell TR, Gross MA, Yunis AA (1978) Modulation of granulopoiesis: opposing roles of prostaglandins F and E. J Lab Clin Med 92:983–990

Miller AM, Weiner RS, Ziboh VA (1986) Evidence for the role of leukotrienes C_4 and D_4 as essential intermediates in CSF-stimulated human myeloid colony formation. Exp Hematol 14:760–765

Miller BA, Scaduto RC Jr, Tillotson DL, Botti JJ, Cheung JY (1988) Erythropoietin stimulates a rise in intracellular free calcium concentration in single early human erythroid precursors. J Clin Invest 82:309–315

Mladenovic J, Kay NE (1988) Erythropoietin induces rapid increases in intracellular free calcium in human bone marrow cells. J Lab Clin Med 112:23–27

Motomura S, Dexter TM (1980) The effect of prostaglandin E, on hemopoiesis in long-term bone marrow cultures. Exp Hematol 8:298–303

Mujovic VM, Fisher JW (1974) The effects of indomethacin on erythropoietin production in dogs following renal artery constriction. I. The possible role of prostaglandins in the generation of erythropoietin by the kidney. J Pharmacol Exp Ther 191:575–580

Nathan DG, Chess L, Hillman DG, Clarke B, Breard J, Merler E, Housman DE (1978) Human erythroid burst-forming unit: T-cell requirement for proliferation in vitro. J Exp Med 147:324–339

Neal WA, Lewis JP, Garver FA, Lutcher CL (1980) The production of prostaglandins with an erythropoietin generating factor(s). Biochem Med 23:55–63

Needleman P, Turk J, Jakschik BA, Morrison AR, Lefkowith JB (1986) Arachidonic acid metabolism. Annu Rev Biochem 55:69–102

Nelson PI, Gross DM, Foley JE, Fisher JW (1978) A concept for control of kidney production of erythropoietin (Ep): the role of prostaglandins (PG) and cyclic nucleotides. Hematologica 63:629–646

Nelson PK, Brookins J, Fisher JW (1983) Erythropoietic effects of prostacyclin (PGI_2) and its metabolite 6-keto-prostaglandin (PG)E_1. J Pharmacol Exp Ther 226:493–499

Oates JA (1982) The 1982 Nobel Prize in physiology or medicine. Science 218: 765–768

Ortega JA, Dukes PP, Ma A, Shore NA, Malakzadeh MH (1984) A clinical trial of prostaglandin E_2 to increase erythropoiesis in anemia of end stage renal disease. A preliminary report. Prostaglandins Leukotrienes Med 14:411–416

Palmberg L, Claesson HE, Thyberg J (1987) Leukotrienes stimulate initiation of DNA synthesis in cultured arterial smooth muscle cells. J Cell Sci 88:151–159

Paulo LG, Wilkerson RD, Roh BL, George WJ, Fisher JW (1973) The effects of prostaglandin E_1 on erythropoietin production. Proc Soc Exp Biol Med 142: 771–775

Pavlovic-Kentera V, Susic D, Milenkovic P, Biljanovic-Paunovic L (1980) Effects of prostaglandin synthetase inhibitors, salt overload and renomedullary dissection on the hypoxia stimulated erythropoietin production in rats. Exp Hematol 8:(8):283–292

Rabinovitch H, Durand J, Rigaud M, Mendy F, Breton JC (1981) Transformation of arachidonic acid into monohydroxy-eicosatetraenoic acids by mouse peritoneal macrophages. Lipids 16:518–524

Radtke HW, Jubiz W, Smith JB, Fisher JW (1980) Albuterol-induced erythropoietin production and prostaglandins release in the isolated perfused dog kidney. J Pharmacol Exp Ther 214:467–471

Reid CDL, Baptista LC, Chanarin I (1981) Erythroid colony growth in vitro from human peripheral blood null cells: evidence for regulation by T-lmmphocytes and monocytes. Br J Haematol 48:155–164

Richter C, Frei B, Cerutti PA (1987) Mobilization of mitochondiral Ca^{2+} by hydroperoxyeicosatetraenoic acid. Biochem Biophys Res Commun 143:609–616

Rigaud M, Durand J, Breton JC (1979) Transformation of arachidonic acid into 12-hydroxy-5,8,10,14-eicosatetraenoic acid by mouse peritoneal macrophages. Biochim Biophys Acta 573:408–412

Rinehart JJ, Zanjani ED, Nomdedeu B, Gormus BJ, Kaplan ME (1978) Cell-cell interaction in erythropoiesis. Role of human monocytes. J Clin Invest 62: 979–986

Rossi GB, Migliaccio AR, Migliaccio G, Lettieri F, DiRosa M, Mastroberardino G, Peschle C (1980) In vitro interactions of PGE and cAMP with murine and human erythroid precursors. Blood 56:74–79

Rouzer CA, Scott WA, Cohn ZA, Blackburn P, Manning JM (1980) Mouse peritoneal macrophages release leukotriene C in response to a phagocytic stimulus. Proc Natl Acad Sci USA 77:4928–4932

Samuelsson B (1983) Leukotrienes: mediators of immediate hypersensitivity reactions and inflammation. Science 230:568–575

Schewe T, Halangk W, Hiebsch C, Rapoport SM (1975) A lipoxygenase in rabbit reticulocytes which attacks phospholipids and intact mitochondria. FEBS Lett 60:149–152

Schooley JC, Mahlmann LJ (1971a) Stimulation of erythropoiesis in the plethoric mouse by cyclic-AMP and its inhibition by anti-erythropoietin. Proc Soc Exp Biol Med 137:1289–1292

Schooley JC, Mahlmann LJ (1971b) Stimulation of erythropoiesis by prostaglandins and its inhibition of anti-erythropoietin. Proc Soc Exp Biol Med 138:523–524

Scott WA, Pawlowski NA, Andreach M, Cohn ZA (1982) Resting macrophages produce distinct metabolites from exogenous arachidonic acid. J Exp Med 155: 535–547.

Siegel MU, McConnell RT, Abrahams SL, Porter NA, Cuatrecasas P (1979) Regulation of arachidonate metabolism via lipoxygenase and cyclooxygenase by 12-HPETE, the product of human platelet lipoxygenase. Biochem Biophys Res Commun 89:1273–1280

Snyder DS, Desforges JF (1986) Lipoxygenase metabolites of arachidonic acid modulate hematopoiesis. Blood 67:1675–1679

Stenke L, Lillemor L, Reizenstein P, Lindgren JA (1987) Leukotriene production by fresh human bone marrow cells: evidence of altered lipoxygenase activation in chronic myelocytic leukemia. Exp Hematol 15:203–207

Susic D, Milenkovic P, Pavlovic-Kentera V (1979) The effect of aspirin on erythropoietin production in the rat. Proc Soc Exp Biol Med 161:476–478

Testa NG, Dexter TM (1977) Long-term production of erythroid precursor cells (BFU) in bone marrow cultures. Differentiation 9:193–195

Torok-Storb B, Hansen JA (1982) Modulation of in vitro BFU-E growth by normal Ia-positive T cells is restricted by HLA-DR. Nature 298:473–474

Torok-Storb B, Martin PG, Hansen JA (1981) Regulation of in vitro erythropoiesis by normal T cells: evidence for two T-cells subsets with opposing function. Blood 58:171–174

Vanderhoek JY, Bryant RW, Bailey JM (1980) 15-hydroxy-5,8,11,13-eicosatetraenoic acid: a potent and selective inhibitor of platelet lipoxygenase. J Biol Chem 255:5996–5998

Vanderhoek JY, Bryant RW, Bailey JM (1982) Regulation of leukocyte and platelet lipoxygenases by hydroxyeicosanoids. Biochem Pharmacol 31:3463–3467

Walden TL, Patchen ML, MacVittie TJ (1988) Leukotriene-induced radioprotection of hematopoietic stem cells in mice. Radiat Res 113:388–395

Werts ED, DeGowin RL, Knapp SA, Gibson DP (1980) Characterization of mouse stromal (fibroblastoid) cells and their association with erythropoiesis. Exp Hematol 8:423–433

White L, Fisher JW, George WJ (1980) Role of erythropoietin and cyclic nucleotides in erythroid cell proliferation in fetal liver. Exp Hematol 8:168–181

Willems C, Stel HV, Van Aken W, Van Mourik JA (1983) Binding and inactivation of prostacyclin (PGI_2) by human erythrocytes. Br J Hematol 54:43–52

Ziboh VA, Lord JT, Blick G, Kursunoglu I, Poitier J, Yunis AA (1977) Alteration of prostaglandin biosynthesis in rat chloroleukemic tumor. Cancer Res 37: 3974–3980

Zuckerman KS (1980) Stimulation of human BFU-E by products of human monocytes and lymphocytes. Exp Hematol 8:924–932

Zuckerman KS (1981) Human erythroid burst-forming units' growth in vitro is dependent on monocytes, but not T lymphocytes. J Clin Invest 67:702–709

CHAPTER 6

Iron Deficiency and Megaloblastic Anemias

L.R. SOLOMON

A. Iron-Deficiency Anemia

I. Introduction

Iron deficiency is a common cause of anemia worldwide (WORLD HEALTH ORGANIZATION 1975). Since iron plays a role in tissue oxygen delivery (as a component of red cell hemoglobin), cellular oxygen utilization (as a component of mitochondrial cytochromes and oxidases), and diverse metabolic processes (as a cofactor for various microsomal and cytoplasmic enzymes), iron deficiency not only limits erythropoiesis but impairs many other systemic functions as well. Moreover, iron deficiency frequently signals the presence of a pathologic source of gastrointestinal blood loss. Thus, recognition of iron deficiency, determination of its cause, and effective iron replacement are particularly important. While the pharmacologic use of iron for both the prevention and treatment of iron deficiency is relatively well defined, iron metabolism is a complex process which is still not completely understood.

II. Iron Metabolism

To maintain iron balance, systemic iron losses must be matched by dietary iron intake and gastrointestinal absorption (Fig. 1). The normal adult man loses 0.6–1.0 mg/day of iron primarily from the gastrointestinal tract (as blood, bile, and mucosal exfoliation) and from the skin (as perspiration, desquamation, and hair loss) (FINCH 1959; GREEN et al. 1968; BOTHWELL et al. 1979). In menstruating women, total iron losses increase to 1.2–1.6 mg/day (FINCH, 1959). Iron requirements are also increased by pregnancy, rapid growth (e.g., infancy, adolescence) (FENTON et al. 1977; DALLMAN et al. 1980; BENTLEY and JACOBS 1975), and certain pathologic states (e.g., blood loss, intravascular hemolysis). In developing countries dietary intake of absorbable iron may not be adequate, while in Western countries, dietary iron intake is often 10–20 fold greater than basal requirements. Although iron losses vary with the iron content of secretions and exfoliated cells (increasing with iron overload and decreasing with iron deficiency) (DURACH et al. 1955; GREEN et al. 1968), these physiologic

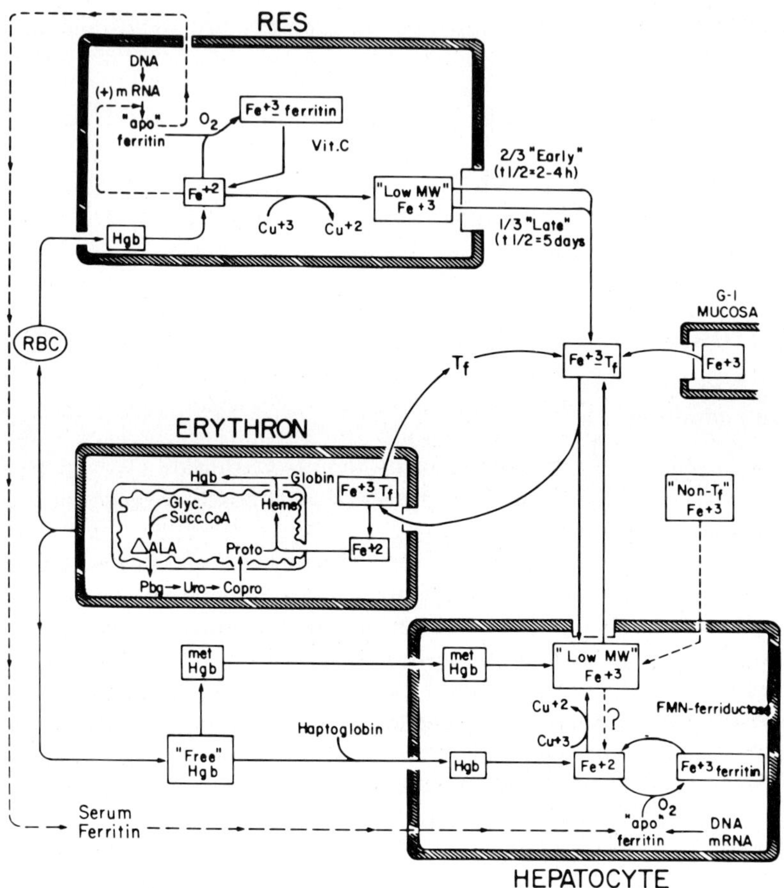

Fig. 1. Iron transport and metabolism. T_f, transferrin; *Vit. C*, vitamin C; "*Low MW*", low molecular weight; *Hgb*, hemoglobin; *G-I*, gastrointestinal; *RES*, reticuloendothelial system: *RBC*, red blood cell; *Glyc*, glycine; *Succ. CoA*, succinyl coenzyme A; *ALA*, δ-aminolevulinic acid; *Pbg*, porphobilinogen; *Uro*, uroporphyrin; *Copro*, coproporphyrin; *Proto*, protoporphyrin; *FMN*, flavin mononucleotide

mechanisms for either iron conservation or the excretion of excess body iron are limited. Thus, iron homeostasis depends primarily on the ability of gastrointestinal iron absorption to respond to changes in systemic iron requirements. (SMITH and PANNACCIULLI 1958). Indeed, in the rat, increased iron demands are met more by increased absorption than by increased mobilization of existing iron stores (COOK et al. 1973).

1. Iron Absorption

Animal tissues contain both heme iron (i.e., porphyrin-bound iron) and nonheme iron, while plant tissues contain only nonheme iron. Both forms are absorbed primarily in the duodenum and the proximal jejunum, but the mechanisms involved and the efficiency of absorption are distinctly different.

a) Nonheme Iron Absorption

Absorption of nonheme iron is particularly dependent on intraluminal factors which include the content of the meal itself, gastric acid, gastric and pancreatic proteases, and mucosal iron-binding proteins. Since nonheme iron in a meal enters a "common pool" (HALLBERG 1981), the chemical composition of the meal determines the nature of the iron complexes formed during digestion. Ferric (trivalent) iron is generally less readily absorbed than ferrous (divalent) iron because of its greater tendency to form oxides, hydroxides, and relatively large and/or insoluble salts with organic and inorganic acid anions (e.g., phosphate, carbonate, and oxalate) in the alkaline milieu of the small intestine (MOORE et al. 1944; HAHA et al. 1945; HEGSTED et al. 1949). Tannates in tea (DISLER 1975a,b; DEALARCON et al. 1979), chelate preservatives such as ethylenediaminetetraacetic acid (EDTA) (COOK and MONSEN 1976a), and plant tissue components such as phosphates and some proteins (HEGSTED et al. 1949; SIMPSON et al. 1978; COOK et al. 1981) form insoluble or poorly absorbable complexes with iron. Decreased absorption of iron bound to plant phytates or plant fibers has also been noted, but findings vary depending on the degree of saturation of phytate with iron and on the type of fiber studied (BJORN-RASMUSSEN 1974; REINHOLD et al. 1975, 1981; SIMPSON et al. 1978; KELSAY et al. 1979; MONNIER et al. 1980; HALLBERG et al. 1986, 1988). Thus, iron deficiency is prevalent in some vegetarian groups but not in others (HARDINAGE and STARE 1954; ANDERSON et al. 1981; DWYER et al. 1982; LATTA and LIEBMAN 1984; BINDRA and GIBSON 1986; HELMAN and DARNTON-HILL 1988). Binding of iron to some concurrently ingested medications (e.g., tetracycline, cholestyramine, and antacids containing sodium bicarbonate or calcium carbonate) (GREENBERGER et al. 1967; NEUVONEN et al. 1970; THOMAS et al. 1972; O'NEILL-CUTTING and CROSBY 1986) or nonfood substances (e.g., starch and clay) (MINNICH et al. 1968; THOMAS et al. 1976) also limits absorption. Coffee decreases iron absorption, but the mechanism of this effect is unclear (MORCK et al. 1983).

In contrast, some food components enhance iron absorption. Ascorbate is particularly effective (CONRAD and SCHADE 1968; DERMAN et al. 1980; HUNGERFORD and LINDER 1983) and can increase absorption of both phytate-bound iron and ferritin iron (a large storage iron complex in animal and plant tissues) (LAYRISSE et al. 1975; MARTINEZ-TORRES et al. 1976; DERMAN et al. 1982; HALLBERG et al. 1988). Ethanol augments ferric iron absorption, perhaps by stimulating gastric acid secretion (CHARLTON et al. 1964). Animal tissues also potentiate iron absorption (LAYRISSE et al. 1968, 1973; MARTINEZ-TORRES and LAYRISSE 1976; COOK and MONSEN 1975, 1976b). Although some amino acids (e.g., histidine, lysine, cysteine) enhance iron absorption, and high molecular weight digests of chicken muscle increase iron solubility in vitro (MARTINEZ-TORRES et al. 1981; SLATEVSKY and CLYDESDALE 1988), the effect of animal tissues on iron absorption is not explained solely by their protein content. Thus, animal proteins in milk, eggs, and cheese do not affect iron absorption (COOK and MONSEN 1976b), but iron in human milk is more available to nursing infants than iron in cow's milk (SAARINEN et al. 1977).

Gastric acid facilitates the dissociation of nonheme iron from the insoluble, nonabsorbable complexes present in many foods. Decreased absorption of both food iron and ferric iron salts in a patients with achlorhydria due to atrophic gastritis, gastric resection, or vagotomy and pyloroplasty can be corrected by either normal gastric juice or hydrochloric acid (STEVENS et al. 1958; COOK et al. 1964; SCHADE et al. 1968; JACOBS et al. 1967; JACOBS and OWEN 1969; BEZWODA et al. 1978; CELADA et al. 1978; MAGNUSSON et al. 1979). Reduction of gastric acid by H_2 antagonists and antacids also decreases dietary nonheme iron absorption, albeit probably not to a clinically significant degree (SKIKNE et al. 1981). An effect of hydrochloric acid on ferrous iron absorption has not been consistently observed (CELADA et al. 1978; JACOBS and OWEN 1969; JACOBS and MILES 1969a,b; HEINRICH 1970).

Neutralized gastric juice may also improve ferric iron absorption in achlorhydric subjects (JACOBS and OWEN 1969), and iron can bind to gastric mucopolysaccharides and to the gastric glycoprotein gastroferrin (DAVIS et al. 1966; SMITH et al. 1969; JACOBS and MILES 1969b,c; GLOVER and JACOBS 1971; SWAN and GLASS 1973; DAVIS et al. 1967; MULTANI et al. 1970). However, the bond between iron and gastric mucopolysaccharides is weak (WYNTER and WILLIAMS 1968; SWAN and GLASS 1973), an effect of neutralifed gastric juice on absorption in vivo has not been consistently observed (COOK et al. 1964; BEZWODA et al. 1978), and the effect of gastroferrin on iron absorption in man has not been directly tested. A role for gastric iron binders in iron absorption is therefore not established.

Bile acids can solubilize iron complexes (JACOBS and MILES 1970), and ligation of the bile duct in rats decreases the absorption of both ferric and ferrous chloride (CONRAD and SCHADE 1968). However, rodent bile is also rich in ascorbate, and direct addition of bile acids to ferrous sulfate solutions has no effect on iron absorption in man (BRISE 1962). Pancreatic proteases enhance the formation of soluble iron complexes, but pancreatic bicarbonate potentiates the formation of insoluble iron oxides and hydroxides (BENJAMIN et al. 1967; KAVIN et al. 1967). While iron absorption is augmented in some subjects with pancreatic insufficiency (DAVIS and BADENOCH 1962; TONZ et al. 1965), the presence of coexistent disorders (e.g., uncorrected iron deficiency and liver disease) complicate the interpretation of these observations (MURRAY and STEIN 1966; MIYAMORI et al, 1976). Moreover, pancreatic secretions do not consistently affect the absorption of ferrous or ferric iron in normal humans, dogs, or rats (KAVIN et al. 1967; MIYAMORI et al. 1976). Thus, it is unlikely that either the gallbladder or the pancreas plays a major role in iron absorption.

Transferrin, the principle iron transport protein in plasma, and transferrin-like proteins have been described in intestinal mucosal cells and in the succus entericus (BROWN and ROTHER 1963; HUEBERS et al. 1971, 1974, 1976; POLLACK and LASKEY 1976; HALLIDAY et al. 1976; BATEY and GALLAGHER 1977; EL-SHOKABI and RUMMEL 1977; SAVIN and COOK 1980; OSTERLOH and FORTH 1981; JOHNSON et al. 1983; OSTERLOH et al. 1985a), but their role in iron absorption is controversial (OSTERLOH et al. 1987a). Thus, only trace amounts of transferrin may be present in the gut lumen (OSTERLOH et al. 1986); enterocytes lack messenger RNA for transferrin synthesis (IDZERDA et al. 1986); neither transferrin nor transferrin receptors have been identified in human duodenal microvilli by immunochemical staining (PARMLEY et al. 1985; OSTERLOH et al. 1986); and transferrin-bound iron may not be readily released to intestinal mucosal cells (COX et al. 1979; SIMPSON et al. 1986; PETERS et al. 1988). However, immunoreactive transferrin has been demonstrated by others in the human intestinal mucosa (MASON and TAYLOR 1978); transferrin synthesized by the liver reaches the intestinal lumen in bile (IDZERDA et al. 1986); and transferrin-bound iron is effectively absorbed in the rat duodenum and jejunum in vitro (HUEBERS et al. 1977, 1983a). While intestinal mucosal transferrin is derived in part from a nonspecific leak of plasma proteins, a more selective process may also be operative (OSTERLOH et al. 1986; JOHNSON et al. 1983). Finally, although absorption of transferrin-bound iron by achlorhydric human subjects is no greater than that of ferric chloride (BEZWODA et al. 1986), this does not preclude a role for *endogenous* mucosal transferrin in the absorption of the unbound iron salt.

Lactoferrin, an immunologically distinct transferrin-like glycoprotein, is present in intestinal, pancreatic and biliary secretions (MASSON et al. 1966; ISOBE and SAKURAMI 1978). Lactoferrin can donate iron to human enterocytes in vitro (COX et al. 1979), and lactoferrin receptors have been described on the jejunal brush border from rabbits and infant monkeys (MAZURIER et al. 1985; DAVIDSON and LONNERDAL 1989). Monkey intestinal receptors bind human and monkey but not bovine lactoferrin, and lactoferrin saturated with iron is more effectively bound than the partially saturated form (DAVIDSON and LONNERDAL 1989). This "species specificity" of lactoferrin may explain why human infants absorb iron more effectively from human milk than from cow's milk (SAARININ et al. 1977). However, lactoferrin decreases ferrous iron absorption when given orally to normal human adults and decreases absorption of iron from ferric nitrolotriacetate in isolated segments of mouse intestine (DEVET and VAN GOOL 1974; SIMPSON et al. 1986). The roles of other structurally and immunologically distinct non-transferrin iron-binding proteins isolated from the intestinal mucosa remain undefined (HILL 1971; WORWOOD and JACOBS 1971; BOULARD et al. 1972;

In contrast, iron loading decreases the release of iron to the circulation but does not suppress mucosal iron uptake (Howard and Jacobs 1972; Thomson and Valberg 1971). Iron deficiency also increases heme iron absorption, perhaps by raising duodenal heme oxygenase activity (Raffin et al. 1974).

Despite extensive study, the factor(s) which signal and/or mediate intestinal mucosal responses to changes in iron requirements remain undefined. Roles for intraluminal gastric, intestinal, and plasma iron binding proteins have been considered. Gastroferrin, which may limit iron absorption, is decreased in iron-deficient human subjects, but this change is not significant when the effect of grastric secretory rates on the iron-binding properties of gastric juice is considered (Luke et al. 1967, 1968; Jacobs and Miles 1969a). Moreover, gastroferrin is not increased in multiply transfused patients with iron overload (Luke et al. 1968). Lactoferrin in intestinal mucus is low in patients with iron overload and increased in normal subjects with low serum iron levels (DeVet and Van Gool 1974). However, the result of frank iron deficiency on intestinal lactoferrin levels has not been described, and whether or not lactoferrin is capable of donating iron to intestinal mucosal cells is uncertain (Cox et al. 1979; Huebers et al. 1983a). The role of transferrin in the intestinal mucus has not been extensively studied. While iron deficiency may increase both transferrin in the intestinal lumen and the capacity of the mucosa to take up transferrin-bound iron (Huebers et al. 1983a), luminal transferrin levels in mice are low and do not increase when iron absorption is stimulated by hypoxia (Simpson et al. 1986).

Intestinal, intracellular, iron-binding proteins may also regulate iron absorption. Transferrin, which may facilitate iron absorption, increases in iron deficiency and decreases with iron overload (El-Shobaki and Rummel 1977; Savin and Cook 1980; Osterloh and Forth 1981; Johnson et al. 1983; Idzerda et al. 1986; Conrad et al. 1987), while ferritin may limit iron overload by "trapping" iron and increasing iron loss with mucosal exfoliation. Decreased mucosal cell ferritin and reduced incorporation of iron into ferritin occurs in iron deficiency, while increased mucosal ferritin has been noted in iron overload (Granick 1946; Charlton et al. 1965; Smith et al. 1968; Bernier et al. 1970; Worwood and Jacobs 1972; Linder et al. 1975; Savin and Cook 1980; Conrad et al. 1987; Whittaker et al. 1989). However, synthesis of apoferritin in response to even small doses of oral iron is the same in mucosal cells from normal and iron-deficient rats (Brittin and Raval 1970, 1971); neither the incorporation of absorbed iron into ferritin nor the total iron content of the intestinal mucosa is increased in rats with iron overload (Richmond et al. 1972; Worwood and Jacobs 1972; Simpson et al. 1986); mucosal cell transferrin and iron levels do not consistently correlate with the changes in iron absorption produced by alterations in iron stores or the rate of erythropoiesis, hypoxia, or inflammation (Chirasiri and Izak 1966; Balcerzak and Greenberger 1968; Schade 1972; Osterloh et al. 1985b, 1986; 1987b; Whittaker et al. 1989); and isolated mucosal cells from iron-deficient rates do not take up iron more avidly than those from normal animals (SAVIN and COOK 1978). Thus, the role of mucosal ferritin in regulating iron absorption is uncertain, and the importance of other as yet unidentified iron-binding proteins in intestinal mucosa cells must be assessed (CONRAD et al. 1987).

Factors affecting the release of iron from intestinal mucosal cells have also been sought without success. Iron deficiency and hypoxia stimulate hepatic transferrin synthesis and increase plasma apotransferrin levels (MCKNIGHT et al. 1980a,b; OSTERLOH et al. 1985b; IDZERDA et al. 1986). Moreover, apotransferrin binds more readily to intestinal mucosal cells than differric transferrin, and both apotransferrin and plasma from iron-deficient rats stimulate the release of iron from rat mucosal cells in vitro (LEVINE et al. 1972; EVANS and GRACE 1974). However, apotransferrin does not stimulate iron absorption in vivo (BEUTLER and BRITTENWEISER 1960; SCHADE et al. 1969; FINCH et al. 1982); saturation of transferrin with iron does not decrease mucosal iron release (WHEBY and JONES 1963); iron is readily released from isolated duodenal loops in the rat even when a plasma-free perfusate is used (JACOBS et al. 1966); and iron absorption is increased in humans and rats with hyportransferrinemia (GOYA et al. 1972; BERNSTEIN 1987). Thus, it is unlikely that plasma apotransferrin regulates mucosal cell iron release. Serum ferritin varies inversely with both total body iron stores and iron absorption (WALTERS et al. 1975). Although intravenous infusion of liver ferritin does not decrease mucosal iron absorption in the rat (GREENMAN and JACOBS 1975), the ferritin used was likely saturated with iron, whereas endogenous circulating ferritin is primarily apoferritin (WORWOOD et al. 1976). Nonetheless, since iron absorption in humans and mice changes more rapidly in response to variations in iron intake than either serum ferritin or the level of iron stores (MUNRO and LINDER 1978; O'NEIL-CUTTING and CROSBY 1987), it is not likely that serum ferritin regulates iron absorption.

2. Iron Transport

In normal subjects, iron in plasma is completely bound to transferrin (Fig. 1). Plasma transferrin is an 80000-dalton monomeric glycoprotein which is synthesized primarily by hepatocytes (JEEJEEBHOY et al. 1975; MORTON and TAVILL 1977; MCKNIGHT et al. 1980a,b), tightly binds ferric iron in conjunction with bicarbonate anion (AISEN et al. 1967; GABER and AISEN 1970; HARRIS and AISEN 1975; ROGERS et al. 1977), and is essential for effective iron delivery to the erythron. Thus, congenital atransferrinemia is characterized by iron-deficiency anemia and absent reticuloendothelial iron stores despite hepatic parenchymal cell iron overload. The anemia does not respond to parenteral iron therapy but improves when intravenous transferrin is administered (GOYA et al. 1972). A similar picture occurs in patients with acquired antibodies against either plasma transferrin or erythroid transferrin receptors (WESTERHAUSEN and MEURET 1977; LARRICK and HYMAN 1984). Several genetic variants of transferrin have been described, but differences in their iron transport properties have rarely been noted (TURNBULL and GIBLETT 1961; YOUNG et al. 1984; WONG and SAHA 1986). However, carbohydrate-deficient transferrin, an acquired variant present in alcoholic subjects, may lead to preferential iron uptake by hepatocytes because of binding to hepatic asialoglycoprotein receptors (BEGUIN et al. 1988; BEHRENS et al. 1988). Ethanol may impair glycosylation of transferrin by reducing hepatic 2,6-sialyltransferase activity (MALAGOLINI et al. 1989). Since rat liver endothelial cells can take up iron-transferrin complexes, desialate the transferrin, and release the intact complex to the space of Disse (TAVASSOLI 1988), asialoglycoprotein receptors may play a role in hepatocyte iron uptake in normal subjects as well.

Glycosylated transferrin binds to specific plasma membrane receptors present in most tissues (GATTER et al. 1983; TESTA 1985). In hepatocytes and reticulocytes, the same receptor binds differic-, monoferric-, and apotranferrin. At neutral pH, binding increases as the saturation of transferrin with iron increases, but at acid pH, apotransferrin is preferentially bound (MORGAN 1963; KLAUSNER et al. 1983a; DAUTRY-VARSAT et al. 1983). Thus, the decrease in pH produced by ethanol metabolism may impair hepatocyte iron uptake (BELOQUI et al. 1986). In contrast, in rat peritoneal macrophage, apotransferrin avidly binds to a receptor site distinct from that for iron-transferrin complexes (NISHISATO and AISEN 1982; SAITO et al. 1986). While this is consistent with the role of reticuloendothelial cells as iron storage sites and plasma iron donors, studies with cultured human monocytes have not confirmed this observation (BAYNES et al. 1987b). Posttranslational glycosylation may increase the affinity of the human erythroid transferrin receptor for transferrin (HUNT et al. 1989).

At the cell surface, some iron can dissociate from transferrin and diffuse into the cell (EGYED 1984; HUNEZ and GLASS 1985). However, in hematopoietic tissues, most iron enters the cell by endocytosis of the intact iron-transferrin complex (MORGAN and APPLETON 1969; BEAMISH et al. 1975; YOUNG and AISEN 1981; KLAUSNER et al. 1983b). The iron-tranferrin complex remains within the resulting endosomal vesicle and does not enter lysosomes as previously believed (OCTAVE et al. 1979, 1982; VAN RENSWOUDE et al. 1982). A decrease in pH then facilitates both dissociation of iron from transferrin and binding of apotransferrin to the endosomal membrane (RAO et al. 1983; TYCKO and MAXFIELD 1982). Apotransferrin is recycled to the circulation when the endosomal vesicle opens into the alkaline milieu at the cell surface (MORGAN and BAKER 1969; MORGAN 1971; MARTINEZ-MEDELLIN and SCHULMAN 1972; BOROVA et al. 1973). Studies using the ferrous iron chelator 2,2-bipyridine suggest that iron in the endosomal vesicle is reduced to the ferrous state and then transferred to the cytosol by a saturable, carrier-mediated process (BAYNES et al. 1988; EGYED 1988). In hepatocytes, uptake of transferrin iron may occur without endocytosis and may be mediated by membrane NADH: ferricyanide oxidoreductase activity (THORSTENSEN 1988).

Transferrin has two physicochemically distinct binding sites (AISEN et al. 1969; AASA 1972; PRICE and GIBSON 1972). A difference in their physiologic function has been suggested (FLETCHER and HUEHNS 1968; FLETSCHER 1969, 1971; HAHN et al. 1975; AWAI et al. 1975; VERHOEF et al. 1978; ZAPOLSKI et al. 1974; VAN BAARLEN et al. 1980; MARX et al. 1982) but not confirmed (OKADA et al. 1979; HUEBERS et al. 1978, 1981, 1984; YOUNG 1982; DIRUSSO et al. 1982; VAN DER HEUL et al. 1981, 1984; DIRUSSO et al. 1985). Rather, observed patterns of iron uptake from transferrin are best explained by the greater binding of diferric transferrin to transferrin receptors and by the "all or none" uptake of iron from iron-transferrin complexes (CHRISTENSEN et al. 1978; HUEBERS et al. 1981a,b,c, 1983b, 1984a, 1985).

Transferrin-mediated iron transport responds to changes in both systemic and cellular iron requirements. Synthesis of transferrin (in the liver) and transferrin binding sites (in human reticulocytes and erythroblasts) increase with iron depletion (MCKNIGHT, 1980a,b; SHUMAK and RACHKEWICH 1984; MUTA et al. 1987), while intracellular heme accumulation limits both reticulocyte iron-transferrin uptake and the release of transferrin iron following endocytosis (PONKA and NEUWIRT 1971; EGYED et al. 1986; PONKA et al. 1988). Transferrin synthesis is also stimulated by estrogens and hypoxia but decreased by starvation and ethanol ingestion. Transferrin depletion occurs in patients with the nephrotic syndrome or protein-losing enteropathies (AISEN 1984).

An iron transport role for ferritin has also been suggested. Ferritin receptors are present on hepatocytes, reticulocytes, and placental cells (BLIGHT et al. 1983; MACK et al. 1983; TAKAMI et al. 1986; ADAMS et al. 1988); erythrophagocytosing Kupffer cells can release ferritin (AISEN et al. 1988); iron-containing ferritin can be transferred from Kupffer cells to hepatocytes in vitro (SIBELLE et al. 1988); and guinea pig reticulocytes can utilize ferritin iron for heme synthesis (BLIGHT and MORGAN 1983). However, serum ferritin contains little or no iron and is cleared slowly from the circulation ($t_{1/2}$ = 50 h) (WORWOOD et al. 1976; WORWOOD 1982). Thus, while ferritin may be involved in *intracellular* iron transport, a physiologic role for ferritin in *systemic* iron transport is unlikely.

Since neither gastrointestinal iron absorption nor reticuloendothelial iron release requirs the presence of apotransferrin (SAITO et al. 1986), non-transferrin-bound iron appears in plasma as low molecular weight complexes when transferrin is completely saturated with iron (HERSHKO 1987). Uptake of non-transferrin-bound iron occurs primarily in hepatocytes by a carrier-mediated mechanism which is insensitive to changes in body iron stores (WRIGHT et al. 1986). Similarly when red blood cell (RBC) destruction is increased, iron in the form of heme or hemoglobin is transported by plasma hemopexin and haptoglobin, respectively, to receptors present exclusively on hepatocytes (HERSHKO et al. 1975; SMITH and MORGAN 1981; KINO et al. 1980).

3. Intracellular Iron Metabolism

Intracellular iron metabolism is not clearly defined (Fig.1). Iron is released from transferrin as the ferrous ion which then complexes with a low molecular weight protein (BAILEY-WOOD et al. 1975; WHITE et al. 1976; JONES et al. 1980) or with small molecules such as amino acids, nucleotides, sugars, or sulfhydryl compounds to form a soluble chelatable pool (HERSHKO et al. 1973; WORKMAN and BATES 1974; JACOBS A 1977; BACON and TAVILL 1984). Release of iron back to the circulation requires reoxidation. Two copper-containing plasma enzymes, ferroxidase I and II, stimulate iron release to plasma transferrin, and a ferroxidase inhibitor in rabbit serum decreases during iron depletion (TOPHAM et al. 1980). Ferroxidase I is identical to ceruloplasmin (OSAKI et al. 1966; RAGAN et al. 1969; ROESER et al. 1970; WILLIAMS et al. 1974). Thus, copper deficiency can decrease serum iron levels and lead to iron-deficient erythropoiesis (FRIEDEN 1983). In the reticuloendothelial cell, iron derived from phagocytosis of senescent red cells is either released rapidly to the circulation ($t_{1/2} < 1\,h$) or incorporated into ferritin and released gradually over several days (FILLET et al. 1974). Entry of iron into the early release pool is increased by iron deficiency and decreased by inflammation.

Heme, the prosthetic group of many iron-containing proteins, is formed in mitochondria from ferrous iron and protoporphyrin IX (JONES and JONES 1969). Both ferrous and ferric iron complexes can enter mitochondria, but all iron is reduced to the ferrous form by an energy-dependent, carrier-mediated process prior to crossing the inner mitochondrial membrane (ROMSLO and FLATMARK 1973; FLATMARK and ROMSCO 1975; BLIGHT and MORGAN 1983). Iron in ferritin may also be available for mitochondrial heme synthesis in the presence of reduced flavins (SPEYER and FIELDING 1979; FUNK et al. 1986). This contrasts with earlier studies suggesting that ferritin in erythroid precursors functions as a terminal storage site for excess iron (ZAIL et al. 1964; PRIMOSIGH and THOMAS 1968; BOROVA et al. 1973).

4. Iron Storage

Apoferritin, the major iron storage protein, has a molecular weight of 450000 daltons, contains 24 subunits derived from two distinct gene products (H&L), and can form a *soluble* complex with up to 4500 iron atoms in the form of ferric oxyhydroxide phosphate (MUNRO and LINDER 1978). Hemosiderin, an *insoluble* complex, probably arises from proteolytic breakdown of ferritin in secondary lysosomes (MUNRO and LINDER 1978). Structurally and immunologically distinct isoferritins are present in different tissues. Iron administration increases ferritin in many tissues in vitro and in vivo (SMITH et al. 1968; LINDER et al. 1970; SUMMERS et al. 1975; VULIMIRI et al. 1977) by stimulating gene transcription as well as by increasing both subunit aggregation and the translation of preformed cytoplasmic messenger RNA (WHITE and MUNRO 1988). The last effect may result from decreased interaction of a particular region of ferritin mRNA with a cytoplasmic protein which normally inhibits its translation (Drysdale and Shafritz 1975; Zahringer et al. 1976; Hentze et al. 1980; Leibold and Munro 1980). Ferritin formation also increases in reticuloendothelial cells after erythrophagocytosis. An effect of iron supply on ferritin degradation has been suggested but not confirmed (Chu and Fineberg 1969; Munro and Drysdale 1970; Millar et al. 1969).

Oxidation and reduction reactions are required for the uptake and release of iron by ferritin. Ferric iron does not complex directly with apoferritin, rather ferrous iron is bound and oxidized to the ferric state by the apoferritin protein (Niederer 1970; Harrison et al. 1977; Baker and Boyer 1986). Conversely, release of iron from ferritin involves reduction to the ferrous ion. In parenchymal cells such as hepatocytes, ferritin iron is reduced by a reduced nicotinamide-adenine dinucleotide-flavin mononucleotide (NADH-FMN) oxidoreductase (Sirivech et al. 1974). Xanthine oxidase can also reduce ferritin iron (Mazur 1965; Topham et al. 1989), but inhibition of this enzyme in vivo with allopurinol does not affect the hepatic nonheme iron content in rats, mice, or men (Kozma et al. 1968; Boyett et al. 1968; Grace et al. 1970). Reticuloendothelial cells in the spleen lack ferriductase activity (Frieden and Osaki 1974) and may utilize ascorbate for the nonenzymatic reductive release of iron from ferritin (Lipschitz et al. 1971). In K562 cells, lysosomal degradation of ferritin protein may mediate storage iron release (Roberts and Bomford 1988).

III. Biochemical and Physiologic Roles of Iron in Mammalian Tissues

Iron participates in many cellular and systemic processes, most often as a component of hemoproteins. Iron availability regulates mitochondrial heme synthesis (Ponka and Schulman 1985), and hemoproteins function in oxygen transport and storage (hemoglobin, myoglobin), electron transport (cytochromes), and oxidation reactions (cytochrome oxidase, cytochrome P-450, catalase, peroxidases, aldehyde oxidases, tryptophan pyrollase). Some nonheme-iron-containing flavoproteins function as oxidases and dehydrogenases (e.g., xanthine oxidase, succinic dehydrogenase, NADH dehydrogenase, α-glycerophosphate dehydrogenase, cytochrome *c* reductase). Nonheme iron in ribonucleotide reductase (Thelander and Reichard 1979) may explain the importance of this metal in nucleic acid synthesis in rapidly proliferating erythroid and nonerythroid cells (Hershko et al. 1970; Hoffbrand et al. 1976a) as well as the appearance of megaloblastic features in some iron-deficient patients (Roberts et al. 1971; Hill et al. 1972). Enzyme changes due to iron deficiency vary in different tissues depending on the turnover rates of both the individual protein and the particular cell type (Jacobs A 1969b).

Iron availability also limits the rates of erythropoiesis (Hillman and Henderson 1969). Moreover, since transferrin receptor expression is increased in neoplastic tissues in vivo (FAULK et al. 1980; KOHGO et al. 1986; KOZLOWSKI et al. 1988) and in mitogen-stimulated lymphocytes in vitro (HUEBERS and FINCH 1987), iron delivery may regulate proliferation of nonerythroid tissues as well (TROWBRIDGE and OMARY 1981). Indeed, some tumor cells have distinct iron transport proteins and can utilize iron in the absence of transferrin (BROWN et al. 1982; FERNANDEZ-POL 1978; BASSET et al. 1986). Iron deficiency can also alter triiodothyronine metabolism and impair temperature regulation (DILLMANN et al. 1980).

IV. Iron-Deficiency Anemia

1. Clinical Aspects

Iron deficiency usually results from increased blood loss (particularly from the gastrointestinal tract) or decreased absorption (Table 1). Despite significant gastrointestinal blood loss, negative tests for occult blood in stool may occur if the bleeding is intermittent or as a result of vitamin C ingestion (JAFFE et al. 1977). While oral iron supplements may cause false-positive

Table 1. Causes of iron deficiency

A. Decreased absorption
   1. Some vegetarian diets
   2. Medications (formation of complexes with iron), e.g., cholestyramine, tetracycline, some antacids
   3. Gastric disorders (decreased acid), e.g., atrophic gastritis, H_2 receptor blockers, gastric surgery
   4. Disorders of the small intestine, e.g., sprue, celiac disease, regional enteritis, surgery
B. Impaired utilization
   1. Decreased transferrin or impaired transferrin function
      a) Hereditary atransferrinemia
      b) Acquired
         1. Antibodies against transferrin
         2. Antibodies against transferrin receptors
   2. Decreased reticuloendothelial iron release, e.g., "inflammation", copper deficiency
C. Increased requirement
   1. Rapid growth, e.g., infancy, early childhood
   2. Pregnancy
   3. Increased erythropoiesis (?), e.g., hemolysis, ineffective erythropoiesis
D. Increased loss
   1. Gastrointestinal bleeding, e.g., peptic ulcers, malignancy, arteriovenous malformations
   2. Menstrual blood loss
   3. Intravascular hemolysis, e.g., sickle cell disease, aortic valve prostheses, paroxysmal nocturnal hemoglobinuria, complement-mediated autoimmune hemolytic anemia
   4. Urinary blood loss
   5. Idiopathic pulmonary hemosiderosis

tests for occult blood in stool, this is rare (LIFTON and KREISLER 1982; LAINE et al. 1988; MCDONNELL et al. 1989). Thus, neither negative tests in iron-deficient subjects nor positive tests in subjects on iron therapy should discourage appropriate diagnostic studies of the gastrointestinal tract.

Iron-deficiency anemia can be asymptomatic or accompanied by weakness and easy fatigability. Limited work capacity and a propensity to develop lactic acidosis in rats and humans (FINCH et al. 1976; OHIRA et al. 1979) may be due to decreased muscle oxygen utilization rather than reduced red cell oxygen transport (FINCH et al. 1979; DAVIES et al. 1984; MCLANE et al. 1981). A link between work capacity and the activities of mitochondrial iron-dependent dehydrogenases has been suggested but not confirmed (FINCH et al. 1979; OHIRA et al. 1982; MACDONALD et al. 1985; CELSING et al. 1988), and it is likely that several mitochondrial iron-related processes are involved. Epithelial changes including koilonychia, angular stomatitis, and papillary atrophy of the tongue may occur, and a role for coexistent vitamin B_6 deficiency in mediating some of these has been suggested (JACOBS and CAVILL 1968). Neurologic symptoms including headache, irritability, decreased attentiveness, and paresthesias may relate to changes in brain oxidative metabolism and dopaminergic functions (YOUDIM and BEN-SHACHAR 1987). However, coexistent lead intoxication should also be considered in appropriate patients since iron deficiency increases intestinal lead absorption (FLANAGAN et al. 1979). Thrombocytosis is common, but thrombocytopenia may occur with severe iron deficiency, and a role for iron in regulating thrombopoiesis has been suggested (KARPATKIN et al. 1974; SCHER and SILBER 1976).

Apotransferrin decreases iron availability to microorganisms, and iron deficiency may increase resistance to bacterial infections (MASAWE et al. 1974; MURRAY et al. 1978). Release of lactoferrin from neutrophils may contribute to local control of infection in a similar manner. However, since iron deficiency impairs both granulocyte function and cell-mediated immunity, susceptibility to certain infections (e.g., *Candida, Herpes*) may actually increase (BUCKLEY 1975; HUEBERS and FINCH 1987). Coexistent deficiencies of other nutrients can also impair host defence mechanisms. Thus, the net clinical impact of iron deficiency on the risk of infection is difficult to assess (BROCK 1986).

2. Diagnosis of Iron Deficiency

Since most patients with iron deficiency require evaluation for the presence of an underlying disorder while administration of iron to patients who are not iron deficient may carry some risk, the diagnosis of iron deficiency must be rigorously established (Table 2). Most often, iron-deficiency anemia is normochromic/normocytic and must be distinguished from the anemia of chronic disease. Microcytosis and hypochromia develop when iron deficiency is more prolonged, and this disorder must then be distinguished

Table 2. Differential diagnosis of iron deficiency

Test	Iron deficiency			Anemia of chronic disease	Thalassemia syndromes	Sideroblastic anemias
	Depleted stores	"Early" anemia	"Late" anemia			
Hemoglobin	NL	↓	↓	↓	NL—↓	↓
Serum ferritin	↓	↓	↓	↑	NL—↑	NL—↑
Serum iron	NL	↓	↓	↓	NL—↑	NL—↑
TIBC	NL	↑	↑	↓	NL	NL
Transferrin saturation	NL	↓	↓	↓	NL—↑	NL—↑
RBC protoporphyrin	NL	NL	↑	NL—↑	NL	↓—NL—↑
Bone marrow iron						
Reticuloendothelial stores	Absent	Absent	Absent	NL—↑	NL—↑	NL—↑
Sideroblasts	NL—↓	↓	↓	↓	NL—↑	"Rings"
RDW	NL	↑	↑	↑	NL	↑
MCV	NL	NL	↓	NL—↓	↓	↓—NL—↑
MCH	NL	NL	↓	NL—↓	↓	↓—NL
Response to iron therapy	(−)	(+)	(+)	(−)	(−)	(−)

TIBC, total iron binding capacity; NL, normal; RBC, red blood cell; RDW, red cell distribution width; MCV, mean corpuscular volume; MCH, mean corpuscular hemoglobin.

from the thalassemia syndromes and, less commonly from other hemoglobinopathies (hemoglobin E), the sideroblastic anemias, copper deficiency, and aluminum intoxication.

There are many pitfalls in the interpretation of noninvasive studies used to diagnose iron deficiency, and no single test is consistently predictive of the status of marrow iron stores particularly in the in-hospital setting (Cook et al. 1976, 1982). As reticuloendothelial iron stores decrease, serum ferritin levels fall (Walters et al. 1973; Cook et al. 1974; Bezwoda et al. 1979a). A low serum ferritin content always indicates iron deficiency, while normal values exclude this diagnosis in otherwise healthy subjects (Lipschitz et al. 1974). However, serum ferritin may be normal or even elevated when iron deficiency is accompanied by inflammation, liver disease, uremia, myocardial infarction, sickle cell crisis, myeloproliferative disorders, or other malignancies (Worwood 1986; Krause and Stolc 1980; Matzner et al. 1980; Halliday and Powell 1984; Brownell et al. 1986). In inflammation, the rise in serum ferritin results from stimulated ferritin synthesis and generally parallels the increase in other acute phase reactants (Konijn and Hershko 1977). Serum ferritin remains elevated for several weeks after an acute inflammatory event (Elin et al. 1977; Birgegard et al. 1978). In contrast, red cell ferritin is low in both iron deficiency and the anemia of chronic disease, increased in thalassemia, and unaffected by coexistent liver disease (Cazzola et al. 1983; Isa et al. 1988; Piperno et al. 1984). Similarly, monocyte ferritin may be a better index of the status of iron stores in hemodialysis patients than serum ferritin (Nuwayri-Salti et al. 1990). However, neither red cell nor monocyte ferritin are measured routinely in clinical labs.

When iron stores are depleted, serum iron falls, and the total iron binding capacity increases. Iron delivery to the marrow limits erythropoiesis when the saturation of transferrin with iron falls below 15% (Bainton and Finch 1962). While occasional microcytes may then be noted on examination of the peripheral smear and the red cell distribution width (RDW) may increase accordingly, the mean corpuscular volume (MCV) and hemoglobin (MCH) do not fall for 1–3 months (Conrad and Crosby 1962; England et al. 1976; Bessman 1980). Persistent iron deficiency also leads to a progressive increase in RBC protoporphyrin. Since inflammation decreases the release of iron to plasma from hepatocytes, reticuloendothelial cells, and intestinal mucosal cells (Lee, 1983), the resulting hypoferremia and desaturation of transferrin leads to "iron-deficient erythropoiesis" indistinguishable from that due to true iron deficiency (Lee et al. 1983; Cazzola et al. 1983; Baynes et al. 1987a; Thompson et al. 1988). Although the serum iron binding capacity usually decreases in inflammation, probably due to increased transferrin catabolism (Aisen 1984), distinguishing iron-deficiency anemia from the anemia of chronic disease not infrequently requires histochemical evaluation of bone marrow aspirates for the presence of reticuloendothelial iron stores which are absent in the former and normal or increased

hemodialysis patients, particularly when phosphate-binding antacids are needed, parenteral iron has also been used in this population (STEWART et al. 1976; HENDLER and SOLOMON 1978; LAWSON et al. 1971; O'NEILL-CUTTING and CROSBY 1986). However, iron absorption in these patients increases appropriately in response to decreases in iron stores, and oral iron supplements are often effective (ESCHBACK et al. 1977; GOKAL et al. 1979; BEZWODA et al. 1981; MILMAN et al. 1976, 1982; PARKER et al. 1979). Intravenous iron initially permits greater iron delivery to both erythroid and nonerythroid tissues than oral iron (HILLMAN and HENDERSON 1969; HENDERSON and HILLMAN 1969) but the net rate of increase in hemoglobin is the same with both routes of iron administration (MCCURDY 1965).

Up to 5 ml of iron dextran can be given by deep intramuscular injection into each buttock using a zigzag approach to prevent skin staining. Because of the risk of anaphylaxis, a test dose of 25 mg of iron should be given 24 h earlier. However, retention of 10%–50% of the dose at the injection site, pain, scarring, and the possible risk of sarcoma (WEINBREN 1978) make intravenous administration more desirable. A dose of 500 mg of iron is diluted with 500 ml of isotonic saline or 5% dextrose. A test dose of 25 mg is infused over 10 min. If there is no reaction 30 min later, the remainder of the dose may be infused over 2–3 h. Although not approved in the USA, administration of the total calculated dose of iron needed (see page 154) as a single infusion is widely practiced. Up to 30% of the iron-dextran stored in reticuloendothelial cells appears to be relatively unavailable. Thus, iron-deficient erythropoiesis may subsequently develop despite the presence of histochemically documented iron stores in bone marrow aspirates (HENDERSON and HILLMAN 1969; CHERNELCH et al. 1969; OLSSON and WEINFELD 1972; OLSSON et al. 1972). Moreover, with chronic use, hepatic and splenic siderosis may be present along with high serum ferritin levels when marrow iron stores are decreased or absent (ALI et al. 1982; CHERNELCH et al. 1969). While parenteral iron acutely decreases absorption of oral iron in rats (MURRAY and STEIN 1972; GRUDEN 1988), the duration of this effect and its relevance to man are unknown.

Parenteral iron may acutely cause transient urticaria and malaise. Fever, headache, arthralgias, myalgia, and generalized lymphadenopathy develop up to 48 h later in 1%–2% of patients and persist for 3–7 days (MEDICAL LETTER 1977; WALLERSTEIN 1969). Joint symptoms may be particularly severe in patients with rheumatoid arthritis (LLOYD and WILLIAMS 1970). Life-threatening acute anaphylactic reactions with hypotension and respiratory compromise occur in 0.1% of patients, while severe delayed reactions occur in 0.4% of patients who tolerate the initial test dose (HAMSTRA et al. 1980; AUERBACH et al. 1983).

B. Megaloblastic Anemias

I. Definition and Differential Diagnosis

The megaloblastic anemias are characterized by abnormal delayed nuclear maturation which results in nuclear-cytoplasmic asynchrony and premature intramedullary destruction of erythroid precursors (ineffective erythropoiesis) (Table 3). Thus, despite often marked erythroid hyperplasia in the bone marrow, the reticulocyte count is low relative to the severity of anemia. Myeloid and megakaryocytic maturation are usually also abnormal, and both neutropenia and thrombocytopenia may result (CHANARIN 1979; PERILLIE et al. 1967). Most often megaloblastic anemia results from vitamin B_{12}- or folic acid deficiency, but drugs or chemicals which directly impair nucleic acid metabolism and primary marrow disorders (e.g., myelodysplastic syndromes) can produce a similar picture (SCOTT and WEIR 1980).

Studies in mitogen-stimulated lymphocytes suggest that a block in the elongation of new DNA daughter strands during DNA synthesis may be the defect common to all causes of megaloblastosis (DAS and HOFFBRAND 1970; HOFFBRAND et al. 1976b; WICKRAMASINGHE and HOFFBRAND 1980), but this has not been confirmed in bone marrow cells (BOND et al. 1982). Nonetheless, marked chromosomal structural changes are present in bone marrow cells from vitamin B_{12} or folate-deficient patients (DAS et al. 1986), and a possible role for vitamin B_{12} and folate deficiency in DNA instability and carcinogenesis has been suggested (BUTTERWORTH et al. 1982; BRANDA et al. 1984; HEIMBURGER et al. 1988; LASHNER et al. 1989). While megaloblastic maturation may lead to the formation of structurally and/or functionally abnormal red cells, granulocytes, and platelets (BALLAS 1978; KAPLAN and BASFORD 1976; CRIST et al. 1980; LEVINE 1973; HAMRELL et al. 1979; SKACEL and CHANARIN 1983; YOUINOU et al. 1982; SCOTT et al. 1982), the mechanism of premature cell death remains undefined.

Table 3. Causes of megaloblastic anemia

- Folic acid deficiency
- Vitamin B_{12} deficiency
- Pharmacologic agents affecting nucleic acid metabolism
  - Antipurines: 6-mercaptopurine, 6-thioguanine, azathioprine
  - Antipyrimidines: 5-fluorouracil, cytosine arabinoside, azauridine
  - Ribonucleotide reductase inhibitors: hydroxyurea
  - Mechanism unknown: arsenic[a]
- Hereditary disorders of nucleic acid metabolism
  - Orotic aciduria
  - Lesch–Nyhan syndrome
- Primary marrow disorders
  - Myelodysplastic disorders: e.g., refractory anemia, sideroblastic anemia
  - Myeloproliferative disorders: e.g., agnogenic myeloid metaplasia, leukemia
  - Multiple myeloma

[a] See Morse et al. 1980.

II. Clinical Manifestations

Since anemia develops slowly, symptoms are often absent or nonspecific, and megaloblastic erythropoiesis is generally suspected because of macrocytes in the peripheral blood and a high MCV. The increase in MCV often precedes the development of anemia (CHANARIN 1976; SAVAGE and LINDENBAUM 1983), but a normal or low MCV and RDW may occur in patients with coexistent iron deficiency or thalassemia or even in anemic patients without other apparent hematologic disorders (PEDERSON et al. 1957; TASKER 1959; PEZZIMENTI and LINDENBAUM 1972; GREEN et al. 1982b; SPIVAK 1982; GRAIG et al. 1985; CARMEL and KARNAZE 1985; MATHEWS et al. 1988; CARMEL et al. 1987; THOMPSON et al. 1989). Iron deficiency also masks the biochemical and morphologic indices of megaloblastosis in the bone marrow (VAN DER WEYDEN et al. 1972). Thus, macrocytosis is not a sensitive marker of megaloblastosis. Moreover, a high MCV is not specific for megaloblastic anemia (MCPHEDRAN et al. 1973). Granulocytes with hypersegmented nuclei are another moderately sensitive, albeit nonspecific, index of megaloblastic hematopoiesis (CHANARIN 1976; EICHACKER and LAWRENCE 1985; THOMPSON et al. 1989), and impaired granulocyte function in patients with vitamin B_{12} deficiency has been suggested but not confirmed (KAPLAN and BASFORD 1976; HAMRELL et al. 1979; KATKA et al. 1983). Hypersegmented granulocytes may persist for 2 weeks after appropriate treatment is instituted (NATH and LINDENBAUM 1979), while macrocytosis gradually resolves over 2–3 months. Although megaloblastic erythroid hyperplasia is characteristically present in bone marrow, erythroid hypoplasia may occur, and megaloblastic myeloid hyperplasia can mimic leukemia (LEVINE and HAMSTRA 1969; PEZZIMENTI and LINDENBAUM 1972). Megaloblastic changes in rapidly proliferating cells in the gastrointestinal tract can cause glossitis, diarrhea, and occasionally nutrient malabsorption (WINAWER et al. 1965). Vitamin B_{12} also plays a role in bone metabolism, but this is of unknown clinical significance (CARMEL et al. 1988b).

Vitamin B_{12} deficiency also affects the cerebrum and the dorsolateral columns of the spinal cord (subacute combined degeneration), resulting in dementia, impaired vibratory and joint position senses (primarily in the legs), and rarely frank paraparesis with urinary and fecal incontinence, Lhermitte's sign (BUTLER et al. 1981), and orthostatic hypotension (WHITE et al. 1981). Neurologic symptoms can develop and progress in the absence of macrocytosis, anemia, or magaloblastic erythropoiesis (JEWESBURY 1954; SMITH 1960; STRACHAN and HENDERSON 1965; KARNAZE and CARMEL 1987). While the folate deficiency commonly present in adults with neuropsychiatric disorders may be secondary to decreased dietary folate intake in this population, folate depletion has been associated with decreased brain neurotransmitter levels, and congenital disorders of folate metabolism are often accompanied by mental retardation and neurologic defects (GRANT et al. 1965; PINCUS et al. 1972; REYNOLDS 1976; CLAYTON et al. 1986; ERBE 1975;

BOTEZ et al. 1979). Thus, folate may also be important for normal neurologic function.

III. Biochemistry of Folic Acid and Vitamin B_{12}

The folate coenzymes directly affect nucleic acid synthesis by mediating the transfer of one-carbon units required for the synthesis of the purine ring (5,10-methenyltetrahydrofolate and 10-formyltetrahydrofolate) and the methyl side chain of the pyrimidine nucleotide, thymidylic acid (5,10-methylenetetrahydrofolate). A rate-limiting role for the latter reaction in mammalian DNA synthesis has been suggested but not confirmed (FRIEDKIN 1963; MATTHEWS et al. 1989). Nonetheless, uracil incorporation into DNA (in place of thymine) is increased in marrow cells from folate-deficient human subjects and in human lymphocytes incubated with folate antagonists (GOULIAN et al. 1980; LAZZATO et al. 1982). Folates also directly influence amino acid metabolism, mediating the interconversion of serine and glycine (5,10-methylenetetrahydrofolate), the formation of homocysteine from methionine (5-methyltetrahydrofolate), and the breakdown of the histidine catabolite, formiminoglutamic acid (FIGLU) (tetrahydrofolate). Intracellular folates exist primarily as polyglutamates, which are more active as coenzymes than the corresponding monoglutamates (SHANE and STOKSTAD 1985). Tetrahydrofolic acid (THF) is the most effective substrate for polyglutamate synthesis (MCGUIRE et al. 1980).

In contrast, vitamin B_{12} affects nucleic acid synthesis indirectly by altering folate and methionine metabolism (Fig. 2). Three mechanisms have been proposed to explain the effects of vitamin B_{12} deficiency on folate metabolism: a methylfolate trap, "formate starvation", and impaired polyglutamate synthesis.

In mammalian tissues, vitamin B_{12} coenzymes participate in only two reactions: methylmalonyl CoA mutase (5′-deoxyasdenosyl B_{12}) and methionine synthetase (methyl B_{12}) (SILBER and MOLDOW 1979; MELLMAN et al. 1977; KOLHOUSE and ALLEN 1977a). The latter reaction is irreversible and provides the only known mechanism for the utilization of *N*-5-methyl-THF (N5MTHF) and, hence, for the regeneration of the other folate coenzymes (NIXON et al. 1973; KUTZBACH and STOKSTAD 1971; TAYLOR et al. 1974; GREEN et al. 1988). Thus, vitamin B_{12} deficiency may decrease DNA synthesis by "trapping" folate in the N5MTHF form and limiting the formation of *N*-5,10-methylene-THF needed for thymidylate synthesis (HERBERT and ZALUSKY 1962). Findings consistent with this "methylfolate trap" hypothesis include: (a) relative or absolute increases in tissue and serum N5MTHF levels in vitamin-B_{12}-deficient animals and humans as well as in L1210 cells cultured in vitamin-B_{12}-deficient media (HERBERT and ZALUSKY 1962; KNOWLES and PRANKERD 1962; STOKSTAD et al. 1966; BROTHERS et al. 1975; SHIN et al. 1975; THENEN and STOKSTAD 1973; SMITH et al. 1974; LUMB et al. 1981; FUJI et al. 1982); (b) failure of exogenous N5MTHF (but not

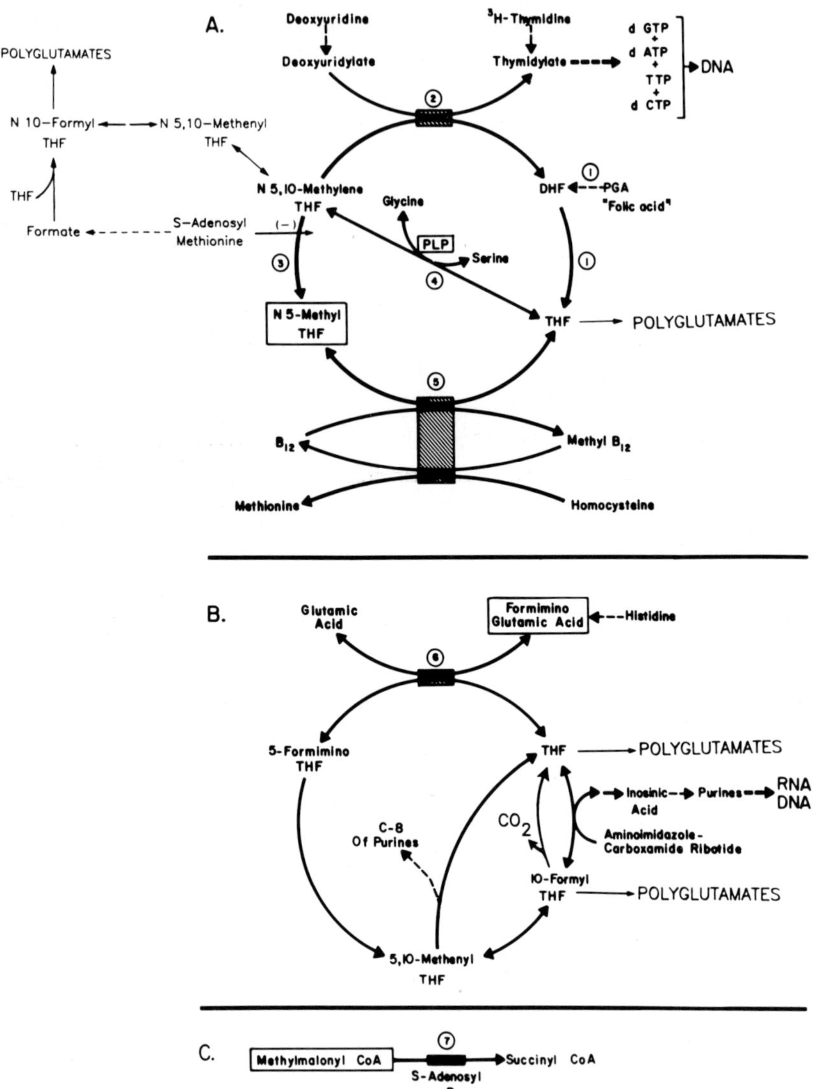

Fig. 2 A-C. Biochemical interrelationships of vitamin B_{12} and the folate vitamers. *THF*, tetrahydrofolate; *DHF*, dihydrofolate; *PGA*, pteroylglutamic acid; *PLP*, pyridoxal 5'-phosphate

pteroylglutamic acid) to support growth of vitamin-B_{12}-depleted L1210 cells (KONDO et al. 1989; CHELLO and BERTINO 1973); (c) decreased clearance of serum N5MTHF but increased clearance of nonmethylated folates in vitamin-B_{12}-deficient subjects (HERBERT and ZALUSKY 1962; NIXON and BERTINO 1972); (d) decreased methionine synthetase activity in the liver of vitamin-B_{12}-deficient rats and in the bone marrow of vitamin-B_{12}-deficient humans (KUTZBACH et al. 1967; GAWTHORNE and SMITH 1974; SAUER and WILLMANNS 1977); and (e) decreased methionine production by megaloblasts from vitamin-B_{12}-deficient patients but not from those with folate deficiency (KASS 1976). Similarly, exposure to nitrous oxide (N_2O) which selectively inactivates methionine synthetase in animal and human tissues by oxidizing the cobalt in methyl-B_{12} from Co(I) to Co(III) also increases plasma and urinary N5MTHF and produces a relative increase in N5MTHF in the liver and bone marrow (DEACON et al. 1980a; CHARNARIN et al. 1985; KANO et al. 1981; KONDO et al. 1981; WILSON and HORNE 1986).

De novo synthesis of thymidylate from deoxyuridylate suppresses the activity of the salvage pathway for the formation of thymidylate from thymidine in normal marrow cells, but this suppression is decreased in marrow cells from subjects with vitamin B_{12} or folate deficiency (KILLMAN 1965). This observation is consistent with the methyl-folate trap hypothesis and is the basis of the deoxyuridine (dU) suppression test which measures the incorporation of radiolabeled thymidine into DNA in either bone marrow cells or peripheral blood lymphocytes before and after incubation with unlabeled dU. However, thymidylate synthetase activity is often normal in megaloblastic marrow cells from subjects with vitamin B_{12} or folate deficiency (SAKAMOTO et al. 1975; MATTHEWS et al. 1989), and thymidylate pools are not lower in megaloblasts than in normoblasts after in vitro incubation with dU (GANESHAGURU and HOFFBRAND 1978). Moreover, thymidine kinase activity is increased in megaloblasts (WICKRAMASINGHE et al. 1975), and the phenomenon of dU suppression appears to result in part from inhibition of thymidine kinase by both dU and thymidylic acid (PELLINEMI and BECK 1980). Nonetheless, abnormal dU suppression in folate-deficient marrows is at least partially corrected in vitro by all folate coenzymes but not by vitamin B_{12}, while abnormal dU suppression in vitamin-B_{12}-deficient marrows is at least partially corrected by vitamin B_{12}, formyl-THF, THF, and folic acid (PGA) but not by N5MTHF (GANESHAGURU and HOFFBRAND 1978; DAS and HERBERT 1978; TAHERI et al. 1982; SKACEL et al. 1983; KANO et al. 1984; WICKRAMASINGHE and MATHEWS 1988). Thus, while the mechanism of dU suppression remains uncertain, this test is a useful biochemical indicator of functional intracellular vitamin B_{12} or folate deficiency.

Contrary to the predictions of the methylfolate trap hypothesis, the clearance of larger doses of N5MTHF from blood is normal in some vitamin-B_{12}-deficient patients, and oxidation of the methyl group of N5MTHF in N_2O-treated rats may occur by a methionine-synthetase-independent pathway (CHANARIN et al. 1980; LUMB et al. 1980, 1985, 1988). Alternatively, then, the decrease in methionine synthesis in vitamin B_{12} deficiency may reduce the availability of formate needed for the synthesis of formyl-THF (CASE and BENEVENGA 1977; CHANARIN et al. 1980, 1985). Findings consistent with this "formate starvation" hypothesis include (a) the

fruit bats develop only neuropathy, and rats and mice suffer no apparent adverse effects. Moreover, the biochemical effects of B12 deficiency vary with the organ system studied (CHENG et al. 1975; SOURIAL and BROWN 1983; CHANARIN et al. 1985), and effects of vitamin B_{12} on mitochondrial metabolism have also been described (MATLIB et al. 1979). Thus, the complex roles of vitamin B_{12} in metabolism remain incompletely understood.

IV. Vitamin B_{12} Deficiency

1. General Considerations

Vitamin B_{12} (cobalamin) is synthesized only by bacteria and consists of a porphyrin ring structure containing monovalent cobalt which is linked to a 5,6-dimethylbenzimidazole ribotide (Fig. 3). Since it is not appreciably concentrated in plants, vitamin B_{12} in the diet is derived almost exclusively from animal tissues and products (e.g., eggs and milk FARQUARSON and ADAMS 1976). Unwashed vegetables grown using human manure as fertilizer also provides an adequate source of B12 which is produced by colonic bacteria (CHANARIN 1979). Although the daily B12 requirement is only 0.5–2.0 µg, a typical nonvegetarian Western diet may provide as little as 3–5 µg/day (CHANARIN 1979; BAKER and MATHAN 1981; HERBERT 1987b). An additional 5–10 µg/day of vitamin B_{12} is excreted in the bile and reabsorbed in the ileum. The diet also contains biologically inactive "analogues" which are either synthesized by intestinal bacteria or produced by chemical modification of active vitamin B_{12} by other dietary components (BRANDT et al. 1977; HERBERT et al. 1978; KONDO et al. 1982; MACKLER et al. 1984; KONDO et al. 1989). These B_{12} analogues can be absorbed in the ileum and have been detected in human plasma and tissues (KOLHOUSE and ALLEN 1977b; KOLHOUSE et al. 1978; KANAZAWA and HERBERT 1983; SHAW et al. 1989). The presence of analogues in human fetal sera but not in the placenta suggests they may also be produced by endogenous vitamin B_{12} metabolism (MUIR and LANDON 1985).

The normal adult body contains 2–5 mg of vitamin B_{12}, most of which is stored in the liver (GRASBECK 1959). The biologically active forms are deoxyadenosyl-B_{12} and methyl-B_{12}. Methyl-B_{12} is the major cobalamin in human plasma, while deoxyadenosyl-B_{12} is the major plasma cobalamin in other animals. Deoxyadenosyl-B_{12} is the principle intracellular cobalamin (KOLHOUSE and ALLEN 1977a; LINNELL and MATHEWS 1984).

2. Vitamin B_{12} Metabolism

a) Vitamin B_{12} Binding Proteins

Vitamin B_{12} absorption and systemic transport are mediated by three distinct types of binding proteins which function to conserve and utilize effic-

COBALAMIN

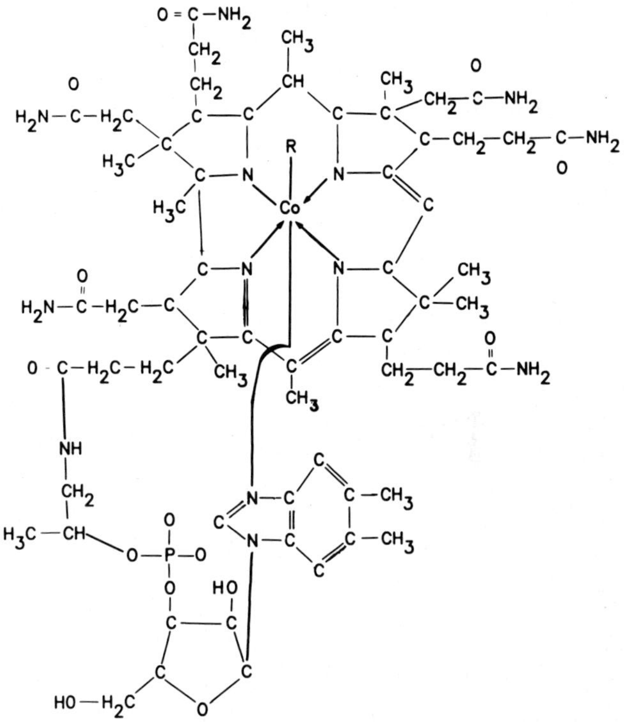

B12 VITAMER	R Group
Cyanocobalamin	CN–
Hydroxocobalamin	HO–
Methylcobalamin	CH_3-
Deoxyadenosylcobalamin	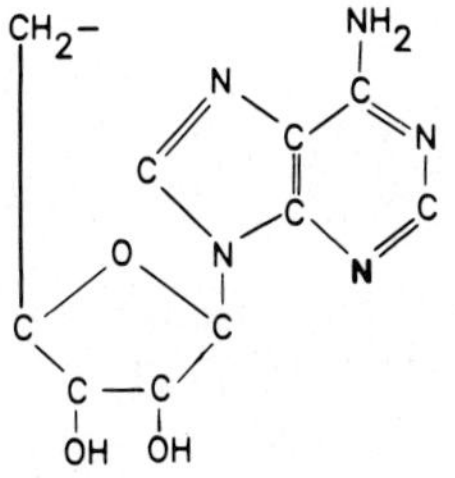 CH_2-

Fig. 3. Structure of the B_{12} vitamers

iently the small amounts supplied in the diet. These proteins may also limit the accumulation of potentially toxic analogues.

Intrinsic factor (IF) is a glycoprotein synthesized by gastric parietal cells which mediates vitamin B_{12} absorption by specific receptors on ileal mucosal cells. IF effectively binds only the microbiologically "active" forms of cobalamin. The presence of antibodies which either block the interaction of IF with vitamin B_{12} or prevent the binding of the vitamin B_{12}-IF complex to ileal receptors suggest that IF has separate domains for these two functions (KAPADIA and DONALDSON 1985). This is supported by the finding of an abnormal IF in a vitamin-B_{12}-deficient child which binds vitamin B_{12} normally but does not promote ileal uptake of vitamin B_{12} (KATZ et al. 1974).

Transcobalamin II (TCII) is a nonglycosylated plasma vitamin B_{12}-binding protein. TCII can also bind vitamin B_{12} analogues in vitro (KOLHOUSE and ALLEN 1977), but TCII-bound analogues have not been detected in human sera except in the setting of vitamin B_{12} deficiency (MRUI and CHANARIN 1983; HERZLICH and HERBERT 1988). Synthesis of TCII can occur in hepatocytes, fibroblasts, macrophages, endothelial cells, and probably ileal enterocytes (SEETHARAM and ALPERS 1982; FEHR and DEVECCHI 1985; HALL et al. 1985; CARMEL et al. 1990). As a result, plasma TCII levels increase in disorders associated with macrophage activation (e.g., Gaucher's disease, inflammatory bowel disease, certain malignancies) and decrease in liver disease (GILBERT and WEINREB 1976; CARMEL and EISENBERG 1977; RACHMILEWITZ et al. 1980; OSIFO et al. 1988). Normally, TCII constitutes only 10%–20% of the vitamin B_{12} binding capacity of plasma, but it is essential for vitamin B_{12} delivery to tissues. Thus, the circulating vitamin B_{12}-TCII complex has a short half-life (5–90 min); receptors for it are present in many tissues; vitamin B_{12} uptake into cells in vitro is stimulated by TCII (MEYER et al. 1974; YOUNGDAHL-TUONER et al. 1979); and hereditary deficiency of TCII or the presence of an abnormal TCII which binds vitamin B_{12} but does not promote vitamin B_{12} uptake results in severe megaloblastic anemia despite the presence of normal serum vitamin B_{12} levels (CARMEL and HERBERT 1969; HITZIG et al. 1974; HAURANI et al. 1979; SELIGMAN et al. 1980). TCII also mediates vitamin B_{12} transport in the brain and placenta, and TCII levels increase during pregnancy (LAZAR and CARMEL 1981; FERNANDES-COSTA and METZ 1979a).

The third class of vitamin B_{12} binders, termed "R" binders (for their rapid electrophoretic mobility), haptocorrin or cobalophilin, are heterogeneous glycoproteins which share an immunologically distinct protein core and avidly bind both vitamin B_{12} and its analogues. R proteins are present in plasma as well as in bile, milk, and gastric and salivary secretions (SANDBERG et al. 1981). The plasma R binders are transcobalamin I (TCI) and transcobalamin III (TCIII). TCI, the major R binder in plasma, is a sialic acid-containing glycoprotein. The presence of high TCI levels in subjects with hepatitis or with hepatic neoplasms suggests that TCI may be produced by the liver (BURGER et al. 1975a; CARMEL 1975; CARMEL and EISENBERG 1977; OSIFO et al. 1988). R binders are also increased in some patients with malignancy, particularly in the presence of liver metastases (CARMEL 1975; CARMEL and EISENBERG 1977). TCIII, which is identical to the R binder noted in granulocytes, is an asialoglycoprotein present at low levels in normal plasma and at higher levels in subjects with granulocytosis and myeloproliferative disorders (GILBERT et al. 1969; CORCINO et al. 1970; CHIKKAPPA et al. 1971; CARMEL 1972; HALL 1976). The TCIII-vitamin B_{12} complex has a half-life of only 5 min and is probably taken up by asialoglycoprotein receptors on hepatocytes (BURGER et al. 1975b). Although 80%–90% of plasma vitamin B_{12} is bound to TCI, the half-life of the vitamin B_{12}-TCI complex is 8–11 days; neither TCI nor TCIII promotes vitamin B_{12} uptake by other cells in vitro, and hereditary deficiency of TCI is not associated with clinical evidence of vitamin B_{12} deficiency despite the presence of low serum vitamin B_{12} levels (CARMEL and HERBERT 1969; MEYER et al. 1974; BURGER et al. 1975; HALL and BEGLEY 1977). Thus, plasma R binders are not essential for tissue vitamin B_{12} delivery. In fact, abnormal or increased R binders can impair vitamin B_{12} availability and produce megaloblastic anemia despite normal serum vitamin B_{12} levels (NEXO et al. 1975; CORCINO et al. 1971). However, R binders may prevent the neurotoxic effects of vitamin B_{12} analogues (SIGAL et al. 1987; CARMEL et al. 1988a).

Immunologically distinct intracellular vitamin-B_{12}-binding proteins in human fibroblasts appear to be the vitamin-B_{12}-dependent apoenzymes, methylmalony-CoA mutase and homocysteine-methionine methyl transferase (ROSENBERG et al. 1975; MELLMAN et al. 1977).

b) Vitamin B_{12} Absorption

In the stomach, acid peptic digestion releases vitamin B_{12} from protein conjugates in food (Fig. 4) (COOPER and CASTLE 1960). Vitamin B_{12} then attaches to R binders present in gastric secretions and saliva. IF released by gastric parietal cells does not bind vitamin B_{12} at acid pH, but the increase in pH in the duodenum and the proteolytic degradation of R binders by pancreatic proteases permits the transfer of vitamin B_{12} to IF (ALLEN et al. 1978a,b). Bile acids inhibit the binding of B12 to IF in vitro, but the physiologic significance of this interaction is unknown (TEO et al. 1981). The IF-vitamin B_{12} complex then binds to specific receptors on ileal mucosal cells (HAGEDORN and ALPERS 1977). This is enhanced by bile acids in vivo and in vitro and decreased by a fall in pH (CARMEL et al. 1969; TEO et al. 1980; SEETHARAM et al. 1983). Bile also contains vitamin B_{12} bound to R binder which is released and reabsorbed through the action of pancreatic proteases and IF (GREEN et al. 1981, 1982a). This enterohepatic circulation recycles as much as 5–10 μg/day of vitamin B_{12}. Because of the limited number of ileal receptor sites, only 1–2 μg of vitamin B_{12} can be absorbed from a single exogenous oral dose by this IF-mediated process (DONALDSON et al. 1973).

It is unclear whether the intact IF-vitamin B_{12} complex enters the enterocyte or whether vitamin B_{12} is released from IF at the cell surface (MARCOULLIS and ROTHENBERG 1981; KAPADIA et al. 1983). In any case, vitamin B_{12} uptake requires calcium but not energy, and IF does not appear

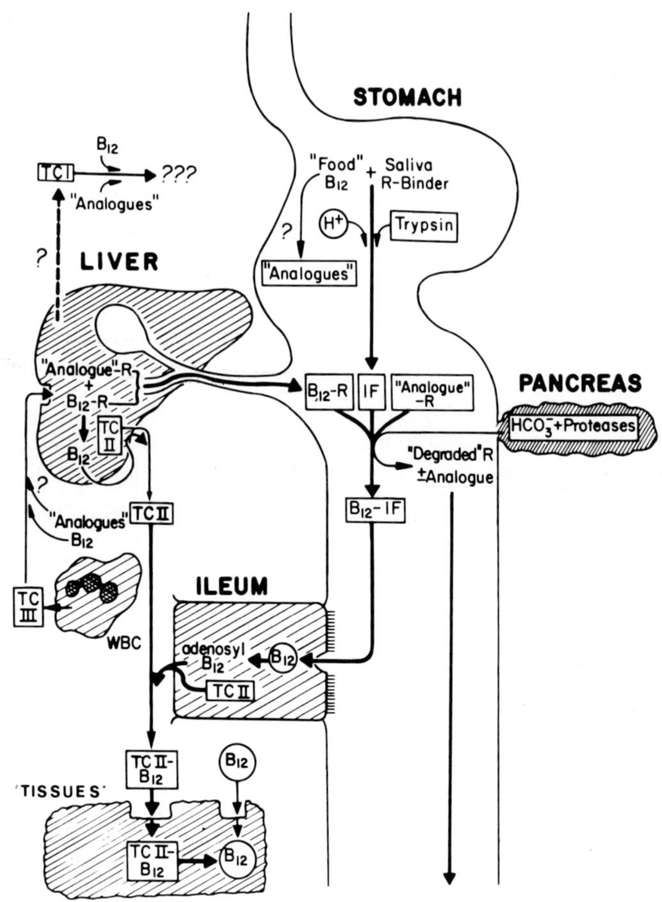

Fig. 4. Absorption and transport of vitamin B_{12}. *IF*, intrinsic factor; *TCI*, transcobalamin I; *TCII*, transcobalamin II; *TCIII*, transcobalamin III; *WBC*, granulocyte

in the portal circulation. Large oral doses of vitamin B_{12} can also be absorbed by passive diffusion in the absence of IF, albeit to a limited degree (WAIFE et al. 1963; CARMEL et al. 1969). The metabolism of vitamin B_{12} within the ileal cell is poorly defined, but this process requires 4–8 h, and vitamin B_{12} appears to localize within mitochondria (PERRY and HOFFBRAND 1970). Vitamin B_{12} then appears in the blood bound to TCII. Intestinal perfusion studies in rats suggest that unbound vitamin B_{12} can directly enter the circulation and attach to unsaturated TCII in plasma, but it is likely that vitamin B_{12} binds to TCII within the enterocyte and enters the blood as the intact TCII-vitamin B_{12} complex (HALL 1975; CHANARIN et al. 1978).

Although vitamin B_{12} analogues cannot combine with IF, they may nonetheless attach to the IF-vitamin B_{12} ileal receptor. However, this interaction is prevented when analogues are complexed with R binders (KANAZAWA et al. 1986). In fact, R binders in bile may facilitate excretion of vitamin B_{12} analogues formed endogenously (KANAZAWA et al. 1983).

c) Transport and Intracellular Metabolism of Vitamin B_{12}

The TCII-vitamin B_{12} complex binds to specific receptors on cell membranes and is internalized en toto by endocytosis which is temperature and energy dependent (YOUNGDAHL-TURNER et al. 1979). Release of vitamin B_{12} from TCII probably occurs in the lysosomal compartment and involves proteolytic degradation of TCII (YOUNGDAHL-TURNER et al. 1978, 1979). Mitochondrial uptake of the TCII-vitamin B_{12} complex has also been suggested but not confirmed (FENTON et al. 1976; GAMS et al. 1976). Unbound cyano-B_{12} can also directly enter cells both in vitro and in vivo, albeit less efficiently (HITZIG et al. 1974; BERLINER and ROSENBERG 1981). Methyl-B_{12} is formed in the cytoplasm by the folate-dependent methyltransferase, while deoxyadenosyl-B_{12} is formed in mitochondria by an adenosyl transferase (QUADROS et al. 1976; FENTON et al. 1976).

3. Causes of Vitamin B_{12} Deficiency

Consumption of a vitamin B_{12}-deficient diet *eventually* produces megaloblastic anemia. Adults ingesting a strict vegetarian diet (e.g., vegans) require up to 20 years to deplete their vitamin B_{12} stores (HARDINAGE and STARE 1954). In fact, a clinically overt vitamin B_{12} deficiency in this population may indicate the presence of a coexistent disorder in vitamin B_{12} absorption (CARMEL 1978a). However, infants breast fed by vitamin-B_{12}-deficient mothers can develop deficiency within the 1st year of life (LAMPKIN et al. 1966; HIGGINBOTTOM et al. 1978).

Vitamin B_{12} deficiency most often results from decreased absorption (HERBERT 1973; Table 4). When intestinal uptake of both dietary vitamin B_{12} and B12 excreted in bile is impaired, signs of deficiency develop in 3–6 years. Malabsorption of food vitamin B_{12} can result from decreased gastric acid and pepsin secretion due to gastric atrophy, surgery for peptic ulcer disease, or the use of histamine H_2 receptor antagonists (DOSCHERHOLMEN and SWAIM 1973; STEINBERG et al. 1980; SLALOM et al. 1982; BELAICHE et al. 1983; POWERS et al. 1989). Histamine H_2 receptor antagonists also decrease IF secretion, but absorption of crystalline vitamin B_{12} is usually not impaired by these drugs since ileal uptake of vitamin B_{12} is not limited until IF secretion is reduced more than 95% (BINDER and DONALDSON 1978; FIELDING et al. 1978; CHANARIN 1979; SLALOM et al. 1982). In contrast, IF deficiency, pancreatic insufficiency, and ileal dysfunction decrease absorption of both food and crystalline vitamin B_{12}. In pernicious anemia, achlorhydria and decreased IF activity are associated with the presence of cytotoxic antibodies directed against the parietal cell membranes as well as with antibodies which either block the interaction of IF with vitamin B_{12} or prevent the binding of

holo-TCII levels) and b) the activity of cellular or systemic vitamin-B_{12}-dependent processes (urinary methylmalonic acid excretion, dU suppression tests, serum homocysteine levels, and reticulocyte response to "physiologic" doses of vitamin B_{12}). Further studies are then indicated to determine whether vitamin B_{12} absorption is impaired (the Schilling test and its variants) and whether pernicious anemia is present (tests for parietal cell and IF antibodies, measures of gastric acid production, serum gastrin levels) (Table 5).

Radioassays to measure serum vitamin B_{12} levels are the tests most widely used to detect deficiency. False normal values in deficient subjects are unusual if assay systems which correct for the presence of inactive vitamin B_{12} analogues are used (KOLHOUSE et al. 1978; KUBASKIK et al. 1980). However, increased TCI levels may mask the presence of vitamin B_{12} deficiency in patients with myeloproliferative disorders and perhaps in patients with liver disease as well (RACHMILEWITZ et al. 1956; JONES et al. 1957; KANAZAWA and HERBERT 1985). False low values in the absence of tissue vitamin B_{12} depletion have been reported in subjects with folate deficiency, pregnancy, oral contraceptive use, rheumatoid arthritis, AIDS, multiple myeloma, TCI deficiency, recent exposure to diagnostic radionuclides, iron deficiency, and occasionally in apparently normal subjects

Table 5. Diagnosis of Nutrient Deficiencies

	Iron	Vitamin B_{12}	Folate
Tissue stores	Ferritin Bone marrow	—	RBC folate
Tissue delivery	Tf saturation	TCII saturation Serum B_{12}	Serum folate
Measures of nutrient function	Hb & MCV Hb response to Fe RBC proto	MCV & Hb Hyperseg. WBC Retic response to B_{12} Serum homocysteine dU suppression Urine MMA	MCV & Hb Hyperseg. WBC Retic response to PGA Serum homocysteine dU suppression
Nutrient absorption	Fe absorption test	Schilling test	PGA absorption test
Underlying disorders	GI studies Urine hemosiderin Sputum hemosiderin	GI studies Gastric acid secretion Serum gastrin Serum pepsinogen IF antibodies	GI studies Drug history

Tf, transferrin; TCII, transcobalamin II; Proto, protoporphyrin; MMA, methylmalonic acid; IF, intrinsic factor; PGA, folic acid; dU, deoxyuridine; Retic, reticulocyte; MCV, mean corpuscular volume; GI, gastrointestinal tract; WBC, white blood cell; RBC, red blood cell; Hb, hemoglobin; Fe, iron.

(ALTZ-SMITH et al. 1981; CHANARIN 1976; SHOJANIA 1982; HERBERT and COLEMAN 1981; SCHILLING et al. 1983; CARMEL and HERBERT 1969; FAIRBANKS and ELVEBACK 1983; ELSBORG et al. 1976; LINDENBAUM 1983a; HITZHUSEN et al. 1986). Although it has been suggested that serum vitamin B_{12} levels fall with age, this has not been confirmed, and low values in elderly patients usually indicate a true deficiency state requiring further evaluation (NILSSON-EHLE et al. 1986. 1989; MATHEWS et al. 1988). A fall in TCII-bound vitamin B_{12} may precede the fall of total serum vitamin B_{12}, and methyl-B_{12} generally decreases to a greater degree than adenosyl-B_{12}, but these assays are not routinely performed (HERZLICH and HERBERT 1988; QUADROS et al. 1988). While microbiologic assays for vitamin B_{12} measure primarily true cobalamins, they are cumbersome, false low values occur in patients receiving antibiotics, and some vitamin B_{12} analogues can support bacterial growth (HERBERT and COLEMAN 1981; LINDENBAUM 1983a).

Tissue deficiency of vitamin B_{12} is established by demonstrating impairment of vitamin-B_{12}-dependent processes. Urinary methylmalonic acid excretion increases with B_{12} deficiency, and serum homocysteine levels increase with either vitamin B_{12} or folate deficiency. Improved methods have increased the reliability and availability of these tests (MATCHAR et al. 1987; STABLER et al. 1988; CHU and HALL 1988). The dU suppression test on bone marrow or peripheral blood lymphocytes also confirms that vitamin B_{12} or folate deficiency is present and distinguishes these disorders from megaloblastosis due to the myelodysplastic syndromes (GOODMAN et al. 1978; MAHMOOD et al. 1979; GARRAND et al. 1980). However, this test is not generally available, and the validity of lymphocyte studies has been questioned (MATTHEWS and WICKRAMASINGHE 1988). Finally, in anemic patients, reticulocytosis after 3–7 days of intramuscular administration of 1–2 µg/day of vitamin B_{12} is diagnostic of vitamin B_{12} deficiency (ADAMS et al. 1953).

In vitamin-B_{12}-deficient subjects, the Schilling test and its variants can establish whether or not malabsorption is present and if it is due to IF deficiency, IF antibodies, failure to liberate vitamin B_{12} from food components or R binders (achlorhydria, pancreatic insufficiency), or ileal dysfunction (STRAUCHEN 1976; BRUGGE et al. 1980; DOSCHERHOLMEN et al. 1983; DAWSON et al. 1984). The diagnosis of pernicious anemia is supported by measurement of serum gastrin and pepsinogen levels, assays for antibodies against IF in serum or gastric juice, and determination of gastric acid secretion (CHANARIN 1979; LINDENBAUM 1983a; SLINGER-LAND et al. 1984; CARMEL 1988a).

5. Management of Vitamin B_{12} Deficiency

Since vitamin B_{12} deficiency most often results from decreased absorption, vitamin B_{12} (in the form of hydroxocobalamin or cyanocobalamin) must usually be administered *parenterally*. Cyanocobalamin has less hematopoietic activity than deoxyadenosyl-B_{12} (SULLIVAN and HERBERT 1965), and hydroxocobalamin must be reduced from Co(III) to Co(I), probably by

NAD-dependent flavoproteins similar to those present in bacteria (WALKER et al. 1969). Retention of hydroxocobalamin at the site of injection and in tissues is greater than that of cyanocobalamin, and this results in more prolonged elevation of serum vitamin B_{12} levels and less urinary vitamin B_{12} loss (ADAMS and KENNEDY 1953; GLASS et al. 1961a,b, 1966; GLASS and LEE 1966; SKOUBY 1966). However, interpatient variation in the metabolism of pharmacologic doses of vitamin B_{12} is great, and the relative advantage of hydroxocobalamin is probably not of practical significance (TUDHOPE et al. 1967).

Regimens used to correct vitamin B_{12} deficiency vary considerably. Doses of cyanocobalamin of 100 µg given *intramuscularly* daily for 2 weeks and then 2 times/week for 1–2 months correct anemia and replenish body stores (BECK 1972). Monthly doses of 100 µg are then required for life. Although the value of more sustained administration of a higher dose (e.g., 200 µg every 2 weeks for 6 months) in patients with neurologic changes has not been established, possible benefits far outweigh the negligible increase in toxicity and cost. Alternatively, daily *oral* doses of 1 mg of cyanocobalamin are sufficiently absorbed in the absence of IF to be effective in some patients with pernicious anemia (BERLIN et al. 1978; CROSBY 1980), and administration of vitamin B_{12} in a *nasal gel* is being studied (COLEMAN et al. 1988). Regular screening to detect gastric cancer in patients with achlorhydria and pernicious anemia is often suggested, although this association remains controversial (ERIKSSON et al. 1981; SVENDSEN et al. 1986).

Sudden death during treatment of patients with severe anemia with parenteral vitamin B_{12} has been noted and related to the development of hypokalemia (LAWSON et al. 1972). However, these deaths may have been due to transfusion-induced hypervolemia (PALVA and KAIPAINEN 1970; LAWSON and PARKER 1976), and an excess mortality has not recently been observed (CARMEL 1988c). Rarely, vitamin B_{12} given parenterally may produce urticarial or anaphylactoid reactions.

Hydroxocobalamin (1 mg/day intramuscularly) may also be used to treat some hereditary forms of methylmalonyl acidemia, and a role for deoxyadenosyl-B_{12} in treating patients with hydroxocobalamin-resistant methylmalonyl acidemia has been proposed (ROSENBERG 1983; BHATT et al. 1986). Hydroxocobalamin may prevent cyanide toxicity during nitroprusside therapy (COTTRELL et al. 1978), but the value of hydroxocobalamin in other disorders possibly related to cyanide toxicity (e.g., optic atrophy due to Leber's disease) is not established (LINNELL and MATHEWS 1984).

V. Folate Deficiency

1. General Considerations

Pteroylglutamic acid (PGA, folic acid) is synthesized from a substituted pterin ring, paraaminobenzoic acid, and L-glutamic acid by bacteria and

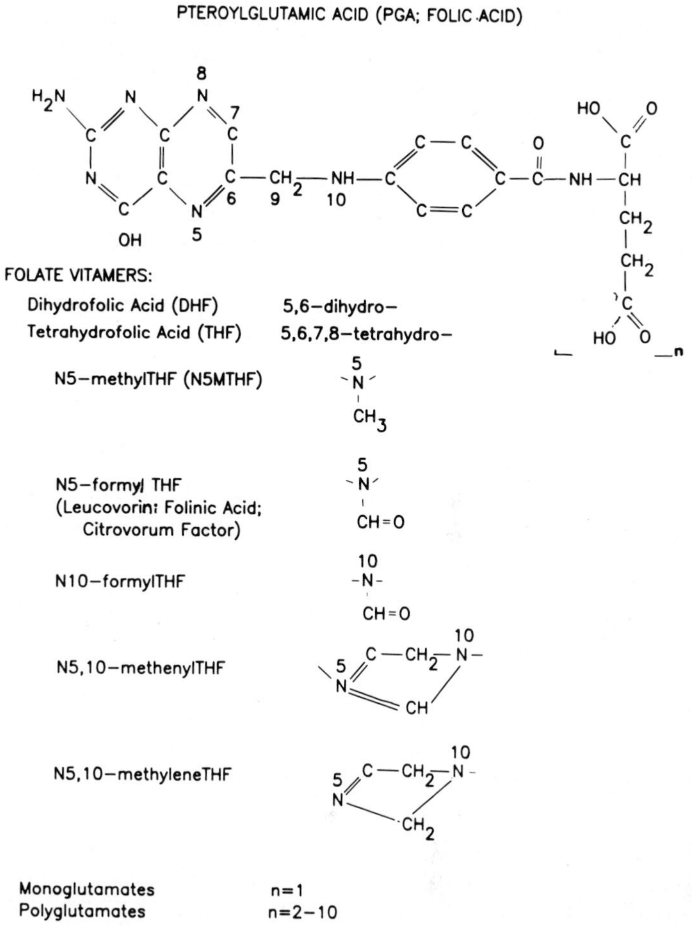

PTEROYLGLUTAMIC ACID (PGA; FOLIC ACID)

FOLATE VITAMERS:

Dihydrofolic Acid (DHF)	5,6–dihydro–
Tetrahydrofolic Acid (THF)	5,6,7,8–tetrahydro–
N5–methylTHF (N5MTHF)	
N5–formyl THF (Leucovorin: Folinic Acid; Citrovorum Factor)	
N10–formylTHF	
N5,10–methenylTHF	
N5,10–methyleneTHF	

Monoglutamates	n=1
Polyglutamates	n=2–10

Fig. 5. Structure of the folate vitamers

green leafy plants. Folate coenzymes are formed from PGA in mammalian tissues by a series of enzymatic reactions (Figs. 2,5) which reduce the pterin ring (DHF; THF); add a one-carbon residue to the nitrogen at position 5 or 10, oxidize or reduce that one-carbon residue (methyl-, methylene-, methenyl- formimino-, and formyl-THF), and add up to 9 more L-glutamate residues in a γ-glutamyl linkage pattern to THF or formyl-THF (folate polyglutamates). The polyglutamate forms are the most active folate coenzymes (MATTHEWS et al. 1987).

The adult male body contains about 7.5 mg of folate, most of which is located in the liver. Approximately 50–100 μg/day of folate is lost in the stool (primarily from bile), and up to 40 μg/day is lost in the urine (CHANARIN 1979; HERBERT 1987b). Since absorption of dietary folates is variable and incomplete, a folate intake of 150–300 μg/day (3 μg/kg) is needed by adults to maintain folate stores (HERBERT 1987b). This requirement is increased by pregnancy, lactation, periods of rapid growth (e.g., infancy), and perhaps by conditions which increase tissue turnover or metabolism (e.g., hyperthyroidism, certain malignancies, hemolytic anemias).

Although folates are abundant in many plant and animal food sources, some folates are readily destroyed by heat (particularly boiling or steaming), ultraviolet light, acid, and oxidants, so that fresh, uncooked fruits and vetetables are the most reliable dietary sources (CHANARIN 1979; HERBERT 1987b). Ascorbate and other reducing agents can protect folate during food preparation and storage. These considerations are of particular importance in the preparation of cow's milk for infant feeding (EK and MAGNUS 1980).

2. Folate Metabolism

a) Folate Absorption

Folate is normally absorbed in the duodenum and proximal jejunum but uptake may occur in the ileum after intestinal resection (Fig. 6) (HEPNER et al. 1968; SAID et al. 1988). Most dietary folates are reduced, methylated polyglutamates which must be converted to monoglutamates prior to absorption. This is accomplished by the action of a zinc-dependent γ-glutamyl carboxypeptidase (folate conjugase) located in the mucosal cell brush border (TAMURA et al. 1978; REISENAUER et al. 1986). Hydrolysis of folate polyglutamates probably occurs at the mucosal cell surface since little conjugase activity is present in bile, pancreatic secretions, or succus entericus (HALSTED et al. 1975; ROSENBERG 1976). Reduced, methylated folates

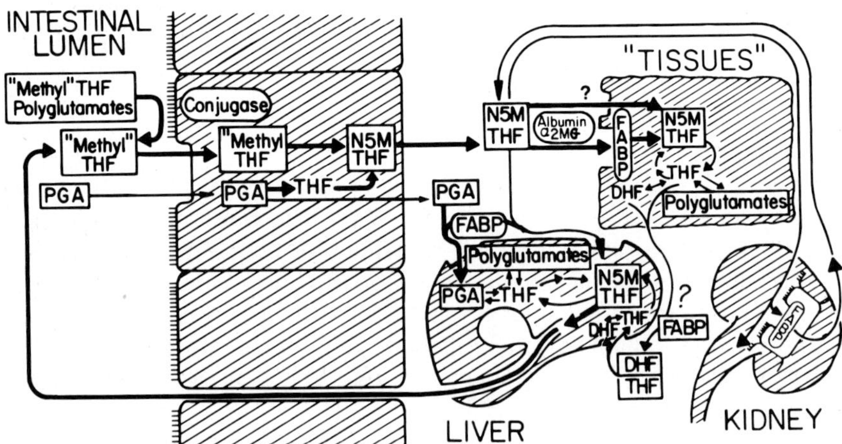

Fig. 6. Absorption and transport of folate vitamers. *PGA*, pteroylglutamic acid (folic acid); *DHF*, dihydrofolic acid; *THF*, tetrahydrofolic acid; *N5MTHF*, *N*-5-methyl-tetrahydrofolic acid; *FABP*, folic acid binding proteins

secreted by the liver into bile must also be reabsorbed in order to maintian tissue folate delivery (PRATT and COOPER 1971; STEINBERG et al. 1979a,b; 1982). Interruption of this folate enterohepatic cycle by external biliary drainage rapidly reduces serum folate levels.

At high concentrations, PGA enters mucosal cells by passive diffusion, but a pH-sensitive, carrier-mediated, active transport mechanism becomes the rate-limiting step in absorption when intraluminal PGA levels are low (STRUM 1981; SELHUB and ROSENBERG 1981; REISENAUER et al. 1986; SAID et al. 1987; DARCY-VRILLON et al. 1988). The same carrier system mediates uptake of all reduced and methylated folates (SAID and STRUM 1983a; SELHUB et al. 1984). Active transport is increased by glucose and cyclic AMP but decreased by alkalinization (GERSON et al. 1971; MACKENZIE et al. 1976; SAID and STRUM 1983b). Although some PGA directly enters the portal blood, most is converted to N5MTHF prior to release into the circulation (WHITEHEAD and COOPER 1967; OLINGER et al. 1973; SELHUB et al. 1973; PERRY and CHANARIN 1973; STEINBERG et al. 1978). N5MTHF is also the major folate which appears in the blood after ingestion of either N5MTHF or N5-formyl-THF (leucovorin) (NIXON and BERTINO 1972; WHITEHEAD et al. 1971; PRATT and COOPER 1971; STRUM et al. 1971). Another specific membrane-associated carrier may mediate the release of folate from the mucosal cell to the blood (SAID and REDHA 1987).

Intraluminal factors may modify folate absorption. Although antacids do not affect folate absorption in rats, PGA absorption in man is decreased by increasing intestinal pH (e.g., gastric atrophy, therapy with bicarbonate, antacids, or H_2 receptor antagonists) (RUSSELL et al. 1979, 1985, 1986, 1988; HOPPNER and LAMPI 1988). Some foods may bind PGA (e.g., fibrous foods), and others may inhibit conjugase activity (e.g., beans, orange juice), but the presence of these interactions and their impact on folate absorption are controversial (KRUMDIECK et al. 1973; TAMURA et al. 1976; KEAGY et al. 1988; BHANDARI and GREGORY 1990). In contrast, folate binding proteins in milk enhance PGA absorption perhaps by permitting uptake at a distinct mucosal cell receptor site (COLMAN et al. 1981; MASON and SELHUB 1988).

Some drugs impair folate absorption by binding dietary folate (e.g., pancreatic extracts, cholestyramine), inhibiting conjugase (e.g., sulfasalazine), or interfering with folate uptake at the mucosal cell surface (e.g., sulfasalazine, diphenylhydantoin, triamterene, bile acids, zinc salts) (RUSSELL et al. 1980; STRUM 1981; SAID et al. 1984c; GRISHNAN et al. 1986; ZIMMERMAN et al. 1986; HALSTED et al. 1989). Although PGA absorption is decreased in chronic alcoholic subjects, ethanol ingestion for up to 2 weeks does not impair PGA absorption in man when other nutrient deficiencies are corrected, and ethanol only slightly decreases PGA absorption in vitro (HALSTED et al. 1967, 1971; HERMOS et al. 1972; STRUM 1981). More prolonged ethanol consumption may damage the intestinal mucosa, decreasing the activities of conjugase and other enzymes and impairing absorption of polyglutamates and/or PGA (GREENE et al. 1974; BAKER et al. 1975;

ROMERO et al. 1981; BLOCKER and THENEN 1987; HALSTED 1989; NAUGHTON 1989; REISENAUER et al. 1989). Effects of oral contraceptives on both PGA absorption and conjugase activity have also been suggested but not confirmed (NECCHELES and SNYDER 1970; STREIFF and GREENE 1970; STEPHENS et al. 1972; SHOJANIA and HORNADY 1973). These nutrient-drug interactions are more likely to be of clinical significance if dietary folate intake is marginal or if other intestinal mucosal abnormalities are present.

b) Transport and Intracellular Metabolism of Folate

Most of the N5MTHF in plasma is loosely bound to proteins (e.g., albumin, α_2-macroglobulin) and is preferentially taken up by extrahepatic tissues (MAKKANNEN et al. 1972; HILLMAN et al. 1978). A small fraction of the circulating folate pool is associated with specific high affinity folic acid binding proteins (FABP). FABP are sialoglycoproteins which bind oxidized folates more avidly than reduced forms (WAXMAN and SCHREIBER 1973b). Serum FABP levels may be increased by pregnancy, oral contraceptive use, chronic ethanol ingestion, folate deficiency, liver disease, inflammation, malignancy, or renal failure (WAXMAN and SCHREIBER 1973b; COLMAN and HERBERT 1976b; FERNANDES-COSTA and METZ 1981; EICHNER and SMILEY 1981; KANE and WAXMAN 1989). FABP are also released from granulocytes during phagocytosis (GILBERT and WAXMAN 1978). The physiologic role of serum FABP is uncertain, but binding to FABP appears to direct folate to the liver in vivo and prevents folate uptake by nonhepatic tissues in vitro (WAXMAN and SCHREIBER 1974; FERNANDES-COSTA and METZ 1979; RUBINOFF et al. 1981). Consistent with this pattern is the observation that reduced folates are extracted primarily by extrahepatic tissues, while oxidized folates are preferentially taken up by the liver (HILLMAN et al. 1978; KIIL et al. 1979). A distinct FABP in umbilical cord serum with a relatively higher binding affinity for N5MTHF may play a role in transplacental folate transport (KAMEN and CASTON 1975).

Specific high affinity folate receptors immunologically related to serum FABP are present on the cell membranes of some mammalian tissues (KANE and WAXMAN 1989). These receptors bind oxidized as well as reduced folates, and receptor expression is increased by folate depletion (SPECTOR and LORENZO 1975; KAMEN and CAPDEVILA 1986; SWEIRY and YUDILEVICH 1988). The receptor-folate complex may enter the cell by endocytosis, and folate release may result from acidification. The intact receptor is then recycled back to the cell surface (KAMEN et al. 1988). In the cytoplasm, N5MTHF is converted to THF by homocysteine-methionine methyltransferase, and polyglutamates are then formed by folypolyglutamate synthetase (MCGUIRE et al. 1980; MCGUIRE and BERTINO 1981). The presence of a receptor for reduced folates on the cell membrane of mouse L1210 leukemia cells distinct from their receptor for oxidized folates has been suggested but not confirmed (HENDERSON et al. 1986, 1987; SITORNAK et al.

1987). However, human red cells may have a different receptor for PGA than for N5MTHF (BRANDA and ANTHONY 1987), and PGA can also enter the red cell by passive diffusion when extracellular concentrations are high (ANTHONY et al. 1989). Some amphipathic drugs (e.g., furosemide, ethacrynic acid, sulfasalazine, phenylbutazone, sulfinpyrazone) inhibit red cell transport of N5MTHF, but the clinical significance of these interactions is unknown (BRANDA and NELSON 1981). Folates may be concentrated and trapped in the red cell as a result of the binding of polyglutamates to hemoglobin (BENESCH et al. 1983).

Free or loosely bound serum folates are also filtered by the renal glomerulus (GORESKY et al. 1963). However, urinary excretion of folate is limited because of reabsorption of folate in the renal tubules. This process may also be mediated by a FABP in the tubule cell brush border (SELHUB et al. 1987a,b). Reabsorbed folate can then return to the blood in the peritubular capillaries. Folate is also enzymatically degraded in tissues, and catabolic products are excreted in the urine (CHANARIN 1979).

3. Causes of Folate Deficiency

Inadequate dietary intake is a common cause of folate deficiency particularly in women, blacks and the elderly (BAILEY et al. 1979; BLUNDELL et al. 1985; SUBAR et al. 1989) (Table 6). Depletion of folate reserves in normal adults consuming a folate-deficient diet requires about 4 months (HERBERT, 1987a; EICHNER et al. 1972).

Decreased absorption of dietary folate can occur in patients with intrinsic diseases of the small intestine (e.g., congenital disorders, celiac disease, sprue, regional enteritis, progressive systemic sclerosis, dermatitis herpetiformis, granulomatous colitis) (LANZKOWSKI 1970; ROSENBERG 1976; KLIPSTEIN 1972; CHANARIN 1979; ELSBORG and LARSON 1979; HENDEL et al. 1987). In addition, drugs can impair folate absorption by binding folate, inhibiting mucosal conjugase activity, or directly damaging the intestinal mucosa. Uremia also decreases N5MTHF absorption in rats, but studies in human subjects with chronic renal insufficiency have not been performed (SAID et al. 1984b). Although many intestinal bacteria actually synthesize folate, overgrowth of intestinal bacteria (e.g., the blind loop syndrome) can occasionally consume dietary folate and limit its absorption (CHANARIN 1979).

Impaired utilization of folate may occur as a result of aging (decreased red cell and hepatocyte uptake of N5MTHF) (ETTINGER and COLMAN 1985; HORNE et al. 1989), congenital deficiencies of folate-dependent or folate-metabolizing enzymes (ERBE 1975; TAURO et al. 1976), a congenital disorder of cellular folate uptake (BRANDA et al. 1978), or drug-induced defects in folate metabolism. Methotrexate, pyrimethamine, pentamidine, trimethoprim, and triamterene can inhibit dihydrofolate reductase and produce megaloblastic anemia (STEBBINS and BERTINO 1976; LINDENBAUM

Table 6. Causes of folic acid deficiency

A. Inadequate dietary intake, e.g., lack of fresh, unprocessed, uncooked foods
B. Decreased absorption
  1. Intraluminal factors
    a) Alkalinization, e.g., gastric atrophy, bicarbonate, H_2 receptor blockers
    b) Drugs (binding folate), e.g., cholestyramine, pancreatic extracts
    c) Bacterial overgrowth
  2. Disorders of the small intestine
    a) Inflammatory disorders, e.g., spruce, coeliac disease, regional enteritis
    b) Drugs, e.g., azulfidine, triamterene, bile acids, zinc salts, diphenylhydantoin (?), ethanol (?)
    c) Miscellaneous, e.g., vitamin B_{12} deficiency, folate deficiency, surgery, uremia(?)
C. Impaired utilization
  1. Hereditary—deficiency of folate-related enzymes
  2. Acquired
    a) Vitamin B_{12} deficiency
    b) Drugs
      1. Dihydrofolate reductase inhibitors, e.g., methotrexate, trimethoprim, pentamidine, pyrimethamine, triamterene
      2. Mechanism uncertain, e.g., diphenylhydantoin, primidone, barbiturates, carbamazepine, valproic acid, ethanol, oral contraceptives (?)
D. Increased requirements
  1. Physiologic—pregnancy, infancy, childhood
  2. Pathologic
    a) Malignancies, e.g., lympho- and myeloproliferative disorders, some solid tumors
    b) Increased metabolism or cell turnover, e.g., hemolytic anemias, psoriasis, hyperthyroidism (?)
E. Increased loss
  1. Hemodialysis
  2. Peritoneal dialysis (?)
  3. Ethanol (?)
  4. Vitamin B_{12} deficiency

1983b). Anticonvulsants (e.g., diphenylhydantoin, phenobarbital, primidone, carbamazepine, valproic acid) may also induce folate deficiency, but their effects on folate metabolism remain poorly defined (SMITH and CARK 1982; LINDENBAUM 1983). Original reports of inhibition of folate polyglutamate absorption by diphenylhydantoin have not been confirmed, and it is more likely that this drug increases folate catabolism (LINDENBAUM 1983). Diphenylhydantoin may also directly inhibit DNA synthesis, and this may in turn indirectly increase folate requirements (TAGUCHI et al. 1977). The effects of oral contraceptives on folate absorption and metabolism are controversial, and these drugs are unlikely to induce frank folate deficiency in the absence of other disorders (STEBBINS and BERTINO 1976; SHOJANIA 1982; LINDENBAUM 1983b).

Folate deficiency is particularly common in alcoholic subjects and results both from decreased dietary intake and impaired metabolism (LINDENBAUM

1980; HILLMANN and STEINBERG 1982). There is little agreement on the mechanisms by which alcohol interferes with folate metabolism. This may be due to differences in the animal models used, the presence or absence of concomitant dietary folate deficiency, and variations in the dose and duration of alcohol administration (McGUFFIN et al. 1975). Thus, ethanol has been reported to (a) decrease the absorption of dietary folates (BAKER et al. 1975; ROMERO et al. 1981; SAID and STRUM 1986; BLOCKER and THENEN 1987; NAUGHTON et al. 1989; REISENAUER et al. 1989), (b) increase urinary folate excretion in a time- and dose-dependent fashion (RUSSEL et al. 1983; TAMURA and HALSTED 1983; McMARTIN et al. 1986a,b; EISENGA et al. 1989), (c) oxidize folate directly as a consequence of ethanol and/or acetaldehyde metabolism (McMARTIN and COLLINS 1983; SHAW et al. 1989b), (d) inhibit folate-related enzymes (BERTINO et al. 1965; BARAK et al. 1985), and (e) interrupt the enterohepatic circulation of folate perhaps by increasing both hepatocyte uptake of N5MTHF and hepatic retention of folate in the form of polyglutamates (McMARTIN et al. 1983; LANE et al. 1976; HILLMAN et al. 1977; 1982; HORNE et al. 1979; STEINBERG et al. 1981, 1982; WILKINSON and SHANE 1982; WEIR et al. 1985). The last mechanism may explain the acute fall in serum folate which follows oral or intravenous ethanol administration and the rapid rise in serum folate which occurs with abstinence (EICHNER and HILLMAN 1973). An acute fall in serum folate may also occur during parental hyperalimentation in the absence of ethanol but the mechanism of this effect is unknown (TENNANT et al. 1981).

Increased folate requirements occur during pregnancy, lactation, and the rapid growth phases of infancy and childhood (HERBERT et al. 1987b). In addition, disorders which are associated with increased metabolic rates or increased tissue turnover (e.g., psoriasis, chronic hemolytic anemias, leukemias) can increase the need for dietary folate (BATRA et al. 1979; CHAN and STOKSTAD 1980; CHANARIN 1979). Although increased clearance of serum folate has also been described in patients with hyperthyroidism, frank folate deficiency in this population has not been consistently observed (LINDENBAUM and KLIPSTEIN 1965; FORD et al. 1989). Paradoxically, folate deficiency has been described in patients with hypothyroidism, but a mechanism for this possible association is unknown (HINES et al. 1968).

Finally, increased folate losses can occur as a result of chronic ethanol abuse (see above), chronic hemodialysis (WHITEHEAD et al. 1968), and perhaps chronic peritoneal dialysis as well (WATSON et al. 1980).

4. Diagnosis of Folate Deficiency

Microbiologic or radioassays to measure serum and red cell folate levels are the tests most commonly used to detect folate deficiency (MILNE and GALLAGHER 1983; HERBERT 1987c). A low serum folate level indicates decreased folate delivery to tissues at the time the sample was taken, but this does not establish that folate tissue stores are depleted. In contrast, a low red cell folate level does not reflect the *current* adequacy of folate delivery but indicates that the tissue folate supply was sufficiently low during the *preceding* 3–4 months to deplete folate stores. Moreover, serum folate levels increase rapidly with folate ingestion or after abstinence from ethanol, while red cell folate levels are increased by iron deficiency or after blood transfusions (CHANARIN 1979). Thus, the information provided by these two measurements is complementary. Although iron deficiency depresses serum folate levels in the absence of folate deficiency, the possibility of coexistent iron and folate deficiency should be considered particularly when hypersegmented neutrophils are noted in the peripheral smear (TOSKES et al. 1974; DAS et al. 1978). Vitamin B_{12} deficiency can depress red cell folate levels, but serum folate levels may be high, normal, or low in this setting.

The presence of *functional* folate deficiency may then be confirmed by the presence of an abnormal dU suppression test, increased excretion of formininoglutamic acid (FIGLU) after an oral histidine load (Fig. 2), increased serum homocysteine levels, or a reticulocyte response to a "physiologic" dose of folic acid (50–100 μg/day of PGA orally or intramuscularly) in anemic patients (WICKRAMASINGHE et al. 1983; and HERBERT 1987b; CHU and HALL 1988). If folate deficiency is present, measurement of urinary folate excretion after an oral dose of [^{3}H] PGA can be used to detect malabsorption of folate monoglutamate (ELSBORG 1981). Although these more costly and laborious tests are seldom necessary, adult celiac disease and other disorders of the small intestine associated with folate malabsorption may be clinically silent. Thus, the gastrointestinal tract should be evaluated in patients with otherwise unexplained folate deficiency (HALLERT et al. 1981). Finally, while large doses of folic acid can improve hematopoiesis in patients with pernicious anemia, they may actually precipitate or accelerate neurologic dysfunction in these patients. Thus, it is also essential to perform studies to exclude the presence of vitamin B_{12} deficiency (Table 5).

5. Management of Folate Deficiency

An oral dose of 1 mg of folic acid (PGA) given 1–3 times per day will *correct* folate-deficient hematopoiesis and replete body folate stores. PGA may be given parenterally when the deficiency is due to malabsorption. As little as 500 μg/day of PGA orally will *prevent* folate deficiency during pregnancy, while supplementation of wine with PGA has been proposed to prevent folate deficiency in chronic alcoholic subjects (KAUNITZ and LINDENBAUM 1977). Although the need for folate supplementation in children with sickle cell disease has been questioned, this practice is likely of value particularly in populations with marginal dietary folate intake (RABB et al. 1983). However, vitamin B_{12} status should also be monitored in these subjects since pernicious anemia may occur at a younger age in blacks than in Caucasians (SINOW et al. 1987). Folic acid may also have a pharmacologic role in improving chromosomal stability in folate-replete subjects with the fragile X syndrome (Branda et al. 1984).

Folinic acid (leucovorin), a reduced folate, is used to lower toxicity after treatment of certain malignancies with high doses of the dihydrofolate reductase inhibitor, methotrexate, or to potentiate the chemotherapeutic effect of 5-fluorouracil. Folinic acid has also recently been recommended to prevent cytopenias in AIDS patients being treated for *Pneumocystis carinii* pneumonia with trimethoprim, a weak dihydrofolate reductase inhibitor (Kinzie and Taylor 1984). However, trimethoprim when used in combination with sulfomethoxazole has direct toxic effects on hematopoiesis (Steinberg et al. 1979b), beneficial effects of folinic acid in this setting have not been confirmed (Stock 1985), and an advantage of folinic acid over PGA has not been demonstrated (Bygbjerg et al. 1988).

Adverse reactions to folic acid therapy are rare and relate primarily to interactions with other drugs or nutrient deficiencies. These include potentiation of neurologic deterioration in patients with vitamin B_{12} deficiency, induction of seizures in some patients receiving anticonvulsant therapy, and possible inhibition of dietary zinc absorption (Butterworth and Tamura 1989; Herbert 1987b; Simmer et al. 1977). Cases of allergic or anaphylactic reactions to oral PGA have also been reported (Sparling and Abela 1985). However, folate ingestion during pregnancy does not appear to be associated with the development of neural tube defects in the fetus as previously suggested (Mills et al. 1989).

References

Aasa R (1972) Reinterpretation of the electron paramagnetic resonance spectra of transferrins. Biochem Biophys Res Commun 49:806–808

Adams JF, Kennedy EH (1953) Hydroxocobalamin: excretion and retention after parenteral doses in anemia and nonanemic subjects with reference to the treatment of vitamin B_{12} deficiency states. Blood 8:450–457

Adams JF, Hume R, Kennedy EH, Pirrie TG, Whitelaw JW, White AM (1953) Metabolic responses to low doses of cyanocobalamin in patients with megaloblastic anaemia. Br J Nutr 22:575–582

Adams PC, Powell LW, Halliday JW (1988) Isolation of human hepatic ferritin receptor. Hapatology 8:719–721

Aisen P (1984) Transferrin metabolism and the liver. Semin Liver Dis 4:193–206

Aisen P (1988) Iron metabolism in isolated liver cells. Ann NY Acad Sci 526:93–100

Aisen P, Aasa R, Malmstrom BG, Vanngard T (1967) Bicarbonate and the binding of iron to transferrin. J Biol Chem 242:2473–2484

Aisen P, Aasa R, Redfield AG (1969) The chromium, manganese and cobalt complexes of transferrin. J Biol Chem 244:4268–4273

Ali M, Fayemi AO, Frascino J, Roigolisi R, Braum EV, Singer R (1982) Failure of serum ferritin levels to predict bone-marrow iron content after intravenous iron-dextran therapy. Lancet 1:652–655

Allen RH, Seetharam B, Podell E, Alpers DH (1978a) Effect of proteolytic enzymes on the binding of cobalamin to R protein and intrinsic factor. J Clin Invest 61:47–54

Allen RH, Seetharam B, Allen NC, Podell E, Alpers DH (1978b) Correction of cobalamin malabsorption in pancreatic insufficiency with a cobalamin analogue that binds with high affinity R protein but not with intrinsic factor. J Clin Invest 61:1628–1634

Altz-Smith M, Miller RK, Cornell PE, Butterworth CE (1981) Low plasma levels of vitamin B_{12} in patients with rheumatoid arthritis. Clin Res 29:858A

Anderson BM, Givson RS, Sabry JH (1981) The iron and zinc status of long-term vegetarian women. Am J Clin Nutr 34:1042–1048

Anthony AC, Kane MA, Krishnan SR, Kincade RS, Verma RS (1989) Folate (pteroylglutamate) uptake in human red blood cells, erythroid precursors and KB cells at high extracellular folate concentrations. Biochem J 260:401–411

Ardeman S, Chanarin I (1965) Steroids and Addisonian pernicious anemia. N Engl J Med 273:1352–1355

Auerbach M, Witt D, Toler W (1983) Complications of total dose infusion of iron dextran. Blood 62[Suppl 1]:35a

Awai M, Chipman B, Brown EB (1975) In vivo evidence for the functional heterogeneity of transferrin-bound iron. II. Studies in pregnant rats. J Lab Clin Med 85:785–796

Bacon BR, Tavill AS (1984) Role of the liver in normal iron metabolism. Semin Liver Dis 4:181–192

Bailey LB, Wagner PA, Christakis GJ, Araujo PE, Appledorf H, Davis CG, Masteryanni J, Dinning JS (1979) Folacin and iron status and hematological findings in predominantly black elderly persons from urban low-income households. Am J Clin Nutr 32:2346–2353

Bailey-Wood R, White GP, Jacobs A (1975) The use of Chang cells cultured in vitro for the investigation of cellular iron metabolism. Br J Exp Pathol 56:358–362

Bainton DF, Finch CA (1964) The diagnosis of iron deficiency anemia. Am J Med 37:62–70

Baird IM, Walters RL, Sutton DR (1974) Absorption of slow-release iron and effects of ascorbic acid in normal subjects and after partial gastrectomy. Br Med J 4:505–508

Baker GR, Boyer RF (1986) Iron incorporation into apoferritin: the role of apoferritin as a ferroxidase. J Biol Chem 261:13182–13185

Baker H, Frank O, Zetterman RK, Rajan KS, ten Hove W, Leevy CM (1975) Inability of chronic alcoholics with liver disease to use food as a source of folates, thiamine and vitamin B_6. Am J Clin Nutr 28:1277–1280

Baker SJ, Mathan VI (1981) Evidence regarding the mimimal daily requirement of dietary vitamin B_{12}. Am J Clin Nutr 34:2423–2433

Balcerzak SP, Greenberger NJ (1968) Iron content in isolated intestinal epithelial cells in relation to iron absorption. Nature 220:270–271

Ballas SK (1978) Abnormal erythrocyte membrane protein pattern in severe megaloblastic anemia. J Clin Invest 63:1097–1101

Bannerman RM, Callender ST, Hardisty RM, Smith RS (1964) Iron absorption in thalassemia. Br J Haematol 10:490–494

Barak AJ, Beckenhauer HC, Tuma DJ (1985) Ethanol feeding inhibits the activity of hepatic N^5-methyltetrahydrofolate-homocysteine methyltransferase in the rat. IRCS Med Sci 13:760–761

Barton JC, Conrad ME, Nuby Y, Harrison L (1978) Effects of iron on the absorption and retention of lead. J Lab Clin Med 92:536–547

Basset P, Quesneau Y, Zwiller J (1986) Iron-induced L-1210 cell growth: evidence of a transferrin-independent iron transport. Cancer Res 47:1644–1647

Batey RG, Gallagher ND (1977) Study of the subcellular localization of ^{59}Fe and iron-binding proteins in the duodenal mucosa of pregnant and nonpregnant rats. Gastroenterology 73:267–272

Batra KK, Watson JE, Stokstad ELR (1979) Effect of dietary thyroid powder on urinary excretion of formiminoglutamic acid and methylmalonic acid. Proc Soc Exp Biol Med 161:589–593

Baumgartner ER, Backmann C, Wick H (1976) Congenital methylmalonic acidemia: a variant of the B_{12} "non-responsive" form with evidence of reduced affinity of methylmalonyl-CoA mutase for its B_{12}-coenzyme. Enzyme 21:553–567

Baynes RD, Bothwell TH, Bezwoda WR, Gear AJ, Atkinson P (1987a) Hematological and iron-related measurements in rheumatoid arthritis. Am J Clin Pathol 87:196–200

Baynes RD, Bukofzer G, Bothwell TH, Bezwoda WR (1987b) Apotransferrin receptors and the delivery of iron from cultured human blood monocytes. Am J Hematol 25:417–425

Baynes RD, Friedman BM, Bukofzer GT, Bothwell TH, Macfarlance BJ, Lampareeli RD (1988) Effect of ferrous and ferric chelators on transferrin-iron-macrophage interactions. Am J Hematol 29:27–32

Beamish MR, Keay L, Okigaki T, Brown EB (1975) Uptake of transferrin bound iron by rat cells in tissue culture. Br J Haematol 31:479–491

Beck WS (1983) Vitamin B_{12} deficiency. In: Williams WJ, Beutler E, Erslev E, Lichtman A (eds) Hematology, 3rd edn. McGraw-Hill, New York, p 446

Beguin Y, Bergmaschi G, Huebers H, Finch CA (1988) The behavior of asialotransferrin in the rat. Am J Hematol 29:204–210

Behrens UJ, Womer TM, Braly LF, Schaffner F, Lieber CS (1988) Carbohydrate-deficient transferrin, a marker for chronic alcohol consumption in different ethnic populations. Alcohol Clin Exp Res 12:427–432

Belaiche J, Cattan D, Zittoun J, Marquet J, Yvart J (1983) Effect of ranitidine on cobalamin absorption. Dig Dis Sci 28:667–668

Beloqui O, Nunes RM, Blades B, Berk PD, Potter BJ (1986) Depression of iron uptake from transferrin by isolated hepatocytes in the presence of ethanol is a pH-dependent consequence of ethanol metabolism. Alcohol Clin Exp Res 10:463–470

Benesch RE, Benesch R, Kwong S, Baugh CM (1983) A pteroylpolyglutamate binds to tetramers in deoxyhemoglobin but to dimers in oxyhemoglobin. Proc Natl Acad Sci USA 80:6202–6205

Benjamin BI, Cortell S, Conrad ME (1967) Bicarbonate-induced iron complexes and iron absorption: one effect of pancreatic secretions. Gastroenterology 53: 389–396

Bentley DP, Jacobs A (1975) Accumulation of storage iron in patients treated for iron deficiency anemia. Br Med J 2:64–66

Berlin R, Berlin H, Brante G, Pilbrant A (1978) Vitamin B_{12} body stores during oral and parenteral treatment of pernicious anaemia. Acta Med Scand 204:81–84

Berliner N, Rosenberg LE (1981) Uptake and metabolism of free cyanocobalamin by cultured human fibroblasts from controls and a patient with transcobalamin II deficiency. Metabolism 30:230–236

Bernier GM, Schade SG, Conrad ME (1970) Ferritin production in the rat small intestine. Br J Haematol 19:361–367

Bernstein SE (1987) Hereditary hypotransferrinemia with hemosiderosis – a murine disorder resembling human atransferrinemia. J Lab Clin Med 110:690–705

Bertino JR, Ward J, Sartorelli AC, Silber R (1965) An effect of ethanol on folate metabolism. J Clin Invest 44:1028

Bessman JD (1980) Heterogeneity of red cell volume, quantitation, clinical considerations and possible mechanisms. Johns Hopkins Med J 146:226–230

Beutler E, Brittenweiser E (1960) The regulation of iron absorption. I. A search for humoral factors. J Lab Clin Med 55:274–280

Bezwoda W, Charlton R, Bothwell T, Torrance J, Mayet F (1978) The importance of gastric hydrochloric acid in the absorption of nonheme food iron. J Lab Clin Med 92:108–116

Bezwoda WR, Bothwell TH, Torrance JD, MacPhail AP, Charlton RW, Kay G, Levin J (1979a) The relationship between marrow iron stores, plasma ferritin concentration and iron absorption. Scand J Haematol 22:113–120

Callender ST, Warner GT (1971) Absorption of "slow iron" measured with a total body counter. Cancer Ther Res 3:591–594

Callender ST, Mallett BJ, Smith MD (1957) Absorption of hemoglobin iron. Br J Haematol 3:186–192

Carmel R (1972) Vitamin B_{12}-binding protein abnormality in subjects without myeloproliferative disease. II. The presence of a third vitamin B_{12}-binding protein in serum. Br J Haematol 22:53–62

Carmel R (1975) Extreme elevation of serum transcobalamin I in patients with metastatic cancer. N Engl J Med 292:282–284

Carmel R (1978a) Nutritional vitamin B_{12} deficiency: possible contributory role of subtle vitamin B_{12} malabsorption. Ann Int Med 88:647–649

Carmel R (1978b) Artefactual radioassay results due to serum contamination by intravenous radioisotope administration: falsely low serum vitamin B_{12} and folic acid results. Am J Clin Pathol 70:364–367

Carmel R (1988a) Pepsinogens and other serum markers in pernicious anemia. Am J Clin Pathol 90:442–445

Carmel R (1988b) Plasma R binder deficiency. N Engl J Med 318:1401

Carmel R (1988c) Treatment of severe pernicious anaemia: no association with sudden death. Am J Clin Nutr 48:1443–1444.

Carmel R, Eisenberg L (1977) Serum vitamin B_{12} and transcobalamin abnormalities in patients with cancer. Cancer 40:1348–1353

Carmel R, Herbert V (1967) Correctable intestinal defect of vitamin B_{12} absorption in pernicious anemia. Ann Int Med 67:1201–1207

Carmel R, Herbert V (1969) Deficiency of vitamin B_{12}-binding alpha globulin in 2 brothers. Blood 33:1–12

Carmel R, Karnaze DS (1985) The deoxyuridine suppression test identifies subtle cobalamin deficiency in patients without typical megaloblastic anemia. J Am Med Assoc 253:1284–1287

Carmel R, Rosenberg AH, Lau KS, Streiff RR, Herbert V (1969) Vitamin B_{12} uptake by human small bowel homogenate and its enhancement by intrinsic factor. Gastroenterology 56:548–555

Carmel R, Sinow RM, Karnaze DS (1987) Atypical cobalamin deficiency: subtle biochemical evidence of deficiency is commonly demonstrable in patients without megaloblastic anemia and is often associated with protein-bound cobalamin malabsorption. J Lab Clin Med 109:454–463

Carmel R, Karnaze DS, Weiner JM (1988a) Neurologic abnormalities in cobalamin deficiency are associated with higher cobalamin "analogue" values than are hematologic abnormalities. J Lab Clin Med 111:57–62

Carmel R, Lau KHW, Baylink DJ, Saxena S, Singer FR (1988b) Cobalamin and osteoclast-specific proteins. N Engl J Med 319:70–75

Carmel R, Neely SM, Francis RB (1990) Human umbilcal vein endothelial cells secrete transcobalamin II. Blood 75:251–254

Cartwright GE, Edwards CQ, Kravitz K, Skolnick M, Amos DB, Johnson A, Buskjaer L (1979) Hereditary hemochromatosis: phenotypic expression of disease. N Engl J Med 301:175–179

Case GL, Benevenga NJ (1977) Significance of formate as an intermediate in the oxidation of the methionine, 5-methyl-L-cysteine and sarcosine methyl carbons to CO_2 in the rat. J Nutr 107:1665–1667

Cazzola M, Dezza L, Bergmaschi G, Barosi G, Bellotti V, Caldera D, Ciriello MM, Quagliani S, Arosio P, Ascari E (1983) Biological and clinical significance of red cell ferritin. Blood 67:1078–1087

Celada A, Rudolf H, Herreros V, Donath A (1978) Inorganic iron absorption in subjects with iron deficiency, achylia gastrica and alcoholic cirrhosis using a whole body counter. Acta Haematol 60:182–192

Celada A, Rudolph H, Donath A (1979) Effect of experimental chronic alcohol ingestion and folic acid deficiency on iron adsorption. Blood 54:906–915

Celsing F, Ekblom B, Sylven C, Everett J, Astrand PO (1988) Effects of chronic iron defiency anaemia on myoglobin content, enzyme activity and capillary density in the human skeletal muscle. Acta Med Scand 223:451–457

Chan M, Stokstad ELR (1980) Metabolic responses of folic acid and related compounds to thyroxine in rats. Biochim Biophys Acta 632:244–253

Chanarin I (1976) Investigation and management of megaloblastic anemia. Clin Haematol 5:747–763

Chanarin I (1979) The megalablastic anemias, 2nd edn. Blackwell Scientific Publications, Oxford

Chanarin I (1982) Disorders of vitamin absorption. Clin Gastroenterol 11:73–85

Chanarin I, Perry J, Lumb M (1974) The biochemical lesion in vitamin B_{12} deficiency in man. Lancet 1:1251–1252

Chanarin I, Muir M, Hughes A, Hoffbrand AV (1978) Evidence for the intestinal origin of transcobalamin II during vitamin B_{12} absorption. Br Med J i: 1453–1455

Chanarin I, Deacon R, Lumb M, Perry J (1980) Vitamin B_{12} regulates folate metabolism by supply of formate. Lancet 2:505–508

Chanarin I, Deacon R, Lumb M, Muri M, Perry J (1985) Cobalamin-folate interrelationships: a critical review. Blood 66:479–489

Chapman RW, Morgan MY, Laulicht M, Hoffbrand AV, Sherlock S (1982) Dig Dis Sci 27:909–916

Charlton RW, Jacobs P, Seftel H, Bothwell TH (1964) Effect of alcohol on iron absorption. Br Med J ii:1427–1429

Charlton RW, Jacobs P, Torrance JD, Bothwell TH (1965) The role of the intestinal mucosa in iron absorption. J Clin Invest 44:543–554

Chello PL, Bertino JR (1973) Dependence of 5-methyl-tetrahydrofolate utilization by L5178Y murine leukemia cells in vitro on the presence of hydroxocobalamin and transcobalamin II. Cancer Res 33:1898–1904

Cheng FW, Shane B, Stokstad ELR (1975) The antifolate effect of methionine on bone marrow of normal and vitamin B_{12} deficient rats. Br J Haematol 31: 323–326

Chernelch M, Winchell HS, Pollycove M, Sargent T, Kusubov N (1969) Prolonged intravenous iron-dextran therapy in a patient with multiple hereditary telangiectasia. Blood 34:691–695

Chikkappa G, Corcino J, Greenberg ML, Herbert V (1971) Correlation between various blood white cell pools and serum B_{12} binding capacities. Blood 37: 142–151

Chirasiri L, Izak J (1966) The effect of acute hemorrage and acute hemolysis on intestinal iron absorption in the rat. Br J Haematol 12:611–622

Christensen AC, Huebers H, Finch CA (1978) Effect of transferrin saturation on iron delivery in rats. Am J Physiol 235:R18–R22

Chu LLH, Fineberg RA (1969) On the mechanism of iron-induced synthesis of apoferritin in HeLa cells. J Biol Chem 244:3847–3854

Chu RC, Hall CA (1988) The total serum homocysteine as an indicator of vitamin B_{12} and folate status. Am J Clin Pathol 90:446–449

Clayton P, Smith I, Harding B, Hyland K, Leonard JV, Leeming RJ (1986) Subacute combined degeneration of the cord, dementia and parkinsonism due to an inborn error of folate metabolism. J Neurol Neurosurg Psychiatry 49:920–927

Colman N, Herbert V (1976) Total folate binding capacity of normal human plasma and variations in uremia, cirrhosis and pregnancy. Blood 48:911–921

Colman N, Hettiarachchy N, Herbert V (1981) Detection of a milk factor that facilitates folate uptake by intestinal cells. Science 211:1427–1429

Colman N, DeMartino L, McAleer E (1988) Long-term treatment of vitamin B_{12} malabsorption with nasal cyanocobalamin gel. FASEB J 2:A1086

Conrad ME, Crosby WH (1962) The natural history of iron deficiency induced by phlebotomy. Blood 20:173–185

Conrad ME, Crosby WH (1963) Intestinal mucosal mechanisms controlling iron absorption. Blood 22:406–415
Conrad ME, Schade SG (1968) Ascorbic acid chelates in iron absorption: a role for hydrochloric acid and bile. Gastronenterology 55:35–45
Conrad ME, Benjamin BI, Williams HL, Foy AL (1967a) Human absorption of hemoglobin iron. Gastronenterology 53:5–10
Conrad ME, Foy AL, Williams HL, Knopse WH (1967b) Effect of starvation and protein depletion on ferrokinetics and iron absorption. Am J Physiol 213: 557–565
Conrad ME, Parmley RT, Osterloh K (1987) Small intestinal regulation of iron absorption in the rat. J Lab Clin Med 110:418–426
Cook JD (1982) Clinical evaluation of iron deficiency. Semin Hematol 19:6–18
Cook JD, Monsen ER (1975) Food iron absorption. I. Use of a semisynthetic diet to study absorption of nonheme iron. Am J Clin Nutr 28:1289–1295
Cook JD, Monsen ER (1976a) Food iron absorption in man. II. The effect of EDTA on absorption of dietary non-heme iron. Am J Clin Nutr 29:614–620
Cook JD, Monsen ER (1976b) Food iron absorption. Am J Clin Nutr 29:859–867
Cook JD, Brown M, Valberg LS (1964) The effect of achylia gastrica on iron absorption. J Clin Invest 43:1185–1191
Cook JD, Hershko C, Finch CA (1973) Storage iron kinetics. V. Iron exchange in the rat. Br J Haematol 25:695–706
Cook JD, Lipschitz DA, Miles LEM, Finch CA (1974) Serum ferritin as a measure of iron stores in normal subjects. Am J Clin Nutr 27:681–687
Cook JD, Finch CA, Smith JN (1976) Evaluation of the iron status of a population. Blood 48:449–455
Cook JD, Morck TA, Lynch CR (1981) The inhibitory effect of soy products on non-heme iron absorption in man. Am J Clin Nutr 34:2622–2629
Cook JD, Lipschitz DA, Skikne BS (1982) Absorption of controlled-release iron. Clin Pharmacol Ther 32:521–539
Cooper BA, Castle WB (1960) Sequential mechanism in the enhanced absorption of vitamin B_{12} by intrinsic factor in the rat. J Clin Invest 39:199–214
Cooper BA, Rosenblatt DS (1987) Inherited defects of vitamin B_{12} metabolism. Ann Rev Nutr 7:291–320
Coppen DE, Davis NT (1988) Studies on the roles of apotransferrin and ceruloplasmin on iron absorption in copper-deficient rats using an isolated vascularly and luminally perfused intestinal preparation. Br J Nutr 60:361–373
Corcino J, Kraus S, Waxman S, Herbert V (1970) Release of vitamin B_{12}-binding protein by human leukocytes in vitro. J Clin Invest 49:2250–2254
Corcino JJ, Zalusky R, Greenberg M, Herbert V (1971) Coexistence of pernicious anemia and chronic myeloid leukemia: an experiment of nature involving vitamin B_{12} metabolism. Br J Haematol 20:511–520
Coronato A, Glass GBJ (1973) Depression of intestinal uptake of radio-vitamin B_{12} by cholestyramine. Proc Soc Exp Biol Med 142:1341–1344
Cortell S, Conrad ME (1967) Effect of endotoxin on iron absorption. Am J Physiol 213:43–47
Cottrell JE, Casthely P, Brodie JD, Patel K, Klein A, Turndorf H (1978) Prevention of nitroprusside-induced cyanide toxicity with hydroxocobalamin. N Engl J Med 298:809–811
Cox TM, Peters TJ (1978) Uptake of iron by duodenal biopsy specimens from patients with iron deficiency anemia and primary hemochromatosis. Lancet 1:123–124
Cox TM, Peters TJ (1979) Kinetics of iron uptake in vitro by human duodenal mucosa: studies in normal subjects. J Physiol 289:469–478
Cox TM, Peters TJ (1980) Cellular mechanisms in the regulation of iron absorption by the human intestine: studies in patients with iron deficiency before and after treatment. Br J Haematol 44:75–86
Cox TM, Mazurier J, Spik G, Montreuil J, Peters TJ (1979) Iron binding proteins and influx of iron across the duodenal brush border. Evidence for specific

lactotransferrin receptors in human small intestine. Biochim Biophy Acta 588: 120–128

Craig GM, Elliot C, Hughes KR (1985) Masked vitamin B_{12} and folate deficiency in the elderly. Br J Nutr 54:613–619

Crist WM, Parmley RT, Holbrook CT, Castleberry RP, Denys FR, Malluk A (1980) Dysgranulopoietic neutropenia and abnormal monocytes in childhood vitamin B_{12} deficiency. Am J Hematol 9:89–107

Crosby WH (1980) Oral cyanocobalamin with intrinsic factor for pernicious anemia. Arch Int Med 140:1582

Dallman PR, Siimes MA, Stekel A (1980) Iron deficiency in infancy and childhood. Am J Clin Nutr 33:86–118

Darcy-Vrillon B, Selhub J, Rosenberg IH (1988) Analysis of sequential events in intestinal absorption of folylpolyglutamate. Am J Physiol 255:G361–G366

Das KC, Herbert V (1978) The lymphocyte as a marker of past nutritional status: persistence of abnormal lymphocyte deoxyuridine (dU) suppression tests and chromosomes in patients with past deficiency folate and vitamin B_{12}. Br J Haematol 38:219–233

Das KC, Hoffbrand AV (1970) Lymphocyte transformation in megaloblastic anemia: morphology and DNA synthesis. Br J Haematol 19:459–468

Das KC, Herbert V, Colman N, Longo DL (1978) Unmasking covert folate deficiency in iron-deficient subjects with neutrophil hypersegmentation: dU suppression tests on lymphocytes and bone marrow. Br J Haematol 39:357–375

Das KC, Mohanty D, Garewal G (1986) Cytogenetics in nutritional megaloblastic anaemia: prolonged persistence of chromosomal abnormalities in lymphocytes after remission. Acta Haematol 76:146–154

Dautry-Varsat A, Ciechanover A, Lodish HF (1983) pH and the recycling of transferrin during receptor-mediated endocytosis. Proc Soc Natl Acad Sci (USA) 80:2263–2266

Davidson LA, Lonnerdal B (1989) Fe-saturation and proteolysis of human lactoferrin: effect on brush-border receptor-mediated uptake of Fe and Mn. Am J Physiol 257:G930–G934

Davies KJA, Donovan CM, Refino CJ, Brooks GA, Packer L, Dallman PR (1984) Distinquishing effects of anemia and muscle iron deficiency on exercise bioenergetics in the rat. Am J Physiol 246:E535–E543

Davis AE, Badenoch J (1962) Iron absorption in pancreatic disease. Lancet 2:6–8

Davis PD, Deller DJ (1966) Effect of a xanthine oxidase inhibitor (allopurinol) on radioiron absorption in man. Lancet 1:470–472

Davis PS, Luke CG, Deller DJ (1966) Reduction of gastric iron-binding protein in haemochromatosis: a previously unrecognized metabolic defect. Lancet 4: 1431–1433

Davis PS, Luke CG, Deller DJ (1967) Gastric iron binding protein in iron chelation by gastric juice. Nature 214:1126

Dawson DW, Sawers AH, Sharma RK (1984) Malabsorption of protein-bound vitamin B_{12}. Br Med J 288:675–678

Dawson RB, Rafal S, Weintraub LR (1970) Absorption of hemoglobin iron: the role of xanthine oxidase in the intestinal heme-splitting reaction. Blood 35:94–103

Deacon R, Lumb M, Perry J, Chanarin I, Minty B, Halsey ML, Nunn JF (1980a) Selective inactivation of vitamin B_{12} in rats by nitrous oxide. Eur J Biochem 104:419–425

Deacon R, Chanarin I, Perry J, Lumb M (1980b) Marrow cells from patients with untreated pernicious anemia cannot use tetrahydrofolate normally. Br J Haematol 46:523–528

DeAizpura HJ, Cosgrove LH, Ungar B, Toh BH (1983) Autoantibodies cytotoxic to gastric parietal cells in serum of patients with pernicious anemia. N Engl J Med 309:625–629

DeAlarcon PA, Donovan M, Forbes GB, Landaw SA, Stockman JA (1979) Iron absorption in thalassemia syndromes and its inhibition by tea. N Engl J Med 300:5–8

Derman DP, Bothwell TH, MacPhail AP, Torrance JD, Bezwoda WR, Charlton RW, Mayet FGH (1980) Importance of ascorbic acid in the absorption of iron from infant foods. Scand J Haematol 25:193–201

Derman DP, Bothwell TH, Torrance TR, MacPhail AP, Bezwoda WR, Charlton RW, Mayet FGH (1982) Iron absorption from ferritin and ferric hydroxide. Scand J Haematol 29:18–24

DeVet BCJM, van Gool J (1974) Lactoferrin and iron absorption in the small intestine. Acta Med Scand 196:393–402

Dillman E, Gale C, Green W (1980) Hypothermia in iron deficiency due to altered triiodothyronine metabolism. Am J Physiol 239:R377–R381

Dirusso SC, Check IJ, Hunder RL (1985) Quantitation of apo-, mono-, and diferric transferrin by polyacrylamide gradient gel electrophoresis in patients with disorders of iron metabolism. Blood 66:1445–1451

Disler PB, Lynch SR, Charlton RW, Torrance JD, Bothwell TH (1975a) The effect of tea on iron absorption. Gut 16:193–200

Disler PB, Lynch SR, Torrance JD, Sayers MH, Bothwell TH, Charlton RW (1975b) The mechanism of the inhibition of iron absorption by tea. S Afr J Med Sci 40:109–116

Donaldson RM (1967) Role of enteric microorganisms in malabsorption. Fed Proc 26:1426–1430

Donaldson RM, Small SM, Robins S, Nathan VI (1973) Receptors for vitamin B_{12} related to ileal surface area and absorptive capacity. Biochim Biophys Acta 311:477–481

Doscherholmen A, Swain WR (1973) Impaired assimilation of egg ^{57}Co vitamin B_{12} in patients with hypochlorhydria and achlorhydria and after gastric resection. Gastroenterology 64:912–919

Doscherholmen A, Silvis A, McMahon J (1983) Dual isotope Schilling test for measuring absorption of food-bound and free vitamin B_{12} simultaneously. Am J Clin Pathol 80:490–495

Dowdle EB, Schechter D, Schenker H (1960) Acute transport of Fe59 by everted segments of rat duodenum. Am J Physiol 198:609–613

Durach RC, Moore CV, Callender S (1955) Studies in iron transport and the excretion of iron as measured by the isotope technique. J Lab Clin Med 45: 499–615

Drysdale JW, Shafritz DA (1975) In vitro stimulation of apoferritin synthesis by iron. Biochem Biophys Acta 383:97–105

Dwyer JT, Dietz WS, Andrews RM, Susking RM (1982) Nutritional status of vegetarian children. Am J Clin Nutr 35:204–216

Eastham EJ, Bell JI, Douglas AF (1977) Iron transport characteristics of vesicles of brush border and basolateral plasma membrane from the rat enterocyte. Biochem J 164:289–294

Eells JT, Black KA, Makar AB, Tedford CE, Tephly CR (1982) The regulation of one-carbon oxidation in the rat by nitrous oxide and methionine. Arch Biochem Biophys 219:316–326

Egyed A (1984) Availability, distribution and kinetics of transferrin receptors of rabbit reticulocytes. Br J Haematol 56:563–570

Egyed A (1988) Carrier mediated iron transport through erythroid cell membrane. Br J Haematol 68:483–486

Egyed A, Fodor O, Lelkes G (1986) Coated pit formation: a membrane function involved in the regulation of cellular iron uptake. Br J Haematol 64:263–269

Eichacker P, Lawrence C (1985) Steroid-induced hypersegmentation in neutrophils. Am J Hematol 18:41–45

Eichner ER, Hillman RS (1973) Effect of alcohol on serum folate level. J Clin Invest 52:584–591

Eichner ER, Smiley CA (1981) Serum folate binding capacity as an index of inflammation and cancer dissemination. Clin Res 29:858A

Eichner ER, Pierce HI, Hillman RS (1972) Folate balance in dietary induced megaloblastic anemia. N Engl J Med 284:933–938
Eisenga BH, Collins TD, McMartin KE (1989) Differential effects of acute ethanol on urinary excretion of folate derivatives in the rat. J Pharm Exp Ther 248: 916–922
Ek J, Magnus E (1980) Plasma and red cell folacin in cow's milk-fed infants and children during the first 2 years of life: the significance of boiling pasteurized cow's milk. Am J Clin Nutr 33:1220–1224
Elin RJ, Wolff SM, Finch CA (1977) Effect of induced fever on serum iron and ferritin concentrations in man. Blood 49:147–153
Elsborg L (1981) The folic acid absorption test compared with other laboratory tests for malabsorption. Acta Med Scand 209:323–325
Elsborg L, Larsen E (1979) Folate deficiency in chronic inflammatory bowel diseases. Scand J Gastroenterol 14:1019–1024
Elsborg L, Lund V, Bastrup-Masden P (1976) Serum vitamin B_{12} levels in the aged. Acta Med Scand 200:309–314
El-Shobaki FA, Rummel W (1977) Mucosal transferrin and ferritin factors in the regulation of iron absorption. Res Exp Med 171:243–253
England JM, Fraser PM (1973) Differentiation of iron deficiency from thalassemia trait by routine blood count. Lancet 1:449–452
England JM, Ward SM, Down MC (1976) Microcytosis, anisocytosis and the red cell indices in iron deficiency. Br J Haematol 34:589–597
Erbe RW (1975) Inborn errors of folate metabolism. N Engl J Med 293:753–757, 807–812
Eriksson S, Clase L, Moquist-Olsson I (1981) Pernicious anemia as a risk factor for gastric cancer. Acta Med Scand 210:481–484
Erlandson ME, Wladen B, Stern G, Hilgartner MW, Wehman J, Smith CH (1962) Studies on congenital hemolytic syndromes. IV. Gastrointestinal absorption of iron. Blood 19:359–378
Eschback JW, Cook JD, Scribner BH, Finch CA (1977) Iron balance in hemodialysis patients. Ann Int Med 87:710–713
Ettinger S, Colman N (1985) Altered relationship between red cell and serum folate in the aged suggesting impaired erythrocyte folate transport. Fed Proc 44:1283
Evans GW, Grace CI (1974) Interaction of transferrin with iron-binding sites on rat intestinal epithelial cell plasma membranes. Proc Soc Exp Biol Med 147: 687–689
Fairbanks VF, Elveback LR (1983) Tests for pernicious anemia: serum vitamin B_{12} assay. Mayo Clin Proc 58:135–138
Fargion S, Piperno A, Panaitopoulos N, Taddei MT, Fiorelli G (1985) Iron overload in subjects with beta-thalassemia trait: role of idiopathic hemochromatosis gene. Br J Haematol 61:487–490
Farquharson J, Adams JF (1976) The forms of vitamin B_{12} in food. Br J Nutr 36:127–136
Faulk WP, Hsi BL, Stevens PJ (1980) Transferrin and transferrin receptors in carcinoma of the breast. Lancet 2:390–392
Fehr J, DeVecchi P (1985) Transcobalamin II: a marker for macrophage histiocyte proliferation. Am J Clin Pathol 84:291–296
Fenton V, Cavill I, Fisher J (1977) Iron stores in pregnancy. Br J Haematol 37: 145–149
Fenton WA, Ambani LA, Rosenberg LE (1976) Uptake of hydroxycobalamin by rat liver mitochondria: binding to a mitochondrial protein. J Biol Chem 251: 6616–6623
Fernandes-Costa F, Metz J (1979a) Transplacental transport in the rabbit of vitamin B_{12} bound to human transcobalamins I, II, and III. Br J Haematol 43:625–630
Fernandes-Costa F, Metz J (1979b) Role of serum folate binders in the delivery of folate to tissues and to the fetus. Br J Haematol 41:335–342

Grace ND, Greenwald MA, Greenberg MS (1970) Effect of allopurinol on iron mobilization. Gastroenterology 59:103–108
Granick S (1946) Ferriton IX: increase of apoferritin in the gastrointestinal mucosa as a direct response to iron feeding. The function of ferritin in the regulation of iron absorption. J Biol Chem 164:737–743
Grant HC, Hoffbrand AV, Wells DG (1965) Folate deficiency and neurological disease. Lancet 2:763–767
Grasbeck R (1959) Calculations on vitamin B_{12} turnover in man. Scand J Clin Lab Invest 11:250–261
Green JM, Ballou DP, Mathews RG (1988) Examination of the role of methylene tetrahydrofolate reductase in incorporation of methyltetrahydrofolate into cellular metabolism. Fed Am Soc Exp Biol 2:42–47
Green R, Charlton R, Seftel H, Bothwell T, Mayet F, Adams B, Finch C, Layrisse M (1968) Body iron excretion in man: a collaborative study. Am J Med 45: 336–353
Green R, Jacobsen DW, Van Tonder SV, Kew MC, Metz J (1981) Enterohepatic circulation of cobalamin in the non human primate. Gastroenterology 81: 773–776
Green R, Jacobsen DW, Van Tonder SV, Kew MC, Metz J (1982a) Absorption of biliary cobalamin in baboons following total gastrectomy. J Lab Clin Med 100:771–777
Green R, Kuhla W, Jacobson R, Johnson C, Carmel R, Beutler E (1982b) Masking of macrocytosis by α-thalassemia in blacks with pernicious anemia. N Engl J Med 307:1322–1325
Greenberger NJ, Ruppert RD, Cuppage FE (1967) Inhibition of intestinal iron transport induced by tetracycline. Gastroenterology 53:590–599
Greenberger NJ, Balcerzak SP, Ackerman GA (1969) Iron uptake by isolated brush borders: changes induced by alteration in iron stores. J Lab Clin Med 73: 711–721
Greene HL, Stifel FB, Herman RH, Herman YF, Rosensweig NS (1974) Ethanol-induced inhibition of human intestinal enzyme activities: reversal by folic acid. Gasteroenterology 67:434–440
Greenman J, Jacobs A (1975) The effect of iron stores on iron absorption in the rat: the possible role of circulating ferritin. Gut 16:613–616
Grishan FK, Said HM, Wilson PC, Murrell JE, Greene HL (1986) Intestinal transport of zinc and folic acid: a mutual inhibitory effect. Am J Clin Nutr 43:258–262
Gruden N (1988) The effect of parenteral iron administration upon iron absorption in young rats. Nutr Rep Intl 38:955–960
Hagedorn CH, Alpers DH (1977) Distribution of intrinsic factor-vitamin B_{12} receptors in human intestine. Gastroenterology 73:1019–1022
Hahn D, Baviera B, Ganzoni AM (1975) Functional heterogeneity of the transport iron compartment. Acta Haematol 53:285–291
Hahn PF, Jones E, Lowe RC, Meneely GR, Peacock W (1945) The relative absorption and utilization of ferrous and ferric iron in anemia as determined with the radioactive isotope. Am J Physiol 139:191–197
Hakami N, Neuman PE, Canellos G, Lazerson P (1971) Neonatal megaloblastic anemia due to inherited transcobalamin II deficiency in 2 siblings. N Engl J Med 285:1163–1170
Hall CA (1975) Transcobalamin I and II as natural transport proteins of vitamin B_{12}. J Clin Invest 56:1125
Hall CA (1976) The failure of granulocytes to produce transcobalamin I (TCI). Scand J Haematol 16:176–182
Hall CA (1981) Congenital disorders of vitamin B_{12} transport and their contributions to concepts. Yale J Biol Med 54:485–495
Hall CA, Begley JA (1977) Congenital deficiency of human R type binding proteins of cobalamin. Am J Human Genet 29:619–626

Hall CA, Green E, Colligan PD, Begley JA (1985) Synthesis of transcobalamin II by cultured human hepatocytes. Biochim Biophys Acta 838:387–389
Hallberg L (1981) Bioavailability of dietary iron in man. Ann Rev Nutr 1:123–147
Hallberg L, Solvell L (1967) Absorption of hemoglobin iron in man. Acta Med Scand 181:335–354
Hallberg L, Ryttinger L, Solvell L (1966) Side effects of oral iron therapy: a double blind study of different iron compounds in tablet form. Acta Med Scand 188 [Suppl 459]:3–10
Hallberg L, Bjorn-Rasmussen E, Howard L, Rossander L (1979) Dietary heme iron absorption. A discussion of possible mechanisms of the absorption promoting effect of meat and for the regulation of iron absorption. Scand J Gastroenterol 14:769–779
Hallberg L, Brune M, Rossander L (1986) Low bioavailability of carbonyl iron in man: studies on iron fortification of wheat flour. Am J Clin Nutr 43:59–67
Hallberg L, Brune M, Rossander L (1988) Iron absorption in man: ascorbic acid and dose-dependent inhibition by phytate. Am J Clin Nutr 49:140–144
Hallert C, Tobiasson P, Walan A (1981) Serum folate determinations in tracing adult coeliacs. Scand J Gastroenterol 16:263–267
Halliday JW, Powell LW (1984) Ferritin metabolism and the liver. Semin Liver Dis 4:207–216
Halliday JW, Powell LW, Mack U (1976) Iron absorption in the rat: the search for possible intestinal mucosal carriers. Br J Haematol 34:237–250
Halsted CH (1989) The intestinal absorption of dietary folates in health and disease. J Am Coll Nutr 8:650–658
Hälsted CH, Griggs RC, Harris JW (1967) The effect of alcoholism on the absorption of folic acid (3H-PGA) evaluated by plasma levels and urine excretion. J Lab Clin Med 69:116–131
Halsted CH, Robles EA, Mezey E (1971) Decreased jejunal uptake of labeled folic acid ^{3}H-PAG) in alcoholic patients: roles of alcohol and nutrition. N Engl J Med 285:701–706
Halsted CH, Baugh CM, Butterworth CE (1975) Jejunal perfusion of simple and conjugated folates in man. Gastroenterology 63:261–269
Hamrell MR, Hochstein P, Carmel R (1979) Leukocyte hexose monophosphate shunt activity during phagocytosis in vitamin B_{12} and folic acid deficiencies. Am J Clin Nutr 32:2265–2268
Hamstra RD, Block MH, Schocket AL (1980) Intravenous iron dextran in clinical medicine. J Am Med Assoc 143:1726–1731
Hardinage MC, Stare FJ (1954) Nutritional studies of vegetarians I. Nutritional, physical and laboratory studies. Am J Clin Nutr 2:73–82
Harriman GR, Smith PD, Horne MK, Fox CH, Koenig S, Lake EE, Lane HC, Fauci AS (1989) Vitamin B_{12} malabsorption in patients with acquired immunodeficiency syndrome. Arch Int Med 149:2039–2041
Harris DC, Aisen P (1975) Iron donating properties of transferrin. Biochemistry 14:262–268
Harrison PM, Banyard SH, Hoare RJ, Russll SM, Trefry A (1977) The structure and function of ferritin. Ciba Found Symp 51:19–35
Haurani FI, Green D, Young K (1965) Iron absorption in hypoferremia. Am J Med Sci 245:537–547
Haurani FI, Hall CA, Rubin R (1979) Megaloblastic anemia as a result of an abnormal transcobalamin II. J Clin Invest 64:1253–1259
Hegsted DM, Finch CA, Kinney TD (1949) The influence of diet on iron absorption. II. The interaction of iron and phosphorus. J Exp Med 90:147–156
Heimburger DC, Alexander CB, Birch R, Butterworth CE, Bailley WC, Krumdieck CL (1988) Improvement in bronchial squamous metaplasia in smokers treated with folated and vitamin B_{12}. J Am Med Assoc 259:1525–1530
Heinrich HC (1970) Gastric intrinsic factor and iron absorption. Lancet 2:1256

Helman AD, Darnton-Hill I (1988) Vitamin and iron stores in new vegetarians. Am J Clin Nutr 45:785–789
Hendel L, Hendel J, Joergenson I (1987) Enterocyte function in progressive systemic sclerosis as estimated by the deconjugation of pteroyltriglutamate to folic acid. Gut 28:435–438
Henderson GB, Suresh MR, Vitols KS, Huennekens FM (1986) Transport of folate compounds in L1210 cells: kinetic evidence that folate influx proceeds via the high affinity transport system for 5-methyltetrahydrofolate and methotrexate. Cancer Res 46:1639–1643
Henderson GB, Tsuji JM, Kumar HP (1987) Transport of folate compounds by leukemic cells: evidence for a single influx carrier for methotrexate, 5-methyltetrahydrofolate and folate in CCRF-CEM human lymphoblasts. Biochem Pharmacol 36:3007–3014
Henderson PA, Hillman RS (1969) Characteristics of iron dextran utilization in man. Blood 34:357–375
Hendler ED, Solomon LR (1978) Use of iron dextran to replace iron loss in chronic hemodialysis patients. Proc Clin Dial Transplant Forum 8:108–112
Hennigar GR, Greene WB, Walker EM, deSaussure A (1979) Hemochromatosis caused by excessive vitamin iron intake. Am J Pathol 96:611–624
Hentze MW, Caughman SW, Roualt TA et al. (1980) Identification and characterization of the iron responsive element for translational regulation of human ferritin mRNA. Science 238:1570–1574
Hepner GW, Booth CC, Cowan J, Hoffbrand AV, Mollin DL (1968) Absorption of crystalline folic acid in man. Lancet 2:302–306
Herbert V (1973) The five possible causes of all nutrient deficiency illustrated by deficiencies of vitamin B_{12} and folic acid. Am J Clin Nutr 26:77–88
Herbert V (1987a) Recommended dietary intakes of folate in humans. Am J Clin Nutr 45:661–670
Herbert V (1987b) Recommended dietary intakes (RDI) of vitamin B_{12} in humans. Am J Clin Nutr 45:671–678
Herbert V (1987c) Making sense of laboratory tests of folate status: folate requirements to sustain normality. Am J Hematol 26:199–207
Herbert V, Coleman N (1981) Evidence humans may use some analogues of B_{12} as cobalamins: pure intrinsic factor radioassay may diagnose clinical B_{12} deficiency where it does not exist. Clin Res 29:317A
Herbert V, Zalusky R (1962) Interrelationship of vitamin B_{12} and folic acid metabolism: folic acid clearance studies. J Clin Invest 41:1263–1276
Herbert V, Jacob E, Wong KTJ, Scott J, Pfeffer RD (1978) Low serum B_{12} levels in patients receiving ascorbic acid in megadoses: studies concerning the effect of ascorbate on radioisotope B_{12} assay. Am J Clin Nutr 31:253–259
Hermos JA, Adams WH, Liu YK, Sullivan LW, Trier JS (1972) Mucosa of the small intestine in folate-deficient alcoholics. Ann Int Med 76:957–965
Herschko C (1975) The fate of circulating hemoglobin. Br J Haematol 29:199–204
Herschko C (1987) Non-transferrin plasma iron. Br J Haematol 66:149–151
Hershko C, Karsai A, Eylon L Izak G (1970) The effect of chronic iron deficiency on some biochemical functions in human hemopoietic tissue. Blood 36:321–329
Hershko C, Cook JD, Finch CA (1973) Storage iron kinetics. III. Study of deferrioxamine action by selective radioiron labels of reticuloendothelial and parenchymal cells. J Lab Clin Med 81:876–886
Herzlich B, Herbert V (1988) Depletion of serum holotranscobalamin II: an early sign of negative vitamin B_{12} balance. Lab Invest 58:332–337
Higginbottom MC, Sweetman L, Nyhan WL (1978) A syndrome of methylmalonic aciduria, homocystinuria, megaloblastic anemia and neurologic abnormalities in a vitamin B_{12} deficient breast-fed infant of a strict vegetarian. N Engl J Med 299:317–323
Hill C (1971) Studies on the mutual interaction of iron and manganese on absorption from chick duodenal segments in situ. Fed Proc 30:236

Hill RS, Pettit JE, Tattersall MHN, Kiley N, Lewis SM (1972) Iron deficiency and dyserythropoiesis. Br J Haematol 23:507–512
Hillman RS, Henderson PA (1969) Control of marrow production by the level of iron supply. J Clin Invest 48:454–460
Hillman RS, Steinberg SE (1982) The effects of alcohol on folate metabolism. Ann Rev Med 33:345–354
Hillman RS, McGuffin R, Campbell C (1977) Alcohol interference with the folate enterohepatic cycle. Trans Assoc Am Physicians 90:145–156
Hillman RS, Steinberg S, Campbel C (1978) Tetrahydrofolate transport: a required pathway in folate metabolism. Clin Res 26:504A
Hillman R, Campbell C, Steinberg S (1982) The role of the folate enterohepatic cycle in the recovery of folate polyglutamate from senescent red cells. Clin Res 30:550A
Hines JD, Halsted CH, Griggs RC, Harris JW (1968) Megaloblastic anemia secondary to folate deficiency associated with hypothyroidism. Ann Int Med 68: 792–805
Hitzhusen JC, Taplin ME, Stephenson WP, Ansell JE (1986) Vitamin B_{12} levels and age. Am J Clin Pathol 85:32–36
Hitzig WH, Dohmann U, Pluss HJ, Vischer D (1974) Hereditary transcobalamin II deficiency: clinical finding in a new family. J Pediatr 85:622–628
Hoffbrand AV, Ganeshaguru K, Hooton WL, Tattersall MHN (1976a) Effect of iron deficiency and desferrioxamine on DNA synthesis in human cells. Br J Haematol 33:517–526
Hoffbrand AV, Ganeshaguru K, Hooton JWL, Tripp E (1976b) Megaloblastic anemia: initiation of DNA synthesis in excess of DNA chain elongations as the underlying mechanism. Clin Haematol 5:727–745
Hoppner K, Lampi B (1988) Antacid ingestion and folate bioavailability in the rat. Nutr Rep Intl 38:539–546
Horne DW, Briggs WT (1980) Effect of dietary and nitrous oxide induced vitamin B_{12} deficiency on uptake of 5-methyltetrahydrofolate by isolated hepatocytes. J Nutr 110:223–230
Horne DW, Briggs WT, Wagner C (1979) Studies on the transport mechanism of 5-methyltetrahydrofolic acid in freshly isolated hepatocytes: effect of ethanol. Arch Biochem Biophys 196:557–565
Horne DW, Patterson D, Said HM (1989) Aging: effect on hepatic metabolism and transport of folate in the rat. Am J Clin Nutr 50:359–363
Howard J, Jacobs A (1972) Iron transport by rat small intestine in vitro effect of body of iron stores. Br J Haematol 23:595–603
Huebers H, Huebers E, Forth W, Rummel W (1971) Binding of iron to a non-ferritin protein in the mucosal cells of normal and iron deficient rats during absorption. Life Sci 10:1141–1148
Huebers H, Huebers E, Rummel W (1974) Dependence of increased iron absorption by iron deficient rats on an elutable component of jejunal mucosa. Hoppe Seylers Z Physiol Chem 355:1159–1167
Huebers H, Huebers E, Rummel W, Crichton RR (1976) Isolation and characterization of iron-binding proteins from rat intestinal mucosa. Eur J Biochem 66: 447–455
Huebers H, Huebers E, Csiba E, Rummel W, Finch CA (1977) Intestinal iron absorption of transferrin bound iron in normal and iron deficient rats. Blood 50:80–87
Huebers H, Huebers E, Csiba E, Finch CA (1978) Iron uptake from rat plasma transferrin by rat reticulocytes. J Clin Invest 62:944–951
Huebers H, Csiba E, Josephson B, Huebers E, Finch C (1981a) Interaction of human diferric transferrin with reticulocytes. Proc Natl Acad Sci USA 78: 621–625
Huebers H, Josephson B, Huebers E, Csiba E, Finch C (1981b) Uptake and release of iron from human transferrin. Proc Natl Acad Sci USA 78:2572–2576

Huebers H, Bauer W, Huebers E, Csiba E, Finch C (1981c) The behavior of transferrin iron in the rat. Blood 57:218–228
Huebers HA, Finch CA (1987) The physiology of transferrin and transferrin receptors. Physiology Rev 67:520–580
Huebers HA, Huebers E, Csiba E, Rummel W, Finch CA (1983a) The significance of transferrin for intestinal iron absorption. Blood 61:283–290
Huebers HA, Csiba E, Huebers E, Finch CA (1983b) Competitive advantage of diferric transferrin in delivering iron to reticulocytes. Proc Natl Acad Sci USA 80:300–304
Huebers HA, Josephson B, Huebers E, Csiba E, Finch CA (1984a) Occupancy of the iron binding sites of human transferrin. Proc Natl Acad Sci USA 81: 4326–4330
Huebers HA, Huebers E, Csiba E, Finch CA (1984b) Heterogeneity of the plasma iron pool: explanation of the Fletcher Huehns phenomenon. Am J Physiol 247:R280–R283
Huebers HA, Csiba E, Huebers E, Finch CA (1985) Molecular advantage of diferric transferrin in delivering iron to reticulocytes: a comparative study. Proc Soc Exp Biol Med 179:222–226
Huebers HA, Beguin Y, Pootrakul P, Einspahr D, Finch CA (1990) Intact transferrin receptors in human plasma and their relation to erythropoiesis. Blood 75:102–107
Hungerford DM, Linder MC (1983) Interactions of pH and ascorbate in intestinal iron absorption. J Nutr 113:2615–2657
Hunt RC, Riegler R, Davis AA (1989) Changes in glycosylation alter the affinity of the human transferrin receptor for its ligand. J Biol Chem 264:9643–9648
Idzerda RL, Huebers H, Finch CA, McKnoght S (1986) Rat transferrin gene expression: tissue specific regulation by iron deficiency. Proc Natl Acad Sci USA 83:3723–3727
Isa L, Jean G, Siolvani A, Arosio P, Taccagni GL (1988) Evaluation of iron stores in patients with alcoholic liver disease: role of red cell ferritin. Acta Haematol 80:85–88
Isobe K, Sakurami T (1978) Studies on iron transport in human intestine by immunoperoxidase technique. The localization of ferritin, lactoferrin and transferrin in human duodenal mucosa. Acta Haematol Jpn 41:1328–1333
Jacob E, Baker SJ, Herbert V (1980) Vitamin B_{12}-binding proteins. Physiol Rev 60:918–960
Jacobs A (1969) An intracellular transit iron pool. Ciba Found Symp 51:91–106
Jacobs A (1977) An intracellular transit iron pool. Ciba Found Symp 51:91–106
Jacobs A, Cavill I (1968) The oral lesions of iron deficiency: pyridoxine and riboflavin status. Br J Haematol 14:291–295
Jacobs A, Miles PM (1969a) The role of gastric secretion in iron absorption. Gut 10:226–229
Jacobs A, Miles PM (1969b) Intraluminal transport of iron from stomach to small intestinal mucosa. Br Med J iv:778–781
Jacobs A, Miles PM (1969c) The iron binding properties of gastric juice. Clin Chim Acta 24:87–92
Jacobs A, Miles PM (1970) The formation of iron complexes with bile and bile constituents. Gut 11:732–734
Jacobs J, Greene H, Gendel BR (1965) Acute iron intoxication. Engl J Med 273: 1124–1127
Jacobs P, Owen GM (1969) Effect of gastric juice on iron absorption in patients with gastric atrophy. Gut 10:488–490
Jacobs P, Bothwell TH, Charlton RW (1966) Intestinal iron transport: studies using a loop of gut with an artificial circulation. Am J Physiol 210:694–700
Jacobs P, Bothwell T, Charlton RW (1967) Role of hydrochloric acid in iron absorption. J Appl Physiol 19:87–88.

Jaffe RM, Kasten B, Young DSK, MacLowry JD (1975) False negative occult blood tests caused by ingestion of ascorbic acid (vitamin C). Ann Int Med 83:824–826

Jeejeebhoy KN, Ho J, Greenberg GR, Philips MJ, Robertson AB, Sodtke U (1975) Albumin, fibrinogen and transferrin synthesis in isolated rat hepatocyte suspensions. A model for the study of plasma protein synthesis. Biochem J 146: 141–155

Jewesbury ECO (1954) Subacute combined degeneration of the cord and achlorhydric peripheral neuropathies without anaemia. Lancet 2:307–312

Johnson BF (1968) Hemochromatosis resulting from prolonged oral iron therapy. N Engl J Med 278:1100–1101

Johnson H, Jacobs P, Purves LR (1983) Iron binding proteins of iron-absorbing rat intestinal mucosa. J Clin Invest 71:1467–1476

Jones MS, Jones OTG (1969) The structural organization of haem synthesis in rat liver mitochondria. Biochem J 113:507–514

Jones PJ, Mills EH, Capps RP (1957) The effect of liver disease on serum vitamin B_{12} concentrations. J Lab Clin Med 49:910–922

Jones RL, Peterson CM, Grady RW, Cerami A (1980) A low molecular weight iron-binding factor from mammalian tissue that potentiates bacterial growth. J Exp Med 151:418–425

Kamen BA, Capdevilla A (1986) Receptor-mediated folate accumulation is regulated by the cellular folate content, Proc Natl Acad Sci USA 83:5983–5987

Kamen BA, Caston D (1975) Purification of folate-binding factor in normal umbilical cord serum. Proc Natl Acad Sci USA 72:4261–4264

Kamen BA, Wang MT, Streckfuss AJ, Peryea X, Anderson RGW (1988) Delivery of folates to the cytoplasm of MA104 cells is mediated by a surface membrance receptor that recycles. J Biol Chem 263:13602–13609

Kanazawa S, Herbert V (1983) Noncobalamin vitamin B_{12} analogues in human red cells, liver and brain. Am J Clin Nutr 37:744–777

Kanazawa S, Herbert V (1985) Total corrinoid, cobalamin (vitamin B_{12}) and cobalamin analogue levels may be normal in serum despite cobalamin depletion in liver in patients with alcoholism. Lab Invest 53:108–110

Kanazawa S, Herbert V, Herzlich B, Drivas G, Manusselis C (1983) Removal of cobalamin analogue in bile by enterohepatic circulation of vitamin B_{12}. Lancet 1:707–708

Kanazawa S, Terada H, Iseki T, Iwasa S, Okuda K, Kondo H (1986) Binding of cobalamin analogs to intrinsic factor-cobalamin receptor and its prevention by R binder. Proc Soc Exp Biol Med 183:333–338

Kane MA, Waxman S (1989) Role of folate binding proteins in folate metabolism. Lab Invest 60:737–746

Kano Y, Sakamoto S, Sakuraya K, Kubota T, Hida K, Suda K, Takaku F (1981) Effect of nitrous oxide on human bone marrow cells and its synergistic effect with methionine and methotrexate on functional folate deficiency. Cancer Res 41:4698–4703

Kano Y, Sakamoto S, Sakuraya K, Kubota T, Taguchi H, Miura Y, Takaku F (1984) Effects of leucovorin and methylcobalamin with N_2O anesthesia. J Lab Clin Med 104:711–717

Kapadia CR, Donaldson RM (1985) Disorders of cobalamin (vitamin B_{12}) absorption and transport. Ann Rev Med 36:93–110

Kapadia CR, Serfilippi D, Voloshin K, Donaldson RM (1983) Intrinsic factor-mediated absorption of cobalamin by guinea pig ileal cells. J Clin Invest 71: 440–448

Kaplan SS, Basford RE (1976) Effect of vitamin B_{12} and folic acid deficiencies on neutrophil function. Blood 47:801–805

Karnaze DS, Carmel R (1987) Low serum cobalamin levels in primary degenerative dementia: do some patients harbor atypical cobalamin deficiency states? Arch Intern Med 147:429–431

Karpatkin S, Garg SK, Freedman ML (1974) Role of iron as a regulator of thrombopoiesis. Am J Med 57:521–525

Kass L (1976) Detection of methionine in pernicious anemia megaloblasts and other types of erythroid preceursors. An J Clin Pathol 63:504–507

Katka K, Seger RA, Matsunaga T, Toivanen A, Hitzig WH (1983) Granulocyte function in pernicious anaemia. Br J Haematol 53:23–30

Katz M, O'Brien R (1979) Vitamin B_{12} absorption studied by vascular perfusion of rat intestine. J Lab Clin Med 94:817–825

Katz M, Lee SK, Cooper BA (1972) Vitamin B_{12} malabsorption due to a biologically inert intrinsic factor. N Engl J Med 287:425–429

Katz M, Mehlman CS, Allen RH (1974) Isolation and characterization of abnormal human intrinsic factor. J Clin Invest 53:1274–1287

Kaunitz JD, Lindenbaum J (1977) The bioavailability of folic acid added to wine. Ann Ind Med 87:542–545

Kavin H, Charlton RW, Jacobs P, Bothwell TH (1967) Effect of the exocrine pancreatic secretion on iron absorption. Gut 8:556–564

Keagy PM, Shane B, Oace SM (1988) Folate bioavailability in humans: effects of wheat bran and beans. Am J Clin Nutr 47:80–88

Kelsay JL, Behall KM, Prather ES (1979) Effect of fiber from fruits and vegetables on metabolic responses of human subjects. II. Calcium, magnesium, iron and silicon balances. Am J Clin Nutr 32:1876–1880

Kill J, Jagerstod M, Elsborg L (1979) The role of liver passage for conversion of pteroylmonoglutamate and pteroyltriglutamate to active folate coenzymes. Gut 49:217–222

Killman SA (1965) Effect of deoxyuridine on incorporation of tritiated thymidine: difference between normoblasts and megaloblasts. Acta Med Scand 175: 483–488

Kino K, Tsunoo H, Higa Y (1980) Hemoglobin-haptoglobin receptor in rat liver plasma membrane. J Biol Chem 255:9616–9620

Kinzie BJ, Taylor JW (1984) Trimethoprim and folinic acid. Ann Int Med 101:565

Klausner RD, van Renswounde J, Ashwell G et al. (1983a) Receptor-mediated endocytosis of transferrin in K562 cells. J Biol Chem 258:4715–4719

Klausner RD, Ashwell G, van Renswoude J et al. (1983b) Binding of apotransferrin to K562 cells: explanation of the transferrin cycle. Proc Natl Acad Sci USA 80:2263–2266

Klipstein FA (1972) Folate in tropical spruce. Br J Haematol 23 [Suppl 1]:119–133

Knowles JP, Prankerd TAJ (1962) Abnormal folic acid metabolism in vitamin B_{12} deficiency. Clin Sci 22:233–238

Kohgo Y, Nishisato K, Kondo H, Tsushima N, Niitsu Y, Urushizaki I (1986) Circulating transferrin receptor in human serum. Br J Haematol 64:277–281

Kolhouse JF, Allen R (1977a) Recognition of two intracellular cobalamin binding proteins and their identification as methylmalonyl-CoA mutase and methionine synthetase. Proc Natl Acad Sci USA 74:921–925

Kolhouse JF, Allen RH (1977b) Absorption, plasma transport and cellular retention of cobalamin analogues in the rabbit. J Clin Invest 60:1381–1392

Kolhouse JF, Hondo H, Allen NC, Podell E, Allen RH (1978) Cobalamin analogues are present in human plasma and can mask cobalamin deficiency because current radioisotope dilution assays are not specific for true cobalamin. N Engl J Med 299:785–792

Kondo H, Osborne ML, Kolhouse JF, Binder MJ, Podell ER, Utley CS, Abrams RS, Allen RH (1981) Nitrous oxide has multiple deleterious effect on cobalomin metabolism and causes decreases in activities of both cobalamin-dependent enzymes in rats. J Clin Invest 67:1270–1283

Kondo H, Binder MJ, Kolhouse JF, Smythe WR, Podell ER, Allen RH (1982) Presence and formation of cobalamin analogues in multivitamin mineral pills. J Clin Invest 70:889–898

Kondo H, Iseki T, Iwasa S, Okuda K, Kanazawa S, Ohto M, Ohuda K (1989) Cobalamin-dependent replication of L1210 leukemia cells and effects of cobalamin analogues. Acta Haematol 81:61–69

Konijn AM, Hershko C (1977) Ferritin synthesis in inflammation: I. Pathogenesis of impaired iron release. Br J Haematol 37:7–16

Kozlowski R, Reilly AG, Sowter D, Robins A, Russel NH (1988) Transferrin receptor expression on AML blasts is related to their proliferative potential. Br J Haematol 69:275–280

Kozma C, Salvador RA, Elion GB (1968) Chronic allopurinol administration and iron storage in mice. Life Sci 7:341–348

Krause JR, Stolc V (1980) Serum ferritin and bone marrow iron stores: II. Correlation with low serum iron and Fe/TIBC ratio less than 15%. Am J Clin Pathol 74:461–464

Krebs HE, Hems R, Tyler B (1976) The regulation of folate and methionine metabolism. Biochem J 158:341–353

Krumdieck CL, Newman AJ, Butterworth CE (1973) A naturally occurring inhibitor of folic acid conjugase (pteroyl-polyglutamyl hydrolase) in beans and other pulses. Am J Clin Nutr 26:460–461

Kubasik NP, Ricotta M, Sine HE (1980) Commercially supplied binders for plasma cobalamin (vitamin B_{12}) analysis – "purified" intrinsic factor, "cobnamide"-blocked R-protein binder and nonpurified intrinsic factor-R protein binder – compared to microbiological assay. Clin Chem 26:598–600

Kushner JP, Edwards CQ, Madone MM, Skolnick MH (1985) Heterozygosity for HLA-linkage hemochromatosis as a likely cause of the hepatic siderosis associated with sporadic porphyria cutanea tarda. Gastroenterology 88:1232–1238

Kutzbach C, Stokstad ELR (1971) Mammalian methylene tetrahydrofolate reductase. Partial purification, properties and inhibition by 5-adenosylmethionine. Biochem Biophys Acta 250:459–477

Kutzbach C, Galloway E, Stokstad ELR (1967) Influence of vitamin B_{12} and methionine on levels of folic acid compounds and folate coenzymes in rat liver. Proc Soc Exp Biol Med 124:801–805

Laine LA, Bentley E, Chandrasoma P (1988) Effect of oral iron therapy on the upper gastrointestinal tract: a prospective evaluation. Dig Dis Sci 33:172–177

Lampkin BC, Shore NA, Chadwick D (1966) Megaloblastic anemia of infancy secondary to maternal pernicious anemia. N Engl J Med 274:1168–1171

Lane F, Goff P, McGuffin R, Hillman RS (1976) Folic acid metabolism in normal, folate deficient and alcoholic man. Br J Haematol 34:489–501

Lanzkowski P (1970) Congenital malabsorption of folate. Am J Med 48:580–583

Larrick JW, Hyman ES (1984) Acquired iron deficiency anemia caused by an antibody against transferrin receptor. N Engl J Med 311:214–218

Lashner BA, Heidenreich PA, Su GL, Kane SV, Hanauer SB (1989) Effect of folate supplementation on the incidence of dysplasia and cancer in chronic ulcerative colitis. Gastroenterology 97:255–259

Latta D, Liebman M (1984) Iron and zinc status of vegetarian and nonvegetarian males. Nutr Rep Int 30:141–149

Lavoie A, Tripp E, Hoffbrand AV (1974) The effect of vitamin B_{12} deficiency on methylfolate metabolism and pteroylpolyglutamate synthesis in human cells. Clin Sci Molec Med 47:617–630

Lawson DH, Parker JLW (1976) Death from severe megaloblastic anemia in hospitalized patients. Scand J Haematol 17:347–352

Lawson DH, Boddy K, King PC, Linton AL, Will G (1971) Iron metabolism in patients with chronic renal failure on regular dialysis treatment. Clin Sci 41: 345–351

Lawson DH, Murray RM, Parker JLW (1972) Early mortality in the megaloblastic anemias. Q J Med 41:1–14

Layrisse M, Martinez-Torres C, Roche M (1968) Effect of the interaction of various foods on iron absorption. Am J Clin Nutr 21:1175–1183
Layrisse M, Martinez-Torres C, Cook JD, Walker R, Finch CA (1973) Iron fortification of food: its measurement by the extrinsic tag method. Blood 41:333–352
Layrisse M, Martinez-Torres C, Renzi M, Leets I (1975) Ferritin iron absorption in man. Blood 45:689–698
Lazar GS, Carmel R (1981) Cobalamin binding and uptake in vitro in the human central nervous system. J Lab Clin Med 97:123–133
Lazzatto L, Falusi AO, Joju EA (1982) Uracil in DNA in megaloblastic anemia. N Engl J Med 305:1156–1157
Lee GR (1983) The anemia of chronic disease. Semin Hematol 20:61–90
Leibold EA, Munro HN (1980) A cytoplasmic protein binds in vitro to a highly conserved sequence in the 5'-untranslated region of ferritin H and L subunit mRNAs. Proc Natl Acad Sci USA 88:2171–2175
Levine DS, Huebers HA, Rubin CE, Finch CA (1988) Blocking action of parenteral desferrioxamine one iron absorption in rodents and men. Gastroenterology 95:1242–1248
Levine PH (1973) A qualitaive platelet defect in severe vitamin B_{12} deficiency: response, hyperresponse and thrombosis after vitamin B_{12} therapy. Ann Int Med 78:533–539
Levine PH, Hamstra RD (1969) Megaloblastic anemia of pregnancy simulating acute leukemia. Ann Int Med 71:1141–1147
Levine PH, Levine AJ, Weintraub L (1972) The role of transferrin in the control of iron absorption: studies on a cellular level. J Lab Clin Med 80:333–341
Lifton LJ, Kreiser J (1982) False positive stool occult blood tests caused by iron preparations. Gastroenterology 83:860–863
Lindenbaum J (1980) Folate and vitamin B_{12} deficiencies in alcoholism. Semin Hematol 17:119–129
Lindenbaum J (1983a) Status of laboratory testing in the diagnosis of megaloblastic anemia. Blood 61:624–628
Lindenbaum J (1983b) Drug-induced folate deficiency and the hematologic effects of ethanol. In: Lindenbaum J (ed) Nutrition in hematology. Churchill Livingstone, New York, pp 33–58
Lindenbaum J, Klipstein FA (1965) Folic acid clearances and basal serum folate levels in patients with thyroid disease. J Clin Pathol 17:666–670
Lindenbaum J, Lieber CS (1975) Effects of chronic ethanol administration on intestinal absorption in man in the absence of nutritional deficiency. Ann NY Acad Sci 252:228–234
Linder MC, Munro HN, Morris HP (1970) Rat ferritin isoproteins and their response to iron administration in a series of hepatic tumors and in normal and regenerating liver. Cancer Res 30:2231–2239
Linder MC, Dunn V, Isaacs E, Jones D, Lim S, Van Volkom M, Munro HN (1975) Ferritin and intestinal iron absorption: pancreatic enzymes and free iron. Am J Physiol 228:196–204
Linnell JC, Mathews DM (1984) Cobalamin metabolism and its clinical aspects. Clin Sci 66:113–121
Lipschitz DA, Bothwell TH, Seftel H (1971) The role of ascorbic acid in the metabolism of storage iron. Br J Haematol 20:155–163
Lipschitz DA, Cook JD, Finch CA (1974) A clinical evaluation of serum ferritin as an index of iron stores. N Engl J Med 290:1213–1216
Lloyd KN, Williams P (1970) Reactions to total dose infusion of iron dextran in rheumatoid arthritis. Br Med J 1:323–325
Luhby AL, Eagle FJ, Roth E, Cooperman JM (1961) Relapsing megaloblasic anemia in an infant due to a specific defect in gastrointestinal absorption of folic acid. Am J Dis Child 102:482–483
Luke CG, Davis PS, Deller DJ (1967) Change in gastric iron-binding protein (gastroferrin) during iron-deficiency anemia. Lancet 2:926–927

Luke CG, Davis PS, Deller DJ (1968) Gastric iron binding in hemochromatosis, secondary iron overload, cirrhosis and diabetes. Lancet 4:844–846

Lumb M, Deacon R, Perry J, Chanarin I, Minty B, Halsey MJ, Nunn JF (1980) The effect of nitrous oxide inactivation of vitamin B_{12} on rat hepatic folate: implications for the methylfolate trap hypothesis. Biochem J 186:933–936

Lumb M, Perry J, Deacon R, Chanarin I (1981) Changes in tissue folates accompanying nitrous oxide-induced inactivation of vitamin B_{12} in the rat. Am J Clin Nutr 34:2412–2417

Lumb M, Perry J, Deacon R, Chanarin I (1982) Urinary folate loss following inactivation of vitamin B_{12} by nitrous oxide in rats. Br J Haematol 51:235–242

Lumb M, Sharer N, Deacon R, Jennings P, Purkiss P, Perry J, Chanarin I (1983) Effects of nitrous oxide-induced inactivation of cobalamin on methionine and *S*-adenosyl methionine metabolism in the rat. Biochim Biophys Acta 756:354–359

Lumb M, Chanarin I, Perry J, Deacon R (1985) Turnover of the methyl moiety of 5-methyltetrahydropteroylglutamic acid in the cobalamin-inactivated rat. Blood 66:1171–1175

Lumb M, Chanarin I, Deacon R, Perry J (1988) In vivo oxidation of the methyl group of hepatic 5-methyltetrahydrofolate. J Clin Pathol 41:1158–1152

Lumb M, Deacon R, Perry J, Chanarin I (1989) Oxidation of 5-methyltetrahydrofolate in cobalamin inactivated rats. Biochem J 258:907–910

MacDonald VW, Charache S, Hathaway PJ (1985) Iron deficiency anemia: mitochondrial glycerophosphate dehydrogenase in guinea pig skeletal muscle. J Lab Clin Med 105:11–18

Mack V, Powell LW, Halliday JW (1983) detection and isolation of a hepatic membrane receptor for ferritin. J Biol Chem 258:4672–4675

MacKenzie IL, Donaldson RM, Trier JS, Mathan VI (1972) Ileal mucosa in familial selective vitamin B_{12} malabsorption. N Engl J Med 286:1021–1025

MacKenzie JF, Russell RI (1976) The effect of pH on folic acid absorption in man. Clin Sci Mol Med 51:363–368

Mackler B, Drivas G, Greenstein R, Herbert V (1984) Colon bacteria are the main source of vitamin B_{12} analogues in human stool and bile and may be necessary for maximal proliferation of such bacteria and for their synthesis of analogues. Clin Res 32:490a

MacPhail AP, Simon MO, Torrance JD, Charlton RW, Bothwell TH, Isaacson C (1979) Changing patterns of dietary iron overload in black South Africans. Am J Clin Nutr 32:1272–1278

Magnusson B, Faxen A, Cederblad A, Rosander L, Kewenter L, Hallberg L (1979) The effect of parietal cell vagotomy and selective vagotomy with pyloroplasty on iron absorption. A prospective randomized study. Scand J Gastroenterol 14: 177–182

Mahmood T, Robinson WA, Hamstra RD, Wallner SF (1979) Macrocytic anemia, thrombocytosis and nonlobulated magakaryocytes: the 5q- syndrome, a distinct entity. Am J Med 66:946–950

Mahoney MJ, Rosenberg LE (1970) Inherited defects of B_{12} metabolism. Am J Med 48:584–593

Majuri R, Kouvonen I, Grasbeck R (1984) Purification of the porcine duodenum haem receptor using a new affinity chromatography medium. In: Protides of the biologic fluids. Pergamon Oxford, pp 229–232

Makkanen T, Pajula RL, Virtanen S, Himanen P (1972) New carrier proteins of folic acid in serum. Acta Haematol 48:145–150

Malagolini N, Dall'Olio F, Serafini-Cessi F, Cessi C (1989) Effect of acute and chronic ethanol administration on rat liver: 2,6-sialyl-transferase activity responsible for sialylation of serum transferrin. Alcohol Clin Exp Res 13:649–653

Manis J, Schechter D (1962) Active transport of iron by intestine. Features of the 2 step mechanism. Am J Physiol 210:694–700

Marcoullis G, Rothenberg SP (1981) Intrinsic factor mediated intestinal absorption of cobalamin in the dog. Am J Physiol 241:294–299

Marcoullis G, Parmentier Y, Nicolas JP, Jimenez M, Gerard P (1980) Cobalamin malabsorption due to nondegradable R protein in human intestine. Inhibited cobalamin absorption in exocrine pancreatic dysfunction. J Clin Invest 61: 430–440

Martinez-Medelin J, Schulman HM (1972) The kinetics of iron and transferrin incorporation into rabbit erythroid cells and the nature of the stromal-bound iron. Biochem Biophys Acta 264:272–274

Martinez-Torres C, Layrisse M (1971) Iron absorption from veal muscle. Am J Clin Nutr 24:531–540

Martinez-Torres C, Renzi M, Layrisse M (1976) Iron absorption by humans of hemosiderin and ferritin. Further studies. J Nutr 106:128–135

Martinez-Torres C, Romano E, Layrisse M (1981) Effect of cysteine on iron absorption in man. Am J Clin Nutr 34:322–327

Marx JJM, Gebbnik JAGK, Nishisato T, Aisen P (1982) Molecular aspects of the binding of absorbed iron to transferrin. Br J Haematol 52:105–110

Masawe AEJ, Muindi JM, Swai GBR (1974) Infections in iron deficiency and other types of anemia in the tropics. Lancet 2:314–317

Mason DY, Taylor CR (1978) Distribution of transferrin, ferritin and lactoferrin in human tissue. J Clin Pathol 31:316–327

Mason JB, Selhub J (1988) Folate binding protein and the absorption of folic acid in the small intestine of the suckling rat. Am J Clin Nutr 48:620–625

Masson PL, Heremans JF, Dive C (1966) An iron-binding protein common to many external secretions. Clin Chim Acta 14:735–739

Matchar DB, Feussner JR, Millington DS, Wilkinson RH, Watson DJ, Gale D (1987) Isotope-dilution assay for urinary methyl-malonic acid in the diagnosis of vitamin B_{12} deficiency. Ann Int Med 106:707–710

Mathews JH, Wickramsinghe SN (1988) The deoxyuridine suppression test performed on phytohaemagglutinin-stimulated peripheral blood cells fails to reflect in vivo vitamin B_{12} or folate deficiency. Eur J Haematol 80:174–180

Mathews JH, Clark DM, Abrahamson GM (1988) Effect of therapy with vitamin B_{12} and folic acid in elderly patients with low concentrations of serum vitamin B_{12} or erythrocyte folate but normal blood counts. Acta Haematol 79:84–87

Mathews JH, Armitage J, Wickramasinghe SN (1989) Thymidylate synthesis and utilization via the de nove pathway in normal and megaloblastic human bone marrow cells. Eur J Haematol 42:396–404

Mathews RG, Ghose C, Green JM, Mathews KD, Dunlap RB (1987) Folylpolyglutamates as substrate inhibitors of folate-dependent enzymes. Adv Enzyme Regul 26:157–171

Mathorn MKS (1971) The influence of hypoxia on iron absorption in the rat. Gastroenterology 60:76–81

Matlib MA, Frenkel EP, Mukherjee A, Henslee J, Srere PA (1979) Enzymatic properties of mitochondria isolated from normal and vitamin B_{12} deficient rats. Arch Biochem Biophys 197:388–395

Matsui SM, Mahoney MJ, Rosenberg LE (1983) The natural history of the inherited methylmalonic acidemias. N Engl J Med 308:847–861

Matzner Y, Konijn AM, Hershko C (1980) Serum ferritin in hematologic malignancies. Am J Hematol 9:13–22

Mazur A, Charlton A (1965) Hepatic xanthine oxidase and ferritin iron in the developing rat. Blood 26:317–322

Mazurier J, Montreuil J, Spike G (1985) Visualization of lactoferrin brush border receptors by ligand blotting. Biochim Biophys Acta 821:453–460

McCurdy PR (1965) Oral and parenteral iron therapy: a comparison. J Am Med Assoc 919:151–161

McDonnell WM, Ryan JA, Seeger DM, Elta GH (1989) Effect of iron on the guaiac reaction. Gastroenterology 96:74–78

McGuffin R, Goff P, Hillman RS (1975) The effect of diet and alcohol on the development of folate deficiency in the rat. Br J Haematol 31:185–192

McGuire JJ, Bertino JR (1981) Enzymatic synthesis and function of folylpolyglutamates. Mol Cell Biochem 28:19–48

McGuire JJ, Hsieh P, Coward JK, Bertino JR (1980) Enzymatic synthesis of folylpolyglutamates: characteristics of the reaction and its products. J Biol Chem 255:5776–5788

McKnight GS, Lee DC, Hemmaplardh D, Finch CA, Palmiter RD (1980a) Transferrin gene expression: effects of nutritional iron deficiency. J Biol Chem 255:144–147

McKnight GS, Lee DC, Palmiter RD (1980b) Transferrin gene expression: regulation of mRNA transcription in chick liver by steroid hormones and iron deficiency. J Biol Chem 255:148–153

McLane JA, Fell RD, McKay RH, Winder WW, Brown EB, Holloszy JO (1981) Physiological and biochemical effects of iron deficiency on rat skeletal muscle. Am J Physiol 241:C47–C54

McMartin KE, Collins TD (1983) Relationship of alcohol metabolism to folate deficiency produced by ethanol in the rat. Pharmacol Biochem Behav 18 [Suppl 1]:257–262.

McMartin KE, Collins TD, Bairnsfather L (1986a) Cumulative excess urinary excretion of folate in rats after repeated ethanol treatment. J Nurt 116:1316–1325.

McMartin KE, Collins TD, Shiao CQ, Vidrine L, Redetzki HM (1986b) Study of dose dependence and urinary folate excretion produced by ethanol in humans and rats. Alcohol Clin Exp Res 10:419–424.

McPhedran P, Barnes MG, Weinstein JS, Robertson JS (1973) Interpretation of electronically determined macrocytosis. Ann Int Med 78:677–683

Medical Letter (1977) Adverse effects of parenteral iron. Med Lett Drugs Ther 19:35–36

Medical Letter (1978) Oral iron. Med Lett Drugs Ther 20:45–47

Mehta BC, Pandya BG (1987) Iron status in α-thalassemia carriers. Am J Hematol 24:137–141

Mellman IS, Youngdahl-Turner P, Willard HF, Rosenberg LE (1977) Intracellular binding of radioactive hydroxocobalamin to cobalamin-dependent apoenzymes in rat liver. Proc Natl Acad Sci USA 74:916–920

Mendel GA (1962) Studies on iron absorption I. The relationship between the rate of erythropoiesis, hypoxia and iron absorption. Blood 18:727–736

Mentzer WC (1973) Differentiation of iron deficiency from thalassemia trait. Lancet 1:882

Metz J, Kelly A, Swett VC, Waxman S, Herbert V (1968) Deranged DNA synthesis by bone marrow from vitamin B_{12} deficient humans. Br J Haematol 14:575–592

Meyer LM, Miller IF, Gizis E, Tripp E, Hoffbrand AV (1974) Delivery of vitamin B_{12} to human lymphocytes by transcobalamin I, II, and III. Proc Soc Exp Biol Med 146:747–750

Middleton EJ, Nagy E, Morrison AB (1966) Studies on the absorption or orally administered iron from sustained release preparations. N Engl J Med 274: 136–139

Millar JA, Cumming RLC, Smith JA, Goldberg A (1969) Effect of actinomycin D, cycloheximide and acute blood loss on ferritin synthesis in rat liver. Biochem J 119:643–649

Mills JL, Rhoads GG, Simpson JL, Cunningham GC, Conley MR, Lassman MR, Walden ME, Depp OR, Hoffman HJ (1989) The absence of a relation between the periconceptual use of vitamins and neural tube defects. N Engl J Med 321:430–435

Milman N (1976) Iron therapy in patients undergoing maintenance hemodialysis. Acta Med Scand 200:315–319

Milman N (1982) Iron absorption measured by whole body counting and the relation to marrow iron stores in chronic uremia. Clin Nephrol 17:77–81

Milne DB, Gallagher SK (1983) Microbiological and radioimmunological assays for folic acid in whole blood compared. Clin Chem 29:2117–2118

Minnich V, Okcuoglu A, Tarcon Y, Arcasoy A, Clin S, Yorukoglu O, Renda F, Demirag B (1968) Pica in turkey. II. Effect of clay on iron absorption. Am J Clin Nutr 21:78–86

Miyamori A, Takebe T Yamagata S (1976) Clinical evaluation of iron metabolism in pancreatic disease. Tohoku J Exp Med 118 [Suppl]:159–172

Monnier L, Colette C, Aquirre L, Mirouze J (1980) Evidence and mechanism for pectin-reduced intestinal inorganic iron absorption in idiopathic hemochromatosis. Am J Clin Nutr 33:1225–1232

Moore CV, Duback R, Minnich V, Roberts HK (1944) Absorption of ferrous and ferric radioiron by human subjects and by dogs. J Clin Invest 23:755–757

Moran RG, Colman PD (1984) Mammalian folyl polyglutamate synthetase: partial purification and properties of the mouse liver enzyme. Biochem 23:4580–4589

Morck TA, Lynch SR, Cook JD (1983) Inhibition of food iron absorption by coffee. Am J Clin Nutr 37:416–420

Morgan EH (1963) Effect of pH and iron content of transferrin on its binding to reticulocyte receptors. Biochim Biophys Acta 762:498–502

Morgan EH (1971) A study of iron transfer from rabbit transferrin to reticulocytes using synthetic chelating agents. Biochim Biophys Acta 224:103–116

Morgan EH, Appleton TC (1969) Autoradiographic localization of ^{125}I-labeled transferrin rabbit reticulocytes. Nature 223:1371–1372

Morgan EH, Baker E (1969) The effect of metabolic inhibitors on transferrin iron uptake and transferrin release from reticulocytes. Biochim Biophys Acta 184:442–454

Morse BS, Conlan M, Giulani DG, Nussbaum M (1980) Mechanism of arsenic-induced inhibition of erythropoiesis in mice. Am J Hematol 8:273–280

Morton AG, Tavill AS (1977) The role of iron in the regulation of hepatic transferrin synthesis. Br J Haematol 36:383–394

Muir M, Chanarin I (1983) Separation of cobalamin analogues in human sera binding to intrinsic factor and to R-type binders. Br J Haematol 54:613–621

Muir M, Landon M (1985) Endogenous origin of microbiologically-inactive cobalamins (cobalamin analogues) in the human fetus. Br J haematol 61: 303–306

Multani JS, Cepurneek CP, Davis PS, Saltman P (1970) Biochemical characterization of gastroferrin. Biochem 9:3970–3976

Munro HN, Drysdale JW (1970) Role of iron in the regulation of ferritin metabolism. Fed Proc 29:1469–1473

Munro HN, Linder MC (1978) Ferritin: structure, biosynthesis and role in iron metabolism. Physiol Rev 58:317–396

Murray MJ, Murray AB (1978) The adverse effect of iron repletion on the course of certain infections. Br Med J 2:1113–1115

Murray MJ, Stein N (1966) Does the pancreas influence iron absorption? A critical review of information to date. Gastroenterology 51:694–700

Murray MJ, Stein N (1968) A gastric factor promoting iron absorption. Lancet 2:614–616

Murray MJ, Stein N (1972) The effect of injected iron on the absorption of iron in iron deficiency. Br J Haematol 23:13–16

Muta K, Nishimura J, Ideguchi H, Umemura T, Ibayshi H (1987) Erythroblast transferrin receptors and transferrin kinetics in iron deficiency and various anemias. Am J Hematol 25:155–163

Nath BJ, Lindenbaum J (1979) Persistence of neutrophil hypersegmentation during recovery from megaloblastic granulopoiesis. Ann Int Med 90:757–760

Nathanson MH, Muir A, McLaren G (1985) Iron absorption in normal and iron-deficient beagle dogs: mucosal iron kinetics. Am J Physiol 249:G439–G448

Naughton CA, Chandler CJ, Duplantier RB, Halsted CH (1989) Folate absorption in alcoholic pigs: in vitro hydrolysis and transport at the intestinal brush border membrane. Am J Clin Nutr 50:1436–1441

Necheles TR, Snyder LM (1970) Malabsorption of folate polyglutamates associated with oral contraceptive therapy. N Engl J Med 282:858–859

Neuvonen PJ, Gothoni G, Hackman R, Bjorksten K (1970) Interference of iron with the absorption of tetracycline in man. Br Med J 4:532–534

Nexo E, Olesen H, Norredam K, Schwartz S (1975) A rare case of megaloblastic anemia caused by disturbances in plasma cobalamin binding proteins in a patient with hepatocellular carcinoma. Scand J Haematol 14:320–327

Niederer W (1970) Ferritin iron incorporation and iron release. Experientia 26: 218–220

Nilsson-Ehle H, Jagenburg R, Landahl S, Lindstedt G, Swolin B, Westin J (1986) Cyanocobalamin absorption in the elderly. Clin Chem 32:1368–1371

Nilsson-Ehle H, Landahl S, Lindstedt G, Netterblad L, Stockbruegger R, Westin J, Ahren C (1989) Low serum cobalamin levels in a population study of 70- and 75-year-old subjects. Dig Dis Sci 34:716–723

Nishisato T, Aisen P (1982) Uptake of transferrin by rat peritoneal macrophage. Br J Haematol 52:631–640

Nixon PF, Bertino JR (1972) Effective absorption and utilization of oral formyltetrahydrofolate in man. N Engl J Med 286:175–179

Nixon PF, Slutsky G, Nahas A, Bertino JR (1973) The turnover of folate coenzymes in murine lymphoma cells. J Biol Chem 248:5932–5942

Norrby A, Arvidsson B, Solvell L (1974) Total absorption of iron and hemoglobin regeneration during 4 weeks of oral iron therapy: a comparative study of 4 different iron doses. Scand J Haematol [Suppl]20:33–53

Nunez MT, Glass J (1985) Iron uptake by reticulocytes: inhibition mediated by monensin and nigersin. J Biol Chem 260:14707–14711

Nuwayri-Salti N, Jabre F, Sa'ab G, Daouk M, Salem Z (1990) Monocyte ferritin as a possible index of bone marrow iron stores in patients on chronic hemodialysis. Nephron 54:7–11

Nyberg W (1960) The influence of *Diphyllobothrium latum* on the vitamin B_{12} intrinsic factor complex: II. In vitro studies. Acta Med Scand 167:189–192

Octave JN, Schneider YJ, Hoffmann P, Trouet A, Crichton RR (1982) Transferrin protein and iron uptake by cultured rat fibroblasts. Eur J Biochem 123:235–240

Ohira Y, Edgerton VR, Gardner GW, Senewiratne B, Barnard RJ, Simpson DR (1979) Work capacity, heart rate and blood lactate response to iron treatment. Br J Haematol 41:365–372

Ohira Y, Hagenauer J, Strause L, Chen C-S, Saltman P, Beinert H (1982) Mitochondrial NADH dehydrogenase in iron-deficient and iron-repleted rat muscle. Br J haematol 52:623–630

Okada A, Jarvis B, Brown EB (1979) In vivo evidence for the functional heterogeneity of transferrin bound iron. Isotransferrins: an explanation of the Fletcher-Huehns phenomenon in the rat. J Lab Clin Med 93:189–198

Okon E, Levij IS, Rachmilewitz EA (1976) Splenectomy, iron overload and liver cirrhosis in B-thalassemia major. Acta Haematol 56:142–150

Olinger EJ, Bertino JR, Binder HJ (1973) Intestinal folate absorption: II. Conversion and retention of pteroylmonoglutamate by jejunem. J Clin Invest 52:2138–2145

Olsson KS, Heedman PA, Staugard F (1987) Preclinical hemochromatosis in a population on a high iron-fortified diet. J Am Med Assoc 239:1999–2000

Olsson SK, Weinfeld A (1972) Availability of iron dextran for hemoglobin synthesis. Acta Med Scand 192:543–549

Olsson SK, Lundvall O, Weinfeld A (1972) Availability of iron stores built up by iron dextrin as studied with desferrioxamine and phlebotomy. Acta Med Scand 192:49–56

O'Neil-Cutting SM, Crosby WH (1986) The effects of antacids on the absorption of simultaneously ingested iron. J Am Med 255:1468–1470

O'Neil-Cutting SM, Crosby WH (1987) Blocking of iron absorption by a preliminary oral dose of iron. Arch Int Med 147:489–491

Osaki S, Johnson DA, Frieden E (1966) The possible significance of the ferrous oxidase activity of ceruloplasmin in normal human serum. J Biol Chem 241: 2746–2751

Osifo BOA, Ayoola A, Parmentier Y, Gerard P, Nicolas JP (1988) Correlation between serum enxymes and serum unsaturated vitamin B_{12} binding proteins in primary liver carcinoma. Enzyme 39:161–166

Osterloh K, Forth W (1981) Determination of transferrin-like immunoreactivity in the mucosal homogenate of the duodenum, jejunum and ileum of normal and iron deficient rats. Blut 43:227–235

Osterloh K, Schumann K, Ehtechami C, Forth W (1985a) Transferrin in isolated cells from rat duodenum and jejunum. Blut 51:41–47

Osterloh K, Simpson RY, Raja K, Snape S, Peters TJ (1985b) Iron absorption and plasma and mucosal transferrin in hypoxic rats. Biochem Soc Trans 13:763–764

Osterloh K, Schumann K, Ehtechami C, Forth W, Snape S, Simpson RJ, Peters TJ (1986) Location and origin of mucosal transferrin in rat small intestine. Biochem Soc Trans 14:118

Osterloh KRS, Simpson RJ, Peters TJ (1987a) The role of mucosal transferrin in intestinal iron absorption. Br J Haematol 65:1–3

Osterloh KRS, Simpson RJ, Snape S, Peters TJ (1987b) Intestinal iron absorption and mucosal transferrin in rats subjected to hypoxia. Blut 55:421–431

Palva IP, Kaipainen WJ (1970) Mortality in megaloblastic anemia. Lancet 2: 1173–1174

Palva IP, Salokannel SJ, Timonen T, Pawa HLA (1972) Drug-induced malabsorption of vitamin B_{12}: IV. Malabsorption and deficiency of B_{12} during treatment with slow-release potassium chloride. Acta Med Scand 191:355–357

Parker PA, Izard MW, Maher JF (1979) Therapy of iron deficiency anemia in patients on maintenance dialysis. Nephron 23:181–186

Parkin JD, Rush B, DeGroot RJ, Budd RS (1974) Iron absorption after splenectomy in hereditary spherocytosis. Aust NZ J Med 4:58–61

Parmley RT, Barton JC, Conrad ME (1985) Ultrastructural localization of transferrin, transferrin receptor and iron-binding sites on human placental and duodenal microvilli. Br J haematol 60:81–89

Pearson WH, Reich MB (1969) Studies of ferritin and a new iron-binding protein found in the intestinal mucosa of the rat. J Nutr 99:137–149

Pedersen J, Lund J, Ohlsen AS, Kristensen HPO (1957) Partial megaloblastic erythropoiesis in elderly achlorhydric patients with mild anemia. Lancet 1: 448–453

Peifer JJ, Lewis RD (1981) Odd-numbered fatty acids in phosphatidylcholine versus phosphatidyl ethanolamine in vitamin B_{12}-deprived rats. Proc Soc Exp Biol Med 167:212–217

Pelliniemi TT, Beck WS (1980) Biochemical mechanisms in the Killman experiment: critique to the "deoxyuridine suppression test." J Clin Invest 71:1183–1190

Perillie PE, Kaplan SS, Finch SC (1967) Significance of changes in serum muramidase activity in megaloblastic anemia. N Engl J Med 277:10–12

Perry J, Chanarin I (1973) Formylation of folate as a step in physiological folate absorption. Br Med J 1:558–559

Perry J, Chanarin I (1977) Abnormal folate polyglutamate ratios in untreated pernicious anemia corrected by therapy. Br J Haematol 35:397–402

Perry J, Hoffbrand AV (1970) Absorption of vitamin B_{12} by the guinea pig: I. Subcellular localization of vitamin B_{12} in the ileal enterocyte during absorption. Br J Haematol 19:369–376

Perry J, Chanarin I, Deacon R, Lumb M (1983) Chronic cobalamin inactivation impairs folate polyglutamate synthesis in the rat. J Clin Invest 71:1183–1189

Peschle C, Jori GP, Marone G, Condorelli M (1974) Independence of iron absorption from rate of erythropoiesis. Blood 44:353–358

Peters TJ, Raja RJ, Simpson RJ, Snape S (1988) Mechanisms and regulation of intestinal iron absorption. Ann NY Acad Sci 526:141–147

Pezzimenti JF, Lindenbaum J (1972) Megaloblastic anemia associated with erythroid hypoplasia. Am J Med 53:748–754

Pincus JH, Reynolds EH, Glaser GH (1972) Subacute combined system degeneration with folate deficiency. J Am Med Assoc 221:496–497

Piperno A, Taddei MT, Sampietro M, Fargion S, Arosio P, Fiorelli G (1984) Erythrocyte ferritin in thalassemia syndromes. Acta Haematol 71:251–256

Pippard MJ, Warner GT, Callender ST, Weatherall DJ (1977) Iron absorption in iron-loading anemia: effect of subcutaneous desferrioxamine infusions. Lancet 2:737–739

Pippard MJ, Warner GT, Callender ST, Weatherall DJ (1979) Iron absorption and loading in B-thalassemia intermedia. Lancet 2:819–821

Pirofsky B, Vaughn M (1968) Addisonian pernicious anemia with positive antiglobulin tests. Am J Clin Pathol 50:459–466

Pirzio-Biroli G, Bothwell TH, Finch CA (1958) Iron absorption. II. The absorption of radioiron administered with a standard meal in man. J Lab Clin Med 51: 37–48

Pollack S, Lasky FD (1976) Guinea pig intestinal iron binding protein. Biochem Biophys Res Commun 70:533–539

Pollack S, Compana T, Acario A (1972) A search for mucosal iron carrier. Identification of mucosal fractions with rapid tunover of Fe59. J Lab Clin Med 80:322–332

Ponka P, Neuwirt J (1971) Regulation of iron entry into reticulocytes. II. Relationship between hemoglobin synthesis and entry of iron into reticulocytes. Biochem Biophys Acta 230:381–392

Ponka P, Schulman HM (1985) Acquisition of iron from transferrin regulates reticulocyte heme synthesis. J Biol Chem 260:14717–14721

Ponka P, Schulman HM, Martinez-Medellin J (1988) Haem inhibits iron uptake subsequent to endocytosis of transferrin in reticulocytes. J Biochem 251: 105–109

Pootrakul P, Rugkiatsakul R, Waki P (1980) Increased transferrin iron saturation in splenectomized thalassemic patients. Br J Haematol 46:143–145

Pootrakul P, Vongsmasa V, La-ongpanich P, Wasi P (1981) Serum ferritin levels in thalassemias and the effect of splenectomy. Acta Haematol 66:244–250

Powell LW (1966) Effects of allopurinol on iron storage in the rat. Ann Rheum Dis 25:697–699

Powers JS, Collins JC, Folk MC, Greene HL (1989) Vitamin B_{12} levels in free-living elderly. Clin Res 37:8A

Pratt RF, Cooper BA (1971) Folates in plasma and bile of man after feeding folic acid-3H and 5-formyltelahydrofolate (folic acid). J Clin Invest 50:455–462

Price EM, Gibson JF (1972) Electron paramagnetic resonance evidence for a distinction between the two iron-binding sites in transferrin. J Biol Chem 247:8031–8035

Primosigh JV, Thomas ED (1968) Studies on the partition of iron in bone marrow cells. J Clin Invest 47:1473–1482

Quadros EV, Matthews DM, Hoffbrand AV, Linnell JC (1976) Synthesis of cobalamin coenzymes by human lymphocytes in vitro and the effects of folates and metabolic inhibitors. Blood 48:609–617

Quadros EV, Rothenberg SP, Polu S (1988) A specific radioimmunoassay for 5′-deoxyadenosyl cobalamin in serum. Br J Haematol 69:551–557

Rabb LM, Grandison Y, Mason K, Hayes RJ, Serjent B, Serjent JR (1983) A trial of folate supplementation in children with homozygous sickle cell disease. Br J Haematol 54:589–594

Rachmilewitz D, Ligumsky M, Rachmilewitz B, Rachmilewitz M, Tarcic N, Schlesinger M (1980) Transcobalamin II level in peripheral blood monocytes – a biochemical marker in inflammatory diseases of the bowel. Gastroenterology 78:43–46

Rachmilewitz M, Aronovitch J, Grossowicz N (1956) Serum concentrations of vitamin B_{12} in acute and chronic liver disease. J Lab Clin Med 48:339–344

Raffin SB, Woo CH, Roost RK, Price DC, Schmid R (1974) Intestinal absorption of hemoglobin: iron-hemoglobin cleavage by mucosal heme oxygenase. J Clin Invest 54:1344–1352

Ragan HA, Nacht S, Lee GR, Bishop CR, Cartwright GE (1969) Effect of ceruloplasmin on plasma iron in copper deficient swine. Am J Physiol 217: 1320–1323

Raja KB, Pippard MJ, Simpson RT, Peters TJ (1986) Relationship between erythropoiesis and the enhanced intestinal uptake of ferric iron in hypoxia in the mouse. Br J Haematol 64:587–593

Raja KB, Simpson RJ, Pippard MT, Peters TJ (1988) In vivo studies on the relationship between iron (Fe^{3+}) absorption, hypoxia and erythropoiesis in the mouse. Br J Haematol 68:373–378

Raja KB, Simpson RJ, Peters TJ (1989) Effect of exchange transfusion of reticulocytes on in vitro and in vivo intestinal iron (Fe^{3+}) absorption in mice. Br J Haematol 73:254–259

Rao K, van Renswoude J, Kempf C et al. (1983) Separation of Fe^{+3} from transferrin in endocytosis: role of the acidic endosome. FEBS Lett 160:213–215

Reinhold JG, Ismail-Beigi F, Faraji B (1975) Fiber vs phytate as determinants of the availability of calcium, zinc and iron in food stuffs. Nutr Rep Inter 12:75–85

Reinhold JG, Carcia JS, Garzon P (1981) Binding of iron by fiber of wheat and maize. Am J Clin Nutr 34:1384–1391

Reisenauer AM, Krumdieck CL, Halsted CL (1977) Folate conjugase: two separate activities in human jejunum. Science 198:196–197

Reisenauer AM, Chandler CJ, Halsted CH (1986) Folate binding and hydrolysis by pig intestinal brush-border membranes. Am J Physiol 251:G481–G486

Reisenauer AM, Buffington CAT, Villanueva JA, Halsted CH (1989) Folate absorption in alcoholic pigs: in vivo intestinal perfusion studies. Am J Clin Nutr 50:1429–1435

Reynolds EH (1976) Neurological aspects of folate and vitamin B_{12} metabolism. Clin Haematol 5:661–695

Richmond VS, Worwood M, Jacobs A (1972) The iron content of intestinal epithelial cells and its subcellular distribution: studies on normal, iron overloaded iron deficient rats. Br J Haematol 23:605–614

Roberts PD, St John DJB, Sinha R, Steward JS, Baird IM, Coghill NF, Morgan JO (1971) Apparent folate deficiency in iron deficiency anaemia. Br J Haematol 20:165–176

Roberts S, Bomford A (1988) Ferrtin iron kinetics and protein turnover in K562 cells. J Biol Chem 263:19181–19187

Roberston JS, Hsia YE, Sailly KS (1976) Defective leukocyte metabolism in human cobalamin deficiency. J Lab Clin Med 87:89–97

Roeser HP, Lee GR, Hacht S, Cartwright GE (1970) The role of ceruloplasmin in iron metabolism. J Clin Invest 53:1527–1533

Rogers TB, Feeney RE, Meares CF (1977) Interaction of anions with iron-transferrin chelate complexes. J Biol Chem 252:8108–8112

Romero JJ, Tamura T, Halsted CH (1981) Intestinal absorption of [^{3}H] folic acid in the chronic alcoholic monkey. Gastroenterology 80:99–102

Romslo I, Flatmark T (1973) Energy-dependent accumulation of iron by isolated rat liver mitochondria. I. General features. Biochim Biochim Biophys Acta 305: 29–40

Rosenberg IH (1976) Absorption and malabsorption of folate. Clin Haematol 5:589–618

Rosenberg LE, Patel L, Lilljequist AC (1975) Absence of an intracellular cobalamin binding protein in cultured fibroblasts from patients with defective synthesis of 5-deoxyadenosylcobalamin and methylcoabalamin. Proc Natl Acad Sci USA 72:4617–4621,

Rosenberg LE (1983) Disorders of propionate and methylmalonate metabolism. In: Stanbury JB, Wygaardeu JB, Fredrickson DS, Goldstein JL, Brown M (eds)

The metabolic basis of inherited disease, 5th edn. McGraw Hill, New York, pp 474–498

Rosenmund A, Geber S, Huebers H, Finch C (1980) Regulation of iron absorption and storage iron turnover. Blood 56:30–37

Rubinoff M, Abrahamson R, Schreiber C, Waxman S (1981) Effect of a folate binding protein on plasma transport and tissue distribution of folic acid. Acta Haematol 65:145–152

Rundles RW, Brewer SS (1958) Hematologic responses in pernicious anemia to orotic acid. Blood 13:99–115

Russell RM, Dhar GJ, Dutta SK, Rosenberg IH (1979) Influence of intraluminal pH on folate absorption: studies in control subjects and in patients with pancreatic insufficiency. J Lab Clin Med 93:428–436

Russell RM, Dutta SK, Oaks EV, Rosenberg IH, Giovetti AC (1980) Impairment of folic acid absorption by oral pancreatic extracts. Dig Dis Sci 25:369–373

Russell RM, Rosenberg IH, Wilson PD, Iber FL, Oaks EB, Giovetti AC, Otradovec CL, Karwoski PA, Press AW (1983) Increased urinary excretion and prolonged turnover time of folic acid during ethanol ingestion. Am J Clin Nutr 38:64–70

Russell RM, Golner BB, Krasinski SO (1985) Impairment of folic acid absorption by post prandial antacid in elderly subjects. Gastroenterology 78:1563

Russel RM, Krasinski SD, Samloff IM, Jacob RA, Hartz SC, Brovender SR (1986) Folic acid malabsorption in atrophic gastritis. Gastroenterology 91:476–482

Russell RM, Golner BR, Krasinski SD, Sadowski JA, Suter PM, Braun CL (1988) Effect of antacid and H2 receptor antagonist on the intestinal absorption of folic acid. J Lab Clin Med 112:458–463

Saarinen UM, Siimes MA, Dallman PR (1977) Iron absorption in infants: high availability of breast milk iron as indicated by the extrinsic tag method of iron absorption and by the concentration of serum ferritin. J Pediatr 91:36–39

Said HM, Redha R (1987) A carrier-mediated transport for folate in basolateral membrane vesicles of rat small intestine. Biochem J 247:141–146

Said HM, Strum WB (1983a) A pH-dependent carrier-mediated system for transport of 5-methyltetrahydrofolate in rat jejunum. J Pharm Exp Ther 226:95–99

Said HM, Strum WB (1983b) Cyclic adenosine-3′5′-monophosphate and folate transport in jejunum. Biochem Biophys Res Commun 115:756–761

Said HM, Strum WB (1986) Effect of ethanol and other aliphatic alcohols on the intestinal transport of folates. Digestion 35:129–135

Said HM, Hollander D, Katz D (1984a) Absorption of 5-methyltetrahydrofolate in rat jejunum with intact blood and lymphatic vessels. Biochim Biophys Acta 775:402–408

Said HM, Vaziri ND, Kariger RK, Hollander D (1984b) Intestinal absorption of 5-methyltetrahydrofolate in experimental uremia. Acta Vitaminol Enzymol 6: 339–346

Said HM, Hollander D, Strum WB (1984c) Inhibitory effect of unconjugated bile acids on the intestinal transport of 5-methyltetrahydrofolate in rat jejunum in vitro. Gut 25:1376–1379

Said HM, Ghishan FK, Redha R (1987) Folate transport by human intestinal brush-border membrane vesicles. Am J Physiol 252:G229–G236

Said HM, Redha R, Tipton W, Nylander W (1988) Folate transport in ileal brush border membrane vesicles following extensive resection of proximal and middle small intestine in the rat. Am J Clin Nutr 47:75–79

Saito K, Nishisato T, Grasso JA, Aisen P (1986) Interaction of transferrin with iron-loaded rat peritoneal macrophages. Br J Haematol 62:275–286

Sakamoto S, Niina M, Takuku F (1975) Thymidylate synthetase activity in bone marrow cells in pernicious anemia. Blood 46:699–704

Saleem A, Irani DR, Bart JB, Alfrey CP (1987) Suppression of hemoglobin H In disorders of iron metabolism. Acta Haematol 77:34–37

Sandberg DP, Begley JA, Hall CA (1981) The content, binding and forms of vitamin B_{12} in milk. Am J Clin Nutr 34:1717–1724

Sauer H, Wilmanns W (1977) Cobalamin dependent methionine synthesis and methylfolate trap in human vitamin B_{12} deficiency. Br J Haematol 36: 189–198

Savage D, Lindenbaum J (1983) Relapses after interruption of cyanocobalamin therapy in patients with pernicious anemia. Am J Med 74:765–772

Savin MA, Cook JD (1978) Iron transport by isolated rat intestinal mucosal cells. Gastroenterology 75:688–694

Savin MA, Cook JD (1980) Mucosal iron transport by rat intestine. Blood 56: 1029–1036

Schade SC, Feick P, Muckerheide M, Schilling RF (1966) Occurrence in gastric juice of antibody to a complex of intrinsic-factor and vitamin B_{12}. N Engl J Med 275:528–531

Schade SG (1972) Normal incorporation of oral into intestinal ferritin in inflammation. Proc Soc Exp Biol Med 119:620–622

Schade SG, Cohen RJ, Conrad ME (1968) Effect of hydrochloric acid on iron absorption. N Engl J Med 279:672–674

Schade SG, Bernier GM, Conrad ME (1969) Normal iron absorption in hypertransferrinaemic rats. Br J Haematol 17:187–190

Scher H, Silber R (1976) Iron responsive thrombocytopenia. Ann Intern Med 84:571–572

Schilling RF, Gohdes PN, Hardie GH (1974) Vitamin B_{12} deficiency after gastric bypass surgery. Ann Int Med 101:501–502

Schilling RF, Fairbanks VF, Miller R, Schmitt K, Smith MJ (1983) Improved vitamin B_{12} assays: a report on two commercial kits. Clin Chem 29:582–586

Scott CS, Bynor AG, Roberts BE (1982) Asynchronous expression of granulocyte membrane receptors in egaloblastic anaemia. Br J Haematol 52:439–443

Scott JM, Weir DG (1980) Drug-induced megaloblastic changes. Clin Haematol 9:587–606

Scott JM, Weir DG (1981) The methylfolate trap. Lancet 2:337–340

Scott JM, Dinn JJ, Wilson P, Weir DG (1981) Pathogenesis of subacute combined degeneration: a result of methyl group deficiency. Lancet 2:334–337

Scott RB, Kramer RB, Burger WF, Middleton FG (1968) Reduced absorption of vitamin B_{12} in 2 patients with folic acid deficiency. Ann Int Med 69:111–114

Seetharan B, Alpers DH (1982) Absorption and transport of cobalamin (vitamin B_{12}). Ann Rev Nutr 3:343–369

Seetharan B, Jimenez M, Alpers DH (1983) Effect of bile and bile acids on binding of intrinsic factor to cobalamin and intrinsic factor-cobalamin complex to ideal receptor. Am J Physiol 245:G72–G77

Selhub J, Rosenberg IH (1981) Folate transport in isolated brush border membrane vesicles from rat intestine. J Biol Chem 256:4489-4493

Selhub JH, Brin H, Grossowicz N (1973) Uptake and reduction of radioactive folate by everted sacs of rat small intestine. Eur J Biochem 33:433–438

Selhub J, Powell GR, Rosenberg IH (1984) Transport of 5-methyltetrahydrofolate. Am J Physiol 246:G515–G520

Selhub J, Emmanouel D, Stavropoulos T, Arnold R (1987a) Renal folate absorption and the kidney folate binding protein. I. Urinary clearance studies. Am J Physiol 252:F750–756

Selhub J, Nakamura S, Carone FA (1987b) Renal folate absorption and kidney folate binding protein. I. Microinfusion studies. Am J Physiol 252:F757–F760

Seligman PA, Steiner DL, Allen RH (1980) Studies of a patient with megaloblastic anemia and an abnormal transcobalamin II. N Engl J Med 303:1209–1212

Senewiratne B, Hettiarachchii J, Senewiratne K (1974) Vitamin B_{12} absorption in megaloblastic anemia. Br J Nutr 32:491–501

Shahid MJ, Abu Haydar N (1967) Absorption of inorganic iron in thalassemia. Br J Haematol 13:713–718

Shane B, Stokstad ELR (1985) Vitamin B_{12}-folate interrelationships. Ann Rev Nutr 5:115–141

Shane B, Watson JE, Stokstad ELR (1977) Uptake and metabolism of [^{3}H] folate by normal and by vitamin B_{12} and methionine deficient rats. Biochim Biophys Acta 497:241–257

Shaw S, Jayatilleke E, Meyers S, Colman N, Herzlich B, Herbert V (1989a) The ileum is the major site of absorption of vitamin B_{12} analogues. Am J Gastroenterol 84:22–26

Shaw S, Jayatilleke E, Herbert V, Colman N (1989b) Cleavage of folates during ethanol metabolism. Biochem J 257:277–280

Sheehan R (1976) Unidirectional uptake of iron across the intestinal brush border. Am J Physiol 231:1438–1444

Sheehan RG, Frenkel EP (1972) The control of iron absorption by the gastrointestinal mucosal cell. J Clin Invest 51:224–231

Shih VE, Coulombe JT, Maties M, Levy HL (1976) Methylmalonic aciduria in the newborn. N Engl J Med 295:1320

Shin YS, Buehring KU, Stokstad ELR (1975) The relationships between vitamin B_{12} and folic acid and the effect of methionine on folate metabolism. Mol Cell Biochem 9:97–108

Shojania AM (1982) Oral contraceptives: effects on folate and vitamin B_{12} metabolism. Can Med Assoc J 126:244–247

Shojania AM, Hornady GL (1973) Oral contraceptives and folate absorption. J Lab Clin Med 82:869–875

Shumak KH, Rachkewich RA (1984) Transferrin receptors on human reticulocytes: variation in site number in hematologic disorders. Am J Haematol 16:23–32

Sibelle J-C, Kondo H, Aisen P (1988) Interactions between isolated hepatocytes and Kupffer cells in iron metabolism: a possible role for ferritin as an iron carrier protein. Hepatology 8:296–301

Sigal SH, Hall CA, Antel P (1987) Plasma R binder deficiency and neurologic disease. N Engl J Med 317:1330–1332

Silber R, Moldow CF (1970) The biochemistry of B_{12} mediated reactions in man. Am J Med 48:549–554

Simmer K, Iles CA, James C, Thompson RPH (1987) Are iron-folate supplements harmful? Am J Clin Nutr 45:122–125

Simon M (1985) Secondary iron overload and hemochromatosis. Br J Haematol 60:1–5

Simon M, Beaumont C, Briere J, Brissot P, Deugnier Y, Edan G, Fauchet R, Garo G, Chandour C, Grolleau J, Grosbois Krempf M, Leblay R, Le Mignon L, Le Prise PY (1985) Is the HLA-linked hemochromatosis allele implicated in idiopathic refractory sideroblastic anaemia? Br J Haematol 60:75–80

Simpson KM, Morris ER, Cook JD (1978) The inhibitory effect of bran on iron absorption. Am J Clin Nutr 34:1469–1478

Simpson RJ, Osterloh KRS, Raja KB, Snape S, Peters TJ (1986) Studies on the role of transferrin and endocytosis in the uptake of Fe^{3+} from iron-nitrilotracetate by mouse duodenum. Biochim Biophys Acta 884:166–171

Sinow RM, Johnson CS, Karnaze DS, Siegel ME, Carmel R (1987) Unsuspected pernicious anemia in a patient with sickle cell disease receiving routine folate supplementation. Arch Int Med 147:1818–1829

Sirivech S, Fieden E, Osaki S (1974) The release of iron from horse spleen ferritin by reducing flavins. Biochem J 143:311–315

Sitornak FM, Goutas LJ, Jacobsen DM, Mines LS, Barrueco JR, Gaumont Y, Kisliuk RL (1987) Carrier-mediated transport of folate compounds in L1210 cells. Biochem Pharmacol 36:1659–1667

Skacel PO, Chanarin I (1983) Impaired chemiluminescence and bactericidal killing by neutrophils from patients with severe cobalamin deficiency. Br J Haematol 55:302–315

Skacel PO, Hewlett AM, Lewis JD, Lumb M, Nunn JF, Chanarin I (1983) Studies on the hematopoietic toxicity of nitrous oxide in man. Br J Haematol 53: 189–200

Skikne BS, Lynch SR, Cook JD (1981) Role of gastric acid in food iron absorption. Gastroenterology 81:1068–1071

Skouby AP (1966) Retention and distribution B_{12} activity, and requirement for B_{12} following parenteral administration of hydroxocobalamin (Vibeden). Acta Med Scand 180:95–101

Slalom IL, Silvis SE, Doscherholmen A (1982) Effect of cimetidine on the absorption of B_{12}. Scand J Gastroenterol 17:129–131

Slatevsky CA, Clydesdale FM (1988) Solubility of inorganic iron as affected by proteolytic digestion. Am J Clin Nutr 47:487–495

Slingerland DW, Cardarelli JA, Burrowe BA, Miller A (1984) The utility of serum gastrin levels in assessing the significance of low serum B_{12} levels. Arch Intern Med 144:1167–1168

Smith A, Morgan WT (1981) Hemopexin-mediated transport of heme into isolated rat hepatocytes. J Biol Chem 256:10902–10909

Smith DB, Cark GF (1982) Interaction between folates and carbamazepine and valproate in the rat. Neurology 32:965–969

Smith DM (1960) Megaloblastic madness. Br Med J 2:1840–1845

Smith JA, Drysdale JW, Goldberg W, Munro HN (1968) The effects of enteral and parenteral iron on ferritin synthesis in the intestinal mucosa of the rat. Br J Haematol 14:79–86

Smith MD, Pannacciulli (1958) Absorption of inorganic iron from graded doses: its significance in relation to iron absorption tests and the mucosal block theory. Br J Haematol 4:428–434

Smith PM, Studley F, Williams R (1969) Postulated gastric factor enhancing iron absorption in haemochromatosis. Br J Haematol 16:443–449

Smith RM, Osborne-White WS, Gawthorne JM (1974) Folic acid metabolism in vitamin B_{12} deficient sheep. Effects of injected methionine on liver constituents associated with folate metabolism. Biochem J 142:105–117

Soliman HA, Olesen H (1976) Folic acid binding by human plasma albumin. Scand J Clin Lab Invest 36:299–304

Solomon LR, Hillman RS, Finch CA (1981) Serum ferritin in refractory anemias. Acta Haematol 66:1–5

Sourial NA, Brown L (1983) Regulation of cobalamin and folate metabolism by methionine in human bone marrow cultures. Scand J Haematol 31:413–423

Sparling R, Abela M (1985) Case report: hypersensitivity to folic acid therapy. Clin Lab Haematol 7:184–185

Spector R, Lorenzo AV (1975) Folate transport by the choroid plexus in vitro. Science 187:540–542

Speyer BE, Fielding J (1979) Ferritin as a cytosol iron transport intermediate in human reticulocytes. Br J Haematol 42:255–267

Spivak J (1982) Masked megaloblastic anemia. Arch Int Med 142:2111–2114

Spurling CL, Sacks MS, Jiji RM (1964) Juvenile pernicious anemia. N Engl J Med 271:995–1003

Stabler SP, Marcell PD, Podell ER, Allen RH, Savage DG, Lindenbaum J (1988) Elevation of total homocysteine in the serum of patients with cobalamin or folate deficiency detected by capillary gas chromatography-mass spectrometry. J Clin Invest 81:466–474

Stebbins R, Bertino J (1976) Megaloblastic anaemia produced by drugs. Clin Haemtol 5:619–629.

Steinberg S, Campbell C, Hillman RS (1978) The physiological behavior of pteroylglutamic acid (Pte Glu). Clin Res 26:586A

Steinberg SE, Campbell CL, Hillman RS (1979a) Kinetics of the normal enterohepatic cycle. J Clin Invest 64:83–88

Steinberg S, Campbell C, Hillman RS (1979b) The effect of trimethoprim sulfamethoxazole on hematopoietic cells. Clin Res 27:80A

Steinberg SE, Campbell CL, Hillman RS (1981) The effect of alcohol on hepatic secretion of methylfolate (CH_3H_4PteGlu) into bile. Biochem Pharmacol 30: 96–98

Steinberg SE, Campbell CL, Hillman RS (1982) The role of the enterohepatic cycle in folate supply to tumour in rats. Br J Haematol 50:309–316

Steinberg WM, King CE, Toskes PP (1980) Malabsorption of protein-bound cobalamin but not unbound cobalamin during cimetidine administration. Dig Dis Sci 25:188–191

Stephens MEM, Craft I, Peters TJ, Hoffbrand AV (1972) Oral contraceptives and folate metabolism. Clin Sci 42:405–414

Stevens AR, Pirzio-Biroli G, Harkins HN, Nyrus LM, Finch CA (1958) Iron metabolism after partial gastrectomy. Ann Surg 149:534–538

Stevens RG, Jones DY, Micozzi MS, Taylor PR (1988) Body iron store and the risk of cancer. N Engl J Med 319:1047–1052

Stewart WK, Fleming LW, Shepard AMM (1976) Hemoglobin and serum iron responses to periodic intravenous iron dextran infusions during maintenance hemodialysis. Nephron 17:121–130

Stock C (1985) Trimethoprim-sulfamethoxazole and folinic acid. Ann Int Med 102:277

Stokstad ELR, Webb RE, Shah E (1966) Effect of vitamin B_{12} and folic acid on the metabolism of formiminoglutamate, formate and propionate in the rat. J Nutr 88:225–232

Strachan RW, Henderson JG (1965) Psychiatric syndromes due to avitaminosis B_{12} with normal blood and marrow. Q J Med 34:303–317

Strauchen JA (1976) An augmented Schilling test for pernicious anemia. Lancet 2:545–547

Streiff RR, Greene B (1970) Drug inhibition of folate conjugase. Clin Res 18:418

Strum WB (1981) Characteristics of the transport of pteroylglutamate and amethopterin in rat jejunum. J Pharm Exp Ther 216:329–333

Strum W, Nixon PF, Bertino JB, Binder HJ (1971) Intestinal folate absorption. I. 5-methyltetrahydrofolic acid. J Clin Invest 50:1910–1916

Subhar AF, Block G, James LD (1989) Folate intake and food sources in the US population. Am J Clin Nutr 50:508–516

Sullivan LW, Herbert V (1965) Studies on the minimum daily requirement for vitamin B_{12}. N Engl J Med 272:340–346

Summers M, White G, Jacobs A (1975) Ferritin synthesis in lymphocytes, polymorphs and monocytes. Br J Haematol 30:425–434

Svendsen JH, Dahl C, Svendsen LB, Christiansen PM (1986) Gastric cancer risk in achlorhydric patients. Scand J Gastroenterol 21:16–20

Swan CH, Glass GB (1973) Iron binding by macromolecular components of human gastric juice. J Lab Clin Med 81:719–732

Sweiry JH, Yudilevich DK (1988) Characterization of folate uptake in guinea pig receptor. Am J Physiol 254:C735–C743

Taguchi H, Laundy M, Reid C, Reynolds EH, Chanaun I (1977) The effect of anticonvulsant drugs on thymidine and deoxyribosenucleic acid synthesis by human marrow cells. Br J Haematol 36:181–187

Taheri MR, Wickremasinghe RG, Jackson BF, Hoffbrand AV (1982) Effect of folate analogues and vitamin B_{12} on provision of thymine nucleotides for DNA synthesis in megaloblastic anemia. Blood 59:634–640

Takami M, Mizumoto K, Kasuya I (1986) Human placental ferritin receptor. Biochim Biophys Acta 884:31–38

Tamura T, Halsted CH (1983) Folate turnover in chronically alcoholic monkeys. J Lab Clin Med 101:623–628

Tamura T, Shin YS, Buehring KU, Stokstad ELR (1976) Bioavailability of folate in man: effects of orange juice supplementation on intestinal conjugase. Br J Haematol 32:123–133

Tamura T, Baer MT, Stokstad ELR (1978) Reduced absorption of folate polyglutamate in zinc-depleted man. Fed Proc 37:493

Tasker PWG (1959) Concealed megaloblastic anaemia. Trans R Soc Trop Med Hyg 53:291–295

Tauro GP, Danks DM, Rowe PB, Van der Weyden MB, Schwarz MA, Collins VL, Neal BW (1976) Dihydrofolate reductase deficiency causing megaloblastic anemia in two families. N Engl J Med 294:466–470

Tavassoli M (1988) The role of liver endothelium in the transfer of iron from transferrin to the hepatocyte. Ann NY Acad Sci 526:83–92

Taylor RT, Hanna ML (1977) Folate dependent enzymes in cultured Chinese hamster ovary cells: folylpolygluamate synthetase and its absence in mutants auxotrophic for glycine and adenosine and thymidine. Arch Biochem Biophys 181:331–344

Taylor RT, Hanna ML, Hutton J (1974) 5-methyltetrahydrofolate homocysteine cobalamin methyltransferase in human bone marrow and its relationships to pernicious anemia. Arch Biochem Biophys 165:787–795

Tennant GB, Smith RC, Leinster SJ, O'Donnell JE, Wardropp CAJ (1981) Acute depression of serum folate in surgical patients during preoperative infusion of ethanol-free parenteral nutrition. Scand J Haematol 27:327–332

Teo NH, Scott JM, Neale G, Weir DG (1980) Effect of bile on vitamin B_{12} absorption. Br Med J 281:831–833

Teo NH, Scott JM, Reed B, Neale G, Weir DG (1981) Bile acid inhibition of vitamin B_{12} binding by intrinsic factor in vitro. Gut 22:270–276

Testa U (1985) Transferrin receptors: structure and function. Curr Top Hematol 5:127–161

Thelander L, Reichard P (1979) Reduction of ribonucleotides. Annu Rev Biochem 48:133–158

Thenen SW, Stokstad ELR (1973) Effect of methionine on specific folate coenzyme pools in vitamin B_{12} deficient and supplemented rats. J Nutr 103:363–370

Thomas FB, Salsbury D, Greenberger NJ (1972) Inhibition of iron absorption by cholestyramine. Demonstration of diminished iron stores following prolonged administration. Dig Dis 17:263–269

Thomas FR, Falko JM, Zuckerman K (1976) Inhibition of intestinal iron absorption by laundry starch. Gastroenterology 71:1028–1032

Thompson WG, Meola T, Lipkin M, Freedman ML (1988) Red cell distribution width, mean corpuscular volume and transferrin saturation in the diagnosis of iron deficiency. Arch Intern Med 148:2128–2130

Thompson WG, Cassino C, Babitz L, Meola T, Berman R, Lipkin M, Friedman M (1989) Hyperpigmented neutrophils and B_{12} deficiency. Acta Haematol 81: 186–191

Thomson AB, Valberg LS (1971) Kinetics of intestinal iron absorption in the rat: effect of cobalt. Am J Physiol 220:1080–1092

Thorstensen K (1988) Hepatocytes and reticulocytes have different mechanism for the uptake of iron from transferrin. J Biol Chem 263:16837–16841

Tikerpae J, Chanarin I (1978) Folate-dependent serine synthesis in lymphocytes from controls and patients with megaloblastic anemia: the effect of therapy. Br J Haematol 38:353–358

Tisman G, Herbert V (1973) B_{12} dependence of cell uptake of serum folate: an explanation for high serum folate and cell folate depletion in B_{12} deficiency. Blood 41:465–469

Tomkin GH (1973) Malabsorption of vitamin B_{12} in diabetic patients treated with phenformin: a comparison with metformin. Br Med J 3:673–675

Tonz O, Weiss S, Strahm WH, Rossi E (1965) Iron absorption in cystic fibrosis. Lancet 2:1096–1099

Topham RW, Woodruff JH, Neatrour GP, Calisch MP, Russo RB, Jackson MR (1980) The role of ferroxidase II and a ferroxidase inhibitor in iron mobilization from tissue stores. Biochem Biophys Res Commun 96:1532–1539

Topham RW, Woodruff JH, Walker MC (1981) Purification and characterization of the intestinal promotor of iron (3+)-transferrin formation. Biochemistry 20: 319–324

Topham R, Goger M, Pearce K, Schultz P (1989) The mobilization of ferritin iron by liver cytosol. Biochem J 261:137–143

Toskes PP, Smith GW, Bensinger TA, Gianella RA, Conrad ME (1974) Folic acid abnormalities in iron deficiency: the mechanism of decreased serum folate levels in rats. Am J Clin Nutr 27:355–361

Trowbridge IS, Omary MB (1981) Human cell surface glycoprotein related to cell proliferation is the receptor for transferrin. Proc Natl Acad Sci USA 78: 3039–3043

Tudhope GR, Swan HT, Spray GH (1967) Patient variation in pernicious anemia as shown in a clinical trial of cyanocobalamin, hydroxocobalamin and cyanocobalamin zinc-tannate. Br J Haematol 13:216–228

Turnbull A, Giblett E (1961) The binding and transport of iron by transferrin variants. J Lab Clin Med 57:450–459

Turnbull A, Cleton F, Finch CA (1962) Iron absorption. IV. The absorption of hemoglobin iron. J Clin Invest 41:1898–1907

Twomey JJ, Jordan PH, Jarrold T, Trubowitz S (1969) The syndrome of immunoglobin deficiency and pernicious anemia. Am J Med 47:340–350

Tycko B, Maxfield FR (1982) Rapid acidification of endocytic vesicles containing alpha-macroglobulin. Cell 28:643–651

Valberg LS, Ghent CN (1985) Diagnosis and management of hereditary hemochromatosis. Ann Rew Med 36:27–37

Valberg LS, Lloyd DA, Ghent CN, Flanagan PR, Sinclair NR, Stiller CR, Chamberlain MJ (1980) Clinical and biochemical expression of the genetic abnormality in idiopathic hemochromatosis. Gastroenterology 79:884–892

Van Baarlen J, Brouwer JT, Leibman A, Aisen P (1980) Evidence for the functional heterogeneity of the two sites of transferrin in vitro. Br J Haematol 46: 417–426

Van der Heul C, Kroos MJ, Van Noort WL, Van Eijk HG (1981) No functional difference of the two iron binding sites of human transferrin in vitro. Clin Sci 60:185–190

Van der Heul C, Kross MJ, Van Noort WL, Van Eijk HG (1984) In vitro and in vivo studies of iron delivery be human transferrins. Br J Haematol 56:571–580

Van der Westhuyzen J, Metz J (1983) Tissue *S*-adenosyl-methionine levels in fruit bats (*Rousettus aegyptiacus*) with nitrous oxide-induced neuropathy. Br J Nutr 50:325–333

Van der Westhuyzen J, Metz J (1984) Betaine delays the onset of neurological impairment in nitrous-oxide-induced vitamin B_{12} deficiency in fruit bats. J Nutr 114:1106–1111

Van der Westhuyzen, J, Fernandez-Costa F, Metz J (1982) Cobalamin inactivation by N_2O produces severe neurologic impariment in fruit bats: protection by methionine and aggravation by folates. Life Sci 31:2001–2012

Van der Westhuyzen J, Cantrill RC, Fernandes-Costa F, Metz J (1983) Effect of a vitamin B_{12} deficient diet on lipid and fatty acid composition of spinal cord myelin in the fruit bat. J Nutr 113:531–537

Van der Weyden M, Rother M, Firkin B (1972) Megaloblastic maturation masked by iron deficiency: a biochemical basis. Brit J Haematol 22:299–307

Van Renswoude JK, Bridges KR, Harford JB et al. (1982) Identification of a non-lysosomal acidic compartment. Proc Natl Acad Sci (USA) 79:6186–6190

Verhoef NJ, Kottenhagen MJ, Mulder HJM, Noordeloos PJ, Leijnse B (1978) Functional heterogeneity of transferrin-bound iron. Acta Haematol 60:21–26

Vulimiri L, Linder MC, Munro HN (1977) Sex difference in distribution and iron responsiveness of the two cardiac ferritins of rat cardiac and skeletal muscle. Biochim Biophys Acta 497:280–287

Young SP (1982) Evidence for the functional equivalence of the iron binding sites of rat transferrin. Biochim Biophys Acta 718:35–41
Young SP, Aisen P (1981) Transferrin receptors and the uptake and release of iron by isolated hepatocytes. Hepatology 1:114–118
Young SP, Bomford A, Madden AD, Garratt RC, Williams R, Evans RW (1984) Abnormal in vitro functions of a variant human transferrin. Br J Haematol 56:581–587
Youngdahl-Turner P, Rosenberg LE, Allen RH (1978) Binding and uptake of transcobalamin II by human fibroblasts. J Clin Invest 61:133–141
Youngdahl-Turner P, Mellman IS, Allen RH, Rosenberg LE (1979) Protein-mediated vitamin uptake: adsorptive endocytosis of transcobalamin II-cobalamin complex by cultured human fibroblasts. Exp Cell Res 118:127–134
Zahringer J, Baliga BS, Munro HN (1976) Novel mechanism for translational control in regulation of ferritin synthesis by iron. Proc Natl Acad Sci USA 73:857–861
Zail SS, Charlton RW, Torrance JD, Bothwell TH (1964) Studies on the formation of ferritin in red cell precursors. J Clin Invest 43:670–680
Zapolski E, Ganz R, Princiotto JV (1974) Biological specificity of the iron binding sites of transferrin. Am J Physiol 226:334–339
Zhang D, Hendricks DG, Mahoney AW, Yu Y (1988) Effect of tea on dietary iron availability in anemic and healthy rats. Nutr Rep Int 37:1225–1235
Zimmerman J, Selhub J, Rosenberg IH (1986) Competitive inhibition of folic acid absorption in rat jejunum by triamterene. J Lab Clin Med 108:272–276

CHAPTER 7

Erythropoietin in the Anemia of End-Stage Renal Disease

R.D. LANGE

A. Assay of Erythropoietin

Erythropoietin (Ep) has been called the hematologists' hormone (KUBANEK 1969). With the advent of genetically engineered hormones, it is now being investigated in the treatment of the anemia of chronic renal disease.

To understand the relationship of Ep to kidney function and to measure its level in the body fluids of patients with renal disease require a reliable method of assay since otherwise the values reported may vary. In 1960, JACOBSON, GURNEY, and GOLDWASSER described the most desirable qualities of the ideal assay as follows:

1. Simple enough to be performed quickly on multiple samples
2. Accurate enough to permit the detection of small differences
3. Sensitive enough to demonstrate consistently and quantitatively the presence of minute amounts

The first Ep assays utilized intact animals but gave unreliable results, until it was found that by increasing the animals' circulating blood volume, endogenous erythropoiesis could be suppressed, and the animals became responsive to injected hormone. The incorporation of radioactive iron into newly formed red blood cells (RBC) simplified the procedure (PLZAK et al. 1955). As a consequence, the ex-hypoxic polycythemic mouse assay involving RBC iron incorporation for many years became the Ep determination method.

However, there were drawbacks:

1. The assay was time consuming and expensive.
2. Further, unless concentration procedures were carried out, the Ep level in the serum of hematologically normal individuals could not be measured. If serum was concentrated by placing it in boiling water, some of the hormone was trapped by the coagulated proteins.
3. Also, some nonEp materials were found to affect the bioassay, including
   a) Cobalt (WHITE et al. 1960)
   b) Testosterone and other androgens (FRIED et al. 1964)
   c) Adrenocorticotropic hormone (ACTH) and tri-iodothyronine (FISHER et al. 1967)
   d) Placental lactogen (JEPSON and LOWENSTEIN 1966)

e) Cyclic AMP (SCHOOLEY and MAHLMANN 1971a; RODGERS et al. 1975)
f) Prostaglandins (SCHOOLEY and MAHLMANN 1971b)
g) Inhibitors (KRZYMOWSKI and KRZYMOWSKA 1962; WHITCOMB and MOORE 1965; LEWIS et al. 1969; LINDEMANN 1971; LORD et al. 1976)

For further information, readers are referred to the reviews of FISHER and GROSS (1977), as well as POPOVIC and ADAMSON (1979).

To overcome some of the difficulties of the in vivo bioassays, in vitro bioassays were devised, based on cultures of spleen fragments, bone marrow, and spleen and fetal liver cells (KRYSTAL et al. 1981a,b; LANGE et al. 1980). Mouse fetal liver cells have been used most extensively (DUNN and LANGE 1980).

The in vitro cultures have, in some cases, suffered from a lack of parallelism with the standard preparations, and the same sources of error described for the bioassay are present in the in vitro assay. These include:

1. Competition with nonradioactive iron, percentage of saturation of transferrin, and high concentrations of human serum (de KLERK et al. 1977; LAPPIN et al. 1985)
2. Growth modulators and hormones, such as insulin (KURTZ et al. 1983a), selenite, and transferrin (GUILBERT and ISCOVE 1976)
3. Stimulators of erythropoiesis, such as prostaglandins (DUKES et al. 1973), hemin (MONETTE and HOLDEN 1982), and steroid hormones (SINGER et al. 1976)
4. Serum inhibitors (see above)

Nevertheless, DUNN and LANGE (1980) found that by modifying the fetal mouse liver assay, a good correlation was obtained with titers measured by a standard, in vivo erythrocythemic mouse technique. However, the in vitro technique detected, on average, approximately 50% more Ep than did the in vivo assay (DUNN et al. 1979).

When it was found in 1964 that antibodies could be produced to Ep, it became the aim of investigators to develop a radioimmunoassay (RIA). This work was hindered for many years by the lack of purified hormone. Ultimately, assays were developed in a number of laboratories, including those of Garcia, Fisher, Cotes, and Goldwasser (GARCIA 1972a,b, 1977; SHERWOOD and GOLDWASSER 1979; REGE and FISHER 1980; GOLDWASSER and SHERWOOD 1981; COTES et al. 1980; COTES 1982, 1983; MATSUBARA et al. 1989; MASON-GARCIA et al. 1990). The principles of the RIA have been detailed by POPOVIC and ADAMSON (1979) as follows:

1. Limited amount of antibody binds approximately 50% of labeled hormone
2. Quantitative competition for antibody binding by nonlabeled hormone
3. Construction of a curve to relate amount of labeled hormone vs. unlabeled hormone bound to antibody

4. Concentration of hormone in an unknown sample can then be obtained from the effect of its competition with a known amount of labeled hormone for a given (limited) number of antibody sites

The antiserum is of quintessential importance in recognizing specific antigens. The in vitro RIA, of course, does not measure biological activity. Nevertheless, COHEN et al. (1985) have found that an excellent correlation exists between the bioassay and the RIA for Ep. They found that the RIA detects biologically active Ep in human serum and urine when it is present in amounts only moderately higher than normal. The assays have been validated by the consistently parallel results found when standard solutions are assayed and by the appropriate results of sera tested before and after the production of anemia or polycythemia (GARCIA et al. 1982).

In looking at the Ep titers in renal disease, those in normal human sera must be determined. The results of published reports of such levels are given in Table 1.

DUNN and LANGE concluded in their 1980 review, "Many assays for Ep exist. None are perfect. Some offer the advantage of convenience of cost over others. Most seem to measure a factor, or factors, which have some or all of the properties expected of an erythroid regulatory hormone. The choice of assay is a matter of personal preference. As long as the selected assay is used carefully throughout the planned investigation and appropriate statistical control is maintained, meaningful results should be obtained."

B. Pathogenesis of the Anemia of Chronic Renal Failure

The pathogenesis of any anemia is a balance between the loss of red blood cells and their production or a combination of the two factors. So it is with the anemia associated with chronic renal disease (ACRF). Table 2 lists the factors which have been ascribed to the pathogenesis of this anemia.

A number of factors have been shown to contribute to a hemolytic component in ACRF and were first described by JOSKE et al. (1956) and confirmed by LOGE et al. (1958) and DESFORGES and DAWSON (1958). Several authors have implicated hypersplenism as a cause of hemolysis and improvement in the anemia by splenectomy (BISCHEL et al. 1971; HARTLEY et al. 1971; BERNE et al. 1973; NEIMAN et al. 1973; ASABA et al. 1977; NAJEAN and MESSIAN 1983). Seven of NAJEAN's patients did not improve.

Extracellular components may cause hemolysis. Copper from the dialysis tubing or as a contaminant is one (MATTER et al. 1969; KLEIN et al. 1972). Other chemicals include nitrates (CARLSON and SHAPIRO 1970) and chloramines (EATON et al. 1973), as well as overheated dialysate and hypophosphatemia (KLOCK et al. 1974).

Turning to intracellular defects as a cause of hemolysis, FORMAN et al. (1973) and ROSENMUND et al. (1975) have called attention to decreased

Table 1. Comparison of erythropoietin titers in serum from hematologically normal individuals utilizing a number of assay methods[a]

Method	Reference	n	mU ep/ml (range or mean ±SEM)	Index of precision
Bioassay				
In vivo	WAGEMAKER et al. (1972)	10	<3.0 ± 4.5[b]	N.D.
	ALEXANIAN (1973)		20[b]	N.D.
	DAVIES et al. (1975)		320 ± 280	N.D.
	SCHULZ et al. (1978)		34	–
	ERSLEV et al. (1979)	11	7.8[c]	N.D.
	CARO et al. (1979)		3.9 ± 2.3[c]	N.D.
	BESSLER et al. (1980)	13	25.8 ± 11	–
	FIRKIN and RUSSELL (1983)		<50	
	SAKATA et al. (1987)		M 15.6 ± 3.6[d]	–
			F 22.9 ± 2.3	–
	EGRIE et al. (1987)		24.5	–
In vitro				
a) Fetal mouse liver cells	DUNN et al. (1977)		240 ± 42	N.D.
	NAPIER et al. (1977)		150 ± 100	0.5 – 0.15
	RADTKE et al. (1978a)	59	136 ± 9	N.D.
	dE KLERK et al. (1978)	F18	29[b,e]	N.D.
		M20	48	N.D.
	KIMZEY et al. (1978)		200 ± 40	N.D.
	DUNN et al. (1979)		50 ± 5[e]	N.D.
	BESSLER et al. (1980)		2120 ± 840	
	NAPIER et al. and EVANS (1980)	24	10.4[f]	
	FIRKIN and RUSSELL (1983)		<50	
	MULLER-WIEFEL (1983b)		11 to 35	
	SAKATA et al. (1985)		87	
	SAKATA et al. (1987)	F	199.5 ± 43	
		M	185.3 ± 41.2	

b) Adult mouse bone marrow	KRYSTAL et al. (1981b)			
	M Raw		520	
	M Treated		790	
	F Raw		490	
	F Treated		730	
c) Mouse spleen cells	PAUL et al. (1987)			
	Raw		8.3	
	Heat-treated		40.2	
Immunological radioimmunoassay				
	GARCIA (1974)		3.7–11.0	N.D.
	LERTORA et al. (1975)		52–84	N.D.
	SCHULZ et al. (1978)		34 ± 2	
	GARCIA et al. (1979)[g]	F	4.3	
		M	4.9	
	REGE and FISHER (1980)	F	25.1	
		M	30.2	
	COTES et al. (1980)	F 73	13.3 ± 0.8	
		M145	13.1 ± 0.5	
	KOEFFLER and GOLDWASSER (1981)	26	14.9 ± 4.2	
	ZAROULIS et al. (1981)[b]	19	29	
	MILLER et al. (1981)	48	18.5 ± 5.0	
	COTES (1982)	46	13.3	
	REGE et al. (1982)		14.7	
	GARCIA et al. (1982)	F	18.8	
		M	17.2	
	EGRIE et al. (1987)		24.0	
	MATSUBARA et al. (1989)		25 ± 5	
	MASON-GARCIA et al. (1990)		6.21 ± 0.43	

[a] Adapted from DUNN and LANGE (1980).
[b] Extrapolated.
[c] Heat treated.
[d] Serum extracted.
[e] Using modified method to take into account potential of ferrokinetic variables.
[f] Serum concentrated.
[g] Pool.

Table 2. Pathogenesis of the anemia associated with uremia accompanying chronic renal disease

Increased red blood cell destruction and blood loss
- A. Hemolysis
  1. Hypersplenism
  2. Extracellular factors, e.g., copper dialysis tubing, nitrates, chloramines, overheated dialysate, hypophosphatemia, uremic toxins
  3. Intracellular defects
     - a) Decreased red blood cell deformability
     - b) Metabolic defects and sodium transport
     - c) Unknown intracellular defects
  4. Microangiopathic factors
- B. Blood loss
  1. Gastrointestinal blood loss due to peptic disease, hemorrhoids, and medication
  2. Loss in dialyzer
  3. Iatrogenic from blood sampling
  4. Menorrhagia

Decreased production of red blood cells
- A. Iron deficiency
- B. Aluminum toxicity
- C. Folic acid and pyridoxine deficiency
- D. Histadine deficiency
- E. Parathyroid hormone intoxication
- F. Inhibitors of erythropoiesis and decrease in Ep's efficiency
- G. Ep deficiency
- H. Infection

Combination – multifactorial

RBC deformability as one cause of intracellular hemolysis. RBCs of uremic patients display a number of metabolic defects (EATON et al. 1973; JACOB et al. 1975; YAWATA et al. 1972) and abnormal sodium transport (SMITH and WELT 1970). Microangiopathic hemolytic anemia has also been described in a few patients but was not a factor in other series (NEFF et al. 1985).

Although hemolysis contributes to the ACRF, it is usually mild and is improved by dialysis (CASTELIANI et al. 1977), which POWELL and ADAMSON (1985) postulate may be related to the removal of toxic products that produce the mechanical or metabolic defects in the erythrocytes. LOGE et al. (1958) found overt hemolysis to be a late phenomenon.

While hemolysis may be found in 70% of uremic patients, actual blood loss occurs in over 20%, and in addition there is loss of blood in priming the dialyzer and in blood samples taken for tests (DESFORGES 1970).

Uremic patients have an increased bleeding tendency. This may be due to a prolonged bleeding time resulting from a defect in platelet factor 3 (HOROWITZ et al. 1970) or reduced platelet adhesion to arterial subendothelium (LIVIO et al. 1982; DEYKIN 1983; LIVIO et al. 1985). Also, the administration of anticoagulants such as heparin and dicumarol may contribute to the tendency to bleed easily.

Gastrointestinal bleeding is common. POINTER et al. (1974) have pointed out the incidence of peptic ulcers due to increased levels of gastrin in uremic patients. The concomitant administration of antacids may lead to constipation and bleeding from hemorrhoids. Menorrhagia occurs in some patients (NEFF et al. 1985). HOCKEN and MARWAH (1971) have estimated that from 1.6 to 4.6 l of blood are lost each year in the dialyzer and in blood sampling.

ACRF is most often described as a hypoproliferative type of anemia. This is most easily demonstrated by measuring the RBC iron incorporation (LOGE et al. 1958). ESCHBACH et al. (1967) found an iron turnover of 0.44 mg/100 ml in their uremic patients vs. 0.6 mg/100 ml in their controls. Morphologically, however, the examination of bone marrow from patients with ACRF may show hypocellularity, normocellularity, or hypercellularity. In 1980, HO-YEN et al. found no significant difference in bone marrow cellularity between controls and patients with ACRF.

In most cases, the RBCs are normocytic and normochromic. However, in some patients the erythrocytes are hypochromic and microcytic as a result of iron deficiency or aluminum toxicity. As mentioned above, blood loss is frequent and ultimately leads to an iron deficiency in some patients. NEFF et al. (1985) in their study of 124 patients found that 22% had ferritin values of 50 ng/ml or less and in 5%, the values were less than 20 ng/ml, indicating a severe depression in bone marrow iron stores. SHORT et al. (1980) noted that in some patients on dialysis a microcytic anemia develops due to aluminum toxicity, and SWARTZ et al. (1987) think that this is a marker of aluminum toxicity.

Megaloblastic anemia may develop occasionally due to a loss of folic acid in the dialysate (HEMMELOFF 1977). Pyridoxine (SJOGREN et al. 1979; KOPPLE et al. 1981) is also lost, and BLUMENKRANTZ et al. (1974) have reported that histidine deficiency may cause ACRF. It should be noted that NEFF et al. (1985) found normal levels of folate and vitamin B_{12} in their study, and the dietician estimated that their patients had adequate intakes of histidine.

Some patients with chronic renal disease (CRD) have active infections. These may, in turn, contribute to the anemia of CRD since patients with chronic diseases due to infection, malignancy, etc., are often mildly anemic. The subject was extensively reviewed in 1966 by CARTWRIGHT.

The anemia of chronic disorders (ACD) bears many similarities to ACRF in its pathogenic mechanisms. The underlying cause is an underproduction of RBCs (CARTWRIGHT 1966), although mildly hemolytic states may be present (CARTWRIGHT and LEE 1971). Many studies have shown this apparent reduction in availability of iron stored in the reticuloendothelial system (RES) for heme synthesis by bone marrow erythroid cells (FREIREICH et al. 1957; BENNETT et al. 1974; DOUGLAS and ADAMSON 1975; HERSHKO et al. 1974). However, at least two investigations have presented evidence against an RES iron blockade (CAVILL et al. 1977; BENTLEY et al. 1979.

Just as in ACRF, Ep has been studied as a possible clue to reticulocytopenia and underproduction of RBCs (NAETS 1975). Several investigators have shown Ep levels to be low in the serum or plasma of patients with ACD (WARD et al. 1969, 1971; DOUGLAS and ADAMSON 1975; ERSLEV et al. 1980). PAVLOVIC-KENTERA and her coworkers in 1979 showed patients with ACD to have an impaired response to Ep. No inhibitors of heme synthesis were found in the sera of 12 patients with ACD. In a recent study, BIRGEGÅRD found an elevated level of Ep in 30 female and 11 male patients with mild ACD (BIRGEGÅRD et al. 1987). They found that the Ep levels correlated with the hemoglobin levels and erythrocyte sedimentation rate (ESR). Thus, with the greater degree of inflammation, the decrease in the hemoglobin level and the increase in the Ep levels demonstrated an ordinary Ep response. BIRGEGÅRD et al. (1987) did not believe that diminished Ep production was the cause of anemia in patients with chronic inflammatory joint disease.

In 1953 SACCHETTI and in 1956 MARKSON and RENNIE described inhibitors of erythropoiesis in the serum of patients with uremia. Since that time, the subject has been under intense investigation with outstanding contributions being made in Fisher's and Wallner's laboratories. The inhibition, in general, has been hypothesized to occur: (a) in opposition to the action of Ep; (b) in decreasing heme synthesis of developing erythroid cells; and/or (c) in decreasing erythroid colony formation by erythroid progenitor cells. Studies have been carried out using human serum and bone marrow cells or the serum and bone marrow of animals made uremic by surgical procedures (WALLNER et al. 1975; FISHER et al. 1978).

I. Inhibition of Erythropoietin Action

FISHER et al. in 1968, found that the plasma from five out of six patients with ACRF produced significant inhibition of erythropoiesis stimulating factor (subsequently named Ep). MORIYAMA and FISHER (1975) also suggested that ACRF serum directly inhibited Ep. In a study of children with renal disease, MCGONIGLE et al. (1985) coincubated Ep in the presence of serum from uremic patients. They found markedly less immunoreactivity in their RIA and, also, less biologic activity in the fetal mouse liver CFU-E assay than when Ep was incubated with normal human sera. These results suggested some alteration in Ep in the presence of uremic serum. However, GALLAGHER et al. (1961) and ERSLEV (1975) were unable to demonstrate that CRF sera directly inactivated Ep. GALLAGHER et al. utilized rabbits made uremic by bilateral nephrectomy, while ERSLEV measured the effect of human CRF sera in the ex-hypoxic mouse assay. ZUCKER et al. (1976) also found no inhibition of Ep. The subject was further investigated by WALLNER et al. (1977) who used both in vitro and in vivo experiments and were unable to find evidence of inhibition or inactivation of Ep by CRF sera. They did demonstrate depression of in vitro heme synthesis by CRF sera and concluded that ACRF sera inhibited erythropoiesis by directly, although reversibly, impairing the ability of erythroblasts to synthesize heme.

II. Inhibition of Heme Synthesis

The inhibition of heme synthesis by erythroid cells was studied in rabbits made acutely uremic by bilateral nephrectomy (Fisher et al. 1977). The sera of these uremic rabbits significantly decreased heme synthesis in normal rabbit bone marrow cells stimulated by Ep. The baseline ^{59}Fe incorporation in unstimulated marrow cells was also decreased in cultures containing sera from uremic rabbits. The sera from uremic rabbits did not inhibit the ^{59}Fe incorporation of polycythemic mice in response to Fe. These authors tested the sera of six uremic patients in a human bone marrow culture system. Three patients' plasmas or sera produced significant inhibition, while the remainder stimulated heme synthesis.

Wallner and his associates have looked at the possible inhibition of heme synthesis by sera from CRF patients in a number of studies. Using a dog bone marrow system, they tested sera from 27 normal subjects and 52 patients with CRF and found less heme synthesis when the CRF sera was incorporated in the system. They felt that the inhibition was, in part, responsible for the ACRF (Wallner et al. 1976). Wallner and Vautrin in 1981 made the important observation that the levels of inhibitor developed and increased as the renal failure worsened. In this study, rabbit bone marrow cells were employed as an indicator of heme synthesis. They also noted a fall in inhibitor level in those patients who had an increase in hematocrit after dialysis. They were able to demonstrate a decrease in erythroid colony formation by marrow as well as a decrease in heme synthesis.

In an interesting study, Linkesch et al. (1978) measured the levels of δ-aminolevulinic acid dehydrase, porphobilinogen deaminase, and ferrochelatase, three heme-synthesizing enzymes, in the sera of uremic patients. All three enzyme levels were decreased in uremic patients. These investigators proposed that the decreased heme biosynthesis in ACRF might be due either to a lack of Ep, leading to a decrease in δ-aminolevulinic acid dehydrase and ferrochelatase, or to the presence of uremic toxins inhibiting Ep and/or the three heme-synthesizing enzymes. Swendseid et al. (1980) have determined the polyamine concentrations in the RBCs and urine of patients with CRF. They found that if the patient's creatinine level was above 6 mg%, the red blood spermidine, but not spermine, concentration was higher.

III. Inhibition of Colony Formation

In acutely uremic rabbits, Moriyama and Fisher (1975) reported that the numbers of erythroid colonies formed from Ep-responsive cells in their marrow was higher than in normal controls. FISHER et al. in their 1977 studies, found that the sera from uremic rabbits did not inhibit CFU-E formation. However, when the studies were repeated in marrow of rabbits 35 days after five-sixth of their kidneys had been removed, a decrease in the number of CFU-E was noted, and their sera had a significant inhibitory effect on colony formation by the CFU-E in normal rabbit bone marrow cultures (OHNO and FISHER 1977). The investigators thought that the findings supported the hypothesis that an inhibitor of the target cell for Ep, the CFU-E, plays an important role in ACRF.

However, MLADENOVIC et al. (1984), employing sheep with CRF surgically produced, did a prospective study to measure the effect of sera on erythroid colony formation of marrow from uremic and normal sheep from the animals pre- and postsurgery. Among 42 sera from five sheep, in only 7 was erythroid colony growth decreased by 20%. These investigators suggested their results refuted the hypothesis that uremic toxins significantly inhibit in vitro erythropoiesis.

A number of studies have been carried out utilizing sera from patients with ACRF, two from Wallner's laboratory. In 1978, WALLNER et al. used mouse bone marrow cells in cultures containing either uremic or normal serum. They found fewer erythroid colonies when uremic serum was included. There was no difference in the size or morphology of colonies, and uremic sera had no effect on white blood cell colony growth in their plasma clot system. WALLNER and VAUTRIN (1981) demonstrated that the inhibition by uremic sera of the ability of mouse marrow cells to form erythroid colonies decreased as the hematocrit of the patient decreased.

FREEDMAN et al. (1983a) studied the effect of uremic serum on erythroid burst formation and CFU-E. That from autologous uremic patients decreased by 63% the BFU-E obtained with serum from 10 anemic patients; the same cells demonstrated a normal or increased BFU-E response to Ep in the presence of normal serum. When uremic serum from 90 patients was cultured with normal human marrow, there was a marked decrease in both BFU-E and CFU-E colony formation. Neither hemodialysis nor peritoneal dialysis of their patients removed the inhibitor.

MCGONIGLE et al. in 1985 did an extensive study on children with renal disease. They found that the degree of inhibition of CFU-E correlated with both the creatinine clearance and hematocrit. They felt that serum inhibition of erythroid progenitor cells in bone marrow was an important factor in the pathogenesis of anemia in children with renal disease.

In a recent study, PAVLOVIC-KENTERA and her associates (1987a) used a mouse bone marrow assay to study 35 patients with ACRF. They found inhibition in all but 1 patient and no difference pre- and postdialysis. They found no inhibition of CFU-GM. In another study, the results indicated that the difference in severity of anemia was due to a difference in production of Ep rather than to the level of inhibitors (PAVLOVIC-KENTERA et al. 1987b). HOTTA et al. (1987) found in their investigations that 20 of 30 uremic sera inhibited erythroid colony growth of human bone marrow cells of the same blood group. Only 1 serum inhibited CFU-GM colony growth. Kushner, in Fisher's laboratory, has recently described the effect of polyamines on erythroid and myeloid colony growth (Kushner et al. 1988; Kushner et al. 1989). They found that predialysis serum from patients with end-stage renal disease exerts a more significant inhibition of erythroid CFU-E than of myeloid CFU-GM. This was also true of the polyamines spermine, spermidine, and putrescine, leading them to conclude that the polyamines may be important uremic toxins, which may contribute to the pathogenesis of the anemia in end-stage renal disease. In two separate case reports, no evidence of inhibitors was found (Hanna et al. 1980; Muto et al. 1987). Delwiche et al. (1986) did an extensive study on hematopoietic inhibitors in uremic sera. They found that although the sera contain inhibitors of colony growth, there was decreased inhibition following dialysis and that the inhibitors lacked specificity.

Intensive efforts have been made to attempt to characterize the inhibitor. The approximate molecular weights are given in Table 3.

The disappearance of inhibitors following dialysis has been variable, but Chandra et al. (1987) reported that one patient's hematocrit markedly improved when treatment was switched from hemodialysis to continuous ambulatory peritoneal dialysis. They postulated that this improvement might be due to a more efficient removal of inhibitors. Eschbach et al. (1970) found that RBC production can improve on dialysis.

Although not every study has demonstrated the presence of inhibitors, most investigators would agree that the serum of some patients contains material that is inhibitory to erythropoiesis. As Freedman and his coinvestigators in 1983 stated, "It seems reasonable to conclude that there are several inhibitors of erythropoiesis in uremic serum, some of which have a molecular size that is too large for removal by conventional forms of dialysis" (Freedman et al. 1983a).

Patients with CRD often have chemical manifestations of secondary hyperparathyroidism. A mild anemia is often seen in hyperparathyroid

Table 3. Characterization of putative inhibitors of erythropoiesis in sera of uremic humans and animals

Inhibitor	Reference
Low molecular weight	Fisher et al. 1977
Spermine	Radtke et al. 1981
Parathyroid hormone	See following section, this chapter
Middle molecular weight	Hotta et al. 1987
with active peptide	Saito et al. 1986
47 000 to >150 000	Freedman et al. 1983a
Ribonuclease	Freedman et al. 1983b
Polar lipid	Wallner and Vautrin 1978

patients (BOXER et al. 1977; FALKO et al. 1976; MALLETTE et al. 1974) and responds to parathyroidectomy. As a consequence, investigators have examined the role of parathyroid hormone (PTH) in ACRD and the effect on the anemia of either subtotal parathyroidectomy or chemical suppression of PTH by vitamin D therapy.

A number of studies found an increase in hematocrit in hemodialyzed patients after parathyroidectomy (LEPOUTRE et al. 1981). In 1978, SHASHA et al. noted an increase in hemoglobin level in four of five patients on hemodialysis following subtotal parathyroidectomy, and a sixth patient improved after therapy with 1α-hydroxycholecalciferol. While the mean increase was not statistically significant in three patients, a significant increase occurred. They quoted the studies of ZINGRAFF, who found improvement in 44 patients (SHASHA et al. 1978). However, POTASMAN and BETTER (1983) recorded that only 50% of the patients improved following the operation, and PODJARNY et al. (1981), who studied 96 long-term hemodialysis patients including 18 before and after parathyroidectomy, noted no correlation between hematocrit levels and biochemical indices of secondary hyperparathyroidism. However, in 44%, the hematocrit rose, and the investigators pointed out that there may be two subgroups of patients. It is of interest that, in a group of patients on continuous ambulatory dialysis followed by ZAPPACOSTA et al. (1982), those patients whose hematocrits increased after a period of dialysis had higher PTH levels than those who did not respond. The evaluation and comparison of these studies are difficult because of variations in parathyroid assay methods, standards, and units.

The mechanism by which an excess of PTH influences erythropoiesis remains an enigma, although some animal studies have shown inhibition (LACOUR et al. 1980). It has been postulated that increased levels of PTH are associated with bone marrow fibrosis, and an inverse relationship between hemoglobin concentration and the degree of endosteal marrow fibrosis has been seen by some investigators. However, other researchers question whether PTH produces bone marrow fibrosis (WEINBERG et al. 1977) and think that it is debatable whether or not the fibrosing effect of PTH is of clinical significance.

Several studies have been made on the effect of PTH on in vitro erythroid colony formation. MEYTES et al. (1981) found that intact parathyroid hormone in concentrations comparable with those found in uremic patients produced a marked and significant inhibition of mouse BFU-E and CFU-GM but not murine marrow CFU-E. They reported that an increased concentration of Ep overcame the inhibition by PTH. DELWICHE et al. (1983) noted that increased concentrations of crude PTH produced a dose-dependent inhibition of BFU-E and CFU-GM but that pure intact hormone preparations did not. These investigators cautioned that the inhibitory effects in culture systems may not be related to the circulating form of PTH.

MCGONIGLE et al. (1984a) have investigated the potential role of PTH as an inhibitor of erythropoiesis in ACRD, using CFU-E and fetal mouse liver cell assays. In nondialyzed patients, they found that the serum level of PTH correlated with the patient's hematocrit and inhibition of colony formation and heme synthesis. However, when the effect of creatinine was controlled, PTH no longer served as a predictor of either hematocrit or erythroid colony formation. A similar lack of correlation was found in dialyzed patients. Thirteen of their patients underwent parathyroidectomy, and although the hematocrit increased in 6, there was no change in serum Ep levels. They found no effect of 1-34 human parathyroid hormone, 1-84 bovine parathyroid hormone, or 1,25-dihydroxycholecalciferol on BFU-E formation. However, 8 μ/ml PTH inhibited and 4.0 ng of 1,25-dihydroxycholecalciferol stimulated CFU-E only in the absence of Ep. These researchers concluded that it was not possible to demonstrate a significant relationship between serum PTH levels and anemia or inhibition of erythropoiesis either before or after long-term dialysis. They concluded that the improvement in anemia after parathyroidectomy is associated with neither an increase in Ep levels nor removal of inhibitors.

In one study, PTH at low concentrations enhanced heme synthesis in the fetal mouse liver culture system, while higher levels inhibited it (Zevin et al. 1981). Dunn and Trent (1981) used this system to reinvestigate the effects of PTH. They found that at PTH concentrations 10–100 times normal a dose-dependent stimulation of erythropoiesis was observed only in the complete absence of Ep. When concentrations of 240 times normal were used, PTH inhibited both endogenous and Ep-mediated heme synthesis. Since these levels were so high, they thought that the hypothesis of PTH being directly responsible for anemia was extremely doubtful.

Caro et al. (1979) also examined the Ep levels in uremic nephric and anephric patients. One group with severe hyperparathyroidism was found to be less responsive to Ep, suggesting the role of PTH in marrow unresponsiveness.

Some investigators have postulated that PTH is an uremic toxin (Massry and Goldstein 1978; Muller-Wiefel et al. 1983), which contributes to: (a) reduced erythropoiesis, (b) hemolysis through its effect on the osmotic fragility of RBC and (c) through increased gastrointestinal blood loss due to its effect on blood platelet aggregating ability.

Other investigators feel that the role of PTH in hematological abnormalities is controversial and that further studies are required to establish PTH as an "universal" toxin in uremia (Klahr and Slatopolsky 1986). It seems obvious that as Muller-Wiefel and his coworkers (1983) state, "In conclusion, the different mechanisms by which PTH might influence renal anemia unfavorably need further elucidation by a comprehensive approach which should not be restricted to the investigation of a single mode of action."

While all of the foregoing may be involved in the pathogenesis of ACRF, Loge et al. (1958) found that there is an invariable depression of erythropoiesis. Subsequent studies have shown that the serum level of Ep in

Table 4. Erythropoietin levels after organ extirpation[a]

Organ removed prjor to Co^{2+} injection	Stimulus	^{59}Fe incorporation[(b)] (%)
None	None	3.7 ± 0.4
None	Co^{2++} (c)	14.4 ± 1.5
Adrenals and gonads	Co^{2++} (c)	15.1 ± 0.9
90% Liver	Co^{2++} (c)	12.4 ± 0.4
Stomach, intestines, spleen, pancreas	Co^{2++} (c)	11.7 ± 1.2
Kidneys	Co^{2++} (c)	4.5 ± 0.7
Thymus	Co^{2++} (c)	16.3 ± 1.6
None	Co^{2++} (d)	6.6 ± 1.1
Kidneys	Co^{2++} (d)	3.3 ± 0.5
Ureter ligation	Co^{2++} (d)	9.8 ± 0.1

[a] Effect of plasma obtained from rats that had been subjected to organ excision and then Co^{2++} stimulation upon the incorporation of ^{59}Fe into the red blood cells of starved rats (from JACOBSON et al. 1959).
[b] Assay of donor plasma in starved rats being percentage of ^{59}Fe incorporation response of recipient to plasma (±SE). [c] 250 μ*M*/kg. [d] 167 μ*M*/kg.

deficient feedback regulation in erythropoiesis in their transplant patients with polycythemia.

The ultimate proof of the importance of Ep in ACRF lies with the hematological improvement which results when therapy with recombinant hormone is instituted. This is detailed in Sect. D.

C. Kidney Production of Erythropoietin

As detailed above, in CRD, decreased Ep production plays a major role in the pathogenesis of the anemia associated with uremia. For over 30 years, since the extirpation experiments of JACOBSON et al. (1957), the kidney has been known to be a major site of Ep production. As shown in Table 4, these investigators were able to stimulate the production of Ep following the extirpation of many organs but not after removal of the kidneys. Rats with a similar degree of urea nitrogen retention after urethral ligation were able to produce Ep. NAETS and HEUSE in 1962 showed that the kidney of dogs was the sole source of Ep. Nephrectomy in starved nephrectomized rats was found to reduce the response to cobalt but not to Ep (SANZARI and FISHER 1963).

ROSSE and WALDMANN (1962) used a parabiotic technique first employed by REISSMANN (1950) to demonstrate definitively the existence of a humoral regulatory mechanism for erythropoiesis and found that radioiron incorporation was less in pairs in which the nephrectomized partner was hypoxic than in pairs in which either the unoperated or ureter-ligated partner was hypoxic (Table 5).

Perfusion studies provided further evidence for the renal source of Ep. Isolated rabbit kidneys were perfused by KURATOWSKA and her associates

Table 5. Studies on the effect of nephrectomy or ureter ligation on the erythropoietic response to anoxia in parabiotic rats

Condition of parabiont	O_2 level	Percentage ^{59}Fe incorporation in red blood cells of pairs (SEM)
Left anephric Right intact	Normal Normal	7.1 (0.2)
Left anephric Right intact	Anoxic Normal	12.6 (1.72)
Left anephric Right intact	Normal Anoxic	19.7 (2.25)
Left ureter ligated Right intact	Anoxic Normal	20.3 (3.28)

From Rosse and Waldmann (1962).

(1961, 1962) with anoxic blood and Tyrode's solution; the perfusate contained erythropoietic stimulating activity. When blood flow as impaired, Nakao (1962) reported an increase in rabbit kidney perfusates. The perfusion of isolated rabbit kidneys by fully oxygenated blood did not influence Ep production, while extremely hypoxic blood caused a significant erythropoietic stimulating activity to appear in the perfusate. In our laboratory, venous blood was used to perfuse dog kidneys in situ (Pavlovic-Kentera et al. 1965) (Fig. 3). The unilateral perfusion was carried out at normal flow rates, and the dogs were artificially ventilated to maintain a constant oxygen saturation. When the perfusion was continued for periods of more than 3 h, increased Ep levels were found in the renal vein blood of the perfused kidney. Similar results, using isolated calf kidneys, have been described (Warter et al. 1962). Erslev reviewed the subject in 1974.

The Ep activity of tissue extracts have been extensively investigated. In early experiments, normal and anemic kidney extracts were found to exert erythropoietic effects (Giono et al. 1962; Milliez et al. 1962; Naets 1960b; Piha 1962; Zangheri et al. 1962). In addition to the direct production of Ep, it was hypothesized that the kidney produced an enzyme, erythrogenin, which interacted with another protein, erythropoietinogen, to form Ep (Contrera and Gordon 1966). Others hypothesized that the kidney produced a proerythropoietin (Peschle and Condorelli 1975). In spite of early studies indicating that Ep could be extracted from kidneys, it remained a matter of controversy (see Jelkman 1986). However, in 1978, Sherwood and Goldwasser found that Ep could be extracted from whole kidney homogenates in isotonic buffered saline. Fried et al. (1981) suggested that the subcellular components needed to be kept in suspension to yield Ep in extract. Other investigators have used different stimuli to produce Ep in kidney extracts, including carbon monoxide, hypotonic hypoxia, bleeding, cobalt, and intrarenal nickel subsulfide (Jelkmann 1986).

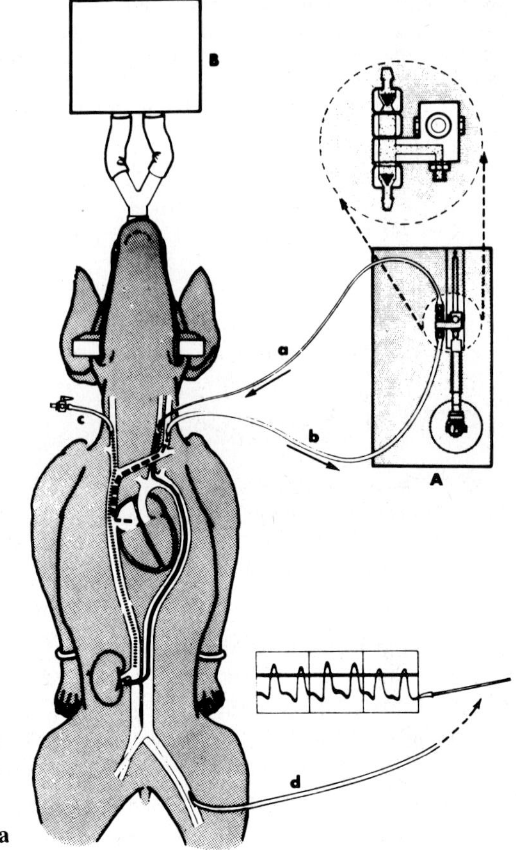
B
a
b
c
d
A

a

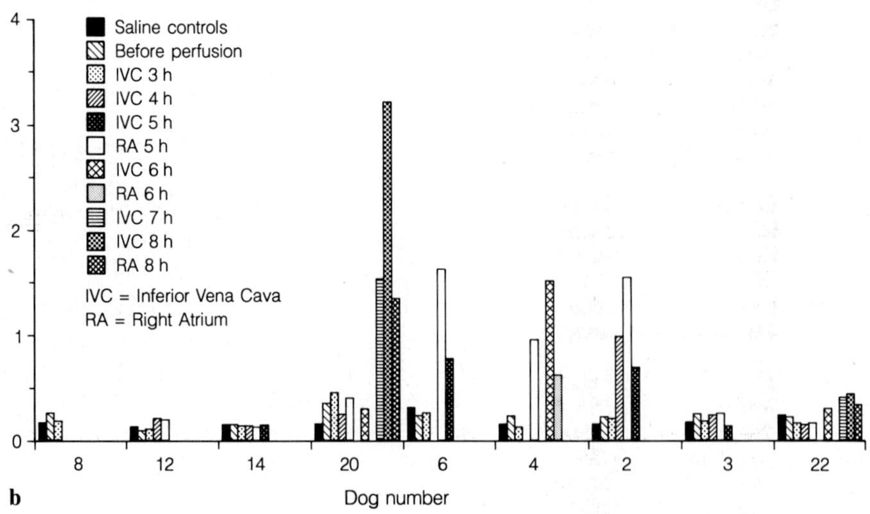
4
3
2
1
0
Saline controls
Before perfusion
IVC 3 h
IVC 4 h
IVC 5 h
RA 5 h
IVC 6 h
RA 6 h
IVC 7 h
IVC 8 h
RA 8 h
IVC = Inferior Vena Cava
RA = Right Atrium
8
12
14
20
6
4
2
3
22
Dog number

b

Since Ep could be extracted from kidneys flushed free of blood, it would seem incontestable that it was contained in the kidney itself and not in trapped plasma (JELKMANN and BAUER 1981).

The presence of Ep in the supernatant of a culture of renal cells provides further evidence for the kidney's contribution to production. OZAWA (1967) contributed one of the first reports of the in vitro production of Ep. He cocultured kidney cortical tissue with bone marrow. Preliminary results of Ep production by bovine kidney cells were reported by McDONALD et al. (1969). In 1972, BURLINGTON et al. reported the use of goat renal glomeruli. The in vitro formation of a protein believed to be Ep by sections of sheep kidney medulla incubated in the presence of 20 naturally occurring amino acids was reported by CHOWDHURY and DATTA (1973). The subject of in vitro production was reviewed by OGLE et al. (1978). They concluded that it was possible to produce, almost routinely, small quantities of Ep in tissue culture.

Clinical medicine has also provided indirect evidence for the renal production of Ep. The low Ep titers in patients with CRD have already been mentioned. It has been seen that the depressed erythropoiesis manifested by low hematocrits is restored by successful kidney transplantation (HOFFMAN 1968). Patients who are anephric have a more depressed erythropoiesis than those in whom the kidneys have been left in place (LAURENT et al. 1974). In approximately 17%, polycythemia develops posttransplantation. This is thought to be due to the production of Ep (WU et al. 1973), but it may stem from other causes (THORLING 1972). Approximately 3% of the patients with renal carcinoma have an associated polycythemia. It should be noted that a variety of other renal lesions may be associated with an elevated red cell mass. The subject was reviewed by MURPHY et al. in 1968.

Ep has been translated in nude mice transplanted with renal carcinoma cells (KATSUOKA 1976; TAMAOKI et al. 1977; TOYAMA et al. 1979; YOSHIMURA et al. 1978; KATSUOKA et al. 1983). MACH et al. (1983) microinjected mRNA extracted from the kidneys of hypoxic rats into frozen oocytes to produce Ep, and in the same year mRNA from the kidneys of anemic baboons was translated (FARBER and ZANJANI 1983). SAITO et al. (1985) reported the translation of mRNA from renal tumor cells maintained in nude mice.

In an interesting group of experiments, HOPFER and coworkers have used intrarenal injections of nickel subsulfide to produce an erythrocytosis in rats and found an increased Ep activity (HOPFER et al. 1979; McCULLY et al. 1982). They later correlated the carcinogenic activity of nickel compounds

---

Fig. 3. a. Technique of right atrial to renal artery perfusion. *A*, Brewer automatic pipetting machine; *B*, Harvard respirators; *a*, perfusion catheter to renal artery; *b*, venous intake from right atrium; *c*, sampling catheter in the inferior vena cava at entry of renal vein; *d*, femoral artery pressure monitor. **b.** Radioiron incorporation into red blood cells of transfused polycythemic mice treated with plasma obtained from the inferior vena cava or right atrium of dogs with localized hypoxia of one kidney (from PAVLOVIC-KENTERA et al. 1965, with permission)

and their potencies for stimulating erythropoiesis (SUNDERMAN and HOPFER 1983). Nine of the 17 particulate nickel compounds led to an increase in hematocrit in their Fischer rats, while 14 led to development of a sarcoma at the injection site. A statistically significant rank correlation ($P < 0.0002$) was observed between the mean hematocrits at 1–4 months after intrarenal injection of nickel compounds and the incidence of sarcoma at 1 year after intramuscular injection.

In 1964, LANGE and PAVLOVIC-KENTERA stated in their review of Ep that "Although the kidney is considered to be the main source of erythropoietin, the cellular site of production is not known." The same statement can be made in 1988. In their 1964 article, they mentioned five potential sites of production:

1. Renal cortex (SOKABE and GROLLMAN 1962)
2. Renal medulla (REISSMANN and NOMURA 1962)
3. Both cortex and medulla (MUIRHEAD et al. 1962)
4. Kidney tubules (FISHER et al. 1963)
5. Renal vasculature (KURATOWSKA et al. 1960)

Most investigators believe that the renal cortex is the most likely site of Ep production. More Ep has been shown to be extracted from the cortical than medullary portions (MUIRHEAD et al. 1968; JELKMAN and BAUER 1981; FRIED et al. 1982). Furthermore, studies showing Ep coming from the medulla may be the result of the hormone originating in tubular fluid.

Four sites of hormone production in the renal cortex have been proposed: juxtaglomerular apparatus, glomerular, tubular, and nonglomerular, nontubular.

1. *Juxtaglomerular apparatus*. OSNES in 1960 reported that when rats were bled there was a decrease in juxtaglomerular granularity and that this was corroborated by the effect of hypoxia and hypertransfusion (HIRASHIMA and TAKAKU 1962; NAKAO 1962). However, GOLDFARB and TOBIAN (1962) were unable to confirm these results.
2. *Glomerular*. There are three lines of investigation which implicate the glomeruli as the site of Ep production.
   a) Immunofluorescent studies: Using antiserum to Ep, a number of investigators have shown intense staining of glomeruli in kidneys of anemic patients and animals or animals stimulated by hypoxia. The first studies were reported by FISHER et al. in sheep in 1965 and confirmed by FRENKEL et al. in 1968. Subsequently, BUSUTTIL et al. reported similar results in human kidneys in 1971 and in hypoxic dog kidneys in 1972. GRUBER et al. used baby rats in 1977. All of these studies were performed before specific or monoclonal antibody was available and now need to be repeated.
   b) Extraction procedures: Isolated glomeruli have been subjected to hypoxia or carbon monoxide with the subsequent production of Ep

(JELKMAN et al. 1983). CARO and ERSLEV in 1984 extracted Ep from isolated glomeruli but found more hormone in their tubular fractions and favored the latter as the source of production.

c) Culture: As previously mentioned, in 1972 BURLINGTON et al. reported that isolated goat kidney glomeruli produced Ep over a period of 7 months, adding further evidence to the importance of the glomerulus as the site of production.

3. *Tubular*

a) Extraction: As mentioned above, CARO and ERSLEV extracted Ep from tubular fractions of the kidney of rats. Recently, SCHUSTER et al. (1987) found Ep mRNA in the tubular fraction but not in glomerular tissue. They concluded that its synthesis takes place in the renal tubule or its interstitium and not in the glomerular tuft.

b) Culture and nude mouse: A tubular cell line was found to produce Ep (CARO et al. 1984). It is thought that renal carcinoma cells are tubular in origin. A number of investigators have found that renal carcinoma cells produce Ep in culture and when they are transplanted into nude mice (SHERWOOD and GOLDWASSER 1976; MURPHY et al. 1970; SHERWOOD and SHOUVAL 1986; SYTKOWSKI et al. 1983; KATSUOKA et al. 1983; HAGIWARA et al. 1984a; OKABE et al. 1985). HAGIWARA et al. (1984b) also found that primary cultures could be formed after the tumor had been maintained in nude mice and that prostaglandin E_2 is important in Ep production and dome formation in the cultures.

4. *Nonglomerular, nontubular*. Recent work using hybridyzation techniques has indicated that Ep is produced in nonglomerular nontubular cells (LACOMBE et al. 1988; KOURY et al. 1987). See the following section.

The cellular site of production remains unknown:

a) In the glomerulus, BUSUTTIL et al. (1971) proposed that the visceral epithelial cells were the most likely candidate as the Ep-producing source. FISHER and BUSUTTIL (1977) later nominated the foot processes of the epithelial cells. MORI et al. (1985) thought it likely that the glomerular epithelial cells were implicated. JELKMANN and his coworkers used rat glomeruli and found evidence that the mesangial cells produced an erythropoiesis stimulating factor (KURTZ et al. 1982). Further, the production was significantly enhanced by lowering the PO_2 or by adding cobalt to their cultures (KURTZ et al. 1983b).

b) The tubular cell thought to produce Ep has not been identified, although MAXWELL et al. (1990), using oligonucleotide gene probes and immunochemical techniques, demonstrated Ep production by kidney tubular cells, as well as the translated product.

c) Recent work from two laboratories has shown that mRNA for Ep is produced in nonglomerular, nontubular cells. Using hybridization by mRNA, they found that cells located in the cortex and outer medulla reacted. They showed evidence that the cells were associated with the peritubular capillary region and were most likely endothelial cells.

LACOMBE et al. presented their results at the 1987 annual meeting of the American Society of Hematology and subsequently published their results (LACOMBE et al. 1988). At the same meeting, KOURY in Bondurant's laboratory described their experiments utilizing an RNA probe which was complementary to an mRNA coding for Ep to examine cells obtained from anemic murine kidneys (KOURY et al. 1987). They found the messenger to be present in the cortical portions of the kidney in nonglomular, nontubular cells. These cells were thought to be a subset of interstitial cells or capillary endothelial cells. In their publication, they issued a caveat in stating that a double reaction using antibodies to specific cell markers was needed, but to date, they have been unsuccessful (KOURY et al. 1988).

d) KOCHEVAR et al. (1990) in Fisher's laboratory have now shown that both glomerular epithelial cells and uncharacterized peritubular cells of anemic human kidneys contain Ep and its mRNA. They concluded that more than one type of renal cell can produce Ep and suggested that the human kidney has a layered system of production.

D. Erythropoietin in Therapy of Renal Anemia

Since Ep is known to be produced in the kidney and low circulating levels of the hormone are present in patients with ACRF, clinicians caring for such patients have looked forward to the day when the hormone would be available for clinical use. Their clinical appetites had been whetted by early human and animal studies using relatively crude Ep preparations.

REISSMANN et al. (1960) found that the injection of Ep produced significant increases in the erythropoiesis of nephrectomized and mercury-bichloride poisoned rats, but the response was substantially smaller than in ureter-ligated or sham-operated controls. NAETS (1960a) at about the same time injected Ep into a nephrectomized dog and observed an augmented cellularity of the marrow as well as increased iron utilization. Rats made uremic by subtotal nephrectomy responded to rat Ep (ANAGNOSTOU et al. 1977). In 1979, VAN STONE and MAX studied the effect of 2 U of sheep plasma Ep daily for 12 days in anemic anephric rats, which were dialyzed peritoneally. The Ep-treated rats had a significantly higher hematocrit than uremic controls which did not receive the hormone. The investigators suggested that, on the basis of their data, Ep was a potentially useful agent for the treatment of ACRF. GRETZ et al. (1987), as a result of their study of uremic rats treated with Ep, issued a caveat to watch for acute renal failure due to increased blood viscosity.

ECSHBACH et al. (1984) reported their research in which sheep were made uremic by subtotal nephrectomy. The injection of Ep-rich sheep plasma corrected the anemia in these sheep and, indeed, made them polycythemic if the injections were continued. These studies reemphasized that

Ep could correct ACRF, and further, that since both normal and uremic sheep had identical erythropoietic responses, no physiologically sig nificant erythropoietic inhibitors were present in the uremic sheep. MLADENOVIC et al. (1985) using the same model showed that the $t_{1/2}$ of Ep was independent of renal function and that Ep could be given infrequently.

In 1972, the Erythropoietin Subcommittee of the American National Institutes of Health hoped to institute a clinical trial of Ep. At the time, there was enough hormone available to treat five patients for 5 days. The trial had to be cancelled when it was discovered that the material contained pyrogens. The following year, it was shown that infusion of Ep-rich (400 ml containing 500 U of Ep) plasma caused a reticulocytosis in three normal subjects (ESSERS et al. 1973, 1975). Two nondialyzed and two dialyzed uremic patients did not respond to this dose. However, when 1870 U of Ep were given to one patient on chronic intermittent dialysis, a marked reticulocytosis ensued.

This research had shown that, in uremic animals and patients, Ep could elicit an erythropoietic response; however, it remained for the advanced technology of molecular biology to make adequate supplies of the hormone available. The seminal event in the clinical use of Ep was the production of the hormone by recombinant DNA technology. Several necessary studies paved the way for this development.

In 1977, human Ep was highly purified from the urine of patients with aplastic anemia (MIYAKI et al. 1977). Utilizing this material, the amino acid sequence was first reported in 1981 (GOLDWASSER 1981) and published by SUE and SYTKOWSKI in 1983. In 1984, YANAGAWA et al. (1984b) described a sequence of 30 amino-terminal residues derived from hormone purified by use of monoclonal antibodies (YANAGAWA et al. 1984a). It differed slightly from the original one. A molecular weight of 34000 had been assigned to the hormone (WANG et al. 1985), and a structural characterization of the urinary hormone was carried out in 1986 (LAI et al. 1986). These investigators determined the primary structure by the protein sequences, located the points of glycosylation, assigned the position of disulfide bonds, and analyzed for secondary structures by circular dichroism.

The results of cloning and expression of human Ep cDNA in *Escherichia coli* was published by LEE-HUANG in 1984. She found that the secreted hormone competed with ^{35}S-labeled, hybrid-selected translation products. This was followed by three other reports of the cloning of cDNA and expression of the human gene (JACOBS et al. 1985; LIN et al. 1985; POWELL et al. 1986), as well as the cloning and expression of the monkey gene (LIN et al. 1986) and mouse gene (SHOEMAKER and MITSOCK 1986; MCDONALD et al. 1986).

JACOBS et al. (1985) remarked that their 166-amino acid sequence differed from the previously published sequences. Since their protein backbone had a M_r of 18398, they assumed that half of the Ep molecule must consist of carbohydrates. LIN and his coworkers (1985) found the gene to contain intervening sequences and five exons, encoding a 27-amino acid signal peptide. They also noted 166 amino acids in the mature protein. When introduced into Chinese hamster ovary cells, the expressed product was biologically active in vivo and in vitro. The Ep gene, together with a marker, were cotransfected into monkey kidney cells and baby hamster kidney cells by POWELL et al. (1986). A hybridization analysis of DNA from human chromosomes provided evidence that the human gene is located on chromosome 7. This has been confirmed by two other groups (WATKINS et al. 1986; LAW et al. 1986). The gene from the cynomolgus monkey was isolated from a kidney cDNA library (LIN et al. 1986) and was found to encode a 168-amino acid mature protein and signal peptide of 24 amino acids. When expressed in Chinese hamster ovary cells, a 34000 M_r, biologically active, glycosylated protein was expressed, which demonstrated over 90% homology to the human gene. SHOEMAKER and MITSOCK (1986) demonstrated the mouse Ep coding sequence to be 80% conserved when compared with the human, and the transcription control region was over 90% conserved between the murine and human genes. BERU et al. (1987) and MCDONALD et al. (1986) also examined the mouse Ep gene for its homology with human and found overall general conservation. They looked at different tissues for gene expression after stressing the animal by bleeding. The message was found only in the kidney.

Four reports have characterized the chemical structure and biological effects of the recombinant hormone (EGRIE et al. 1986; DAVIS et al. 1987; SASAKI et al. 1987; GOTO et al. 1988). EGRIE and associates (1986) found the recombinant hormone to be biologically active. DAVIS et al. (1987) used physicochemical techniques, including circular dichroism, luminescence spectroscopy, gel filtration, and sedimentation equilibrium, to characterize human Ep produced in Chinese hamster ovary cells. They showed a conformation identical with the natural product but found an M_r of 30400 ± 400 and a carbohydrate content of 39%. SASAKI and his coworkers (1987) looked at the carbohydrate structure of human recombinant Ep (rHuEp) also expressed in Chinese hamster ovary cells. They found the carbohydrate moiety of the recombinant hormone to be quite similar to the urinary hormone except for the degree of sialylation. The major carbohydrate units were found to be tetraantennary saccharides with or without *N*-acetyl lactosamine repeats. GOTO et al. (1988) observed that the carbohydrates attached to the Ep peptide were responsible for the different biological activities.

The means were now at hand to produce enough hormone to use clinically. The first reports of the clinical use of rHuEp appeared in 1986 and early 1987 (WINEARLS et al. 1986; ESCHBACH et al. 1987). These trials had been preceded by pharmokinetic studies of intravenous (IV) and subcutaneous (SC) injections of rHuEp in 32 normal men. In these studies, an erythroid response was found after either IV or SC injections, and no adverse reactions occured. In particular, there were no changes in hemodynamic parameters or in the systolic or diastolic blood pressures.

The original phase I and II studies mentioned above have been followed by the treatment of over 500 patients worldwide (ADAMSON et al. 1987). Almost universally, treatment with rHuEp has been succeeded by a reticulocytosis and an increase in hemoglobin and hematocrit. These parameters demonstrate a dose-response relationship. MCMAHON et al. (1987) at the American Society of Hematology reported on the pharmokinetics of IV and SC administered recombinant Ep in normal men. They did not find any changes in the hemodynamic parameters of blood pressure.

Most of the patients requiring transfusions to maintain their red blood counts were able to forego further transfusions. Accompanying these changes was an increase in ferrokinetics with a decrease in serum ferritin (STUTZ et al. 1987; ESCHBACH and ADAMSON 1987), and indeed, the only patients who failed to have a RBC response have an iron deficiency. In one study, the erythroid progenitors (BFU-E, CFU-E) decreased when the patients were being treated with Ep; however, the number of cells in S phase increased (REID et al. 1987).

Ep has been shown to have an effect not only on erythroid progenitors but also on megakaryocytes and platelet formation (ISHIBASHI et al. 1987). In addition, patients with uremia have prolonged bleeding times and reduced platelet adhesion to arterial subendothelium (LIVIO et al. 1982; DEYKIN 1983; LIVIO et al. 1985). The treatment with Ep was followed by a decrease in the bleeding time and an improvement in platelet adhesion (MOIA et al. 1987; MANNUCCI et al. 1987). In one study, the mean platelet count increased from 209 to 239 with $P < 0.01$ (BOMMER et al. 1987). JACQUOT et al. (1988) have added desmopressin to Ep to improve further the hemostatic defect.

In addition to the hematologic effects, most patients describe an increased feeling of well-being (CASATI et al. 1987) with a reduction in asthenia and fatigue and a stimulation of appetite (BOMMER et al. 1987). Of BOMMER's male patients, three reported improved sexual function. Six of their seven patients had amelioration of their Raynaud's phenomenon as the hematocrits improved. In general, blood chemical values remain unchanged, but CASATI et al. (1987) found a rise in serum potassium level. However, ESCHBACH and ADAMSON (1987), in their report on 247 treated patients, uncovered no increases in blood urea nitrogen (BUN), creatinine, or potassium values and, significantly, no formation of antibodies to Ep.

In CASATI's (1987) series of 14 patients, 3 noted bone pain, fever, sweating, abdominal cramps, and "flu-like" symptoms within 2 h after Ep injection. The symptoms disappeared in 10–12 h. The most serious complications are related to vascular events. Among ESCHBACH and ADAMSON's (1987) 247 patients, 13 suffered cerebral seizures. Thrombosis of arteriovenous fistulas has been reported (CASATI et al. 1987; WINEARLS et al. 1986; AHMAD and HAND 1987). Frequently, a rise in blood pressure is noted, which may be due to an increase in viscosity from the greater RBC mass (NEFF et al. 1971) or to an increase in arterial resistance (COLEMAN 1972). NEFF, in particular, observed an elevation in peripheral vascular resistance and diastolic hypertension when his dialysis patients were transfused to increase their hematocrits from 20% to 40% over a 3-week period. TOMSON et al. (1988) and EDMUNDS and WALLS (1988) have reported cases of hypertensive encephalopathy in Ep-treated patients. However, JACQUOT et al. (1987) found no increased risk in their hemodialyzed patients treated with Ep. MAYER et al. (1988) stated that patients on hemodialysis with nearly normal hematocrits are not at higher risk for untoward cardiovascular events and that the rise in blood pressure in hypotensive patients improved their quality of life. One of the major advances in dialysis therapy has been the technique of high flux hemodialysis and hemofiltration (WALCZYK and GOLPER 1987). Since maximum dialysis efficiency requires higher rates of blood flow, the increased hematocrit following Ep therapy may lead to an increase in dialysis time, which may be contraproductive in some patients.

The dosages of rHuEp used have varied widely. In the most recent report of ESCHBACH and ADAMSON, the initial doses were 150–300 U/kg given 3 times a week. A dose of approximately 100 U/kg administered IV 3 times a week is satisfactory in most patients for maintenance therapy. Since iron stores decrease with an increased level of erythropoiesis and as many patients have a degree of iron insufficiency, iron supplements need to be given. Patients on antihypertensive medication require close blood pressure monitoring, and their antihypertensive medications may have to be increased. The tendency towards thromboembolism also must be watched carefully.

The evidence that rHuEp can successfully be used to increase the hematocrit of uremic patients on hemodialysis is incontestable. This has been supported in several symposia and review articles published recently (KURTZMAN ed. 1989; ESCHBACH ed. 1989; FISHER 1989; GRABER and KRANTZ 1989; KEOWN (1989); ECSHBACH et al. 1989). Its success is now leading to trials in other anemic patients, such as those with the anemia of chronic disorders like rheumatoid arthritis (MEANS et al. 1987; GRABER and KRANTZ 1989), and as fetal hemoglobin formation is stimulated in baboons (AL-KHATTI et al. 1987), it shows promise in the therapy of sickle cell anemia patients. It has also been found to be useful in patients with AIDS treated with zidovudine (FISCHL et al. 1990), as well as accelerating erythropoiesis perioperatively, thus possibly reducing the requirements for homologous blood transfusions (LEVINE et al. 1989).

In 1987, ERSLEV concluded his editorial with the following statement, "Even if erythropoietin does not eliminate anemia but only ameliorates it, rEpo must now be ranked as yet another new and important therapeutic agent made available through the wizardry of molecular biology."

E. Conclusions

This chapter has briefly reviewed the methods used for the assay of Ep and called attention to the fact that the values found in the literature depend on the method used for assay. The earliest assays were based on biological methods, whereas most current studies use RIAs.

Although many factors, such as hemolysis, blood loss, and multiple causes for decreased production of RBCs, contribute to the pathogenesis of ACRF, the principle cause of the anemia remains the decreased production of Ep.

The evidence for the kidney production of Ep is based on extirpation experiments, extraction procedures, clinical medical reports of low Ep levels in uremic patients, and the production of Ep in vitro by culture of Ep-producing cells. The most recent studies have presented suggestions that the Ep-producing cells are nonglomerular and nontubular and are most likely endothelial in origin.

A seminal event in the therapeutic use of Ep in uremic patients has been the development of recombinant hormone. Ep has now been used in the treatment of thousands of dialyzed patients with almost universal improvement in the ACRF. The bleeding tendency of some patients decreased after treatment. Most patients have had no untoward effects, although in a few, hypertensive encephalopathy episodes have been noted. Due to increased iron requirements, supplements should be used.

Acknowledgments. I greatly appreciate the editorial assistance of Mr. F.J. Miller, the stenographic work of Ms. Lucy Simpson, and the staff of the Preston Medical Library for aid in checking the bibliography.

References

Adamson JE, Teehan BP, Krantz SB (1987) Clinical experience with erythropoietin in pre-dialysis patients: reports from three centers. Symposium on recent advances in the treatment and prevention of amemia, Dec 4th. Washington, DC (unpublished)

Ahmad R, Hand M (1987) Recombinant erythropoietin for anemia of chronic renal failure. N Engl J Med 317:169–170

Alexanian R (1973) Erythropoietin excretion in bone marrow failure and hemolytic anemia. J Lab Clin Med 82:438–445

Al-Khatti A, Fritsch E, Papayannopolou T, Stamatoyannopoulos G (1987) Erythropoietin stimulates fetal hemoglobin in macaques and produces an additive Hb F induction in baboons treated with hydroxyurea. Blood 70[Suppl 1]:146a(441)

Anagnostou A, Barone J, Kedo A, Fried W (1977) Effect of erythropoietin therapy on the red cell volume of uraemic and non-uraemic rats. Br J Haematol 37:85–91

Asaba H, Bergstrom J, Lundgren G (1977) Hypersequestration of ^{51}Cr-labelled erythrocytes as a criterion for splenectomy in regular hemodialysis patients. Clin Nephrol 8:304–307

Bennett RM, Holt PJL, Lewis SM (1974) Role of the reticuloendothelial system in the anaemia of rheumatoid arthritis. A study using the ^{59}Fe-labelled dextran model. Ann Rheum Dis 33:147–152

Bentley DP, Cavill I, Ricketts C, Peake S (1979) A method for the investigation of reticuloendothelial iron kinetics in man. Br J Haematol 43:619–624

Berne TV, Bischel MD, Payne JE, Barbour BH (1973) Selective splenectomy in chronic renal failure. Am J Surg 126:271–276

Beru N, McDonald J, Goldwasser E (1987) Expression of the erythropoietin gene. Blood Cells 13:263–268

Besarab A, Caro J, Jarrell BE, Francos G, Erslev AJ (1987) Dynamics of erythropoiesis following renal transplantation. Kidney Int 32:526–536

Bessler H, Notti I, Djaldetti M (1980) Quantitative determination of human plasma erythropoietin using embryonic mouse liver erythroblasts. Acta Haematol 63:204–210

Birgegård G, Hallgren R, Caro J (1987) Serum erythropoietin in rheumatoid arthritis and other inflammatory arthritides: relationship to anaemia and effect of anit-inflammatory treatment. Br J Haematol 65:479–483

Bischel MD, Neiman RS, Berne TV, Telfer N, Lukes RJ, Barbour BH (1971) The elimination by splenectomy of blood transfusion requirements, leucopenia and thrombocytopenia in a patient of RTD. Proc Eur Dial Transplant Assoc 8:81

Blumenkrantz MJ, Shapiro DJ, Swendseid ME, Kopple JD (1974) The effect of histidine supplementation of the anemia of uremia. Proc Clin Dial Transplant Forum 4:152–155

Bommer J, Muller-Buhl E, Ritz E, Eifert J (1987) Recombinant human erythropoietin in anaemic patients on haemodialysis. Lancet 1:392

Bonomini V, Orsoni G, Stefoni S, Vangelista A (1979) Hormonal changes in uremia. Clin Nephrol 11:275–280

Boxer M, Ellman L, Gelter R, Wang C (1977) Anemia in primary hyperparathyroidism. Arch Int Med 137:588–593

Brown R (1965) Plasma erythropoietin in chronic uraemia. Br Med J 2:1036–1038

Burlington H, Cronkite EP, Reincke U, Zanjani ED (1972) Erythropoietin production in cultures of goat renal glomeruli. Proc Natl Acad Sci USA 69: 3547–3550

Busuttil RW, Roh RL, Fisher JW (1971) The cytological localization of erythropoietin in the human kidney using the fluorescent antibody technique. Proc Soc Exp Biol Med 137:327–330

Busuttil RW, Roh BL, Fisher JW (1972) Localization of erythropoietin in the glomerulus of the hypoxic dog kidney using a fluorescent antibody technique. Acta Haematol 47:238–242

Carlson DJ, Shapiro FL (1970) Methemoglobinemia from well water nitrates. A complication of home dialysis. Ann Int Med 73:757–759

Caro J, Erslev AJ (1984) Biologic and immunologic erythropoietin in extracts from hypoxic whole rat kidneys and in their glomerular and tubular fractions. J Lab Clin Med 103:922–931

Caro J, Brown S, Miller O, Murray T, Erslev AJ (1979) Erythropoietin levels in uremic, nephric and anephric patients. J Lab Clin Med 93:449–458

Caro J, Hickey J, Erslev AJ (1984) Erythropoietin production by an established kidney proximal tubule cell line ($LLCPK_1$). Exp Hematol 12:357 (abstr)

Cartwright GE (1966) The anemia of chronic disorders. Semin Hematol 3:351–375

Cartwright GE, Lee GR (1971) The anaemia of chronic disorders. Br J Haematol 21:147–150

Casati S, Passerini P, Compise MR, Graziani G, Cesana B, Perisic M, Ponticelli C (1987) Benefits and risks of protracted treatment with human recombinant erythropoietin in patients having haemodialysis. Br Med J 295:1017–1020

Casteliani A, Cristinelli L, Mileti M, Brandi F (1977) Beneficial and detrimental effects of hemodialysis on uremic anemia. Kidney Int 11:142 (abstr)

Cavill I, Ricketts C, Napier JAF (1977) Erythropoiesis in the anaemia of chronic disease. Scand J Hematol 19:509–512

Chandra M, Miller ME, Garcia JF, Mossey RT, McVicar M (1985) Serum immunoreactive erythropoietin levels in patients with polycystic kidney disease as compared with other hemodialysis patients. Nephron 39:26–29

Chandra M, McVicar M, Clemons G, Mossey RT, Wilkes BM (1987) Role of erythropoietin in the reversal of anemia of renal failure with continuous ambulatory peritoneal dialysis. Nephron 46:312–315

Chowdhury RR, Datta AG (1973) Studies on the in vitro formation of erythropoietin in sheep kidney medulla and the effect of cobalt thereon. Biochem Biophys Res Commun 52:1329–1337

Cohen RA, Clemons G, Ebbe S (1985) Correlation between bioassay and radioimmunoassay for erythropoietin in human serum and urine concentrates. Proc Soc Exp Biol Med 179:296–299

Coleman TG (1972) Hemodynamics of uremic anemia. Circulation 45:510–511

Contrera JF, Gordon AS (1966) Erythropoietin: production by a particulate fraction of rat kidney. Science 152:653–654

Cotes PM (1982) Immunoreactive erythropoietin in serum. 1. Evidence for the validity of the assay method and the physiological relevance of estimates. Br J Haematol 50:427–438

Cotes PM (1983) Erythropoietin. In: Gray CH, James VHT (eds) Hormones in blood. Academic, London, pp 195–218

Cotes PM, Brozovic B, Mansell M, Samson DM (1980) Radioimmunoassay of erythropoietin (Ep) in human serum. Validation and application of an assay system. Exp Hematol 8[Suppl 8]:292 (abstr)

Cotes PM, Canning CE, Goines Dos RD (1982) Modification of a radioimmunoassay for serum erythropoietin to provide increased sensitivity and investigate non-specific serum responses. In: Hunter WM, Carrie JET (eds) Immunoassays in clinical chemistry. Churchill Livingstone, Edinburgh, pp 106–112, 124–127

Davies S, Glynne-Jones E, Bisson M, Bisson P (1975) Plasma erythropoietin assay in patients with chronic renal failure. J Clin Pathol 28:875–878

Davis JM, Arakawa T, Strickland TW, Yphantis DA (1987) Characterization of recombinant human erythropoietin produced in Chinese hamster ovary cells. Biochemistry 26:2633–2638

de Klerk G, Otten-Kruiswijk C, Goudsmit R (1977) Factors in human serum influencing its dose-response curve in the bioassay for erythropietin using mouse fetal liver cells. Br J Haematol 35:672 (abstr)

de Klerk G, Hart AAM, Kruiswijk C, Goudsmit R (1978) Modified method of erythropoietin (ESF) bioassay in vitro using mouse fetal liver cells. II. Measurement of ESF in human serum. Blood 52:569–577

de Klerk G, Wilmink JM, Rosengarten PCJ, Vet RJWM, Goudsmit R (1982) Serum erythropietin (ESF) titers in anemia of chronic renal failure. J Lab Clin Med 100:720–734

Delwiche F, Garrity MJ, Powell JS, Robertson RP, Adamson JW (1983) High levels of the circulating from of parathyroid hormone do not inhibit in vitro erythropoiesis. J Lab Clin Med 102:613–620

Delwiche F, Segal GM, Eschbach JW, Adamson JW (1986) Hematopoietic inhibitors in chronic renal failure: lack of in vitro specificity. Kidney Int 29:641–648

Desforges JF (1970) Anemia in uremia. Arch Int Med 126:808–811

Desforges JF, Dawson JP (1958) The anemia of renal failure. Arch Int Med 101:326–332

Deykin D (1983) Uremic bleeding. Kidney Int 24:698–705

Douglas SW, Adamson JW (1975) The anemia of chronic disorders. Studies of marrow regulation and iron metabolism. Blood 45:55–65

Dukes PP, Shore NA, Hammond D, Ortega JA, Data MC (1973) Enhancement of erythropoiesis by prostaglandins. J Lab Clin Med 82:704–712

Dunn CDR, Do N (1979) The stability of erythroid stimulating activity in normal human serum. Biochem Med 21:190–195

Dunn CDR, Lange RD (1980) Erythropoietin assay and characterization. In: Roath

S (ed) Topical reviews in hematology 1. John Wright and Sons, Bristol, pp 1–32

Dunn CDR, Trent D (1981) The effect of parathyroid hormone on erythropoiesis in serum free cultures of fetal mouse liver cells. Proc Soc Exp Biol Med 166: 556–561

Dunn CDR, Preston J, Lange RD (1977) Serum erythropoietin titers during bed rest. In: Johnson PC, Mitchell C (eds) Final report of Johnson Space Center/ Methodist Hospital 28-day bed rest simulation of skylab, vol. II. The Lyndon B Johnson Space Center, Houston, publ numb NAS 9-14578, p D60

Dunn CDR, Lange RD, Jones JB (1979) Evidence that the fetal mouse liver cell assay detects erythroid regulatory factors (ERF) not measured with a standard in vivo assay. Exp Hematol 7:519–523

Eaton JW, Kolpin CF, Swafford HS, Kjellstrand C-M, Jacob HS (1973) Chlorinated urban water: a cause of dialysis- induced hemolytic anemia. Science 181: 463–464

Edmunds ME, Walls J (1988) Letter to editor. Lancet I:352

Egrie JC, Strickland TW, Lane J, Aoki K, Cohen AM, Smalling R, Trail G, Lin FK, Browne JK, Hines DK (1986) Characterization and biological effects of recombinant human erythropoietin. Immunobiology 172:213–224

Egrie JC, Cotes PM, Lane J, Gaines Das RE, Tam RC (1987) Development of radio-immunoassays for human erythropoietin using recombinant erythropoietin as tracer and immunogen. J Immounol Methods 99:235–241

Erslev AJ (1974) In vitro production of erythropoietin by kidneys perfused with a serum-free solution. Blood 44:77–85

Erslev AJ (1975) The effect of uremic toxins on the production and metabolism of erythropoietin. Kidney Int 7:S129–S133

Erslev A (1987) Erythropoietin coming of age. N Engl J Med 316:101–103

Erslev AJ, Caro J (1987) Erythropoietin titers in response to anemia or hypoxia. Blood Cells 13:207–216

Erslev AJ, McKenna PJ, Capelli JP, Hamburger RJ, Cohn HE, Clark JE (1968) Rate of red cell production in two nephrectomized patients. Arch Int Med 122:230–235

Erslev AJ, Caro J, Kansu E, Miller O, Cobb E (1979) Plasma erythropoietin in polycythemia. Am J Med 66:243–247

Erslev AJ, Caro J, Miller O, Silver R (1980) Plasma erythropoietin in health and disease. Ann Clin Lab Sci 10:250–257

Eschbach JW (ed) (1989) Recominant human erythropoietin therapy: overall approach to the anemia of chronic renal failure. Am J Kidney Dis 14[Suppl]: 1–25

Eschbach JW, Adamson JW (1973) Improvement in the anemia of chronic renal failure with fluoxymesterone. Ann Int Med 78:527–532

Eschbach JW, Adamson JW (1987) Correction of the anemia of hemodialysis (HD) patients with recombinant erythropoietin (rHuEpo). Blood 70[Suppl 1]: 134a(392)

Eschbach JW Jr, Funk D, Adamson J, Kuhn I, Scribner BH, Finch CA (1967) Erythropoiesis in patients with renal failure undergoing chronic dialysis. N Engl J Med 276:653–658

Eschbach JW, Adamson JW, Cook JD (1970) Disorders of red blood cell production in uremia. Arch Intern Med 126:812–815

Eschbach JW, Mladenovic J, Garcia JF, Wahl PW, Adamson JW (1984) The anemia of chronic renal failure in sheep: response to erythropoietin-rich plasma in vivo. J Clin Invest 74:434–441

Eschbach JW, Egrie JC, Downing MR, Browne JK, Adamson JW (1987) Correction of the anemia of end-stage renal disease with recombinant human erythropoietin. Results of a combined phase I and II clinical trial. N Engl J Med 316:73–78

Eschbach JW, Abdulhadi MH, Browne JK, Delano BG, Downing MR, Egrie JC et al. (1989) Recombinant human erythropoietin in anemic patients with end-stage renal disease. Results of a phase III multicenter clinical trial. Ann Int Med 111:992–1000

Essers U, Muller W, Brunner E (1973) Zur Wirkung von Erythropoietin bei Gesunden und bei Patienten mit chronischer Uramie. Klin Wochenschr 51: 1005–1009

Essers U, Muller W, Heintz R (1975) Effect of erythropoietin in normal men and in patients with renal insufficiency. Proc Eur Dial Transplant Assoc 11:398–402

Falko JM, Guy JT, Smith RE, Mazzaferri EL (1976) Primary hyperparathyroidism and anemia. Arch Intern Med 136:887–889

Farber NM, Zanjani ED (1983) Translation of mRNA from anemic baboon kidney into biologically active erythropoietin. Exp Hematol 11[Suppl 14]:57 (abstr)

Firkin FC, Russell SH (1983) Influence of human serum components on measurement of erythropoietin biological activity in vitro. Studies with a rabbit bone marrow bioassay procedure. Scand J Haematol 31:349–358

Fischl M, Galpin JE, Levine JD, Groopman JE, Henry DH, Kennedy P. Miles S, Robbins W, Starrett B, Zalusky R, Abels RJ, Tsai HC, Rudnick SA (1990) Recombinant human erythropoietin for patients with AIDS treated with zidovudine. N Engl J Med 322:1488–1493

Fisher JW (chair) (1989) NKF position paper. Statement on the clinical use of recombinant erythropoietin in anemia of end-stage renal disease. Am J Kidney Dis 14:163–169

Fisher JW, Busuttil RS (1977) Sites of production of erythropoietin. In:Fisher JE (ed) Kidney hormones, vol II. Academic Press, London, pp 165–186

Fisher JW, Gross DM (1977) Hormonal influence on erythropoiesis: anterior pituitary, adrenocortical, thyroid, growth and other hormones. In: Fisher JE (ed) Kidney hormones, vol II. Academic Press, London, pp 415–435

Fisher JW, Knight DB, Couch C (1963) The influence of several diuretic drugs on erythropoietin formation. J Pharmacol Exp Ther 141:113–121

Fisher JW, Taylor G, Porteous DD (1965) Localization of erythropoietin in glomeruli of sheep kidney by fluorescent antibody technique. Nature 205:611–612

Fisher JW, Roh BL, Halvorsen S (1967) Inhibition of erythropoietic effects of hormones by ertythropoietin antisera in mildly plethoric mice. Proc Soc Exp Biol Med 126:97–100

Fisher JW, Hatch FE, Roh BL, Allen RC, Kelley BJ (1968) Erythropoietin inhibitor in kidney extracts and plasma from anemic uremic human subjects. Blood 31:440–452

Fisher JW, Modder BH, Foley JE, Ohno Y, Rege AB (1977) The role of erythropoietin and inhibitors of erythropoiesis in the mechanism of the anemia of renal insufficiency. In: Fisher JE (ed) Kidney hormones, vol II. Academic, London, pp 551–570

Fisher JW, Ohno Y, Barona J, Martinez M, Rege AB (1978) Role of erythropoietin and inhibitors of erythropoiesis in the anemia of renal insufficiency. Dialysis and Transplantation 7:472–481

Forman S, Bischel M, Hochstein P (1973) Erythrocyte deformability in uremic hemodialyzed patients. Ann Intern Med 79:841–843

Freedman MH, Cattran DC, Saunders EF (1983a) Anemia of chronic renal failure: inhibition of erythropoiesis by uremic serum. Nephron 35:15–19

Freedman MH, Saunders EF, Cattran DC, Rabin EZ (1983b) Ribonuclease inhibition of erythropoiesis in anemia of uremia. Am J Kidney Dis 2:530–533

Freireich EJ, Miller A, Emerson CP, Ross JF (1957) The effect of inflammation on the utilization of erythrocyte and transferrin bound radioiron for red cell production. Blood 12:972–983

Frenkel EP, Suki W, Baum J (1968) Some observations on the localization of erythropoietin. Ann NY Acad Sci 149:292–293

Fried W (1975) Erythropoietin and the kidney. Nephron 15:327–349

Fried W, De Gowin R, Gurney CW (1964) Erythropoietic effect of testosterone in the polycythemic mouse. Proc Soc Exp Biol Med 117:839–842

Fried W, Barone-Varelas J, Berman M (1981) Detection of high erythropoietin titers in renal extracts of hypoxic rats. J Lab Clin Med 97:82–86

Fried W, Barone-Varelas J, Barone T (1982) The influence of age and sex on erythropoietin titers in the plasma and tissue homogenates of hypoxic rats. Exp Hematol 10:472–477

Gallagher NI, McCarthy JM, Hart KT, Lange RD (1959) Evaluation of plasma erythropoietic-stimulating factors in anemic uremic patients. Blood 14:662–667

Gallagher NI, McCarthy JM, Lange RD (1960) Observations on erythropoietic-stimulating factor (ESF) in the plasma of uremic and nonuremic anemic patients. Ann Intern Med 52:1201–1212

Gallagher NI, McCarthy JM, Lange RD (1961) Erythropoietin production in uremic rabbits. J Lab Clin Med 57:281–289

Garcia JF (1972a) The radioimmunoassay of human plasma erythropoietin. In: Gordon AS, Peschle C, Condorelli M (eds) Regulation of erythropoiesis. Il Ponte, Milan, pp 132–153

Garcia JF (1972b) Radioimmunoassay of erythropoietin. In: Symposium on Radioimmunoassay and related procedures in clinical medicine and research, vol 1. Int Atomic Energy Agency, Vienna, pp 275–287

Garcia JF (1977) Assays for erythropoietin. In: Fisher JE (ed) Kidney hormones, vol II. Academic, London, p 7

Garcia JF, Sherwood J, Goldwasser E (1979) Radioimmunoassay of erythropoietin. Blood Cells 5:405–419

Garcia JF, Ebbe SN, Hollander L, Cutting HO, Miller ME, Cronkite EP (1982) Radioimmunoassay of erythropoietin: circulating levels in normal and polycythemic human beings. J Lab Clin Med 99:624–635

Giono H, Manoussos G, Dormand Y, Thuillier Y (1962) Étude chez le rat de l'activité erythropoietique d'un extrait renal. Therapie 17:349–354

Goldfarb B, Tobian L (1962) The interrelationship of hypoxia, erythropoietin and the renal juxtaglomerular cell. Proc Soc Exp Biol Med 111:510–511

Goldwasser E (1981) Erythropoietin: progress report 1981. American Society of Hematology Annual Meeting (unpublished)

Goldwasser E, Sherwood JB (1981) Radioimmunoassay of erythropoietin. Br J Haematol 48:359–363

Goto M, Akai K, Murakami A, Hashimoto C, Tsuda E, Ueda M, Kawanishi G, Takahashi N, Ishimoto A, Chiba H, Sasaki R (1988) Production of recombinant human erythropoietin in mammalian cells: host cell dependency of the biological activity of the cloned glycoprotein. Biotechnology 6:67–71

Graber SE, Krantz SB (1989) Erythropoietin biology and clinical use. Hematol Oncol Clin North Am 3:369–400

Gretz N, Lasserre JJ, Meisinger E, Strauch M, Waldherr R, Kraft K, Weidler A (1987) Potential side-effects of erythropoietin. Lancet 1:46

Gruber DF, Zucali JR, Wleklinski J, LaRussa V, Mirand EA (1977) Temporal transition in the site of rat erythropoietin production. Exp Hematol 5:399–407

Guilbert LJ, Iscove NN (1976) Partial replacement of serum by selenite transferrin, albumin and lecithin in haemopoietic cell cultures. Nature 263:594–595

Gurney CW, Jacobson LO, Goldwasser E (1958) The physiologic and clinical significance of erythropoietin. Ann Intern Med 49:363–370

Hagiwara M, Chen I-L, McGonigle R, Beckman B, Kasten FH, Fisher JW (1984a) Erythropoietin production in a primary culture of human renal carcinoma cells maintained in nude mice. Blood 63:828–835

Hagiwara M, McNamara DB, Chen I-L, Fisher JW (1984b) Role of endogenous prostaglandin E2 in erythropoietin production and dome dormation and human renal carcinoma cells in culture. J Clin Invest 74:1252–1261

Hanna W, Dunn CDR, Smith LN (1980) The anemia of uremia: erythropoietin and bone marrow culture studies. J Tenn Med Assoc 73:492–493

Hartley LC, Innis MD, Morgan TO, Clunie GJA (1971) Splenectomy for anemia in patients on regular haemodialysis. Lancet 2:1343–1345

Hemmeloff AKE (1977) Folic acid status of patients with chronic renal failure maintained by dialysis. Clin Nephrol 8:510–513

Hershko C, Cook JD, Finch CA (1974) Storage iron kinetics. VI. The effect of inflammation on iron exchange in the rat. Br J Haematol 28:67–75

Hirashima K, Takaku F (1962) Experimental studies on erythropoietin. II. The relationship between juxtaglomerular cells and erythropoietin. Blood 20:1–8

Hocken AG, Marwah PK (1971) Iatrogenic contribution to anaemia of chronic renal failure. Lancet 1:164–165

Hoffman GC (1968) Human erythropoiesis following kidney transplantation. Ann NY Acad Sci 149:504–508

Hopfer SM, Sunderman FW, Fredrickson TN, Morse EE (1979) Increased serum erythropoietin activity in rats following intrarenal injection of nickel subsulfide. Res Commun Chem Pathol Pharmacol 23:155–170

Ho-Yen DO, Saleem N, Fleming LW, Stewart WK, Goodall HB (1980) Bone marrow cellularity and iron stores in chronic renal failure. Acta Haematol 64:265–270

Horowitz HI, Stein IM, Cohen BD, White JG (1970) Further studies on the platelet inhibitory effect of guanidino-succinic acid and its role in uremic bleeding. Am J Med 49:336–345

Hotta T, Maeda H, Suzuki I, Chung TG, Saito A (1987) Selective inhibition of erythropoiesis by sera from patients with chronic renal failure. Proc Soc Exp Biol Med 186:47–51

Ishibashi T, Koziol JA, Burstein SA (1987) Human recombinant erythropoietin promotes differentiation of murine megakaryocytes in vitro. J Clin Invest 79: 286–289

Jacob HS, Eaton JW, Yawata Y (1975) Shortened red blood survival in uremic patients: beneficial and deleterious effects of dialysis. Kidney Int 2[Suppl]: 139–143

Jacobs K, Shoemaker C, Rudersdorf R, Neill SD, Kaufamn RJ, Mufson A, Seehra J, Jones SS, Hewick R, Fritsch EF, Kawakita M, Shimizu T, Miyaki T (1985) Isolation and characterization of genomic and cDNA clones of human erythropoietin. Nature 313:806–810

Jacobson LO, Goldwasser E, Fried W, Plzak L (1957) Role of the kidney in erythropoiesis. Nature 179:633–634

Jacobson LO, Goldwasser E, Gurney CW, Fried W, Plzak L (1959) Studies of erythropoietin: the hormone regulating red cell production. Ann NY Acad Sci 77:551–573

Jacobson LO, Gurney CW, Goldwasser E (1960) The control of erythropoiesis. Adv Intern Med 10:297–327

Jacquot Ch, Ferragu-Haquet M, Lefebvre A, Berthelot J-M, Peterlongo F, Castaigne JP (1987) Recombinant erythropoietin and blood pressure. Lancet 2:1083

Jacquot C, Masselot JP, Berthelot JM, Peterlongo F, Castaigne JP (1988) Addition of desmopressin to recombinant human erythropoietin in treatment of haemostatic defect of uraemia. Lancet 1:420

Jelkmann W (1986) Renal erythropoietin: properties and production. Rev Physiol Biochem Pharmacol 104:139–215

Jelkmann W, Bauer C (1981) Demonstration of high levels of erythropoietin in rat kidneys following hypoxia. Pflugers Arch 392:34–39

Jelkmann W, Kurtz A, Bauer C (1983) Extraction of erythropoietin from isolated renal glomeruli of hypoxic rats. Exp Hematol 11:581–588

Jepson J, Lowenstein L (1966) Erythropoiesis during pregnancy and lactation in the mouse. II. Role of erythropoiein. Proc Soc Exp Biol Med 121:1077–1081

Joske RA, McAlister JM, Prankerd TAJ (1956) Isotope investigations of red cell production and destruction in chronic renal disease. Clin Sci 15:511–522

Katsuoka Y, Baba S, Hata M, Tazaki H (1976) Transplantation of human renal cell carcinoma to nude mice: as an intermediate of in vivo and in vitro studies. J Urol 115:373–376

Katsuoka Y, McGonigle R, Rege AB, Beckman B, Fisher JW (1983) Erythropoietin production in human renal cell carcinoma cells passaged in nude mice and in tissue culture. Gann 74:534–541

Keown PA (1989) Canadian erythropoietin study group: recombinant human erythropoietin: from concept to clinic. Transplant Proc 21[Suppl 2]:49–53

Kimzey SL, Johnson PC, Dunn CDR (1978) The influence of space flight on erythrokinetics in man. Final report of the spacelab mission development test, vol 1. Scientific experiments. The Lyndon B Johnson Space Center, publ numb JSC-13950, Houston, p 309

Klahr S, Slatopolsky E (1986) Toxicity of parathyroid hormone in uremia. Annu Rev Med 37:71–78

Klein WJ Jr, Metz EN, Price AR (1972) Acute copper intoxication. A hazard of hemodialysis. Ann Intern Med 129:578–582

Klock JC, Williams HE, Mentzer WC (1974) Hemolytic anemia and somatic cell dysfunction in severe hypophosphatemia. Arch Intern Med 134:360–364

Koch KM, Radtke HW (1978) Absolute and relative erythropoietin deficiency in renal anemia. Contrib Nephrol 13:60–68

Kochevar J, Stanek JA, Mason-Garcia M, Fisher JW (1990) Glomerular and interstitial cell sites of erythropoietin production in anemic human kidneys. Clin Res 38:235A (abstr)

Koeffler HP, Goldwasser E (1981) Erythropoietin radioimmunoassay in evaluating patients with polycythemia. Ann Intern Med 94:44–47

Kopple JD, Mercurio K, Blumenkrantz MJ, Jones MR, Tallos J, Roberts C, Card B, Saltzman R, Casciato DA, Swendseid ME (1981) Daily requirement for pyridoxine supplements in chronic renal failure. Kidney Int 19:694–704

Koury ST, Bondurant MC, Koury MJ (1987) Localization of cells containing erythropoietin messanger RNA in the kidneys of anemic mice using in situ hybridization. Blood 1[Suppl]:176a(558)

Koury ST, Bondurant MC, Koury MJ (1988) Localization of erythropoietin synthesizing cells in murine kidneys by in situ hybridization. Blood 71:524–527

Krystal G, Eaves AC, Eaves CJ (1981a) A quantitative bioassay for erythropoietin using mouse bone marrow. J Lab Clin Med 97:144–157

Krystal G, Eaves Ac, Eaves CJ (1981b) Determination of normal human serum erythropoietin levels using mouse bone marrow. J Lab Clin Med 97:158–169

Krzymowski T, Krzymowska H (1962) Studies on the erythropoiesis inhibiting factor in the plasma of animals with transfusion polycythemia. Blood 19:38–44

Kubanck B (1969) Erythropoietin: the hematologist's hormone. Horm Metab Res 1:151–156

Kuratowska Z, Lewartowski B (1962) Studies on the active principle released by hypoxic kidney into Tyrode's solution. In: Jacobson LO, Doyle M (eds) Erythropoiesis. Grune and Stratton, New York, p 101

Kuratowska Z, Lewartowski B, Michalak E (1960) Studies on production of erythropoietin by isolated hypoxic kidney. Bull Acad Pol Sci (Serie Biol) 8:77–80. Cited in: Waldmann TA, Rosse WF (1962) Sites of formation of erythropoietin. In: Jacobson LO, Doyle M (eds) Erythropoiesis. Grune and Stratton, New York, p 87

Kuratowska Z, Lewartowski B, Michalak E (1961) Studies on the production of erythropoietin by isolated perfused organs. Blood 18:527–534

Kurtz A, Jelkmann W, Bauer C (1982) Mesangial cells derived from rat glomeruli produce an erythropoiesis stimulating factor in cell culture. FEBS Lett 137: 129–132

Kurtz A, Jelkmann W, Bauer C (1983a) Insulin stimulates erythroid colony formation independently of erythropoietin. Br J Haematol 53:311–316

Kurtz A, Jelkmann W, Sinowatz F, Bauer C (1983b) Renal mesangial cell cultures as a model for study of erythropoietin production. Proc Natl Acad Sci USA 80:4008–4011

Kurtzman NA (ed) (1989) Recombinant human erythropoietin therapy. Semin Nephrol 9[Suppl 1]:1–34

Kushner D, Nguyen L, Beckman B, Fisher JW (1988) Differential effects of spermine and spermidine on erythroid and granulocytic/macrophage colony growth. Clin Res 36:16A (abstr)

Kushner D, Nguyen L, Beckman B, Fisher JW (1989) Differential sensitivity of bone marrow erythroid (CFU-E) and myelocytic (CFU-GM) cells to polyamines and serum from patients with renal disease. FASEB J 3:A1192 (abstr 5612)

Lacombe C, Bruneval P, Da Silva JL, Camilleri JP, Bariety J, Tambourin P, Varet B (1987) Expression of the erythropoietin gene in the hypoxic adult mouse. Blood 70[Suppl 1]:176a(559)

Lacombe C, Da Silva J-L, Bruneval P. Fournier J-G, Wendling F, Casadevall N, Camilleri J-P, Bariety J, Varet B, Tambourin P (1988) Peritubular cells are the site of erythropoietin synthesis in the murine hypoxic kidney. J Clin Invest 81:620–623

LaCour B, Basile C, Drueke T (1980) Hyperparathyroidism and red cell production. Kidney Int 18:137

Lai P-H, Everett R, Wang F-F, Arakawa T, Goldwasser E (1986) Structural characterization of human erythropoietin. J Biol Chem 261:3116–3121

Lange RD, Gallagher NI (1962) Clinical and experimental observations on the relationship of the ability to erythropoietin production. In Jacobson LO and Doyle M (eds.) Erythropoiesis Grune and Stratton, New York pp 361–373

Lange RD, Ichiki AT (1977) Immunological studies of erythropoietin. In: Fisher JW (ed) Kidney hormones. II. Erythropoietin. Academic, London, pp 111–149

Lange RD, Pavlovic-Kentera V (1964) Erythropoietin. Prog Hematol 4:72–96

Lange RD, Chen JP, Dunn CDR (1980) Erythropoietin assays: some new and different approaches. Exp Hematol 8[Suppl 8]:197–223

Lappin TRJ, Elder GE, McKibbin SH, McNamee PT, McGeown MG, Bridges JM (1985) The effect of transferring saturation on the estimation of erythropoietin by the mouse spleen cell microassay. Exp Hematol 13:1007–1013

Laurent C, Wittek M, Vereerstraeten P, Toussaint C, Naets JP (1974) Red cells life span, splenic sequestration and transfusion requirements in chronic renal failure treated by hemodialysis. Effects of bilateral nephrectomy. Clin Nephrol 2:35–40

Law MR, Cai G-Y, Lin F-K, Wei Q, Huang S-Z, Hartz JH, Morse H, Lin C-H, Jones C, Kao F-T (1986) Chromosomal assignment of human erythropoietin gene and its DNA polymorphism. Proc Natl Acad Sci USA 83:6920–6924

Lee-Huang S (1984) Cloning and expression of human erythropoietin cDNA in *Escherichia coli*. Proc Natl Acad Sci USA 81:2708–2712

Lepoutre E, Moulront S, Proye C, Bauters F (1981) Insuffisance renale avec anemie sévère interel de la parathyroidectomie. Nouv Press Med 10:2669

Lertora JJL, Dargon PA, Rege AB, Fisher JW (1975) Studies on a radioimmunoassay for human erythropoietin. J Lab Clin Med 86:140–151

Levine EA, Gould SA, Rosin AL, Sehgal LR, Egrie JC, Sehgal HL, Levine HD, Moss GS (1989) Perioperative recombinant human erythropoietin. Surgery 106:432–438

Lewis JP, Neal WA, Moores RR, Gardner E Jr, Alford DA, Smith LL, Wright C-S, Welch ET (1969) A protein inhibitor of erythropoiesis. J Lab Clin Med 74: 608–613

Lin F-K, Suggs S, Lin C-H, Browne JK, Smalling R, Egrie JC, Chen KK, Fox GM, Martin F, Stabinsky Z, Badrawi SM, Lai P-H, Goldwasser E (1985) Cloning and expression of the human erythropoietin gene. Proc Natl Acad Sci USA 82: 7580–7584

Lin F-K, Lin C-H, Lai P-H, Browne JK, Egrie JC, Smalling R, Fox GM, Chen KK, Castro M, Suggs S (1986) Monkey erythropoietin gene: cloning, expression and comparison with the human erythropoietin gene. Gene 44:201–209

Lindemann R (1971) Erythropoiesis inhibiting factor (EIF). I. Fractionation and demonstration of urinary EIF. Br J Haematol 21:623–631

Linkesch W, Stummvoll HK, Wolf A, Muller M (1978) Heme synthesis in anemia of the uremic state. Isr J Med Sci 14:1173–1176

Livio M, Gotti E, Marchesi D, Mecca G, Remuzzi G, de Gaetano G (1982) Uraemic bleeding: role of anaemia and beneficial effect of red-cell transfusions. Lancet 2:1013–1015

Livio M, Benigni A, Remuzzi G (1985) Coagulation abnormalities in uremia. Semin Nephrol 5:82–90

Loge JP, Lange RD, Moore CV (1958) Characterization of the anemia associated with chronic renal insufficiency. Am J Med 24:4–18

Lord BI, Mori KJ, Wright EG, Lajtha LG (1976) An inhibitor of stem cell proliferation in normal bone marrow. Br J Haematol 34:441–445

Mach B, Ucla C, Fisher J, Zanjani ED (1983) Translation of mRNA from kidneys of hypoxic rats into biologically active erythropoietin following microinjection into frog oocytes. Clin Res 31:484A

Maezawa M, Takaku F, Muto Y, Mizoguchi H, Miura Y (1978) A case of intrarenal artery stenosis associated with erythrocytosis. Scand J Haematol 21:278–282

Mallette LE, Bilezikian JP, Heath DA, Aurbach GD (1974) Primary hyperparathyroidism: clinical and biochemical features. Medicine 53:127–146

Mann DL, Donati RM, Gallagher NI (1968) Relationship of renal mass to erythropoietin production. Lab Invest 19:406–411

Mannucci PM, Moia M, Casati S, Ponticelli C (1987) Recombinant human erythropoietin (rHuEpo) improves hemostatic abnormalities in uremics. Blood 70[Suppl 1]:138a(408)

Markson JL, Rennie JB (1956) The anemia of chronic renal insufficiency: the effect of serum from azotemic patients on maturation of erythroblasts in suspension cultures. Scott Med J 1:320–322

Mason C, Thomas TH (1984) A model for erythropoiesis in experimental chronic renal failure. Br J Haematol 58:729–740

Mason-Garcia M, Beckman BS, Brookins JW, Powell JS, Lanham W, Blaisdell S, Keay L, Li S-C, Fisher JW (1990) Development of a new radioimmunoassay for erythropoietin using recombinant erythropoietin Kidney Int 38:1–7

Massry SG, Goldstein DA (1978) Role of parathyroid hormone in uremic toxicity. Kidney Int [Suppl]8:S39–S42

Matsubara K, Yoshimura T, Kamachi S, Fukushima M, Hino M, Mori H (1989) Radioimmunoassay for erythropoietin using anti-recombinant erythropoietin antibody with high affinity. Clin Chim Acta 185:177–184

Matter BJ, Pederson J, Psimenos G, Lindeman RD (1969) Lethal copper intoxication in hemodialysis. Trans Am Soc Artif Intern Organs 15:309–315

Maxwell AP, Labbin TRJ, Johnston CF, Bridges JM, McGeown MG (1990) Erythropoietin production in kidney tubular cells. Br J Haematol 74:535–539

Mayer G, Stefenelli T, Cada EM, Thum J, Stummvoll HJ, Graf H (1988) Letter to editor. Lancet 1:351–352

McCully KS, Sunderman FW Jr, Hopfer SM, Kevorkian CB, Reid MC (1982) Effects of unilateral nephrectomy on erythrocytosis and arteriosclerosis induced in rats by intrarenal injection of nickel subsulfide. Virchows Arch [A] 397: 251–259

McDonald JD, Lin F-K, Goldwasser E (1986) Cloning, sequencing and evolutionary analysis of the mouse erythropoietin gene. Mol Cell Biol 6:842–848

McDonald TP, Martin DH, Simmons ML, Lange RD (1969) Preliminary results of erythropoietin production by bovine kidney cells in culture. Life Sci 8:949–954

McGonigle RJS, Wallin JD, Husserl F, Deftos LJ, Rice JC, O'Neill WJ Jr, Fisher JW (1984a) Potential role of parathyroid hormone as an inhibitor of erythropoiesis in the anemia of renal failure. J Lab Clin Med 104:1016–1026

McGonigle RJS, Wallin JD, Shadduck RK, Fisher JW (1984b) Erythropoietin deficiency and inhibition of erythropoiesis in renal insufficiency. Kidney Int 25:437–444

McGonigle RJS, Boineau FG, Beckman B, Ohene-Frempong K, Lewy JE, Shadduck RK, Fisher JW (1985) Erythropoietin and inhibitors of in vitro

erythropoiesis in the development of anemia in children with renal disease. J Lab Clin Med 105:449–458
McMahon RG, Ryan M, Phillips JH Jr, Abels R, Wilk K, Rudnick SA (1987) Safety and multiple dose pharmacokinetic profile of intravenous and subcutaneous recombinant human erythropoietin (rHuEpo) in normal subjects: a double-blind, placebo controlled study. Blood 70[Suppl 1]:139a(412)
Means RT, Olsen NJ, Krantz SB, Graber SE, Dessypris EN, Stone WJ, Pincus TP, O'Neil V (1987) Treatment of the anemia of rheumatoid arthritis with recombinant human erythropoiein: clinical and in vitro results. Blood 70[Suppl 1]: 139a(413)
Meytes D, Bogin E, Ma A, Dukes PP, Massry SG (1981) Effect of parathyroid hormone on erythropoiesis. J Clin Invest 67:1263–1269
Miller ME, Garcia JF, Cohen RA, Cronkite EP, Moccia G, Acevedo J (1981) Diurnal levels of immunoreactive erythropoietin in normal subjects and subjects with chronic lung disease. Br J Haematol 49:189–200
Milliez P, Lagrue G, Tcherdakoff P, Boivin P (1962) Reins et erythropoiese. Infom Med Paramed 14:1–9
Miyaki T, Kung CK-H, Goldwasser E (1977) Purification of human erythropoietin. J Biol Chem 252:5558–5564
Mladenovic J, Eschbach JW, Garcia JF, Adamson JW (1984) The anaemia of chronic renal failure in sheep: studies in vitro. Br J Haematol 58:491–500
Mladenovic J, Eschbach JW, Koup JR, Garcia JF, Adamson JW (1985) Erythropoietin kinetics in normal and uremic sheep. J Lab Clin Med 105:659–663
Moia M, Vizzotto L, Cattaneo M, Mannucci PM, Casati S, Ponticelli C (1987) Improvement in the haemostatic defect of uraemia after treatment with recombinant human erythropoietin. Lancet 2:1227–1229
Monette FC, Holden SA (1982) Hemin enhances the in vitro growth of primitive erythroid progenitor cells. Blood 60:527–530
Mori S, Saito T, Morishita Y, Saito K, Urabe A, Wakabayashi T, Takaku F (1985) Glomerular epithelium as the main locus of erythropoietin in human kidney. Jpn J Exp Med 55:69–70
Moriyama Y, Fisher JW (1975) Effects of erythropoietin on erythroid colony formation in uremic rabbit bone marrow cultures. Blood 45:659–664
Muirhead EE, Kosinski M, Jones F, Reno E (1962) Erythropoietin and the state of renal tissue. Blood 20:782 (abstr)
Muirhead EE, Leach BE, Fisher JW, Kosinski M (1968) Renal transplantation and extacts and erythropoiesis. Ann NY Acad Sci 149:135–142
Muller-Wiefel DE, Sharer K (1983) Serum erythropoietin levels in children with chronic renal failure. Kidney Int 24[Suppl 15]:S70–S76
Muller-Wiefel DE, Mehls O, Sharer K (1983) The role of hyperparathyroidism in the pathogenesis of renal anemia. Eur J Pediatr 141:63–65
Murphy GP, Mirand EA, Johnston GS, Gibbons RP, Schirmer HKA, Scott WW (1968) Erythropoietin alterations in human genitourinary disease states: correlation with experimental observations. J Urol 99:802–810
Murphy GP, Brendler H, Mirand EA (1970) Erythropoietin release from renal carcinomas grown in tissue culture. Res Commun Chem Pathol Pharmacol 1:617–626
Muto S, Asano Y, Hosoda S, Shionoya S, Miura Y, Urabe A, Takaku F (1987) Polycythemia of end-stage renal failure: no inhibition of erythropoiesis by uremic serum and markedly increased serum erythropoietin level. Nephron 46:34–36
Naets JP (1960a) The role of the kidney in erythropoiesis. J Clin Invest 39:102–110
Naets JP (1960b) Erythropoietic factor in kidney tissue of anemic dogs. Proc Soc Exp Biol Med 103:129–132
Naets JP (1975) Hematologic disorders in renal failure. Nephron 14:181–194

Naets JP, Heuse AF (1962) Effect of anaemic anoxia on erythropoiesis of nephrectomized dog. Nature 195:190

Naets JP, Garcia JF, Toussaint C, Buset M, Wakes D (1986) Radioimmunoassay of erythropoietin in chronic uraemia or anephric patients. Scand J Haematol 37:390–394

Najean Y, Messian O (1983) Anemie de l'insuffisance renale traitié par hemodialyse periodique. III. Effect de la splenectomie. Étude rétrospective de 25 cas. La Presse Medicale 12:2307–2310

Nakao K (1962) Studies on erythropoietin. Acta Haematol Jpn 25:253–279

Napier JAF, Evans J (1980) Erythropoietin assay using fetal mouse liver cell cultures: a modified technique using semi-automatic harvesting of I125 deoxyuridine labelled erythroblasts. Clin Lab Haematol 2:13–19

Napier JAF, Dunn CDR, Ford TW, Price V (1977) Pathophysiological changes in serum erythropoiesis stimulating activity. Br J Haematol 35:403–409

Neff MS, Kim KE, Persoff M, Onesti G, Swartz C (1971) Hemodynamics of uremic anemia. Circulation 43:876–883

Neff MS, Goldberg J, Slifkin RF, Eiser AR, Calamia V, Kaplan M, Baez A, Gupta S, Mattoo N (1985) Anemia in chronic renal failure. Acta Endocrinol 271[Suppl 1]:80–86

Neiman RS, Bischel MD, Lukes RJ (1973) Hypersplenism in the uremic hemodialyzed patient: pathology and proposed pathophysiologic mechanisms. Am J Clin Pathol 60:502–511

Ogle JW, Lange RD, Dunn CDR (1978) Production of erythropoietin in vitro: review. In Vitro 14:945–950

Ohno Y, Fisher JW (1977) Inhibition of bone marrow erythroid colony-forming cells (CFU-E) by serum from chronic anemic uremic rabbits. Proc Soc Exp Biol Med 156:56–59

Okabe T, Urabe A, Kato T, Chiba C, Takaku F (1985) Production of erythropoietin-like activity by human renal and hepatic carcinomas in cell culture. Cancer Res 43:1415–1419

Ortega JA, Malekzadeh MH, Dukes PP, Ma A, Pennisi AV, Fine RN, Shore NA (1977) Exceptionally high serum erythropoietin activity in an anephric patient with severe anemia. Am J Hematol 2:299–306

Osnes S (1960) Influence of the pituitary on erythropoietic principle produced in the kidney. Br Med J 1:1153–1157

Ozawa S (1967) Erythropoietin from kidney cells cultured in vitro. Keio J Med 16:193–203

Paul P, Rothmann SA, Zydiak L, Beck GJ (1987) Improved assessment of bioactive erythropoietin in human sera using a modified tritiated-thymidine incorporation assay. Exp Hematol 15:382–388

Pavlovic-Kentera V, Hall DP, Bragassa C. Lange RD (1965) Unilateral renal hypoxia and production of erythropoietin. J Lab Clin Med 65:577–588

Pavlovic-Kentera V, Ruvidic R, Milenkovic P, Marinkovic D (1979) Erythropoietin in patients with anaemia in rheumatoid arthritis. Scand J Haematol 23:141–145

Pavlovic-Kentera V, Djukanovic L, Beljanovic-Paunovic L, Stojanovic N, Milenkovic P (1987a) Inhibitors of erythropoiesis in patients with chronic renal failure. In: Najman A, Guigan M, Garin NC, Mary JY (eds) The inhibitors of hematopoiesis. Colloque INSERM. Libbey London, Paris pp 133–136

Pavlovic-Kentera V, Clemons GK, Djukanovic L, Biljanovic-Paunovic L (1987b) Erythropoietin and anemia in chronic renal failure. Exp Hematol 15:785–789

Penington DG (1961) The role of the erythropoietic hormone in anaemia. Lancet 1:301–306

Peschle C, Condorelli M (1975) Biogenesis of erythropoietin: evidence for proerythropoietin in a subcellular fraction of kidney. Science 190:910–912

Piha RS (1962) Demonstration of erythropoietic activity in body fluids, organs and tissues, Ann Acad Sci Fenn [A] 98:1–40

Plzak LF, Fried W, Jacobson LO, Bethard WF (1955) Demonstration of stimulation of erythropoiesis by plasma from anemic rats using ^{59}Fe. J Lab Clin Med 46:671–678

Podjarny E, Rathaus M, Korzets Z, Blum M, Zevin D, Bernheim J (1981) Is anemia of chronic renal failure related to secondary hyperparathyroidism? Arch Intern Med 141:453–455

Pointer VH, Flegel U, Schmidt P, Zazarnik J, Kopsa H, Waldhouse W (1974) Gastrin in Serum von Patienten mit Uramie während der Hamodialyse. Klin Wochenschr (Wein) 86:696–699

Pololi-Anagnostou L, Westenfelder C, Anagnostu A (1981) Marked improvement of erythropoiesis in an aneprhic patient. Nephron 29:277–279

Popovic WJ, Adamson JW (1979) Erythropoietin assay: present status of methods, pitfalls and results in polycythemic disorders. CRC Crit Rev Clin Lab Sci 10:57–97

Potasman I, Better OS (1983) The role of secondary hyperparathyroidism in the anemia of chronic renal failure. Nephron 33:229–231

Powell JS, Adamson JW (1985) Hematopoiesis and the kidney. In: Seldin DW, Giefisch G (eds) The kidney: physiology and pathophysiology. Raven Press, New York, pp 847–866

Powell JS, Berkner KL, Leko RV, Adamson JW (1986) Human erythropoietin gene: high level expression in stably transfected mammalian cells and chromosome location. Proc Natl Acad Sci USA 83:6465–6469

Radtke HW, Erbes PM, Fassbinder W, Koch KM (1978a) Serum erythropoietin measurements using the fetal mouse liver cell culture: the importance of reduction of variation in the specific activity of radioiron-transferrin. Exp Hematol 6:468–472

Radtke HW, Erbes PM, Schippers E, Koch KM (1978b) Serum erythropoietin concentration in anephric patients. Nephron 22:361–365

Radtke HW, Claussner A, Erbes PM, Scheuerman EH, Schoeppe W, Koch KM (1979) Serum erythropoietin concentration in chronic renal failure: relationship to degree of anemia and excretory renal function. Blood 54:877–884

Radtke HW, Rege AB, La Marche MB, Bartos D, Bartos F, Campbell RA, Fisher JW (1981) Identification of spermine as an inhibitor of erythropoiesis in patients with chronic renal failure. J Clin Invest 67:1623–1629

Raich PC, Korst DR (1978) Plasma erythropoietin levels in patients undergoing long term hemodialysis. Arch Pathol Lab Med 102:73–75

Rege AB, Fisher JW (1980) Radioimmunoassay for erythropoietin. Exp Hematol 8[Suppl 7]:60 (abstr)

Rege AB, Brookins J, Fisher JW (1982) A radioimmunoassay for erythropoietin: serum levels in normal human subjects and patients with hemopoietic disorders. J Lab Clin Med 100:829–843

Reid CDL, Fidler J, Winearls CG, Oliver DO, Cotes PM (1987) The response of erythroid progenitors to administered recombinant human erythropoietin in haemodialysed renal failure patients. Blood 70[Suppl 1]:142a(422)

Reissmann KR (1950) Studies on the mechanism of erythropoietic stimulation in parabiotic rats during hypoxia. Blood 5:372–380

Reissmann KR, Nomura T (1962) Erythropoietin formation in isolated kidneys and liver. In: Jacobson LO, Doyle M (eds) Erythropoiesis. Grune and Stratton, New York, pp 71–77

Reissmann KR, Nomura T, Gunn RW, Brosius F (1960) Erythropoietic response to anemia or erythropoietin injection in uremic rats with or without functioning renal tissue. Blood 16:1411–1423

Rejman ASM, Grimes AJ, Cotes PM, Mansell MA, Jaekes AM (1985) Correction of anemia following renal transplantation: serial changes in erythropoietin absolute reticulocyte count and red-cell creatine levels. Br J Haematol 16:421–431

Rodgers GM, Fisher JW, George WJ (1975) Increase in hematocrit, hemoglobin and red cell mass in normal mice after treatment with cyclic AMP. Proc Soc Exp Biol Med 148:380–382

Rosenmund A, Binswanger U, Straub PW (1975) Oxidative injury to erythrocytes, cell rigidity, and splenic hemolysis in hemodialyzed uremic patients. Ann Intern Med 82:460–465

Rosse WF, Waldmann TA (1962) The role of the kidney in the erythropoietin response to hypoxia in parabiotic rats. Blood 19:75–91

Sacchetti C (1953) Physiopathologie des erythroblasts dans l'anémie des azotémies chroniques. Acta Haematol (Basel) 9:97–106

Saito A, Suzuki I, Chung TG, Okamoto T, Hotta T (1986) Separation of an inhibitor of erythropoiesis in "middle molecules" from hemodialysate from patients with chronic renal failure. Clin Chem 32:1938–1941

Saito T, Saito K, Trent DJ, Dragnac PS, Andrews RB, Farkas WR, Dunn CDR, Etkin LD, Lange RD (1985) Translation of messenger RNA from a renal tumor into a product with the biological properties of erythropoietin. Exp Hematol 13:23–28

Sakata S, Enoki Y, Tomita S, Kohzuki H (1985) In vitro erythropoietin assay based on erythroid colony formation in fetal mouse liver cell culture. Br J Haematol 61:293–302

Sakata S, Enoki Y, Nakatani A, Kohzuki H, Ohga U, Shimizu S (1987) Plasma erythropoietin assay by a fetal liver cell culture method with special reference to effective elimination of erythroid colony inhibitor(s) in plasma. Exp Hematol 15:226–233

Sanzari NP, Fisher JW (1963) The influence of cobalt and sheep erythropoietin on radioactive iron incorporation in RBC of starved intact and nephrectomized rats. Blood 21:729–738

Sasaki H, Bothner B, Dell A, Fukuad M (1987) Carbohydrate structure of erythropoietin expressed in Chinese hamster ovary cells by a human erythropoietin cDNA. J Biol Chem 262:12059–12076

Shasha, Eingraff J, Drueke T, Bordier P, Man NK, Jungers P (1976) Subtotal parathyroidictomy in chronic dialysis patients. (Abstr) Proc 2nd Int Workshop on Phosphate, Heidelberg, Germany, p 77

Schooley JC, Mahlmann LJ (1971a) Stimulation of erythropoiesis in the plethoric mouse by cyclic AMP and its inhibition by antierythropoietin. Proc Soc Exp Biol Med 137:1289–1292

Schooley JC, Mahlmann LJ (1971b) Stimulation of erythropoiesis in plethoric mice by prostaglandins and its inhibition by antierythropoietin. Proc Exp Biol Med 138:523–524

Schulz E, Modder B, Rath K (1977) Verhalten von Plasma – Erythropoietin (ESF) und Hamatokrit unter dem Einfluß der Dauerdialyse – Behandlung. Klin Wochenschr 55:65–69

Schulz E, Modder B, Fisher JW (1978) Role of erythropoietin in anemia of renal insufficiency in man and in an experimental uremic rabbit model. Contrib Nephrol 13:69–80

Schuster SJ, Wilson JH, Erslev AJ, Caro J (1987) Physiologic regulation and tissue localization of renal erythropoietin messenger RNA. Blood 70:316–318

Shalhoub RJ, Rajan U, Kim VV, Goldwasser E, Kark JA, Antoniou LD (1982) Erythrocytosis in patients on long-term hemodialysis. Ann Intern Med 97: 686–690

Shasha SM, Better OS, Winaver J, Chaimovitz C, Barzilai A, Erlik D (1978) Improvement in the anemia of hemodialyzed patients following subtotal parathyroidectomy. Isr J Med Sci 14:328–332

Sherwood JB, Goldwasser E (1976) Erythropoietin production by human renal carcinoma cells in culture. Endocrinology 99:504–510

Sherwood JB, Goldwasser E (1978) Extraction of erythropoietin from normal kidneys. Endocrinology 103:866–870

Sherwood JB, Goldwasser E (1979) A radioimmunoassay for erythropoietin. Blood 54:885–893

Sherwood JB, Shouval D (1986) Continuous production of erythropoietin by an established human renal carcinoma cell line: development of the cell line. Proc Natl Acad Sci USA 83:165–169

Shoemaker CB, Mitsock LD (1986) Murine erythropoietin gene: cloning, expression and human gene homology. Mol Cell Biol 6:849–858

Short AIK, Winney RJ, Robson JS (1980) Reversible microcytic hypochromic anaemia in dialysis patients due to aluminum intoxication. Proc Eur Dial Transplant Assoc 17:226–233

Simon P, Boffa G, Ang KS, Menault M (1982) Polycythemia in a haemodialyzed anephric patient with hepatitis. Demonstration of erythropoietin secretion. Nouv Presse Med 11:1401–1403

Singer JW, Samuels AI, Adamson JW (1976) Steroids and hematopoiesis. I. The effect of steroids on in vitro erythroid colony growth: structure/activity relationships. J Cell Physiol 88:127–134

Sjogren L, Thysell H, Lindholm T (1979) The influence of vitamin B6 supplementation on the bone marrow morphology in patients on regular haemodialysis treatment. A double blind study. Scand J Urol Nephrol 13:101–103

Smith EKM, Welt LG (1970) The red blood cell as a model for the study of uremic toxins. Arch Intern Med 126:827–830

Sokabe H, Grollman A (1962) Localization of blood pressure regulating and erythropoietic functions in rat kidney. Am J Physiol 203:991–994

Stutz B, Rhyner K, Vogtli J, Binswanger U (1987) Erfolgreiche Behandlung der Anämie bei Hamodialyse – Patienten mit rekombinierten humanem Erythropoietin. Schweiz Med Wochenschr 117:1397–1402

Sue JM, Sytkowski AJ (1983) Site-specific antibodies to human erythropoietin directed toward the NH_2-terminal region. Proc Natl Acad Sci USA 80: 3651–3655

Summerfield GP, Gyde OHB, Forbes AMW, Goldsmith HJ, Bellingham AJ (1983) Haemoglobin concentration and serum erythropoietin in renal dialysis and transplant patients. Scand J Haematol 30:389–400

Sunderman FW, Hopfer SM (1983) Correlation between carcinogenic activities of nickel compounds and their potencies for stimulating erythropoiesis in rats. In: Sarkar B (ed) Biological aspects of metals and metal-related diseases. Raven, New York, pp 171–181

Swartz R, Dambrouski J, Burnatoska-Hledin M, Mayor G (1987) Microcytic anemia in dialysis patients: reversible marker of aluminum toxicity. Am J Kidney Dis 9:217–223

Swendseid ME, Panaqua M, Kopple JD (1980) Polyamine concentrations of red cells and urine of patients with chronic renal failure. Life Sci 26:533–539

Sytkowski AJ, Richie JP, Bicknell KA (1983) New human "renal cell" line established from a patient with erythrocytosis. Cancer Res 43:1415–1419

Tamaoki N, Hata J, Izumi S, Ueyama Y, Toyama K (1977) Systemic effects of human renal cell carcinoma on nude mice: polycythemia, anemia, hypovolemia, and hepatomegaly. In: Normura T, Ohsawa M, Tamaoki N, Fujiwara K (eds) Proceedings of the second international workshop on nude mice. University of Tokyo Press, Tokyo, p 417

Thevenod F, Radtke HW, Gruztmacher P, Vincent E, Koch KM, Schoeppe W, Fassbinder W (1983) Deficient feedback regulation of erythropoiesis in kidney transplant patients with polycythemia. Kidney Int 24:227–232

Thorling EB (1972) Paraneoplastic erythrocytosis and inappropriate erythropoietin production. Scand J Haematol [Suppl]17:111–116

Tomson CRV, Venning MC, Ward MK (1988) Blood pressure and erythropoietin. Lancet 1:351

Toyama K, Fujiyama N, Suzuki H, Chen TP, Tamaoki N, Ueyama Y (1979) Erythropoietin levels in the course of a patient with erythropoietin-producing renal cell carcinoma and transplantation of this tumor in nude mice. Blood 54:245–253

Urabe A, Saito T, Fukamachi H, Kubota M, Takaku F (1987) Serum erythropoietin titers in the anemia of chronic renal failure and other hematological states. Int J Cell Cloning 5:202–208

Van Stone JC, Max P (1979) Effect of erythropoietin on anemia of peritoneally dialyzed anephric rats. Kidney Int 15:370–375

Wagemaker G, Van Eijk HG, Leijnse B (1972) A sensitive bio-assay for the determination of erythropoietin. A modification of the post-hypoxic polycythemic mice assay. Clin Chim Acta 36:357–361

Walczyk MH, Golper TA (1987) Correction of the anemia of end-stage renal disease with recombinant human erythropoietin. N Engl J Med 317:249

Walle AJ, Wong GY, Clemons GK, Garcia JF, Niedermayer W (1987) Erythropoietin–hematocrit feedback circuit in the anemia of end-stage renal disease. Kidney Int 31:1205–1209

Wallner SF, Vautrin RM (1978) The anemia of chronic renal failure: studies of the effect of organic solvent extraction of serum. J Lab Clin Med 92:363–369

Wallner SF, Vautrin RM (1981) Evidence that inhibition of erythropoiesis is important in the anemia of chronic renal failure. J Lab Clin Med 97:170–178

Wallner SF, Ward HP, Vautrin R, Alfrey AC, Mishell J (1975) The anemia of chronic renal failure: in vitro response of bone marrow to erythropoietin. Proc Soc Exp Biol Med 149:934–944

Wallner SF, Kurnick JE, Ward HP, Vautrin R, Alfrey AC (1976) The anemia of chronic renal failure and chronic diseases: in vitro studies of erythropoiesis. Blood 47:561–569

Wallner SF, Kurnick JE, Vautrin R, Ward HP (1977) The effect of serum from uremic patients on erythropoietin. Am J Hematol 3:45–55

Wallner SF, Vautrin RM, Kurnick JE, Ward HP (1978) The effect of serum from patients with chronic renal failure on erythroid colony growth in vitro. J Lab Clin Med 92:370–375

Wang FF, Kung CK-H, Goldwasser E (1985) Some chemical properties of human erythropoietin. Endocrinology 116:2286–2292

Ward HP, Gordon B, Pickett JC (1969) Serum levels of erythropoietin in rheumatoid arthritis. J Lab Clin Med 74:93–97

Ward HP, Kurnick JE, Pisarczyk MJ (1971) Serum level of erythropoietin in anemias associated with chronic infection, malignancy, and primary hematopoietic disease. J Clin Invest 50:332–335

Warter J, Martz J, Hammon B (1962) Research on hemopoietin (erythropoietin). I. Erythropoietic potency of the wash liquid from the isolated and hypoxic calf kidney. CR Soc Biol 156:897–900

Watkins PC, Eddy R, Hoffman N, Stanislovitis P, Beck AK, Galli J, Vellucci V, Gusella JF, Shows TB (1986) Regional assignment of the erythropoietin gene to human chromosome region 7pter-q22. Cytogenet Cell Genet 42:214–218

Weinberg SG, Lubin A, Wiener SN, Deoras MP, Ghose MK, Kopelman RC (1977) Myelofibrosis and renal osteodystrophy. Am J Med 63:755–764

Whitcomb WH, Moore MZ (1965) The inhibitory effect of plasma from hypertransfused animals on erythrocyte iron incorporation in mice. J Lab Clin Med 66:641–651

White WF, Gurney CW, Goldwasser E, Jacobson LO (1960) Studies on erythropoietin. Recent Prog Horm Res 16:219–262

Winearls CG, Oliver DO, Pippard MJ, Reid C, Downing MR, Cotes PM (1986) Effect of human erythropoietin derived from recombinant DNA on the anaemia of patients maintained by chronic haemodialysis. Lancet 2:1175–1177

Wu KK, Gibson TP, Freeman RM, Bonney WW, Fried W, DeGowin RL (1973) Erythrocytosis after renal transplantation. Its occurrence in two recipients of kidneys from the same cadaveric donor. Arch Intern Med 132:898–902

Yanagawa S, Hirade K, Ohnota H, Sasaki R, Chiba H, Ueda M, Goto M (1984a) Isolation of human erythropoietin with monoclonal antibodies. J Biol Chem 259:2707–2710

Yanagawa S, Yokoyama S, Hirade K, Sasaki R, Chiba H, Ueda M, Goto M (1984b) Hybridomas for production of monoclonal antibodies of human erythropoietin. Blood 64:357–364

Yawata Y, Kjellstrand C, Buselmeier T, Howe R, Jacob H (1972) Hemolysis in dialyzed patients. Tap water induced red blood cell metabolic deficiency. Trans Am Soc Artif Int Organs 18:301–304, 310

Yoshimura S, Tamaoki N, Ueyama Y, Hata J (1978) Plasma protein production by human tumors xenotransplanted in nude mice. Cancer Res 38:3474–3478

Zangheri EO, Suarez JR, Fernandez FO, Campana H, Silva JC, Ponce FE (1962) Erythropoietic action of tissue extracts. Nature 194:938–939

Zappacosta AR, Caro J, Erslev A (1982) Normalization of hematocrit in patients with end stage renal disease on continuous ambulatory peritoneal dialysis. Am J Med 72:53–57

Zaroulis CG, Hoffman BJ, Kourides IA (1981) Serum concentrations of erythropoietin measured by radioimmunoassay in hematologic disorders and chronic renal failure. Am J Hematol 11:85–92

Zevin D, Levi J, Bessler J, Djalditti M (1981) Effect of parathyroid hormone and 1,25 dihydroxy-vitamin D3 on RNA and heme synthesis by erythroid precursors. Miner Electrolyte Metab 6:125–129

Zucker S, Lysik RM, Mohammad G (1976) Erythropoiesis in chronic renal disease. J Lab Clin Med 88:528–535

CHAPTER 8

Humoral Control of Thrombocytopoiesis

T.P. McDonald

A. Introduction

It is well established that a thrombocytopoiesis stimulating factor (TSF or thrombopoietin) is a major controlling factor of megakaryocytopoiesis and thus thrombocytopoiesis. During the past 30 years there have been intermittent periods of active research on the hormone, with most of the decisive work occurring during the past 15 years. It should be noted that the study has been difficult, largely because of the lack of suitable assays and stable sources of the hormone. Only during the past decade have reliable assays been developed and potent sources identified. Therefore, with these assays and sources, definitive studies on the presence and characterization of the hormone have now been published and will be discussed in this review. In this chapter, a model for megakaryocytopoiesis and its controlling factors, to include the megakaryocyte-colony stimulating factor (meg-CSF) and thrombopoietin, are presented. Since thrombopoietin is the major controlling factor of in vivo blood platelet production, it will be considered in greater detail than the other factors. Its biology, mode of action, immunology, site of production, purification, and chemical characterization will be reviewed in some detail. Although the effects of thrombopoietin on megakaryocytopoiesis appear to be similar to those of other humoral factors with their control of specific hematopoietic lineages, there are some aspects of platelet production mechanisms that need additional discussion, e.g., the effects of hypoxia and its ability to interrupt thrombocytopoiesis and the stimulating effects of erythropoietin and other growth factors on megakaryocytopoiesis and thrombocytopoiesis. The clinical aspects of thrombopoietin, to include several disease states that are known to be associated with increased or decreased thrombopoietin titers, will be briefly mentioned, along with a brief summary and views of its future in clinical medicine.

B. Model for Megakaryocytopoiesis

A model for megakaryocytopoiesis (McDonald 1987) that appears to be in agreement with most published works in the field is presented in Fig. 1. In this model, cells of the megakaryocytic lineage can be subdivided into a

secrete large quantities of acetylcholinesterase and that the addition of acetylcholinesterase to cultures suppresses the cells responsible for forming megakaryocytic colonies (Burstein et al. 1980). This finding has led to the hypothesis that autoregulation may occur in rodents by local modulation of the concentration of acetylcholinesterase of megakaryocyte origin. Other data presented by Paulus et al. (1981) support the hypothesis that the secretion of acetylcholinesterase by megakaryocytes controls the proliferation of progenitors. In vivo, the injection of neostigmine (an inhibitor of acetylcholinesterase) into mice significantly elevated the percentage of small acetylcholinesterase positive (SAChE+) cells in the marrow of mice (McDonald et al. 1985a). Data from Kalmaz et al. (1987) showed that when fetal mouse liver cells (FMLC) were used in vitro to study the effects of acetylcholinesterase or neostigmine, the number of megakaryocytes rose with increasing doses of neostigmine compared with control cultures, supporting the findings previously presented by McDonald et al. (1985a). Therefore, all these results suggest that acetylcholinesterase produced by mature megakaryocytes inhibits megakaryocytopoiesis in rodents, both in vitro and in vivo. Chemicals from mature megakaryocytes of other species may also exert an effect on megakaryocytopoiesis, but their identity is not yet known.

III. Thrombopoietin

1. Background and Historical Aspects

The idea that thrombocytopoiesis is controlled by a humoral regulator, thrombopoietin, was developed in the mid-1950s from studies that were being performed on a RBC regulator, erythropoietin. The first paper on the subject was written by Yamamoto (1957), and the name "thrombopoietin" was proposed by Kelemen et al. (1958) the following year. Since this time, several review articles on the development of knowledge of thrombopoietin have been published (Abildgaard and Simone 1967; Cooper 1970; Ebbe 1974, 1976; Gewirtz 1986; Levin and Evatt 1979; McDonald 1974b, 1977a, 1981a,b, 1987, 1988a; Odell 1974).

Urine, serum, and plasma from thrombocytopenic animals and patients were found to contain thrombopoietin (Dassin et al. 1983; Enomoto et al. 1980; Evatt et al. 1974; Evatt and Levin 1969; Grossi et al. 1987; Hill and Levin 1986; Levin et al. 1982; McDonald 1981b, 1987; Nakeff and Roozendaal 1975; Odell et al. 1961; Penington 1970; Vannucchi et al. 1986, 1988). Thrombopoietin has also been shown to be present in body fluids of patients with thrombocytosis (McDonald 1975; Shreiner et al. 1980). Moreover, media from human embryonic kidney (HEK) cell cultures have been identified as another potent source of thrombopoietin which is more stable than that from in vivo sources (Cullen and McDonald 1986; Kalmaz and McDonald 1981a,b, 1982, 1985; McDonald 1980, 1981b,

1987; McDonald et al. 1975, 1987a; McDonald and Kalmaz 1983a; McDonald and Nolan 1979; Raha et al. 1985).

Thrombocytopoiesis-stimulating factor (TSF) from HEK cell culture media is free of erythropoietin (McDonald et al. 1975), and although the crude media contains a granulocyte-colony stimulating factor (G-CSF), TSF and G-CSF are clearly separate entities (McDonald and Shadduck 1982). There are many similarities in thrombopoietin from plasma of thrombocytopenic animals and TSF from HEK cells (McDonald 1981a,b, 1987). A megakaryocyte stimulating factor (MSF) with a molecular weight of 15000 has been described (Greenberg et al. 1987; Tayrien and Rosenberg 1987). MSF was isolated from both HEK cell culture medium and plasma from thrombocytopenic rabbits. It was shown to stimulate the synthesis of platelet factor 4 in alpha granules of megakaryocytes and to increase the rate of cytoplasmic maturation during megakaryocyte development. There appear to be many similarities between this factor and thrombopoietin (McDonald 1988a), and the data that exist so far indicate that the two are probably identical. However, amino acid sequencing will be required for absolute proof of identity.

2. Assays

In early work, thrombopoietin was assayed by platelet counting (de Gabriele and Penington 1967; Odell et al. 1961; Spector 1961); however, this was neither reliable nor sufficiently sensitive to measure the effects of altered thrombocytopoiesis in rodents. Additional work has involved measurements of alterations in platelet labeling with radioisotopes (Evatt and Levin 1969; McDonald 1973b, 1977a), changes in platelet sizes (Levin et al. 1982; McDonald 1980; Weiner and Karpatkin 1972; Weintraub and Karpatkin 1974), an immunoassay (McDonald 1973a), alterations and measurement of megakaryocytes in vivo (Cullen and McDonald 1986; McDonald and Kalmaz 1983a) and in vitro (Grant et al. 1987; Leven and Yee 1987; Williams et al. 1982), and determination of the number of SAChE+ cells in the marrow of rodents (Kalmaz and McDonald 1982) for the assay of thrombopoietin. In some of these studies, the thrombopoietin recipient animals were pretreated, i.e., splenectomized (Odell et al. 1961), transfused with platelets (Evatt and Levin 1969; McDonald et al. 1976b), or injected with platelet-specific antiserum (McDonald 1973b; Penington 1970), in an attempt to increase their sensitivity to the hormone. Of the several attempts to find the optimum conditions for the assay of thrombopoietin, mice in rebound thrombocytosis appear to be more sensitive to exogenous thrombopoietin preparations than are normal mice (McDonald 1981a). A sensitive assay for thrombopoietin that utilizes measurement of SAChE+ cells in the marrow of mice was described by Kalmaz and McDonald (1982). This assay technique was able to detect smaller doses of thrombopoietin than the rebound-thrombocytotic mouse and may prove to be useful for further studies when assaying for small amounts of thrombopoietin is needed. However, the SAChE+ cell assay is time consuming, requiring long hours of microscope time. The immunothrombocythemic mouse assay is preferred because of its reliability, sensitivity, and rapidity compared with other available methods (Clift and McDonald 1979; McDonald 1973b, 1977a,b; McDonald et al. 1979a). Improvements in the original assay procedure including establishing the most sensitive route and number of injections of thrombopoietin, the selection of the mouse sex and strain, and a comparison of [^{35}S]sodium sulfate versus [^{75}Se]selenomethionine have been made (McDonald 1981a). At the present time, a RIA for thrombopoietin is under development.

3. Site of Production

The precise site of thrombopoietin production is unknown. However, thrombocytopenia has been reported in up to 50% of patients with chronic renal disease (Rath et al. 1957), and thrombopoietin titers were shown to be reduced in patients with chronic renal failure (Gafter et al. 1987). Additional work in rodents points to the kidney as at least one site of production of the hormone (Fig. 1).

Krizsa (1971) showed that the kidney was necessary for the appearance of a factor which was termed "post-hemorrhagic thrombopoietic factor." Platelet counts of rats were reduced by bleeding, and thrombocytopoietic activity was assayed by platelet counting in recipient rats. Thrombocytopoietic activity was not found in the serum of donor rats after nephrectomy but was present in the serum of rats with intact kidneys. Moreover, the thrombocytopoietic factor could be produced in rats after other organs, such as the spleen, adrenal glands, and pituitary, had been removed. Other workers have shown that both bleeding and antiplatelet serum action release large amounts of thrombopoietin into the circulation (Odell et al. 1961). Although it may be argued that it is the erythropoietin in the plasma of bled animals that causes the increase in platelet counts of recipient rats, it does not appear that large enough quantities of erythropoietin could have been produced to cause this rise. For example, several workers (Evatt et al. 1976; McDonald et al. 1987b; McDonald and Clift 1979) showed that at least 5, and in some experiments, 15 units of erythropoietin were required to stimulate platelet production in normal mice. It should also be noted that X-irradiation, bleeding, or phenylhydrazine treatment releases a maximum of about 0.5 unit of erythropoietin per milliliter of plasma in rodents (Erslev et al. 1980; McDonald et al. 1970), which is too small an amount to alter platelet counts of animals injected with plasma from bled rats. It seems possible, therefore, that Krizsa (1971) was measuring a factor that was produced by bleeding and was largely thrombocytopoietic in nature (Odell et al. 1962).

In additional studies, the kidney was found to be necessary for the appearance of thrombopoietin in plasma of rats after production of acute thrombocytopenia with platelet-specific antisera (McDonald 1976b). In this work, extracts of plasma from normal rats, rats injected with rabbit antirat platelet serum, nephrectomized rats, and nephrectomized rats injected with antiserum were tested in the immunothrombocythemic mouse assay for the presence of thrombopoietin. Only an extract of plasma from unoperated rats made thrombocytopenic by an injection of antiserum gave positive results for thrombopoietin. In agreement with this work, Klener et al. (1977) showed that vinblastine treatment caused significant increases in serum thrombopoietin activity in animals. The vinblastine-induced increase was abolished by bilateral nephrectomy but was not affected by bilateral ligation of the ureters. Klener et al. (1977) concluded that the kidney is probably a major source of the serum thrombocytopoietic factor.

In support of these findings, McDonald et al. (1975) reported the detection of thrombopoietin in the media of HEK cell cultures. Thrombopoietin production seems to be localized in the kidney, since FMLC cultures (Zucali et al. 1977) and adult livers from other species (Ogle et al. 1978) did not have demonstrable thrombopoietin levels. Other experiments (Ogle et al. 1978) showed that kidneys from adult animals could also produce thrombopoietin. Therefore, the hypothesis that the kidney is necessary for thrombopoietin production appears to have been confirmed by these in vitro data.

Another, more recent study demonstrated not only that bilaterally nephrectomized rats failed to show an increase in the number of megakaryocyte precursor cells (SAChE+) after being made thrombocytopenic but that other anephric rats which were not given antiplatelet serum had decreased percentages of SAChE+ cells compared with untreated control rats (McDonald and Kalmaz 1983b). These findings indicate the importance of the kidney for the day-to-day production of thrombopoietin for the maintenance of the number of SAChE+ cells in the marrow of rodents. It was also interesting to note that unilateral nephrectomy and ligation of the ureters had little effect on altering the percentages of SAChE+ cells in the marrow of rodents, suggesting that surgical stress and uremia do not interfere significantly with the release and action of thrombopoietin.

In a study by Gafter et al. (1987), platelet counts were reduced, and mild thrombocytopenia was frequently found in patients with chronic renal failure. Thrombopoietic activity was lowered in the plasma of seven thrombocytopenic patients with kidney failure, as measured by [^{75}Se] selenomethionine incorporation into platelets of recipient mice. These workers concluded that the cause for the platelet count reduction was probably insufficient thrombopoietic activity.

Although there is some evidence that the kidney is important for platelet production in humans (Gafter et al. 1987; Rath et al. 1957), anephric man is not usually markedly thrombocytopenic. Therefore, it seems possible that in humans extrarenal sites for thrombopoietin production may play a significant role. However, the data outlined here and elsewhere (McDonald 1981a) illustrate that in rodents the intact kidney is required for thrombopoietin production. It is interesting to note that the primary source of erythropoietin appears to be the kidney of both dogs and man (Naets 1958; Naets and Wittek 1968), but significant extrarenal sites for erythropoietin production are found in rodents (Erslev et al. 1980). Thrombopoietin, on the other hand, appears to be produced exclusively in the kidney by rodents (McDonald 1981a) but may be produced at extrarenal sites in other species. This interesting disagreement in production sites of these two hormones is presently only theoretical; additional work will be required to clarify the precise site(s) of production of thrombopoietin in both animals and man.

4. Antibodies to Thrombopoietin

In the past, polyclonal antibodies against thrombopoietin from thrombocytopenic sheep and humans have been raised in rabbits (McDonald 1973a, 1974a, 1978c). Recently, monoclonal antibodies (McDonald et al. 1986a) were raised in mice against human urinary thrombopoietin. The data indicate that antibodies made against thrombopoietin from human urinary or sheep plasma sources can neutralize the biological activity of both HEK-cell thrombopoietin (McDonald 1978c; McDonald et al. 1986a) and endogenously produced thrombopoietin in mice (McDonald, 1974a). Thrombopoietin activity, when assayed in the immunothrombocythemic mouse assay, can be neutralized in vitro by the addition of serum obtained from rabbits previously immunized with thrombopoietin-rich preparations from sheep (McDonald 1974a), humans (McDonald 1978c), and HEK-cell culture media (McDonald 1978c). When injected into normal mice, antithrombopoietin serum did not directly affect platelets; however, a depression in thrombocytopoiesis was observed a few days later (McDonald 1974a). It was concluded that injections of an antibody developed against thrombopoietin into normal mice interrupted thrombocytopoiesis by reducing endogenous thrombopoietin levels. A monoclonal antibody made against human urinary thrombopoietin was shown to reduce the bioactivity of thrombopoietin extracted from HEK-cell culture media (McDonald et al. 1986a) when tested in the immunothrombocythemic mouse assay. These data indicate that thrombopoietin is required for the day-to-day maintenance of platelet counts (McDonald 1974a) and that antibodies made against one source of thrombopoietin can detect (McDonald et al. 1977b) or neutralize the biological activity of others (McDonald 1974a, 1978c; McDonald et al. 1986a).

5. Purification

a) Methods for Purification

Thrombopoietin has been partially purified by use of several chromatographic and selective precipitation techniques, i.e., ion exchange chromatography (EVATT et al. 1979; McDONALD et al. 1985b, 1986b, 1987a), gel filtration chromatography (EVATT et al. 1979; McDONALD et al. 1985b, 1986b, 1987a), diethylaminoethyl (DEAE) and size exclusion-high performance liquid chromatography (SE-HPLC) (McDONALD et al. 1985b; VANNUCCHI et al. 1988), reverse phase (RP)-HPLC (McDONALD et al. 1988), affinity chromatography using immobilized lectins (HILL and LEVIN 1986; McDONALD et al. 1981), ammonium sulfate precipitation (EVATT et al. 1974, 1979; HILL and LEVIN 1986; McDONALD et al. 1985b, 1986b; McDONALD and NOLAN 1979; VANNUCCHI et al. 1988), and ethanol precipitation (McDONALD et al. 1974). Previous studies have utilized a five-step procedure (McDONALD et al. 1985b, 1986b, 1987a), and recently a four-step procedure was described consisting of Sephadex column chromatography, ethanol precipitation, sodium dodecyl sulfate polyacrylamide gel electrophoresis (SDS-PAGE), and RP-HPLC for the purification of TSF (McDONALD et al. 1988). With the aid of Tween 20, the final product maintained its biological activity for several weeks at −76°C. The purified thrombopoietin was very potent and migrated on SDS-PAGE and chromatofocused as a homogeneous product.

b) Characterization of the Molecule

These purification techniques have helped our understanding of the chemical characteristics of thrombopoietin. The fact that TSF precipitates at >40% ethanol and at 60%–80% ammonium sulfate concentrations (EVATT et al. 1974, 1979; GROSSI et al. 1987; HILL and LEVIN 1986; McDONALD and NOLAN 1979) indicates that the molecule is very hydrophilic. It is probably a glycoprotein, based upon its binding characteristics to both anion and cation exchange resins (EVATT et al. 1979; McDONALD et al. 1985b, 1986b, 1987a) and its affinity for wheatgerm agglutinin and concanavalin A (HILL and LEVIN 1986; McDONALD et al. 1981). Thrombopoietin has been shown to be stable during β-mercaptoethanol and SDS treatment (McDONALD et al. 1985b, 1986b, 1987a), and it maintains its biological activity after treatment with endoglycosidases F and H (McDONALD 1988b). Thrombopoietin exists in trace amounts in both plasma from thrombocytopenic animals (HILL and LEVIN 1986; McDONALD et al. 1974) and crude HEK cell culture media (McDONALD 1987; McDONALD et al. 1985b, 1986b, 1987a). Recently, it was found that if thrombopoietin was protected by Tween 20, a relatively stable molecule was produced, supporting the conclusion that it is a glycoprotein (McDONALD et al. 1988). The fact that thrombopoietin is stable against β-mercaptoethanol (McDONALD et al.

1985b, 1986b, 1987a) may indicate that disulfate bridges are not necessary for its biological activity. Also, thrombopoietin appears to be extensively glycosylated (McDonald et al. 1981; McDonald 1988a), but since its activity was unaffected by endoglycosidases F and H (McDonald 1988b), glycosylation of thrombopoietin by complex carbohydrates that are probably linked through asparagine to the protein backbone does not appear to be necessary for thrombocytopoietic activity.

It was recently shown that the molecular weight (MW) of thrombopoietin varies depending upon the method of separation used. Boiling the preparations for 10 min in the presence of denaturing reagents before applying to SDS-PAGE yielded a 15000 MW protein band that contained most of the thrombopoietin bioactivity (McDonald et al. 1988). However, if this 15000 MW thrombopoietin was processed under nondenaturing conditions, it self-associated to yield a 30000 MW protein. This finding is in agreement with the work previously done by Tayrien and Rosenberg (1987), who showed that a purified 15000 MW protein that stimulates megakaryocytopoiesis in vitro has a remarkable tendency to self-associate under nondenaturing conditions. Normally, thrombopoietin probably exists as a dimer with a MW of ~30000.

The isoelectric pH of highly purified thrombopoietin has been measured to be 4.47 (McDonald et al. 1988). An isoelectric pH of about 4.7 for partially purified thrombopoietin was previously noted (McDonald et al. 1985b), but the protein used in the earlier study was impure. Therefore, the actual value is probably near 4.5, which is slightly lower than that of serum albumin but higher than that of human urinary erythropoietin (Puchmann et al. 1978).

Earlier, it was shown that thrombopoietin from HEK cell culture media (McDonald et al. 1981, 1985b, 1986b, 1987a; McDonald and Nolan 1979) and plasma from thrombocytopenic animals (Evatt et al. 1974, 1979; Hill and Levin 1986; McDonald et al. 1974) are not dialyzable. The factor from HEK cell culture media does not deteriorate in either ammonium sulfate or Sephadex fractions during 4–5 weeks of storage at −76°C (McDonald and Nolan 1979), and it is relatively heat stable (McDonald et al. 1981). Thrombopoietin will withstand lyophilization (McDonald et al. 1981, 1985b, 1986b, 1987a; McDonald and Nolan 1979) and does not deteriorate at pH of 1–8 (McDonald et al. 1981). However, digestion of thrombopoietin with trypsin (McDonald et al. 1981; Vannucchi et al. 1988) or cyanogen bromide (McDonald 1988b) destroys its biological activity, indicating that the molecule requires a primary protein structure involving methionine for biological activity.

6. Effects on Megakaryocytopoiesis

a) In Vitro Effects

Thrombopoietin has been shown to potentiate magakaryocyte colony formation in the presence of meg-CSF; it causes a small, but measurable, increase in colonies of murine bone marrow and fetal mouse liver cells and is important in the maintenance of SAChE+ cells in vitro.

Potentiation of meg-CSF. WILLIAMS and coworkers (1979, 1982, 1984) have demonstrated the formation of murine megakaryocyte colonies in semisolid cultures and proposed that two factors are required – a growth stimulus, meg-CSF, and another factor (which they called "potentiator") – to achieve full megakaryocyte development. In vitro, meg-CSF is required for colony induction and cell division, whereas the potentiator influences DNA and acetylcholinesterase content and cell size of developing mouse megakaryocytes (WILLIAMS et al. 1984). In many of these studies, thrombopoietin has been identified as one of the megakaryocyte potentiators in vitro, e.g., thrombopoietin from HEK cells will stimulate megakaryocytic colony formation when added with a murine myelomonocytic leukemic cell line (WEHI-3CM) materials (WILLIAMS et al. 1984). Thrombopoietin from HEK cells is the only known in vitro potentiator that also stimulates blood platelet production in animals. As shown by WILLIAMS et al. (1984), a small number of colonies will develop after adding WEHI-3CM-conditioned material alone. In these experiments, thrombopoietin by itself did not significantly stimulate megakaryocyte colony formation, but synergism between thrombopoietin and the factor in WEHI-3CM-conditioned media was observed, with optimal activity found at about 12 μg of crude thrombopoietin per culture of 1×10^5 murine bone marrow cells. The data indicate that in the in vitro system used by WILLIAMS and coworkers (1984), TSF caused an increase in the number of megakaryocytic colonies. However, its main effect was probably on the nonmitotic pool of megakaryocytes because an increase in the maturation of these cells led to elevated platelet production (WILLIAMS et al. 1984).

Megakaryocytic Colonies. Several studies have shown that thrombopoietin by itself will not increase the number of megakaryocytic colonies in vitro (reviewed by LEVIN 1983), while other studies have shown positive effects (FREEDMAN et al. 1981; KALMAZ and MCDONALD 1981b). The culture of megakaryocytes in vitro is very complex, and standardization of the techniques that have been used is lacking (MCDONALD 1987), leading to inconsistent results. However, the experiments of KALMAZ and MCDONALD (1981b) showed that crude thrombopoietin preparations from HEK cell culture medium, when added to plasma clots containing 1×10^5 murine bone marrow cells, increased the total number of megakaryocytes in a linear fashion. In addition, megakaryocytes per colony and megakaryocytic colonies per culture were also increased by thrombopoietin in a dose-response relationship. Therefore, thrombopoietin stimulated not only the total number of megakaryocytes in cultures, it also increased the number of megakaryocytic colonies and their size. These data were confirmed by Hoffman and coworkers (1986), who showed that a more highly purified preparation of thrombopoietin promoted megakaryocytic colony formation in a serum-free assay system.

Recently, Keller et al. (1988) found that a plasma fraction from thrombocytopenic rabbits that stimulates platelet production in vivo will also stimulate megakaryocytopoiesis in vitro. Although the data showed that plasma-derived thrombopoietin had no effect on the size of the colonies, it stimulated differentiation of megakaryocyte precursors from unidentifiable to identifiable cells.

When considering all experiments together, it appears that thrombopoietin by itself probably does not have marked effects on the number of megakaryocytic colonies in vitro. However, when used in conjunction with meg-CSF, it causes increased development of megakaryocytes, leading to platelet production.

Fetal Mouse Liver Cells. In addition to bone marrow, FMLC have also been used as target cells for the study of thrombopoietin and its in vitro effects on megakaryocytopoiesis (Kalmaz and McDonald 1985). Both Nicola and Johnson (1982) and Vainchenker et al. (1979) found significant megakaryocytopoiesis with platelet production using FMLC in vitro, but neither of these studies used thrombopoietin as a stimulus. However, the studies by Kalmaz and McDonald (1985) did use partially purified thrombopoietin. The results showed that 1 μg of a crude preparation of thrombopoietin per culture increased the number of acetylcholinesterase-positive cells twofold after 6 days compared with suitable controls. Increasing the dose of thrombopoietin led to additional stimulation of the number of acetylcholinesterase-positive cells. As shown previously (Kalmaz and McDonald 1981b, 1985), thrombopoietin influences the number and size of megakaryocytic colonies of both murine bone marrow and FMLC. These data indicate that the hormone not only affects platelet production but may also have an effect on the cellular proliferation of early megakaryocytes.

SAChE+ Cell Formation. In vitro, thrombopoietin stimulates the formation and growth of SAChE+ cells. Long and coworkers (1982a,b) have shown that the density of cells that respond to thrombopoietin is in the range that corresponds to SAChE+ cells, and growth of these cells will not occur without thrombopoietin. Therefore, the most immature subpopulation of SAChE+ cells will, in the presence of thrombopoietin, grow into large, mature, single megakaryocytes. In support of these findings, Nakeff et al. (1975) earlier showed a rise in the isolated recognizable megakaryocytes in plasma clot cultures after the addition of serum from thrombocytopenic mice. Other studies (Kalmaz and McDonald 1981b), using in vitro techniques, found an increase in single megakaryocytes of mouse bone marrow after stimulation with thrombopoietin from HEK cell cultures.

b) In Vivo Effects

Several studies have shown that injections of thrombopoietin into mice will increase megakaryocyte size and number, markedly improve the number of SAChE+ cells, elevate the rate of megakaryocyte endomitosis, and increase megakaryocyte maturation. The hormone also has a positive effect on the number of megakaryocytic colonies in the spleens of bone-marrow-reconstituted mice.

Megakaryocyte Size and Number. Increases in megakaryocyte size (EBBE et al. 1968; LEVINE et al. 1982) and number (ODELL et al. 1962) have been found to be excellent indicators of megakaryocytopoietic stimulation. Although there appears to be independence in the microenvironmental control of megakaryocyte number and size in vitro (EBBE et al. 1985), it should not be surprising that both thrombopoietin from HEK cell culture medium and endogenously produced thrombopoietin will stimulate megakaryocyte size and number in mice (CULLEN and MCDONALD 1986; MCDONALD and KALMAZ 1983a). After thrombopoietin injection, the number and size of megakaryocytes of murine bone marrow were elevated. In the work by MCDONALD and KALMAZ (1983a), the results showed a 6% increase in megakaryocyte number on day 1 after thrombopoietin therapy, a 65% rise on day 2, and a 48% elevation on day 3 compared with suitably treated control mice. Endogenously produced thrombopoietin (caused by an injection of rabbit antimouse platelet serum, RAMPS) resulted in an increase in megakaryocyte numbers by 11% on day 1, 66% on day 2, and 100% on day 3 compared with values of other mice injected with normal rabbit serum. The relative sizes of megakaryocytes from the same mice showed highly significant increases after both thrombopoietin and RAMPS treatment on days 1–3 (MCDONALD and KALMAZ 1983a). In another study, using the same specimens but re-evaluated by a more sophisticated technique utilizing stereologic theory and a modification of correction factors of HARKER (1968), the relative sizes and numbers of megakaryocytes were also found to be increased by thrombopoietin treatment (CULLEN and MCDONALD 1986).

SAChE+ Cells. We now know that SAChE+ cells are early cells in the megakaryocytic series and that they appear to be sensitive indicators of changes in thrombocytopoiesis (JACKSON 1973). SAChE+ cells are elevated in vivo by thrombocytopenia (JACKSON 1973; KALMAZ and MCDONALD 1981a; LEPORE et al. 1984) and decreased by thrombocytosis (LONG and HENRY 1979). Previous data indicated that injection of thrombopoietin from HEK cells and thrombocytopenic mice and humans causes a transitory increase in the percentage of SAChE+ cells in the marrow of mice (KALMAZ and MCDONALD 1981a, 1982; VANNUCCHI et al. 1988). In addition to a rapid

into the newly formed platelets. This apparent discrepancy, therefore, can be resolved on physiological bases.

b) Platelet Sizes

Previous work (Weiner and Karpatkin 1972; Weintraub and Karpatkin 1974) showed that the effects of thrombopoietin can be measured in animals by determining changes in platelet sizes. Recent research demonstrated that a measurable increase in average platelet size may also occur after stimulation of thrombocytopoiesis by thrombopoietin (Levin et al. 1982; McDonald 1980; Vannucchi et al. 1988). It was shown that thrombopoietin from HEK cell culture media will increase platelet sizes of mice (McDonald 1980). For controls, other mice were injected with saline. At 2 days after injection, the mice were sacrificed, their platelets harvested, and platelet sizes determined using previously published techniques (McDonald 1976a). Compared with values of mice injected with saline, highly significant increases in average platelet sizes were found in mice injected with thrombopoietin.

In other studies (Levin et al. 1982), platelet sizes were measured at 64 h after injection of the first of 4 equally divided doses of thrombopoietin that had been extracted from the plasma of thrombocytopenic rabbits. Levin and coworkers (1982) found increases in platelet sizes, indicating that both sources of thrombopoietin, i.e., thrombopoietin from HEK cell culture media and from plasma of thrombocytopenic rabbits, will increase platelet sizes in mice. These data are in agreement with previous work (Weiner and Karpatkin 1972; Weintraub and Karpatkin 1974) showing that injections of plasma from thrombocytopenic guinea pigs would increase platelet sizes of recipient animals.

c) Isotope Incorporation

Several previous studies have shown that thrombopoietin increases the percentage of both [^{35}S]sodium sulfate and [^{75}Se]selenomethionine incorporation into platelets of mice (Clift and McDonald 1979; Cooper 1970; Levin and Evatt 1979; McDonald, 1981a). As shown earlier, different thrombopoietin preparations increased %^{35}S incorporation into platelets of mice in rebound thrombocytosis. In one investigation (McDonald et al. 1977a), plasma from thrombocytopenic mice whose thrombocytopenia was produced by platelet-specific antisera or by X-irradiation and thrombopoietin from HEK cell culture media were tested. All sources of TSF gave highly significant increases in %^{35}S incorporation into platelets of recipient mice, indicating the presence of thrombopoietin. In addition, several previous studies have shown dose-response relationships between thrombopoietin from HEK cell culture media and %^{35}S incorporation into platelets of assay mice (McDonald 1987). In these studies, a linear correlation over a broad dose range was observed.

D. Other Factors Affecting Thrombocytopoiesis

I. Effects of Hypoxia

Hypoxia has been shown to cause marked thrombocytopenia in laboratory animals (BIRKES et al. 1975; COOPER and COOPER 1977; JACKSON and EDWARDS 1977; LANGDON and McDONALD 1977; McDONALD 1978a,b). The thrombocytopenia has been associated with reduced platelet production (COOPER and COOPER 1977; LANGDON and McDONALD 1977; McDONALD 1978a), while normal platelet survival values have been found (JACKSON and EDWARDS 1977). The hypoxic-induced thrombocytopenia was not caused by excess sequestration of platelets by an enlarged spleen (BIRKES et al. 1975; LANGDON and McDONALD 1977) or expanding blood volumes (McDONALD et al. 1978a). The effect of hypoxia does not appear to be on thrombocytopoiesis directly, since stimulated RBC prodution was required for reduced platelet production (LANGDON and McDONALD 1977; McDONALD 1978a). For example, RBC transfusion of mice prior to making them thrombocytopenic by injection of RAMPS did not impair their rebound-thrombocytotic patterns (McDONALD 1978a). However, when mice were returned to hypoxic environments after being made thrombocytopenic, marked inhibition of platelet production occurred, indicating that it is the hypoxia (and not the presence of elevated RBC) that decreases platelet production in mice (McDONALD 1978a). Also, exposure of BALB/c mice (which have a defective erythropoietin production mechanism) to hypoxia resulted in unaltered platelet counts and normal RBC counts (LANGDON and McDONALD 1977).

Other work (McDONALD 1978b) showed that platelet production in ex-hypoxic mice was reduced when compared with the results of mice recovering from thrombocytopenia induced with RAMPS, probably because of diminished quantities of megakaryocyte precursor cells (SAChE+ cells) in the marrow of ex-hypoxic mice (McDONALD et al. 1986c). The finding that the number of SAChE+ cells is decreased in mouse bone marrow by hypoxia indicates that megakaryocyte precursor cells are likewise fewer and lends support to the stem-cell competition theory (Fig. 1).

It was shown previously (McDONALD et al. 1979b) that hypoxia decreased platelet production by action on a precursor cell or a primitive population of megakaryocytes without altering the ability of mice to produce thrombopoietin. In this work, 24 h of hypoxia prior to or immediately after stimulation of platelet production by RAMPS reduced platelet production rates 3 days later, indicating that the effect of hypoxia is on a precursor cell or on an early megakaryocyte. However, if thrombocytopoiesis was stimulated by antiserum injections 24–48 h before exposure to hypoxia, there was little or no effect on platelet production rates. These findings demonstrate that hypoxia does not directly influence the differentiated megakaryocyte pool or its production of platelets.

The quantity of SAChE+ cells in bone marrow was elevated at 2 days of hypoxia (McDONALD et al. 1986c), but thereafter, their number was significantly reduced. The reason for the increase at this early time period is not known, but this finding may be related to the biphasic platelet response previously observed (JACKSON and EDWARDS 1977). It had been shown (McDONALD et al. 1978a) that the total circulating platelet count and mass of mice were increased at this early time period, lending support to the claim that it is a true increase in platelet numbers in the circulation. However, the percentage of ^{35}S incorporation into platelets and platelet sizes did not show a concurrent increase (McDONALD et al. 1978a). These findings may indicate that the increase in platelet counts was not the result of a true thrombocytopoiesis. It was hypothesized that megakaryocytes may "shed" platelets into the circulation in response to the stress of hypoxia, similar to the platelet release mechanism(s) of postsurgical thrombocytosis. These mature, platelet-producing megakaryocytes may, in the process of "shedding" platelets, release substances that cause an increase in the number of SAChE+ cells.

In a recent study, the relative number and size of megakaryocytes in both the bone marrow and spleen were evaluated (CULLEN and McDONALD 1989). The data show that the number of megakaryocytes decreased after 14 days of hypoxia by more than 80% in both the bone marrow and spleen. Splenic volumes and megakaryocyte concentrations were altered by hypoxia, and the absolute number of splenic megakaryocytes cycled throughout the experiment. PETURSSON and CHERVENICK (1987) reported similar results; they measured nucleated cells in murine bone marrow and spleens by flow cytometry following isobaric hypoxia. The work of CULLEN and McDONALD (1989) showed that mean marrow megakaryocyte diameter increased after 10 days of hypoxia and was inversely related to the absolute megakaryocyte number in the spleen. Changes in megakaryocyte diameter and number with hypoxia suggest a compensatory mechanism for increasing platelet production, which may be regulated separately in the bone marrow and spleen (LAYENDECKER and McDONALD 1982).

The above findings indicate that hypoxia decreases platelet production by action on an early precursor cell (Fig. 1), possibly the multipotential stem cell, and that hypoxia-induced thrombocytopenia is probably caused by stem-cell competition between the erythrocytic and the megakaryocytic cell lines (LANGDON and McDONALD 1977).

II. Effects of Erythropoietin and Other Growth Factors

Crude erythropoietin preparations, when administered in high doses, will stimulate thrombocytopoiesis in mice (EVATT et al. 1976; McDONALD and CLIFT 1979). Moreover, recombinant erythropoietin (rEp) has been shown to stimulate megakaryocyte colony formation and differentiation in vitro (CLARK and DESSYPRIS 1986; DESSYPRIS et al. 1987; DUKES et al. 1986a,b;

Ishibashi et al. 1987) and megakaryocytopoiesis and thrombocytopoiesis in vivo (Dukes et al. 1986a,b; McDonald et al. 1987b). Other factors including interleukin-3 (IL-3) and granulocyte macrophage-colony stimulating factor (GM-CSF) are known to stimulate megakaryocytopoiesis in cultures (Burstein 1986; Mazur et al. 1987; Oon and Williams 1987; Quesenberry et al. 1985), whereas interferon (IFN) inhibits megakaryocyte colony formation in vitro (Dukes et al. 1980).

McDonald et al (1987b) showed that rEp, like thrombopoietin, given under appropriate conditions, will stimulate platelet production in mice. Although it is not as effective as thrombopoietin in augmenting thrombocytopoiesis in mice, when administered in multiple doses it significantly increases %^{35}S incorporation values into platelets. In earlier work using crude erythropoietin preparations, high levels of the hormone stimulated thrombocytopoiesis in mice (Evatt et al. 1976; McDonald and Clift 1979). The finding that rEp elevates platelet production in mice complements and extends previous in vitro studies showing that it has an effect on murine megakaryocyte colony formation. Clark and Dessypris (1986) claimed that the in vitro effect was exerted during the early stages of colony development; however, significant increases in the diameters and ploidies of the megakaryocytes were recently reported (Ishibashi et al. 1987). rEp potentiates the growth of human marrow CFU-M, and this influence seems to be exerted during the early stages of megakaryocyte development in vitro (Dessypris et al. 1987). Its mechanism of action on platelet production is not clear. However, the available data appear to support the hypothesis that thrombopoietin and erythropoietin may be similar structurally. For example, the hormones have been shown to compete for combining sites on the surfaces of differentiating megakaryocytes and/or progenitor cells (Fraser et al. 1987). This hypothesis is compatible with the observed increases in megakaryocytic colonies (Clark and Dessypris 1986) and elevations in size and ploidy of megakaryocytes that are produced in vitro (Ishibashi et al. 1987) following rEp treatment. Thrombocytosis is found frequently as a concomitant feature of certain anemias when elevated levels of erythropoietin are present (Jackson et al. 1974). These findings further support the results presented above that erythropoietin can influence platelet production.

IL-3 has been shown to act as a megakaryocyte stimulator of murine bone marrow, similar to meg-CSF (Oon and Williams 1987; Quesenberry et al. 1985; Sparrow et al. 1987; Williams et al. 1985), and it causes megakaryocyte differentiation (Ishibashi and Burstein 1986). Also, GM-CSF was shown to have megakaryocyte colony stimulating activity (Quesenberry et al. 1985). More recently, Metcalf and coworkers (1986) and Robinson et al. (1987) demonstrated that recombinant GM-CSF augments the effect of IL-3 on megakaryocyte colony formation. Robinson et al. (1987) established that GM-CSF, as a multilineage growth factor, had definite megakaryocyte-colony stimulating activity. In addition, Oon and

Williams (1987) found that the in vitro megakaryocyte stimulating activities of TSF and rIL-3 were synergistic when tested at low concentrations. The data indicate that TSF, GM-CSF and IL-3 may be important in the regulation of megakaryocytopoiesis in vitro. It is unknown, however, whether IL-3 and/or GM-CSF will stimulate thrombocytopoiesis in vivo (Clark and Kamen 1987; Metcalf 1985; Sieff 1987).

Dukes et al. (1980) used a plasma clot system to show that naturally occurring preparations of IFN would inhibit mouse megakaryocytic progenitor cells. More recently, recombinant IFN-α and IFN-γ have been noted to inhibit human megakaryocytopoiesis in vitro (Ganser et al. 1987). The inhibition of megakaryocytopoiesis by IFN-α may be due to direct effects on hematopoietic progenitor cells, whereas the effects of IFN-γ on megakaryocytes were thought to be caused indirectly by accessory cells.

E. Clinical Aspects of Thrombopoietin

Previous studies have shown a relationship between plasma, serum, or urine thrombopoietin content and several disease states (Adams et al. 1978; Baynes et al. 1987; Choi et al. 1968; Eyster et al. 1986; Grossi et al. 1987; Hirsh et al. 1980; McClure and Choi 1968; McDonald 1975; McDonald et al. 1985c; McDonald and Green 1977; Nickerson et al. 1980; Pinto et al. 1985; Shreiner et al. 1980), pointing to the fact that thrombopoietin may play a causative role.

As expected, thrombopoietin titers were found to be increased in several patients with thrombocytopenia (Choi et al. 1968; McClure and Choi 1968; McDonald 1975; Shreiner et al. 1980). These investigations demonstrated elevated thrombopoietin levels in the urine, sera, or plasma of thrombocytopenic patients with acute myelocytic leukemia, eosinophilic leukemia, chronic erythroleukemia, chronic and acute idiopathic thrombocytopenic purpura, alcoholism with splenomegaly, carcinoma of the lung, multiple myeloma, aplastic anemia, renal failure, infectious mononucleosis, and others. Interestingly, several other patients with similar degrees of thrombocytopenia did not have elevated thrombopoietin titers, and it appears that either the levels of thrombopoietin were too low for measurement, or the increased megakaryocyte number found in the bone marrow of many of these thrombocytopenic patients represents utilization of the hormone by the target cells. In support of this theory, Choi et al. (1968) noted elevated thrombopoietin titers in patients with acute, but not chronic, idiopathic thrombocytopenic purpura, with elevated numbers of megakaryocytes in the marrow. However, it is possible, but not likely, that these cells are less responsive to the hormone than are megakaryocytes in the marrow of normal patients.

Thrombocytopenia due to a lack of thrombopoietin has also been described (Hirsh et al. 1980; McDonald et al. 1985c; McDonald and

GREEN 1977). HIRSH et al. (1980) reported a patient with acquired hypomegakaryocytic thrombocytopenic purpura without elevated thrombopoietin titers. It was postulated that the lack of thrombopoietin may have led to the thrombocytopenia. Also, two patients with decreased thrombopoietin titers and chronic thrombocytopenia whose platelet counts were transiently increased repeatedly by infusions of normal human plasma were examined (JOHNSON et al. 1971; MIURA et al. 1984b; SCHULMAN et al. 1960, 1965). Both had elevated thrombopoietin titers 1 h after plasma transfusion (McDONALD et al. 1985c; McDONALD and GREEN 1977). The similarities in the two patients were remarkable. Most likely, they had chronic thrombocytopenia because of thrombopoietin deficiencies, and they both had microangiopathic hemolytic anemia since childhood; these abnormalities were markedly improved with plasma transfusions. Although unexplained, large multimers of Factor VIII/von Willebrand's factor were found when platelet counts were normal and decreased when platelet counts were low. Deficiency of a plasma factor that is necessary for thrombopoietin production appeared to be the cause of these chronic thrombocytopenic conditions.

In addition to increased thrombopoietin levels in thrombocytopenic subjects, patients with thrombocytosis have also been shown to have elevated thrombopoietin titers (McDONALD 1975; NICKERSON et al. 1980; PINTO et al. 1985; SHREINER et al. 1980). The mechanism is probably similar to secondary polycythemia being caused by elevated levels of erythropoietin (ERSLEV et al. 1979). In the work by SHREINER et al. (1980), about one-half of the thrombocytotic patients that were tested had elevated thrombopoietin titers. McDONALD (1975) found that urine fractions from thrombocytotic patients contained the hormone, and NICKERSON et al. (1980) described two patients with hepatoblastoma, thrombocytosis, and high α-ferroproteins with elevated plasma thrombopoietin titers. Moreover, extracts of a liver tumor from one of the patients contained the platelet-stimulating factor, suggesting that in some circumstances tumors may produce thrombopoietin.

Patients with acute megakaryoblastic leukemia and translocation of chromosome 3q21 were shown to have elevated thrombopoietin titers (BERNSTEIN et al. 1986; PINTO et al. 1985). It was hypothesized that the abnormal platelets from leukemic patients might not be recognized by the thrombocytopoiesis regulating system, or alternatively, leukemic cells themselves may produce the hormone, resulting in positive stimulation of platelet production. This mechanism may occur by activation of an oncogene in the leukemic cells on chromosome 3q, which might be involved in thrombopoietin production and/or regulation.

Finally, examples of low or absent thrombopoietin titers and thrombocytosis have also been found. EYSTER et al. (1986) reported low thrombopoietin titers in a family with essential thrombocythemia with possible dysregulation of an early cell in the megakaryocytic cell line leading to a more rapid mobilization of progenitor cells into mature, platelet-producing megakaryocytes.

Other instances of thrombopoietin being related to disease states include the measurement of thrombopoietin production, platelet counts, and platelet sizes in the grey collie dog with cyclic hematopoiesis (McDonald et al. 1976a). The results show that platelet sizes and thrombopoietin levels cycled in relation to platelet counts. Platelet sizes varied inversely with the platelet count and the levels of thrombopoietin; the highest thrombopoietin values were found at the beginning of active thrombocytopoiesis. It should also be noted that patients with cyclic hematopoiesis and cyclic thrombocytopoiesis have also been described (Adams et al. 1978). Although the grey collies are important for studying the mechanisms of platelet sensors and thrombopoietin release, the causes of thrombopoietin release and action are as yet unknown.

In summary, thrombopoietin levels have been found to be normal, elevated, or decreased in both thrombocytopenic and thrombocythemic disease states. Clarification of the role of this hormone in patients with platelet-production problems will be the subject of future work.

F. Future of Thrombopoietin

The existence and action of thrombopoietin and its control of blood platelet production in both animals and humans seem quite clear. Moreover, it does not appear to be the result of a panic mechanism but is required for the day-to-day maintenance of platelet counts. Figure 1 shows a model for megakaryocytopoiesis including the controlling factors, meg-CSF, and thrombopoietin. There is some evidence that points to autoregulation of megakaryocytopoiesis, and this will no doubt be the subject of future research from several different laboratories. Although several studies have been devoted to the determination of the site of production of thrombopoietin, much work remains before absolute proof will be obtained. Both the development of assays and the creation of antibodies against the hormone are promising tools to meet this goal. However, the ideal system for the assay of TSF is still not available. Hopefully, within the next few years, a radioimmunoassay for thrombopoietin will be developed that will aid sig-

Table 1. Summary of effects of thrombopoietin on thrombocytopoiesis

In vitro, thrombopoietin elevates:	
I.	Number of megakaryocytic colonies, size of colonies, and number and maturation of single megakaryocytes
II.	Division and maintenance of small acetylcholinesterase positive cells
In vivo, thrombopoietin increases:	
I.	Platelet counts, platelet sizes, and isotopic incorporation into platelets
II.	Megakaryocyte size and number, megakaryocyte endomitosis and maturation, and megakaryocytic spleen colonies in mice with reconstituted bone marrow
III.	Number of small acetylcholinesterase-positive precursor cells of mouse bone marrow

nificantly in the purification, identification, and establishment of its site(s) of production. However, at the present time, the rebound-thrombocythemic mouse assay appears to be the most sensitive and reliable one available. Table 1 summarizes the known effects of thrombopoietin on megakaryocytopoiesis and thrombocytopoiesis both in vitro and in vivo. As shown, there have been several studies showing that thrombopoietin will stimulate megakaryocytes to make increased numbers of new platelets.

Since poietins are not as lineage specific as was originally thought, it should be no surprise to learn that erythropoietin, IL-3, GM-CSF, and perhaps others will stimulate megakaryocytopoiesis both in vitro and in vivo. However, hypoxia causes the release and action of erythropoietin, which has been shown to shunt stem cells from the megakaryocytic cell line into the erythroid series. This interesting contradiction will require additional work for its resolution. If these findings are correct, it should be possible in the future to treat animals with large doses of thrombopoietin and cause anemia. Although thrombopoietin is just now beginning to be studied in clinical cases, there is sufficient evidence to indicate that it may play a critical role in many patients who are suffering from platelet production disorders. Thrombopoietin's involvement in diseases appears in some cases to be direct, either in deficiency or in excess, on platelet production, and it may be diagnostic.

Finally, we are now at a point in the study of this important hormone that the development of recombinant thrombopoietin should be attempted. Since thrombopoietin has been purified to homogeneity and monoclonal antibodies have been developed, experiments to clone its gene should be forthcoming. After successful cloning and production, large amounts of recombinant thrombopoietin will be helpful in clarifying its mode of action and will no doubt prove therapeutic for several patients with various hematological disorders caused by bone marrow transplantation, chemotherapy, radiotherapy, etc.

Acknowledgments. This work was supported by a grant from the National Heart, Lung, and Blood Institute (HL14637). I am grateful to Marilyn Cottrell and Rose Clift for expert technical assistance, to Wanda Aycock and Joyce Stringfield for excellent secretarial support, and to many collaborators both past and present for their contributions to the work summarized in this review.

References

Abildgaard CF, Simone JV (1967) Thrombopoiesis. Semin Hematol 4:424–452

Adams WH, Liu YK, Sullivan LW (1978) Humoral regulation of thrombopoiesis in man. J Lab Clin Med 91:141–147

Baynes RD, Bothwell TH, Flax H, McDonald TP, Atkinson P, Chetty N, Bezwoda WR, Mendelow BV (1987) Reactive thrombocytosis in pulmonary tuberculosis. J Clin Pathol 6:676–679

Bernstein R, Bagg A, Pinto M, Lewis D, Mendelow B (1986) Chromosome 3q21 abnormalities associated with hyperactive thrombopoiesis in acute blastic transformation of chronic myeloid leukemia. Blood 68:652–657

Bertoncello I, Bradley TR, Hodgson GS (1981) Characterization and enrichment of macrophage progenitor cells from normal and 5-fluorouracil treated mouse bone marrow by unit gravity sedimentation. Exp Hematol 9:604–610

Birks JW, Klassen LW, Gurney CW (1975) Hypoxia-induced thrombocytopenia in mice. J Lab Clin Med 86:230–238

Burstein SA (1986) Interleukin-3 promotes maturation of murine megakaryocytes in vitro. Blood Cells 11:469–484

Burstein SA, Adamson JW, Harker LA (1980) Megakaryocytopoiesis in culture: modulation by cholinergic mechanisms. J Cell Physiol 103:201–208

Choi SI, McClure PD, Vranic M (1968) Thrombopoietin activity in idiopathic thrombocytopenia purpura, Br J Haematol 15:345–350

Clark DA, Dessypris EN (1986) Effects of recombinant erythropoietin on murine megakaryocytic colony formation in vitro. J Lab Clin Med 108:423–429

Clark SC, Kamen R (1987) The human hematopoietic colony-stimulating factors. Science 236:1229–1237

Clift R, McDonald TP (1979) A comparison of (^{35}S) sodium sulfate and (^{75}Se) selenomethionine as platelet labels for the assay of thrombopoietin. Proc Soc Exp Biol Med 162:380–382

Cooper GW (1970) The regulation of thrombopoiesis. In: Gordon AS (ed) Regulation of hematopoiesis, vol 2. Appleton-Century-Crofts, New York, p 1611

Cooper GW, Cooper B (1977) Relationships between blood platelet and erythrocyte formation. Life Sci 20:1571–1580

Cullen WC, McDonald TP (1986) Comparison of stereologic techniques for the quantification of megakaryocyte size and number. Exp Hematol 14:782–788

Cullen WC, McDonald TP (1989) Effects of isobaric hypoxia on murine medullary and splenic megakaryocytopoiesis. Exp Hematol 17:246–251

Dassin E, Bourebia J, Najean Y, Rosset AM (1983) Partial purification of a thrombocytopoiesis-stimulating factor present in the serum of thrombocytopenic rats. Acta Haematol 69:249–253

deGabriele G, Penington DG (1967) Regulation of platelet production: thrombopoietin. Br J Haematol 13:210–215

Dessypris EN, Gleaton JH, Armstrong OL (1987) Effect of human recombinant erythropoietin on human marrow megakaryocyte colony formation in vitro. Br J Haematol 65:265–269

Dukes PP, Izadi P, Ortega JA, Shore NA, Gomperts E (1980) Inhibitory effect of interferon on mouse megakaryocytic progenitor cells in culture. Exp Hematol 8:1048–1056

Dukes PP, Egrie JC, Strickland TW, Browne JK, Lin FK (1986a) In vitro and in vivo megakaryocytopoietic effects of recombinant erythropoietin. Exp Hematol 14:469 (abstr)

Dukes PP, Egrie JC, Strickland TW, Browne JK, Lin FK (1986b) Megakaryocyte colony stimulating activity of recombinant human and monkey erythropoietin. In: Levine R, Williams N, Levin J, Evatt B (eds) Megakaryocyte development and function, vol 215. Alan R Liss, New York, p 105

Ebbe S (1974) Thrombopoietin. Blood 44:605–608

Ebbe S (1976) Biology of megakaryocytes. In: Spaet TH (ed) Progress in hemostasis and thrombosis. Grune and Stratton, New York, p 211

Ebbe S, Phalen E (1979) Does autoregulation of megakaryocytopoiesis occur? Blood Cells 5:123–138

Ebbe S, Stohlman F Jr, Overcash J, Donovan J (1968) Megakaryocyte size in thrombocytopenic and normal rats. Blood 32:383–392

Ebbe S, Adrados C, Phalen E (1985) Independence of megakaryocyte number and size in long-term cultures of normal mouse marrow. Exp Hematol 13:817–820

Enomoto K, Kawakita M, Kishimoto S, Katayama N, Miyake T (1980) Thrombopoiesis and megakaryocyte colony stimulating factor in the urine of patients with aplastic anaemia. Br J Haematol 45:551–556

Erslev AJ, Caro J, Kansu E, Miller O, Cobbs E (1979) Plasma erythropoietin in polycythemia. Am J Med 66:243–247

Erslev AJ, Caro J, Kansu E, Silver R (1980) Renal and extrarenal erythropoietin production in anaemic rats. Br J Haematol 45:65–72

Evatt BL, Levin J (1969) Measurement of thrombopoiesis in rabbits using ^{75}selenomethionine. J Clin Invest 48:1615–1626

Evatt BL, Shreiner DP, Levin J (1974) Thrombopoietic activity of fractions of rabbit plasma: studies in rabbits and mice. J Lab Clin Med 83:364–371

Evatt BL, Spivak JL, Levin J (1976) Relationships between thrombopoiesis and erythropoiesis: with studies of the effects of preparations of thrombopoietin and erythropoietin. Blood 48:547–558

Evatt BL, Levin J, Algazy KM (1979) Partial purification of thrombopoietin from the plasma of thrombocytopenic rabbits. Blood 54:377–388

Eyster ME, Saletan SL, Rabellino EM, Karanas A, McDonald TP, Locke LA, Luderer JR (1986) Familial essential thrombocythemia. Am J Med 80:497–502

Fraser JK, Tan AS, Lin F-K, Berridge MV (1987) Erythropoietin receptors on megakaryocytes. Exp Hematol 15:496 (abstr)

Freedman MH, McDonald TP, Saunders EF (1981) Differentiation of murine marrow megakaryocyte progenitors (CFUm): humoral control in vitro. Cell Tissue Kinet 14:53–58

Gafter U, Bessler H, Malachi T, Żevin D, Djaldetti M, Levi J (1987) Platelet count and thrombopoietic activity in patients with chronic renal failure. Nephron 45:207–210

Ganser A, Carlo-Stella C, Greher J, Völkers B, Hoelzer D (1987) Effect of recombinant interferons alpha and gamma on human bone marrow-derived megakaryocytic progenitor cells. Blood 70:1173–1179

Gewirtz AM (1986) Human megakaryocytopoiesis. Semin Hematol 23:27–42

Grant BW, Nichols WL, Solberg LA, Yachimiak DJ, Mann KG (1987) Quantitation of human in vitro megakaryocytopoiesis by radioimmunoassay. Blood 69: 1334–1339

Greenberg SM, Kuter DJ, Rosenberg RD (1987) In vitro stimulation of megakaryocyte maturation by megakaryocyte stimulatory factor. J Biol Chem 262:3269–3277

Grossi A, Vannucchi AM, Rafanelli D, Ferrini PR (1987) Biological characterization of partially purified human urinary thrombopoietin. Haematologica 72:291–295

Harker LA (1968) Megakaryocyte quantitation. J Clin Invest 47:452–457

Hill R, Levin J (1986) Partial purification of thrombopoietin using lectin chromatography. Exp Hematol 14:752–759

Hirsh EH, Vogler WR, McDonald TP, Stein SF (1980) Acquired hypomegakaryocytic thrombocytopenic purpura: occurrence in a patient with absent thrombopoietic stimulating factor. Arch Intern Med 140:721–723

Hoffman R, Mazur E, Bruno E, Floyd V (1981) Assay of an activity in the serum of patients with disorders of thrombopoiesis that stimulates formation of megakaryocytic colonies. N Engl J Med 305:533–538

Hoffman R, Yang HH, Bruno E, Straneva JE (1985) Purification and partial characterization of a megakaryocyte colony-stimulating factor from human plasma. J Clin Invest 75:1174–1182

Hoffman R, Straneva J, Yang H, Bruno E, Brandt J, Lu L, Geissler D (1986) Humoral regulation of cellular events occurring during megakaryocytopoiesis. Exp Hematol 14:417 (abstr)

Iscove NN, Roitsch CA, Williams N, Guilbert LJ (1982) Molecules stimulating early red cell, granulocyte, macrophage and megakaryocyte precursors in culture: similarity in size, hydrophobicity and charge. J Cell Physiol [Suppl]1: 67–78

Ishibashi T, Burstein SA (1986) Interleukin 3 promotes the differentiation of isolated single megakaryocytes. Blood 67:1512–1514

Ishibashi T, Koziol JA, Burstein SA (1987) Human recombinant erythropoietin promotes differentiation of murine megakaryocytes in vitro. J Clin Invest 79: 286–289

Jackson CW (1973) Cholinesterase as a possible marker for early cells of the megakaryocyte series. Blood 42:413–421

Jackson CW, Edwards CC (1977) Biphasic thrombopoietic response to severe hypobaric hypoxia. Br J Haematol 35:233–244

Jackson CW, Simone JV, Edwards CC (1974) The relationship of anemia and thrombocytosis. J Lab Clin Med 84:357–368

Johnson CA, Abildgaard CF, Schulman I (1971) Functional studies of young versus old platelets in a patient with chronic thrombocytopenia. Blood 37:163–171

Kalmaz GD, McDonald TP (1981a) Effects of antiplatelet serum and thrombopoietin on the percentage of small acetylcholinesterase-positive cells in bone marrow of mice. Exp Hematol 9:1002–1010

Kalmaz GD, McDonald TP (1981b) The effects of thrombopoietin on megakaryocytopoiesis of mouse bone marrow cells in vitro. In: Evatt B, Levine R, Williams N (eds) Megakaryocyte biology and precursors: in vitro cloning and cellular properties. Elsevier North Holland, New York, p 77

Kalmaz GD, McDonald TP (1982) Assay for thrombopoietin: a new, more sensitive method based on measurement of the small acetylcholinesterase-positive cell. Proc Soc Exp Biol Med 170:213–219

Kalmaz GD, McDonald TP (1985) Effect of thrombopoietin on in vitro production of megakaryocytes from fetal mouse liver cells. Proc Soc Exp Biol Med 180: 50–56

Kalmaz GD, Kumakawa N, Kumakawa T, McDonald TP, Bessman JD (1987) Effects of neostigmine on in vitro production of megakaryocytes from fetal mouse liver cells. Exp Hematol 15:493 (abstr)

Kawakita M, Miyake T, Kishimoto S, Ogawa M (1982) Apparent heterogeneity of human megakaryocyte colony and thrombopoiesis-stimulating factors: studies on urinary extracts from patients with aplastic anemia and idiopathic thrombocytopenic purpura. Br J Haematol 52:429–438

Kelemen E, Csèrhati I, Tanos B (1958) Demonstration and some properties of human thrombopoietin in thrombocythemic sera. Acta Haematol (Basel) 20: 350–355

Keller KL, Rolovic Z, Evatt BL, Sewell ET, Ramsey RB (1988) The effects of thrombopoietic activity of rabbit plasma fractions on megakaryocytopoiesis in agar cultures. Exp Hematol 16:262–267

Kimura H, Burstein SA, Thorning D, Powell JS, Harker LA, Fialkow PJ, Adamson JW (1984) Human megakaryocytic progenitors (CFU-M) assaying in methylcellulose: physical characteristics and requirements for growth. J Cell Physiol 118:87–96

Klener P, Marcibal O, Donner L, Kornalik F (1977) Serum thrombopoietic activity following administration of vinblastine. Scand J Haematol 19:287–292

Krizsa F (1971) Study on the development of posthaemorrhagic thrombocytosis in rats. Acta Haematol (Basel) 46:228–231

Langdon JR, McDonald TP (1977) Effects of chronic hypoxia on platelet production in mice. Exp Hematol 5:191–198

Layendecker SJ, McDonald TP (1982) The relative roles of the spleen and bone marrow in platelet production in mice. Exp Hematol 10:332–342

Lepore DA, Harris RA, Penington DG (1984) Megakaryoblast precursors in rodent bone marrow: specificity of acetylcholinesterase staining. Br J Haematol 58: 473–481

Leven RM, Yee MK (1987) Megakaryocyte morphogenesis stimulated in vitro by whole and partially fractioned thrombocytopenic plasma: a model system for the study of platelet formation. Blood 69:1046–1052

Levin J (1983) Murine megakaryocytopoiesis in vitro: an analysis of culture systems used for the study of megakaryocyte colony-forming cells and of the characteristics of megakaryocyte colonies. Blood 61:617–623

Levin J, Evatt BL (1979) Humoral Control of thrombopoiesis. Blood Cells 5:105–121

Levin J, Levin FC, Hull DF III, Penington DG (1982) The effects of thrombopoietin on megakaryocyte-CFC, megakaryocytes, and thrombopoiesis: with studies of ploidy and platelet size. Blood 60:989–998

Levine RF, Hazzard KC, Lamberg JD (1982) The significance of megakaryocyte size. Blood 60:1122–1131

Long MW, Henry RL (1979) Thrombocytosis-induced suppression of small acetylcholinesterase-positive cells in bone marrow of rats. Blood 54:1338–1346

Long MW, Williams N, Ebbe S (1982a) Immature megakaryocytes in the mouse: physical characteristics, cell cycle status, and in vitro responsiveness to thrombocytopoietic stimulatory factor. Blood 59:569–575

Long MW, Williams N, McDonald TP (1982b) Immature megakaryocytes in the mouse: in vitro relationship to megakaryocyte progenitor cells and mature megakaryocytes. J Cell Physiol 112:339–344

Mazur EM (1987) Megakaryocytopoiesis and platelet production: a review. Exp Hematol 15:340–350

Mazur EM, South K (1985) Human megakaryocyte colony-stimulating factor in sera from aplastic dogs: partial purification, characterization and determination of hematopoietic cell lineage specificity. Exp Hematol 13:1164–1172

Mazur EM, Cohen JL, Wong GG, Clark SC (1987) Modest stimulatory effect of recombinant human GM-CSF on colony growth from peripheral blood human megakaryocyte progenitor cells. Exp Hematol 15:1128–1133

McClure PD, Choi SI (1968) Thrombopoietin and erythropoietin levels in idiopathic thrombocytopenic purpura and iron-deficiency anaemia. Br J Haematol 15: 351–354

McDonald TP (1973a) The hemagglutination-inhibition assay for thrombopoietin. Blood 41:219–233

McDonald TP (1973b) Bioassay for thrombopoietin utilizing mice in rebound-thrombocytosis. Proc Soc Exp Biol Med 144:1006–1012

McDonald TP (1973c) Regulation of thrombopoiesis. Medicina 33:459–466

McDonald TP (1974a) Immunological studies of thrombopoietin. Proc Soc Exp Biol Med 147:513–518

McDonald TP (1974b) Immunoassay and bioassay for thrombopoietin. In: Baldini MG, Ebbe S (eds) Platelets: production, function, transfusion, and storage. Grune and Stratton, New York, p 81

McDonald TP (1975) Assay of thrombopoietin utilizing human sera and urine fractions. Biochem Med 13:101–110

McDonald TP (1976a) A comparison of platelet size, platelet count, and platelet ^{35}S incorporation as assays for thrombopoietin. Br J Haematol 34:257–267

McDonald TP (1976b) Role of the kidneys in thrombopoietin production. Exp Hematol 4:27–31

McDonald TP (1977a) Annotation: assays for thrombopoietin. Scand J Haematol 18:5–12

McDonald TP (1977b) Effects of different routes of administration and injection schedules of thrombopoietin on ^{35}S incorporation into platelets of assay mice. Proc Soc Exp Biol Med 155:4–7

McDonald TP (1978a) Platelet production in hypoxic and RBC-transfused mice. Scand J Haematol 20:213–220

McDonald TP (1978b) A comparison of platelet production in mice made thrombocytopenic by hypoxia and by platelet specific antisera. Br J Haematol 40:299–309

McDonald TP (1978c) Neutralizing antiserum to thrombopoietin. Proc Soc Exp Biol Med 158:557–560

McDonald TP (1980) Effect of thrombopoietin on platelet size of mice. Exp Hematol 8:527–532

McDonald TP (1981a) Annotation: assay and site of production of thrombopoietin. Br J Haematol 49:493–499

McDonald TP (1981b) Thrombopoietin and its control of thrombocytopoiesis and megakaryocytopoiesis. In: Evatt B, Levine R, Williams N (eds) Megakaryocyte biology and precursors: in vitro cloning and cellular properties. Elsevier North Holland, New York, p 39

McDonald TP (1987) Regulation of megakaryocytopoiesis by thrombopoietin. Ann NY Acad Sci 509:1–24

McDonald TP (1988a) Thrombopoietin: its biology, purification, and characterization. Exp Hematol 16:201–205

McDonald TP (1988b) Current status of thrombopoietin. In: Tavassoli M, Abraham N, Ascensao E, Zanjani E, Levine A (eds) Molecular biology of hemopoiesis. Plenum, New York, p 245

McDonald TP, Clift R (1979) Effects of thrombopoietin and erythropoietin on platelet production in rebound-thrombocytotic and normal mice. Am J Hematol 6:219–228

McDonald TP, Green D (1977) Demonstration of thrombopoietin production after plasma infusion in a patient with congenital thrombopoietin deficiency. Thromb Haemost 37:577–579

McDonald TP, Kalmaz GD (1983a) Effects of thrombopoietin on the number and diameter of marrow megakaryocytes of mice. Exp Hematol 11:91–97

McDonald TP, Kalmaz GD (1983b) Nephrectomy abolishes the increase in small acetylcholinesterase-positive immature rat megakaryocytes induced by acute thrombocytopenia. Proc Soc Exp Biol Med 174:131–136

McDonald TP, Nolan C (1979) Partial purification of a thrombopoietic-stimulating factor from kidney cell culture medium. Biochem Med 21:146–155

McDonald TP, Shadduck RK (1982) Comparative effects of thrombopoietin and colony-stimulating factors. Exp Hematol 10:544–550

McDonald TP, Lange RD, Congdon CC, Toya RE (1970) Effect of hypoxia, irradiation and bone marrow transplantation on erythropoietin levels in mice. Radiat Res 42:151–163

McDonald TP, Cottrell M, Clift R, Lane K (1974) Purification and assay of thrombopoietin. Exp Hematol 2:355–361

McDonald TP, Clift R, Lange RD, Nolan C, Tribby IIE, Barlow GH (1975) Thrombopoietin production by human embryonic kidney cells in culture. J Lab Clin Med 85:59–66

McDonald TP, Clift R, Jones JB (1976a) Canine cyclic hematopoiesis: platelet size and thrombopoietin level in relation to platelet count. Proc Soc Exp Biol Med 153:424–428

McDonald TP, Clift R, Nolan C, Tribby IIE (1976b) A comparison of mice in rebound-thrombocytosis with platelet-hypertransfused mice for the assay of thrombopoietin. Scand J Haematol 16:326–334

McDonald TP, Cottrell M, Clift R (1977a) Hematologic changes and thrombopoietin production in mice after X-irradiation and platelet-specific antisera. Exp Hematol 5:291–298

McDonald TP, Cottrell M, Nolan C, Walasek O (1977b) Immunologic similarities of thrombopoietin from different sources. Scand J Haematol 18:91–97

McDonald TP, Cottrell M, Clift R (1978a) Effects of short-term hypoxia on platelet counts of mice. Blood 51:165–175

McDonald TP, Cottrell M, Congdon CC, Walasek O, Barlow GH (1978b) Stimulation of megakaryocytic spleen colonies in mice by thrombopoietin. Life Sci 22:1853–1858

McDonald TP, Clift R, Cottrell M (1979a) Assay for thrombopoietin: a comparison of time of isotope incorporation into platelets and the effects of different strains and sexes of mice. Exp Hematol 7:289–296

McDonald TP, Cottrell M, Clift R (1979b) Effects of hypoxia on thrombocytopoiesis and thrombopoietin production of mice. Proc Soc Exp Biol Med 160:335–339

McDonald TP, Andrews RB, Clift R, Cottrell M (1981) Characterization of a thrombocytopoietic-stimulating factor from kidney cell culture medium. Exp Hematol 9:288–296

McDonald TP, Cottrell M, Clift R (1985a) Regulation of megakaryocytopoiesis by acetylcholinesterase. Exp Hematol 13:437 (abstr)

McDonald TP, Cottrell M, Clift R, Khouri JA, Long MD (1985b) Studies on the purification of thrombopoietin from kidney cell culture medium. J Lab Clin Med 106:162–174

McDonald TP, Miura M, Koizumi S (1985c) Thrombopoietin production in a patient with chronic thrombocytopenia after plasma infusion. Thromb Res 38:353–359

McDonald TP, Clift R, Cottrell M (1986a) Monoclonal antibodies to human urinary thrombopoietin. Proc Soc Exp Biol Med 182:151–158

McDonald TP, Clift R, Cottrell M, Long MD (1986b) Further studies on the purification and assay of thrombopoietin. In: Levine RF, Williams N, Levin J, Evatt BL (eds) Megakaryocyte development and function. Alan R Liss, New York, p 215

McDonald TP, Cullen WC, Cottrell M, Clift R (1986c) Effects of hypoxia on the small acetylcholinesterase-positive megakaryocyte precursor in bone marrow of mice. Proc Soc Exp Biol Med 183:114–117

McDonald TP, Clift R, Cottrell M, Long MD (1987a) Recovery of thrombopoietin during purification. Biochem Med Metab Biol 37:335–343

McDonald TP, Cottrell MB, Clift RE, Cullen WC, Lin FK (1987b) High doses of recombinant erythropoietin stimulate platelet production in mice. Exp Hematol 15:719–721

McDonald TP, Clift RE, Cottrell MB, Long MD (1988) A four-step procedure for a rapid purification of thrombopoietin. Exp Hematol 16:488 (abstr)

Messner HA, Jamal N, Izaguirre C (1982) The growth of large megakaryocyte colonies from human bone marrow. J Cell Physiol [Suppl]1:45–51

Metcalf D (1985) The granulocyte-macrophage colony-stimulating factors. Science 229:16–22

Metcalf D, Begley CG, Johnson GR, Nicola NA, Vadas MA, Lopez AF, Williamson DJ, Wong GG, Clark SC, Wang EA (1986) Biologic properties in vitro of a recombinant human granulocyte-macrophage colony stimulating factor. Blood 67:37–45

Miura M, Jackson CW, Lyles SA (1984a) Increases in circulating megakaryocyte growth-promoting activity in the plasma of rats following whole-body irradiation. Blood 63:1060–1066

Miura M, Koizumi S, Nakamura K, Ohno T, Tachinami T, Yamagami M, Taniguchi N, Kinoshta S, Abildgaard CF (1984b) Efficacy of several plasma components in a young boy with chronic thrombocytopenia and hemolytic anemia who responds repeatedly to normal plasma infusions. Am J Hematol 17:307–319

Miura M, Jackson CW, Steward SA (1988) Increase in circulating megakaryocyte growth-promoting activity (meg-GPA) following sublethal irradiation is not related to decreased platelets. Exp Hematol 16:139–144

Miyake T, Kawakita M, Enomoto K, Murphy MJ Jr (1982) Partial purification and biological properties of thrombopoietin extracted from the urine of aplastic anemia patients. Stem Cells 2:129–144

Naets JP (1958) Erythropoiesis in nephrectomized dogs. Nature 181:1134–1135

Naets JP, Wittek M (1968) Erythropoiesis in anephric man. Lancet 1:941–943

Nakeff A, Daniels-McQueen S (1976) In vitro colony assay for a new class of megakaryocyte precursor: colony forming unit megakaryocyte (CFU-M). Proc Soc Exp Biol Med 151:587–590

Nakeff A, Roozendaal KJ (1975) Thrombopoietin activity in mice following immune-induced thrombocytopenia. Acta Haematol (Basel) 54:340–344

Nakeff A, Dicke KA, van Noord MJ (1975) Megakaryocytes in agar cultures of mouse bone marrow. Semin Haematol 8:4–21

Nickerson HJ, Silberman TL, McDonald TP (1980) Hepatoblastoma, thrombocytopoiesis, and increased thrombopoietin. Cancer 45:315–317

Nicola NA, Johnson GR (1982) The production of committed hemopoietic colony-forming cells from multipotential precursor cells in vitro. Blood 60:1019–1029

Odell TT Jr (1974) Megakaryocytopoiesis and its response to stimulation and suppression. In: Baldini MG, Ebbe S (eds) Platelets: production, function, transfusion and storage. Grune and Stratton, New York, p 11

Odell TT, Boran DA (1977) The mitotic index of megakaryocytes of mice after acute thrombocytopenia. Proc Soc Exp Biol Med 155:149–151

Odell TT Jr, McDonald TP, Detwiler TC (1961) Stimulation of platelet production by serum of platelet-depleted rats. Proc Soc Exp Biol Med 108:428–431

Odell TT Jr, McDonald TP, Asano M (1962) Response of rat megakaryocytes and platelets to bleeding. Acta Haematol (Basel) 27:171–179

Odell TT, McDonald TP, Shelton C, Clift R (1979) Stimulation of mouse megakaryocyte endomitosis by plasma from thrombocytopenic rats. Proc Soc Exp Biol Med 160:263–265

Ogle JW, Dunn CDR, McDonald TP, Lange RD (1978) The in vitro production of erythropoietin and thrombopoietin. Scand J Haematol 21:188–196

Oon SH, Williams N (1987) Immature megakaryocytes in the mouse: synergistic response to megakaryocyte potentiator, thrombopoietic stimulatory factor and interleukin 3. Leukemia 1:772–776

Paulus JM, Maigne J, Keyhani E (1981) Mouse megakaryocytes secrete acetylcholinesterase. Blood 58:1100–1106

Penington DG (1970) Isotope bioassay for "thrombopoietin". Br Med J 1:606–608

Petursson SR, Chervenick PA (1987) Effects of hypoxia on megakaryocytopoiesis and granulopoiesis. Eur J Haematol 39:267–273

Pinto MR, King MA, Goss GD, Bezwoda WR, Fernandes-Costa F, Mendelow B, McDonald TP, Dowdle E, Bernstein R (1985) Acute megakaryoblasic leukaemia with 3q inversion and elevated thrombopoietin (TSF): an autocrine role for TSF? Br J Haematol 61:687–694

Puschmann M, Thorn W, Yen Y (1978) Partial purification procedure for human urinary erythropoietin by preparative isotachophoresis. Res Exp Med (Berl) 173:293–296

Quesenberry PJ, Ihle JN, McGrath E (1985) The effect of interleukin 3 and GM-CSA-2 on megakaryocyte and myeloid clonal colony formation. Blood 65: 214–217

Raha S, Wesemann W, McDonald TP (1985) Isolation of mouse megakaryocytes: I. Separation of two fractions enriched in different maturational stages. Eur J Cell Biol 37:111–116

Rath CE, Mailliard JA, Schreiner GE (1957) Bleeding tendency in uremia. N Engl J Med 257:808–811

Robinson BE, McGrath HE, Quesenberry PJ (1987) Recombinant murine granulocyte macrophage colony-stimulating factor has megakaryocyte colony-stimulating activity and augments megakaryocyte colony stimulation by interleukin 3. J Clin Invest 79:1648–1652

Schulman I, Pierce M, Lukens A, Currimbhoy Z (1960) Studies on thrombopoiesis. I. A factor in normal human plasma required for platelet production: chronic thrombocytopenia due to its deficiency. Blood 16:943–957

Schulman I, Abildgaard CF, Cornet JA, Simone JV, Currimbhoy Z (1965) Studies on thrombopoiesis. II. Assay of human plasma thrombopoietic activity. J Pediatr 66:604–612

Shreiner DP, Weinberg J, Enoch D (1980) Plasma thrombopoietic activity in humans with normal and abnormal platelet counts. Blood 56:183–188

Sieff CA (1987) Hematopoietic growth factors. J Clin Invest 79:1549–1557

Sparrow R, Swee-Huat D, Williams N (1987) Haemopoietic growth factors stimulating murine megakaryocytopoiesis: interleukin-3 is immunologically distinct from megakaryocyte-potentiator. Leuk Res 2:31–36

Spector B (1961) In vivo transfer of a thrombopoietic factor. Proc Soc Exp Biol Med 108:146–149

Straneva JE, Yang HH, Hui SL, Bruno E, Hoffman R (1987) Effects of megakaryocyte colony-stimulating factor on terminal cytoplasmic maturation of human megakaryocytes. Exp Hematol 15:657–663

Straneva JE, Briddell RA, McDonald TP, Yang HH(1988) Thrombocytopoiesis stimulating factor (TSF) in aplastic anemia serum accelerates cytoplasmic maturation of human megakaryocytes. Exp Hematol 16:513 (abstr)

Tayrien G, Rosenberg RD (1987) Purification and properties of a megakaryocyte stimulatory factor present both in the serum-free conditioned medium of human embryonic kidney cells and in thrombocytopenic plasma. J Biol Chem 262: 3262–3268

Vainchenker W, Guichard J, Breton-Gorius J (1979) Growth of human megakaryocyte colonies in culture from fetal, neonatal, and adult peripheral blood cells: ultrastructural analysis. Blood Cells 5:25–42

Vainchenker W, Chapman J, Deschamps JF, Vinci G, Bouguet J, Titeux M, Breton-Gorius J (1982) Normal human serum contains a factor(s) capable of inhibiting megakaryocyte colony formation. Exp Hematol 10:650–660

Vannucchi AM, Grossi A, Rafanelli D, Dilollo S, Bertani C, Ferrini PR (1986) Partial purification of a thrombopoietic stimulating activity from human urine. In: Levine RF, Williams N, Levin J, Evatt BL (eds) Megakaryocyte development and function. Alan R Liss, New York, p 221

Vannucchi AM, Grossi A, Rafanelli D, Ferrini PR, Ramponi G (1988) Partial purification and biochemical characterization of human plasma thrombopoietin. Leukemia 2:236–240

Weiner M, Karpatkin S (1972) Use of the megathrombocyte to demonstrate thrombopoietin. Thromb Diath Haemorrh 28:24–30

Weintraub AH, Karpatkin S (1974) Heterogeneity of rabbit platelets. II. Use of the megathrombocyte to demonstrate a thrombopoietic stimulus. J Lab Clin Med 83:896–901

Williams N, Levine RF (1982) The origin, development and regulation of megakaryocytes. Br J Haematol 52:173–180

Williams N, McDonald TP, Rabellino EM (1979) Maturation and regulation of megakaryocytopoiesis. Blood Cells 5:43–55

Williams N, Eger RR, Jackson HM, Nelson DJ (1982) Two-factor requirement for murine megakaryocyte colony formation. J Cell Physiol 110:101–104

Williams N, Jackson H, Iscove NN, Dukes PP (1984) The role of erythropoietin, thrombopoietic stimulating factor, and myeloid colony-stimulating factors on murine megakaryocyte colony formation. Exp Hematol 12:734–740

Williams N, Sparrow R, Gill K, Yasmeen D, McNiece I (1985) Murine megakaryocyte colony stimulating factor: its relationship to interleukin 3. Leuk Res 9: 1487–1496

Yamamoto S (1957) Mechanism of the development of thrombocytosis due to bleeding. Acta Haematol (Jpn) 20:163–178

Yang HH, Bruno E, Hoffman R (1986) Studies of human megakaryocytopoiesis using an anti-megakaryocyte colony-stimulating factor antiserum. J Clin Invest 77:1873–1880

Zucali JR, McDonald TP, Gruber DF, Mirand EA (1977) Erythropoietin, thrombopoietin, and colony stimulating factor in fetal mouse liver culture media. Exp Hematol 5:385–391

CHAPTER 9

Arachidonic Acid Metabolism, Platelets, and Thromboembolic Disease*

D.M. KERINS and G.A. FITZGERALD

A. Arachidonic Acid Metabolism

I. Introduction

Arachidonic acid (C20:5;n-6) is a polyunsaturated 20 carbon fatty acid that contains 4 double bonds, at the 5, 8, 11 and 14 positions and is the most abundant fatty acid in the phospholipid component of cell membranes. Interest in arachidonic acid has been fostered by the biologically active compounds into which it may be converted; the variety of these compounds has led to the introduction by Corey of the term "eicosanoid" as a generic title.

Arachidonic acid may be converted by three routes, the cyclooxygenase and lipoxygenase pathways and via the action of cytochrome P-450. Synthesis of the eicosanoids depends on the prior release of arachidonic acid from cell membranes (BAKHLE 1983). Arachidonic acid is released from the sn-2 position in the phospholipid pool by the action of phospholipase A_2. Alternatively, arachidonate may be formed via phospholipase-C-catalyzed release of diacylglycerol. Phospholipase A_2 appears to be the predominant regulator of arachidonate release in whole cell systems (SMITH et al. 1985). The eicosanoids produce a variety of effects throughout the body; in the cardiovascular system they act as local mediators of platelet-vascular interactions, vessel tone and inflammatory processes.

II. The Cyclooxygenase Pathway

Following the deesterification of free arachidonic acid, the first step in the formation of thromboxane (TX) A_2, prostacyclin (PGI_2) and the "classic" prostaglandins (PGE_2, PGE_2, $PGF_{2\alpha}$, and PGD_2) is the formation of an unstable endoperoxide, 15-hydroperoxy-9, 11-endoperoxide (PGG_2), via the

* Dr. KERINS is a recipient of a Merck Sharp and Dohme International Fellowship in Clinical Pharmacology. This work was supported by grants (HL30400 and GMI5431) from the National Institutes of Health and from Daiichi Seiyaku. Dr. FITZGERALD is an Established Investigator of the American Heart Foundation and the William Stokes Professor of Experimental Therapeutics.

reported concentrations of 6-keto-$PGF_{1\alpha}$ of less than 3 pg/ml in human plasma using a GC-MS assay. These concentrations are less than the threshold required for inhibition of ex vivo platelet aggregation (FITZGERALD et al. 1979). In addition, the same group of authors were able to confirm that mechanical distension or irritation of the veins was capable of stimulating the local release of prostacyclin in vivo (RITTER et al. 1983), indicating the physiological potential for local prostacyclin biosynthesis.

PGI_2 stimulates the release of cAMP in target tissues; it is the increase in concentration of this second messenger that inhibits platelet aggregation (GORMAN et al. 1977; TATESON et al. 1977). PGE_1 and PGD_2 also act to stimulate cAMP production, but PGI_2 produces an increase that is both more marked in magnitude and longer in duration (GORMAN et al. 1977). Whereas PGI_2 and PGE_1 may act at shared receptors in human platelets (DUTTA-ROY and SINHA 1987), there is evidence that they activate different subpopulations in human erythroleukemia cells: thus, PGE_1 but not PGI_2 activates phospholipase D_2 (WU et al. 1991). In addition to its antiplatelet effects, PGI_2 is a potent vasodilator, but it differs from the other vasodilator eicosanoids in its lack of clearance across the pulmonary circulation (DUSTING et al. 1977). Infusion of 11β-[^{3}H]PGI_2 over 24 h revealed that most of the administered radioactivity was excreted in urine. Analysis of the radiolabelled metabolites in the urine identified 16 compounds. Of these, 2,3-dinor-6-keto-$PGF_{1\alpha}$ was the most abundant (BRASH et al. 1983).

III. Shunting of Endoperoxides

Up to the stage of formation of the endoperoxide PGH_2, both the platelet and the endothelial cells share a common synthetic pathway. However, distal to this step, synthesis becomes relatively specific to the particular cell type. The platelet, for example, forms mainly TXA_2 and the endothelial cell, prostacyclin. In view of the proximity of platelets and endothelial cells, this raises the possibility of an interaction occurring between the endoperoxides at these sites. Such an interaction was demonstrated initially in 1976 by BUNTING et al. They found that indomethacin-treated rings of celiac or mesenteric arteries developed an antiaggregatory substance when incubated with platelet-rich plasma. When the rings were incubated in buffer, no such inhibition occurred. They proposed that the formation of this activity, subsequently identified as prostacyclin, by arterial walls in vivo can be dependent on the supply of prostaglandin endoperoxides by platelets. Direct proof of this hypothesis was provided by MARCUS et al. (1980), who showed that in the presence of platelets preincubated with [^{3}H]arachidonic acid, thrombin stimulated unlabelled endothelial cell suspensions to produce radiolabelled 6-keto-$PGF_{1\alpha}$. No such product was formed when the endothelial cells were pretreated with aspirin. In contrast, suspensions of platelets radiolabelled with arachidonic acid and endothelial cells pretreated with aspirin produced significant quantities of labelled 6-keto-$PGF_{1\alpha}$. In the absence of an endoperoxide source, aspirin-treated endothelial cells were unable to form PGI_2. In contrast, the transfer of endothelial cell endoperoxides to platelets does not occur. SCHAFER et al. (1984) labelled cultured bovine aortic endothelial cells with [^{3}H]arachidonic acid; when these cells were stimulated with the calcium ionophore, A23187, in the presence of aspirin-treated and washed platelet suspensions, no radiolabelled TXB_2 was formed. Thus, the transfer of prostaglandins between platelets and endothelial cells is unidirectional. However, these experiments were performed in the absence of flow albumin, and other components of plasma which might influence the stability of intermediate compounds in this process (FITZPATRICK and WYNALDA 1982).

This diversion of endoperoxides to the formation of other eicosanoid products under conditions of thromboxane synthesis inhibition is illustrated in Fig. 2. From a pharmacological standpoint, it offers the possibility of broadening the spectrum of platelet inhibition from preventing TXA_2-dependent aggregation, as with aspirin, to inhibiting the effects of all recognized platelet agonists by augmenting the formation of prostacyclin.

Evidence of such a transcellular metabolism of prostaglandin endoperoxides in man has recently been demonstrated (NOWAK and FITZGERALD 1989). These authors utilized a microquantitative assay to measure the eicosanoids in 40 μl samples of blood from a template bleeding time incision. Following the administration of a thromboxane synthase inhibitor, production of PGI_2 as well as PGE_2, PGF_2 and PGD_2 increased, reflecting a transcellular metabolism of arachidonic acid at the platelet-vascular interface in man.

IV. The Lipoxygenase Pathway

In addition to the cyclooxygenase pathway, the platelet is also capable of metabolizing arachidonic acid via a 12-lipoxygenase (Fig. 4). Tissues differ not only in the site at which oxygen is inserted by lipoxygenases, but also in the stereospecificity of its insertion, i.e., the production of 12*S* and 12*R* products (BRASH 1989). While lipoxygenation of arachidonic acid in platelets leads to the formation of 12*S*-hydroxy-5,8,10,14-eicosatetraenoic acid (12*S*-HETE) 12-*R*-HETE is the major product of corneal epithelial cells. Polymorphonuclear leukocytes form 5-HETE and cultured endothelial cells produce 5-HETE, 11-HETE, and 15-HETE. The presence of lipoxygenase activity in platelets was demonstrated by HAMBERG and SAMUELSSON (1974) and by NUGTEREN (1975); this was one of the earliest sites at which such activity was found in animal tissue. As a chemo-attractant for human polymorphonuclear leukocytes, the 12*R*-HETE stereoisomer was more potent than 12*S*-HETE (CUNNINGHAM and WOLLARD 1987). The platelet 12-lipoxygenase has recently been clones (FUNK et al. 1990). The deduced amino acid sequence is 85% homologous with the 12-hypoxygenate of porcine leucocytes (YOSHIMOTO et al. 1990).

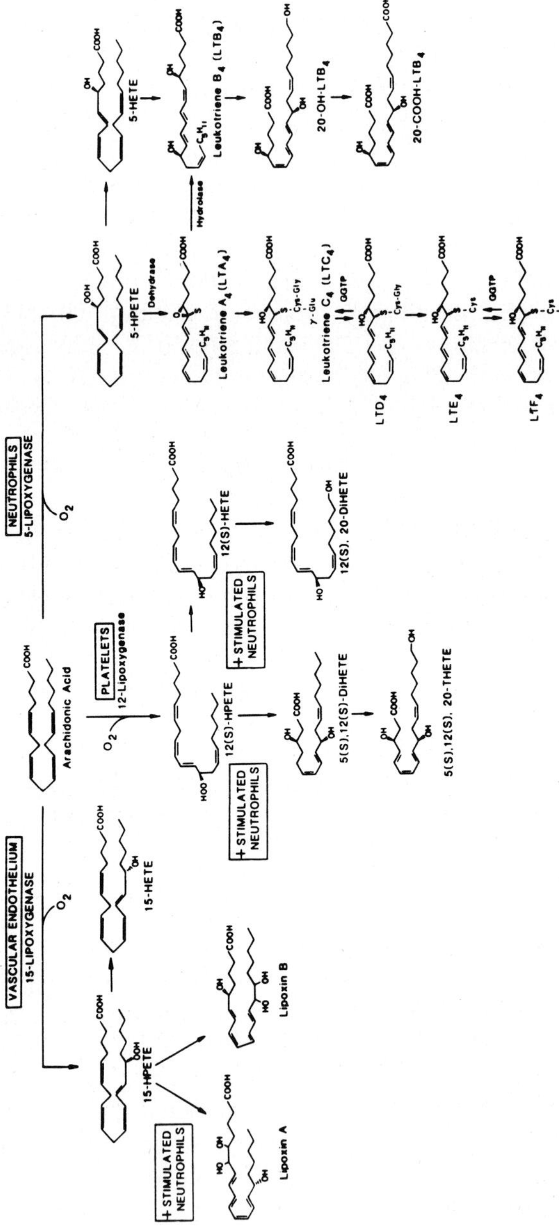

Fig. 4. Metabolism of arachidonic acid by lipoxygenase enzymes. (From WYNGARDEN and SMITH 1988)

In the platelet, arachidonic acid is initially converted to the 12-hydroperoxyeicosa-5,8,10,14-tetraenoic acid (12-HPETE). The next step in the synthetic pathway is reduction by a peroxidase to 12-HPETE (TAYLOR and MORRIS 1983). The 12-lipoxygenase is activated over a time course that is both later in onset and more prolonged in duration than that of cyclooxygenase (HAMBERG and HAMBERG 1980). A further difference between the cyclooxygenase and 12-lipoxygenase pathways is the lack of inhibition of the latter by aspirin (MARCUS 1984). Both 12-HETE and 12-HPETE are capable of stimulating neutrophil chemotaxis, with a greater chemotactic activity observed with 12-HPETE (GOETZL et al. 1980). Both compounds also enhance neutrophil expression of C3b receptors. These compounds may also play a part in tumor metastasis; HONN et al. (1988) reported that exogenous 12*S*-HETE but not 12*R*-HETE, 5-HETE, or 15-HETE was capable of stimulating the adhesion of Lewis lung carcinoma cells to endothelium, subendothelium, and fibronectin. This adhesion was mediated, at least in part, by expression of the glycoprotein IIb/IIIa adhesion molecule (GpIIb/IIIa) on the tumor cells. It has been suggested by BRASH (1985) that 12-lipoxygenase acts to eliminate free arachidonic acid from platelet membranes and facilitate the shape changes that occur during platelet activation. HAMMARSTROM and FALARDEAU (1977) demonstrated that 12-HPETE but not 12-HETE was capable of inhibiting the conversion of PGG_2 to TXB_2 by thromboxane synthase. 12-HPETE is formed during platelet aggregation (HAMBERG and SAMUELSSON 1975) and has been proposed by HAMMARSTROM and FALARDEAU (1977) to serve as a regulator of thromboxane synthesis in vivo. MARCUS et al. (1987) have demonstrated that unstimulated neutrophils can convert 12-lipoxygenase products of stimulated platelets to 12,20-diHETE by a cytochrome-P-450-dependent process. MACLOUF and his coworkers (1989) provided evidence of a further cell-cell interaction, whereby the presence of platelets in a neutrophil-rich suspension greatly increased the stimulated production of sulfidopeptide leukotrienes. Within the leukocyte, 5-lipoxygenase activity leads to the production of 5-HPETE which is converted to the sulfidopeptide leukotrienes, as reviewed by LEWIS and AUSTEN (1984). MEHTA and her colleagues (1986) have demonstrated that the leukotrienes LTC_4, LTD_4, and LTE_4 have no direct effects on platelet aggregation but potentiate the effects of subthreshold concentrations of epinephrine or thrombin. LTC_4, LTD_4, and LTE_4 have vasoconstricting effects; their influence can be inhibited utilizing peptido-leukotriene antagonists (EGAN et al. 1989). Such tools may enable the determination of the contribution of products of the lipoxygenase pathway to a variety of inflammatory processes.

V. The Epoxygenase Pathway

In addition to the cyclooxygenase and lipoxygenase pathways, it has been recognized more recently that arachidonic acid can be metabolized via

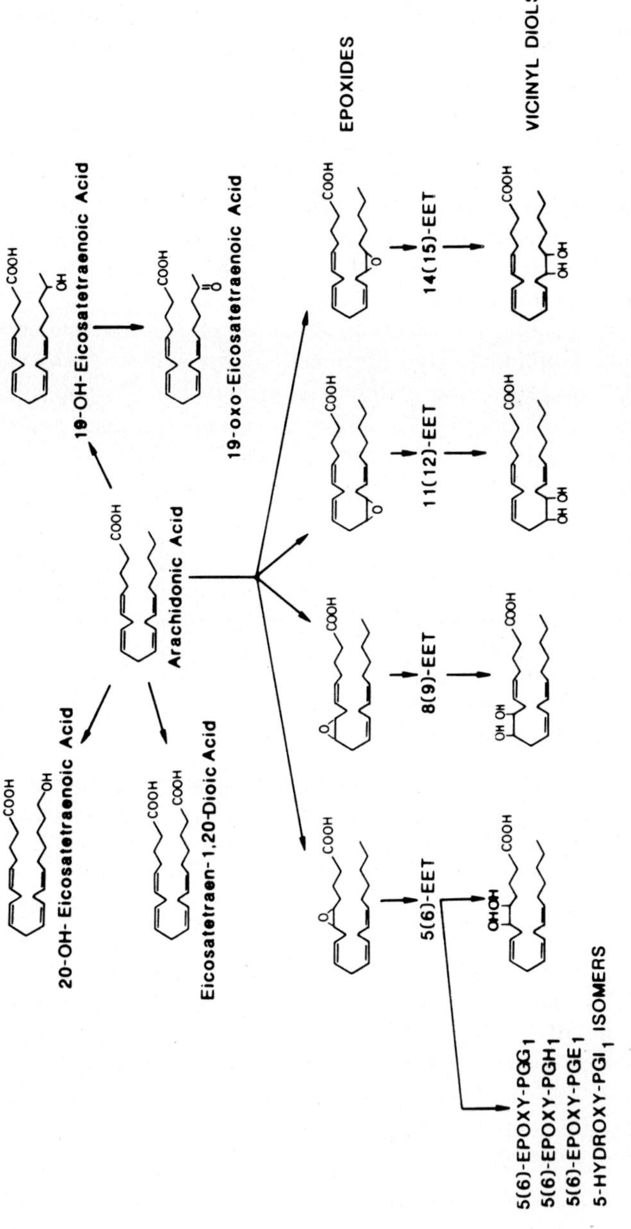

Fig. 5. Metabolism of arachidonic acid by cytochrome P-450 (From WYNGARDEN and SMITH 1988)

cytochrome P-450 (Fig. 5). This was demonstrated by CAPDEVILA et al. (1981) for liver microsomal preparations. The reaction obeyed the stoichiometry of a monooxygenase reaction and resulted in the formation of products of W-oxidation and W-1-oxidation of arachidonic acid. Epoxidation of arachidonic acid by hepatic monooxygenases results in the formation of a series of four epoxyeicosatrienoic acids (EETs), the 5,6-, 8,9-, 11,12-, and 14,15-EETs (OLIW et al. 1982). The epoxides may, in turn, give rise to the formation of the corresponding dihydroxyeicosatrienoic acids. These EETs have been demonstrated to have a variety of effects in vitro. Synthetic 5,6-EET is capable of stimulating pituitary cells in culture to release somatostatin (CAPDEVILA et al. 1983); EETs have also been reported to inhibit renal Na^+ K^+-ATPase activity (SCHWARTZMAN et al. 1985). In terms of influences on vascular tone, PROCTOR et al. (1987) examined the vasoactivity of purified synthetic EETs on the intestinal microcirculation. The order of potency was 5,6-EET > 8,9-EET = 11,12-EET > 14,15-EET. In the rat caudal artery, the only form to produce detectable vasodilation was 5,6-EET, with a potency similar to that of acetylcholine; the corresponding dihydroxyeicosatrienoic acid (DHET) was inactive (CARROLL et al. 1987). SCHWARTZMAN et al. (1989) have recently demonstrated that the vasoconstriction caused by 20-HETE is dependent on further metabolism to its cyclooxygenase metabolites, 20-OH-PGG_2 and 20-OH-PGH_2. Increased EET biosynthesis has been demonstrated in patients with pregnancy induced hypertension; a condition characterized by abnormalities in blood pressure, renal and hemostatic function (CATELLA et al. 1990).

VI. Pharmacology of Antiplatelet Agents

There is more experience with aspirin both in the experimental and clinical domains than with any other antiplatelet drug. Aspirin produces its inhibitory effects by the acetylation of cyclooxygenase (ROTH et al. 1975; ROTH and MAJERUS 1975), a component of prostaglandin endoperoxide G/H synthase, an enzyme that has been isolated, sequenced, and expressed from sheep vesicular glands by DEWITT et al. (1989). The enzyme in platelets (FUNK et al. 1990) derives from the same gene (YOKOYAMA and TANABE 1989). RAZ et al. (1988) and BAILEY et al. (1989), have presented biochemical evidence to suggest that there might be more than one cyclooxygenase gene or that more than one product might arise from a single gene via differential splicing. Thus, while one product appears to be constitutively expressed, a second one seems to be regulated by growth factors (BAILEY et al. (1989) and interleukins (RAZ et al. 1988). Recently, XIE et al. (1991) have identified a second cyclooxygenate gene in chick fibroblasts. An intron which separates the leader sequence from the coding region is spliced out when cells are stimulated to divide. Messages for both cyclooxygenated have been detected in endothelial cells.

Aspirin inhibits cyclooxygenase activity by acetylation of the serine residue at position 529 in human platelets but does not influence the hydroperoxidase activity. Production of a mutant PGG/H synthase with the replacement of this serine residue by alanine (DEWITT et al. 1990) does not result in an alteration in inhibition by the nonsteroidal antiinflammatory agent flurbiprofen but abolishes aspirin-induced inhibition. The authors conclude that aspirin produces its inhibitory action by stearically inhibiting arachidonic acid entry to the active site. Studies by PAN CHEN and MARNETT (1989) indicate that the heme prosthetic group of PGG/H synthase is essential for acetylation by aspirin.

Aspirin produces inhibitory effects on cyclooxygenase in both platelets and endothelial cells. The resultant acetylation is irreversible and can only be overcome by further synthesis of the enzyme, which is possible in the endothelial cell but not for the anucleate platelet. This difference in response raises the possibility for selective inhibition of platelet cyclooxygenase and TXA_2 production with preservation, relatively or absolutely, of endothelial cell prostacyclin synthesis. PATRIGNANI et al. (1982) studied the dose-response relationship of oral aspirin and TXB_2 production during whole blood clotting in healthy volunteers. They reported a linear relationship between single doses of aspirin and inhibition of TXB_2 production (correlation $r = 0.92$, $P < 0.01$). Cumulative inhibition was observed with repeated administration of 0.45 mg/kg day, 36% after the first dose, 70% after the second, 87% after the third, and 95% after the fourth. However, this did not affect urinary excretion of PGE_2, $PGF_{2\alpha}$, or 6-keto-$PGF_{1\alpha}$. WEKSLER et al. (1985) randomized 20 male patients, scheduled for coronary artery bypass grafting, to either aspirin 20 mg daily over the week prior to surgery or to placebo. On the morning of surgery, platelet aggregation was inhibited in the group treated with the low-dose aspirin, as was serum TXB_2 generation, to less than 10% of the control value. The authors assessed the ability of vascular tissue isolated at the time of surgery to generate PGI_2 when incubated with arachidonic acid. PGI_2 production was reduced by roughly 60% in aortic tissue and by about 50% in saphenous vein. Despite the inhibition of platelet function, perioperative blood loss was not detectably increased. In contrast, a previous study by WEKSLER et al. (1983) demonstrated that a single dose of aspirin of 80 mg produced a nonsignificant (mean 19%) decrease in venous production of PGI_2 and an approximately 40% reduction in the capacity to produce PGI_2 by arterial specimens.

One potential mechanism of inhibition of platelet thromboxane biosynthesis is the presystemic inhibition of platelets exposed to aspirin in the intestinal capillaries and portal vessels prior to hepatic metabolism. Hepatic clearance of aspirin may lower concentrations sufficiently to prevent a sytemic effect on endothelial production of prostacyclin. PEDERSEN and FITZGERALD (1984) noted a presystemic component to the action of aspirin at doses as low as 20 and 40 mg. More recently, a controlled release preparation of aspirin 75 mg, formulated according to these principles, maximally inhibited platelet T_xA_2 while preserving the augmentation in PGI_2 biosynthesis evoked by systemic infusion of bradykinin (CLARKE et al. 1991).

This concept raises the possibility that variation in rate as well as dose of aspirin administration may enhance the selectivity of this drug for the platelet.

Studies of low-dose aspirin performed to date have utilized a dosage in excess of that which may produce selective inhibition of thromboxane. The effect on PGI_2 biosynthesis was not determined in any of these trials; however, it is likely that it was decreased in all.

Other targets for drug action are more distal to the formation of the endoperoxides and involve committed steps in thromboxane synthesis and action. The literature on the response to thromboxane synthase inhibitors in experimental models is extensive; such agents are currently being assessed in man for a variety of thromboembolic conditions. One advantage is their ability to divert the precursor prostaglandin endoperoxides towards the endothelium, resulting in the increased formation of PGI_2, PGE_2, and PGD_2. AIKEN et al. (1981) showed that the response to a thromboxane synthase inhibitor in a canine model of coronary thrombosis was dependent on endogenous prostacyclin production. However, the endoperoxides are themselves capable of acting on the thromboxane receptor. Such a disadvantage does not apply to agents that inhibit the action of thromboxane at the thromboxane/endoperoxide receptor. Indeed, the combination of thromboxane receptor antagonists with thromboxane synthetase inhibitors may overcome stimulation of the receptor by the prostaglandin endoperoxides as demonstrated recently in vivo by GRESELE et al. (1987) and FITZGERALD et al. (1988b). Compounds are also under clinical development which combine features of both thromboxane synthesis inhibition and thromboxane receptor antagonism in a single agent (DECLERK et al. 1989a,b).

Platelet inhibition can be achieved by the use of antiaggregatory prostaglandins, such as the naturally occurring PGI_2, PGE_1, or PGD_2 or their synthetic analogues, which act via the stimulation of platelet cAMP production. These compounds are limited by the requirement to administer them by the intravenous route, but orally active compounds are currently under development (KERINS et al. 1990). Agents that inhibit platelet phosphodiesterase, such as dipyridamole, act to reduce the catabolism of cAMP and result in platelet inhibition in vitro; however, the clinical results of the currently available compounds has been disappointing, probably due to inadequate oral bioavailability (FITZGERALD 1987).

Platelet activation may also result from a decrease in the production of endogenous thromboregulators (for discussion see MARCUS 1990). Decreased formation of endothelium-derived relaxing factor (EDRF) by vein grafts may contribute to their higher frequency of occlusion (LÜSCHER et al. 1989). Future research into the role of such thromboregulators may provide a target for pharmacological manipulation.

GpIIb/IIIa is expressed on the surface of activated platelets where it serves as a receptor for fibrinogen and other adhesive molecules. The efficacy of antibodies (COLLER 1985) and small peptides (GAN et al. 1988;

GARSKY et al. 1989) directed against this receptor has been demonstrated in a variety of animal models (HANSON et al. 1988; FITZGERALD and FITZGERALD 1989). DI MINNO et al. (1985) have reported that the antiplatelet agent ticlopidine, which is under extensive investigation, depends on the induction of a functional state of thrombasthenia by inhibition of the GpIIb/IIIa receptor.

B. Thromboembolic Disease

I. Introduction

The potent influences of eicosanoids both on the platelet and on vascular smooth muscle tone, as evidenced by studies in vitro, suggests a potential role for these compounds in thrombotic disease. Conditions under which platelets play a role and pharmacological modification of their activity has clinical importance include unstable angina, acute myocardial infarction, coronary artery bypass grafting, coronary angioplasty, valvular replacement, carotid arterial disease and stroke. TXA_2 is also of potential importance in transplant rejection, in the nephrotoxicity of cyclosporine and in the reduction in placental blood flow in pregnancy-induced hypertension.

II. Unstable Angina

Unstable angina is a clinical condition which may precede acute myocardial infarction. In an autopsy study of 25 cases of sudden death due to acute coronary thrombosis, 15 had experienced unstable angina (FALK 1985). All but 1 of these 15 patients had morphological evidence of repetitive episodes of thrombus formation/fragmentation in the form of a layered epicardial thrombus consisting of material of differing age and/or peripheral microemboli and/or microembolic infarcts (FALK 1985). A larger study of patients with sudden ischemic cardiac death at postmortem examination (DAVIES et al. 1986) revealed platelet masses downstream of an atheromatous plaque over which thrombus had developed. In addition, DAVIES and coworkers (1986) reported a significant increase from roughly 20% to 45% in the incidence of intramyocardial platelet emboli in patients with unstable angina.

In contrast to its beneficial effect in patients with unstable angina, the evidence for the efficacy of aspirin in the presence of chronic stable angina is much less pronounced. A single oral dose of 650 mg aspirin, administered 15 h previously, did not delay the onset of symptoms of exercise-induced angina or influence the product of heart rate and blood pressure at the onset of angina or the extent of ST segment change at the onset of angina in a group of 13 patients with stable angina pectoris (DAVIS et al. 1978). Similar negative results were obtained (ROBERTSON et al. 1981; CHIERCHIA et al. 1982) for patients with coronary artery spasm. It is of interest that aspirin (4 g per day for 2 days) aggravated the symptoms of 4 patients with Prinzmetal's variant angina (MIWA et al. 1983). MAHONY (1989) studied 6 patients with angiographically documented three-vessel coronary artery disease and assessed the degree of myocardial ischemia utilizing ambulatory Holter monitoring. Aspirin resulted in a reduction in spontaneous episodes of ischemia in terms of their frequency, number and duration.

Direct visualization of intracoronary vessels has been performed employing angioscopic techniques (SPEARS et al. 1983; INOUE et al. 1987). Angioscopy of patients with unstable angina revealed the presence of complex plaques and thrombi (SHERMAN et al. 1986), some of which were not detected by angiography. Biochemical evidence that platelet activation occurs during unstable angina was given by FITZGERALD et al. (1986); they demonstrated an increase in the urinary excretion of 2,3-dinor-TXB_2 and also in the metabolite of prostacyclin, 2,3-dinor-6-keto-$PGF_{1\alpha}$ in such patients. The increase in the excretion of these metabolites exhibited a close temporal relationship to episodes of chest pain and was in contrast to the lack of any increase in patients with chronic stable angina (FITZGERALD et al. 1986). In contrast, VEJAR et al. (1988) did not find such a relationship and reported that elevations in urinary excretion of 11-dehydro-TXB_2 were not directly related to electrocardiographic features of ischemia. Consistent with a role for platelet activation as an important mediator of outcome in patients with unstable angina, there have been three clinical trials indicating an unequivocal reduction in both myocardial infarction and death in patients treated with aspirin and/or heparin.

The earliest of these trials was performed by the Veterans Administration Cooperative Study Group (LEWIS et al. 1983). Patients were recruited into the study within 48 h of hospital admission, were randomized to receive either 324 mg of aspirin or placebo daily and were treated for 12 weeks. During the period of drug administration, ex vivo platelet aggregation was assessed. The study end-points were defined as death or acute myocardial infarction. A total of 1266 patients with unstable angina were investigated. Over the 12-week study period the combined incidence of death or acute myocardial infarction was 5% (31 of 625) in the aspirin group as compared with 10.1% (65 of 641) in the placebo group; this represented a 51% reduction and was statistically highly significant ($P = 0.0005$).

Aspirin reduced the frequency of the primary end-points, acute myocardial infarction and nonfatal infarction, by 55% (22 vs. 50) and 51% (21 vs. 44), respectively, both being statistically significant. The influence on mortality alone was insignificant, with a trend to a reduction with aspirin therapy (10 vs. 21; $P = 0.054$). Although not planned for in the study protocol, follow-up data were available at 1 year for 86% of the patients. The mean mortality for the aspirin-treated group was 43% less than in the placebo group, that is, a reduction to 5.5% from 9.6% ($P = 0.008$).

The results of the Veterans Administration study, which by design was

Table 1. Comparison of clinical trials of antiplatelet therapy in the setting of unstable angina

	THEROUX et al. (1988)	LEWIS et al. (1983)	CAIRNS et al. (1985)
Number	479	1266	555
Sex ratio (M:F)	2.5	a	2.7
Treatment groups	Asp/Hep	Asp	Asp/Sul
Dose of aspirin/day	650 mg	324 mg	1300 mg
Delay from symptom onset	<8 h	<48 h	8 days
Treatment phase	6 days	12 weeks	2 years
Benefit: death + MI	76%	51%	50.8%

Asp, aspirin; Sul, sulfinpyrazone; Hep, heparin; MI, myocardial infarction.
[a] All patients were male.

confined to males, was subsequently confirmed for both sexes and expanded by the Canadian Multicenter Trial (CAIRNS et al. 1985). Here, patients were recruited within 8 days of hospitalization and were followed over a period of up to 2 years. A total of 555 patients were randomized to either aspirin (325 mg four times daily) or placebo plus sulfinpyrazone (200 mg four times daily) or placebo. The primary analysis of effect was planned on the basis of the occurrence of either cardiac death or nonfatal infarction. Analysis of this study was not two-tailed. Either cardiac death or nonfatal myocardial infarction occurred in a total of 53 patients.

The authors did not find any benefit of sulfinpyrazone, either alone or in combination with aspirin. In contrast, aspirin led to a risk reduction of 50.8%; 17 events occurred in the aspirin-treated groups in comparison with 36 in the untreated groups ($P = 0.008$). Aspirin led to a dramatic 70.6% risk reduction in cardiac death, from 22 in placebo-treated patients to 6 in those treated with aspirin ($P = 0.004$). Events not included in the primary analysis were those in patients who had stopped the study medication for more than 28 days, had outcomes in the postoperative phase of coronary artery bypass, or had normal vessels or minimal disease on coronary angiography. When such events were included and analyzed on an intention-to-treat basis there was a 30% reduction in the risk for both cardiac death and nonfatal outcome ($P = 0.072$) and a 56% reduction for cardiac death ($P = 0.009$). Thus, by an intention-to-treat analysis, aspirin did not have a significant effect on the combination of fatal and nonfatal cardiac events. There was also no significant influence of aspirin on total mortality when the data were analyzed using a two-tailed statistical analysis.

A third study of aspirin in the setting of unstable angina was performed by THEROUX et al. (1988). This study differed from those of LEWIS et al. (1983) and CAIRNS et al. (1985) in that it examined the very acute phase of unstable angina. The patients entered the study at a mean time of 7.9 ± 8.0 h after the last episode of pain, and the study was completed within 6 ±

3 days. It compared therapy with aspirin at an initial dose of 650 mg followed by 325 mg twice daily with heparin, 5000 units as a bolus followed by an infusion of 1000 units per h and modified according to the coagulation time and a combination of both agents. The defined end-points of the study were refractory angina, myocardial infarction and death. Patients were excluded if they had used aspirin on a regular basis prior to admission. A total of 479 patients were recruited. The study was initially planned for a targeted sample size of 696 patients; however, it was terminated prematurely at the time of the first interim analysis of data by the policy board. In the group of patients receiving double placebo, refractory angina occurred in 22.9%, myocardial infarction in 11.9%, and death in 1.7%. The incidence of myocardial infarction was reduced in all treatment groups, to 3.3% with aspirin ($P = 0.012$), to 0.8% with heparin ($P < 0.0001$) and to 1.6% by the combination of aspirin with heparin ($P = 0.001$). There were no deaths among any of the patients receiving active study drugs. Heparin, but not aspirin, was associated with a reduction in the incidence of refractory angina. Thus, this study was unable to address the influences of these agents on either cardiovascular or total mortality. There were no statistically significant differences between the three treatment groups with respect to the outcome for any of the study end-points. There was only a slight trend towards improvement with the combination of aspirin and heparin over aspirin alone. An ongoing trial now compares treatment with aspirin alone to that with heparin alone.

These three studies of patients with unstable angina differed in several key aspects (Table 1). Patients were admitted over different time intervals from the onset of their symptoms: In the Canadian trial patients were entered within 8 days of hospitalization, in the Veterans Administration Cooperative trial within 48 h of admission; this interval was further reduced in the trial of THEROUX et al. (1988) to 24 h. Patients were also followed up over differing periods of time from 6 days to 2 years. The study of LEWIS et al. (1983), in contrast with the other trials, was confined to men. The RISC Group (1990) examined the response to aspirin and heparin in men with unstable angina or non-Q-wave myocardial infarction. Some 796 patients were randomized to receive aspirin (75 mg daily), heparin administered by intermittent 6-hourly bolus, both treatments or neither. Heparin alone had no effect on the end-points of myocardial infarction or death. The only group to exhibit a reduction in these indices over the initial 5-day period of heparin administration was that treated with both aspirin and heparin. However, the benefit was limited. Events occurred in 3 of 210 patients on heparin and aspirin in contrast with 7 of 189 on aspirin and 12 of 189 control patients. Any additional benefit of adding heparin to aspirin appeared to be confined to the earliest period of evaluation, that is, 5 days after randomization. These data indicate that chronic administration of 75 mg aspirin is effective in reducing myocardial infarction and death in the setting of unstable angina.

In conclusion, these trials demonstrated a benefit of aspirin therapy for the end-points of cardiac death and myocardial infarction among patients with unstable angina pectoris. On comparison of these results, patients admitted earlier in relationship to the onset of their symptoms of unstable angina had a slightly greater reduction in mortality. Despite variation in the dosage of aspirin between 75 mg and 1300 mg daily, there does not appear to be a dose-response relationship between aspirin and benefit. The possibility of an enhanced benefit from a selective dose of aspirin that would preserve prostacyclin production remains to be tested in the setting of unstable angina.

The only therapy that was associated with a reduction in episodes of chest pain was anticoagulation with heparin. This finding is reinforced further by the lack of effect of aspirin on chest pain in patients with stable angina pectoris. The benefits of antiplatelet therapy appeared to be greater in the study of THEROUX et al. (1988); however, this study was terminated prematurely, an action which would tend to exaggerate the magnitude of a favorable response. Subgroup analysis of the Canadian Multicenter Trial would suggest that the response to antiplatelet therapy was greater for men than women, but the population of females was smaller, and there is no strong evidence to suggest why this should occur. This hypothesis remains to be addressed by prospective study.

III. Acute Myocardial Infarction

When arteriographic studies are performed carefully (DEWOOD et al. 1980), they provide evidence consistent with thrombosis in the majority of patients during the early stages of acute myocardial infarction. Intermittent coronary occlusion may occur in this condition (HACKETT et al. 1987) and may be exacerbated or even caused by platelet activation or ameliorated by local production of prostacyclin. Biochemical evidence of increased formation of both thromboxane and prostacyclin has been provided by FITZGERALD et al. (1986), HAMM et al. (1986), and HENRIKSSON et al. (1986).

1. Secondary Prevention

Studies of antiplatelet therapy in patients with myocardial infarction have commenced at varying times from the onset of the infarction. This is of potential importance as SHERRY (1980) has highlighted the time-dependent nature of the death rate in untreated patients after myocardial infarction. Studies in which treatment was initiated within the first 24 h were performed by ELWOOD and WILLIAMS (1979) and the ISIS-2 COLLABORATIVE GROUP (1988). ELWOOD and WILLIAMS studied 1705 patients and found no difference in mortality at 1 month between those randomized to a single dose of aspirin 325 mg and placebo. However, the second International Study of Infarct Survival (ISIS-2) was of sufficient size to establish definitively the efficacy of aspirin in preventing death in patients who have suffered a recent myocardial infarction. The design of this study assessed the response to aspirin alone (162.5 mg/daily) for 1 month, streptokinase alone (1 500 000 units intravenously), both agents, or both placebos in a total of 17 187 patients. Treatment was initated on the day of infarction. There was a 23% reduction in the 5-week mortality from 11.8% to 9.4% among all patients treated with aspirin ($2P < 0.00001$; 95% confidence interval 15%–30%). Comparison of the four groups revealed that the reduction in mortality for aspirin (21%) was similar to that for streptokinase (23%). An interesting finding was that the beneficial effects on mortality of combined aspirin and streptokinase, a 42% reduction, was similar to the sum of the effects of each individual agent.

In contrast to these trials, in which patients were entered at an early stage, there was a large range in the delay between entry of the earliest and the latest patients in many of the studies of secondary prevention of myocardial infarction. Another source of variation between these studies involved the dose of aspirin administered to the actively treated patients.

Amongst the earliest retrospective studies was that performed by ELWOOD et al. in 1974. In all, 1239 men were randomized to receive aspirin (300 mg daily) or placebo, at varying intervals from the time of their infarction; 51% were entered after 6 weeks. The results were inconclusive and revealed a nonsignificant trend towards a reduction in mortality with aspirin. The Coronary Drug Project Research Group study was initially designed to evaluate several agents in the prophylaxis of recurrent myocardial infarction. On termination of the portions of this study involving estrogen (5 mg and 2.5 mg per day) and dextrothyroxine (6 mg per day), a population of volunteers was identified who were subsequently reallocated to the Coronary Drug Project Aspirin Study (1976). A minimum of 6.5 months passed from discontinuation of the prior study drug before patients entered the aspirin study. Due to the study design, the interval from myocardial infarction and entry was considerable and greater than 5 years in roughly three-quarters of the patients. A total of 1529 patients were randomized to receive either aspirin (972 mg daily) or placebo. A nonsignificant reduction was found for overall mortality, coronary death and nonfatal myocardial infarction, despite a 30% decrease in overall mortality which did not reach conventional levels of statistical significance.

The Anturane Reinfarction Trial (1978) compared sulfinpyrazone (Anturane) 200 mg four times daily with placebo in 1475 patients of both sexes, admitted within a 25–35-day window after their infarction. Sulfinpyrazone is a reversible cyclooxygenase inhibitor of poor biochemical selectivity (PEDERSEN and FITZGERALD 1985). There was a 48.5% reduction in the annual death rate from 9.5% to 4.9% ($P = 0.011$). However, the trial was discontinued prematurely by the policy committee at a time when the average period of patient observation was only 8.4 months. A later report Anturane Reinfarction Trtal (1980) demonstrated a 74% reduction in sudden death in the group treated with sulfinpyrazone for the early period following the infarct. However, the Food and Drug Administration, (FDA) issued a critique of this trial (Temple and Pledger 1980), in which it was demonstrated that the reported classification of cause of death strengthened the apparent response to sulfinpyrazone; the FDA reinterpreted the results to demonstrate no more than a favorable trend towards increased overall survival.

A further study performed by the Medical Research Council Epidemiology Unit in Wales and reported by Elwood and Sweetnam in 1979 of aspirin (900 mg daily) in 1682 men and women reported a nonsignificant reduction in both total and coronary mortality. In this trial the majority of patients were admitted within 7 days of their infarct.

The German-Austrian Multicenter Prospective Trial (Breddin et al. 1979) compared patients who had survived their infarct for 30-42 days and were randomized to aspirin (1500 mg per day), phenprocoumon (an anticoagulant used widely in those countries at the time of study design in 1970 as an agent in the secondary prevention of myocardial infarction), and placebo. Following 2 years of observartion, a trend was seen towards a reduction in death from all causes, cardiovascular mortality and reinfarction in the aspirin group compared will either control group.

The Aspirin Myocardial Infarction Study Research Group (AMIS) (1980) reported an increase in total mortality from 9.7% in the placebo group to 10.8% in the aspirin (1000 mg/day) group; there was a trend towards a reduction in nonfatal reinfarction. There were baseline differences between the groups that favored the placebo group. Overall, a total of 4524 patients were entered between 8 weeks and 5 years after their infarction. In view of the incidence of side effects in the aspirin group and the lack of benefit, the authors advised against aspirin use.

Two studies were performed by the Persantine-Aspirin Relnfarction Study (PARIS) research group, the first was reported in 1980 and the second, in 1986 (Klimt et al. 1986). In the earlier study, 2026 patients were recruited and randomized to aspirin 324 mg three times daily, dipyridamole 75 mg plus aspirin 324 mg daily, or both placebos. No group received dipyridamole alone. Some 810 patients were entered into each of the active treated groups and 406 to the placebo group. The interval between myocardial infarction and entry varied from 2 months to 5 years, with a follow-up period of 41 months. The primary end-points were total mortality, coronary mortality and coronary incidence. Compliance in this study was similar to that in other studies in this area and ranged from an estimated 70% for the group taking both active drugs to 74% for the placebo group. There was a trend towards a benefit for all end-points with no differences between the group receiving aspirin and dipyridamole when compared with the group receiving aspirin alone. The reduction in coronary mortality was 21% for aspirin alone and 24% for the combination. A difficulty in the interpretation of such studies is illustrated by the post hoc finding that patients randomized within 6 months of infarction showed the largest benefit; however, this applied to only 20% of the patients studied.

In view of the trends detected in PARIS I and the apparent reduction in mortality in the subgroup enrolled in the early postinfarct phase, the PARIS II study was undertaken. Patients were enrolled closer in time to their index infarction, between 4 weeks and 4 months. Only two groups were studied, a placebo group and one receiving aspirin 330 mg in a combined preparation with dipyridamole 75 mg on a three times daily regimen. Despite the absence of a difference between the actively treated groups in the PARIS I study, no group was allocated to aspirin alone. A total of 3128 patients were recruited and the end-points were those of PARIS I with the addition of a follow-up examination at the end of 1 year and at the end of the study period. In contrast to other studies of similar dimension in this setting, a statistically significant reduction of coronary incidence was detected at 1 year (30%) and at the end of the study (24%) for the dipyridamole plus aspirin group. The reductions in the other end-points were not statistically significant.

The French Enquête de Prévention Secondaire de l'Infarctus du Myocarde (EPSIM 1982) compared aspirin (1500 mg daily) with oral anticoagulation in 1303 men and women. Patients were assessed for eligibility within 1 week of myocardial infarction; however, they were entered at an average of 11.4 days. Follow-up was over a mean of 29 months. The primary end-point was death and this did not differ between the two groups. Total mortality was 8.4% among both groups. There was a trend towards an increase in reinfarction among the aspirin-treated group (5% vs. 3%).

The Cottbus Reinfarction Study (Hoffmann and Forster 1987) compared low doses of aspirin (30 mg and 60 mg) with 1000 mg daily. However, the method of allocation was not random: Patients from one group of hospitals were administered low-dose aspirin [30 mg for those recruited over the 1st year ($n = 179$) and 60 mg for the subsequent 20 months ($n = 245$)], and those from a second group of hospitals received high-dose aspirin (1000 mg, $n = 277$); there was no placebo group. Apart from a comparison of antecedent risk factors, no effort was made to compare hospital course, treatment during the acute phase, or in-hospital mortality between the two groups of hospitals. The patients were allocated to these doses at 3 weeks after their infarction. The 30 mg daily regimen reduced reinfarction by 58% and the 60 mg by 50% ($P < 0.01$).

The Antiplatelet Trialists' Collaboration (1988) performed an overview of 25 trials of antiplatelet therapy in patients with histories of transient ischemic attacks, occlusive stroke, unstable angina, or myocardial infarction. Such an overview was undertaken as it enabled inclusion of larger numbers of patients and could also provide information from studies that would not usually be referred to, i.e., they did not confine themselves to studies with unusually promising or unpromising results. The outcomes of 22 of the 25 studies favored antiplatelet therapy. In this analysis, the odds of suffering a vascular event were reduced by 25% ($P < 0.0001$).

In conclusion, the majority of the trials of antiplatelet therapy in the secondary prevention of myocardial infarction demonstrated a trend towards improved outcome. Most failed to demonstrate a significant difference due to a lack of statistical power. The influence of sample size may be inferred from the similarity of the outcome of the metaanalysis of the smaller studies with that of the 17 187 patients enrolled in the ISIS-2 study. The size of ISIS-2 permitted detection of a 23% reduction in vascular mortality with a probability of $2P < 0.00001$. These results suggest that the individual studies included in the Antiplatelet Trialists Group overview were too small to detect the magnitude of the reduction in coronary risk achieved with aspirin. The detection of benefit in patients with unstable angina required trials of modest size. This may be because the population is less dilute with respect to potential benefit for aspirin than that studied in the typical secondary prevention trial (REILLY and FITZGERALD 1987). Indeed, the magnitude of reduction of deaths by aspirin in unstable angina (roughly 50%) seems greater than that in the secondary prevention of myocardial infarction (roughly 25%).

The issue of the ideal dosage of aspirin for the prevention of coronary thrombosis has not been finalized and many of the earlier studies utilized regimens that are associated with an excessive incidence of side effects. The results of the Cottbus Reinfarction Study would suggest that benefits may be seen with doses as low as 30 mg per day. More conclusively, the results of ISIS-2 demonstrate that a dose of 160 mg per day, or less, is likely to be sufficient. However, at a dosage of 160 mg aspirin would be expected to depress prostacyclin formation. The potential benefit of a further reduction in dosage in terms of both dose-related side effects and efficacy remains to be demonstrated. For the present, 160 mg of aspirin has been shown to be of conclusive benefit in this patient population.

The impact of these studies on clinical practice is reflected by the increase in the routine use of antiplatelet therapy for acute myocardial infarction in Great Britain (R. Collins, personal communication) from 11% in 1987 to 86% in 1989. A similar 87% of the patients recruited in GISSI-2 (1990) received aspirin and 96% of those in the International Study Group (1990) trial. An outstanding issue is whether equivalent benefit might be expected in men and women. Most of these trials enrolled both sexes. However, the proportion of female patients was of the order of 14%. There is no convincing evidence that the pharmacokinetics or pharmacodynamics of aspirin differ between men and women.

2. Coronary Thrombolysis

Thrombolytic therapy is established importance for patients with acute myocardial infarction (MARDER and SHERRY 1988). This treatment is directed towards the dissolution of the underlying thrombus of occluded coronary arteries that is present in the majority of patients (DeWood et al. 1980). Platelets may limit outcome during myocardial infarction by inducing vasoconstriction and by the formation of platelet thrombi. However, in the setting of thrombolytic therapy, platelet activation may produce a more specific limitation by the release from activated platelets of plasminogen activator inhibitor (PAI-1) (Erikson et al. 1984) and of α_2-antiplasmin (Joist et al. 1976). There are experimental data to suggest that platelet activation does indeed act as a factor that may limit the response to fibrinolytic agents, both by delaying reperfusion and by inducing reocclusion (Golino et al. 1988; Fitzgerald et al. 1989). In addition, there are biochemical results from clinical studies that platelet activation occurs in the setting of coronary thrombolysis, using streptokinase (Fitzgerald et al. 1988a) and with tissue-type plasminogen activator (Kerins et al. 1989), as reflected by the increased urinary excretion of metabolites of TXA_2.

Sharma and his colleagues (1988) examined the combination of intracoronary PGE_1, a platelet inhibitory prostaglandin and the thrombolytic agent streptokinase, in patients with acute myocardial infarction. The addition of PGE_1 accelerated reperfusion of the occluded coronary artery and improved patency by day 10.

Verheugt et al. (1988) reported on the influence of aspirin (100 mg) administered orally immediately after intravenous streptokinase. Some 24 patients received aspirin and 26, placebo. Reinfarction occurred in 1 patient in the aspirin-treated group and in 6 in the placebo group ($P = 0.11$).

At the present time, the only reliable assessment of antiplatelet therapy in combination with a thrombolytic agent is the ISIS-2 (1988) trial, to which reference has already been made. However, in addition to the results on outcome, this study also presented evidence on the safety or otherwise of the combination of these two forms of therapy. The most obvious complication curtailing the application of such adjuvant therapy would be an increase in the rate of bleeding events. The incidence of minor bleeding, such as oozing from puncture sites, microscopic hematuria, blood-streaked vomit or sputum was 2.3% ± 0.3% in the presence of streptokinase alone and 2.8% ± 0.3% for both agents together. The combination of both streptokinase and aspirin was associated with a 0.3% ± 0.1% (NS) excess of major bleeds; 11 patients who were randomized to both placebos required blood transfusion in contrast to 24 of those who received both agents. An uncontrolled portion of this study was an enquiry as to the intention to administer anticoagulant therapy; this was asked at the time of randomization. The excess of bleeds was more influenced by the clinician's decision to use heparin: For patients who received streptokinase, the excess of any bleeding event was 5.3% ± 0.27% with intravenously given heparin, 2.6% ± 0.12% with subcutaneous administration and 1.5% ± 0.14% without any intended use of heparin. There were 25 strokes among those treated with both streptokinase and aspirin in contrast with 45 for the double placebo group. Issues regarding the value and the minimal dose of aspirin required as an effective adjunct to t-PA have been raised by the Heparin Aspirin Reperfusion Trial

(HART, HSIA et al. 1990). The combination of tissue-plasminogen activator (t-PA) plus intravenous heparin (at a dose sufficient to maintain the partial thromboplastin time at 1½, to 2 times baseline) resulted in infarct-related artery patency of 82% at 7–24 h; in contrast the patency was 52% in the group treated with tissue-type plasminogen activator (t-PA) plus aspirin 80 mg ($P < 0.0001$). After 7 days, the patency of initially patent vessets was 95% for the aspirin-treated group and 88% for the heparin-treated group (NS). The adequacy of inhibition of cyclooxygenase by 80 mg aspirin was not assessed in this study and indeed, the authors incorrectly extrapolated that inhibition that would result from this dose of aspirin based on the published data of PATRIGNANI et al. (1982) for the effect of single doses of 6, 12, 25, 50, and 100 mg of aspirin on serum TXB_2 generation at 24 h after aspirin administration. At 50 mg of aspirin, the inhibition of serum TXB_2 generation was of the order of 75% and at 100 mg it was 95% ± 4% (PATRIGNANI et al. 1982). Their conclusion that "inadequate inhibition of cyclooxygenase activity is thus unlikely to be the basis of the lower patency rate among the patients receiving aspirin" should be viewed with caution in the absence of confirmatory biochemical data.

Table 2. Comparison of trials of prophylactic aspirin usage among physicians

	British study (PETO et al. 1988)		American study (STEERING COMMITTEE 1989)	
Patient characteristics				
Sex	Male		Male	
Age >60 years	53%		25%	
Smokers (current)	30%		11%	
Smokers (ex)	45%		39%	
Study design				
Dose of aspirin	500 or 300 mg/day		325 mg alternate days	
Placebo control	No		Yes	
Blinded	No		Double-blind	
Number	5139		22071	
Duration	72 months		60.2 months	
Compliance				
Compliance (aspirin)	70%		86%	
Compliance (placebo)	98%		86%	
Outcome[a]				
	Aspirin	Control	Aspirin	Control
Fatal MI	47.3 (NS)	49.6	1.8 ($P = 0.007$)	4.8
Nonfatal MI	42.5 (NS)	43.3	23.6 ($P < 0.00001$)	39.2

[a] Event rate per 10 000 person years.
MI, myocardial infarction.

3. Primary Prevention

The potential for aspirin in the prevention of myocardial infarction in asymptomatic subjects has long been recognized. Over 30 years ago CRAVEN (1956) described his experiences of suggesting regular aspirin consumption to his friends and patients. Over 8000 men adopted a regimen of 5–10 g of aspirin daily and he was impressed by the absence of any cases of detectable coronary or cerebral thrombosis.

The Boston Collaborative Drug Surveillance Group reported its findings in a single report covering two separate retrospective studies of aspirin usage in patients with acute myocardial infarction (1974). In one of these studies, regular use of the medication was determined in patients admitted to medical wards. They identified 325 patients with acute myocardial infarction and 3807 controls. Less than 1% of their patients with infarction gave a history of regular aspirin consumption versus 4.9% of the control group, resulting in an estimated crude relative risk of 0.18 in the aspirin-treated group. The second portion of this study questioned patients from medical and surgical wards but excluded those who had been in hospital during the prior 3 months. This gave a crude relative risk of 0.53 (90% confidence intervals, 0.33–0.84). Both of the Boston studies included nonfatal infarctions only. Neither estimated the dose of aspirin taken, the duration of such consumption, or the occurrence of side effects.

A case control study of regular aspirin use and coronary deaths was also performed by HENNEKENS et al. (1978). They studied married men who died of coronary heart disease following hospital admission; information was also collected on an equal number of living controls matched for age, sex, marital status and neighborhood. Their 568 case control pairs did not show any evidence for a preventive role of aspirin in coronary heart disease.

Two trials of aspirin in the primary prevention of mortality from myocardial disease have been reported recently (Table 2). Both were conducted using male physicians, one in the USA (Steering Committee of the Physicians' Health Study Research Group, 1989) and the other in Britain (PETO et al. 1988). In the American trial, aspirin 325 mg on alternate days was administered to 11037 physicians, and 11304 received placebo. The study was terminated before its scheduled end, firstly because of the beneficial effects of aspirin on nonfatal and fatal myocardial infarction, with relative risks of 0.34 (95% confidence interval, 0.15–0.75) and 0.59 (0.47–0.74), respectively and secondly, because it was decided that the low event rate would prevent the study from reaching a definitive result with respect to its primary aim, the reduction of cardiovascular mortality. There was a nonsignificant increase in total stroke with a relative risk of 1.22 (0.93–1.60, $P = 0.32$). Total deaths were the same in the placebo and aspirin-treated groups. Two interesting subgroup findings were reported; firstly, that the benefit was observed only in those over the age of 50 years ($P = 0.02$)

and secondly, that despite a consistent benefit of aspirin with all levels of cholesterol, it was greatest at a low level.

The British study differed in numbers, a total of 5139 doctors of whom two-thirds were randomized to aspirin, in the use of a higher dosage of aspirin (500 mg of soluble or 325 mg enteric-coated aspirin daily) and in the absence of placebo tablets for the control group. Differences also existed in the event rates of the study end-points. In contrast to the American study, there were no differences in fatal or nonfatal myocardial infarction incidence; the combined 95% confidence intervals were 0.73–1.24. Daily aspirin intake reduced the frequency of transient ischemic episodes by about half, but there was an excess of strokes, although this increase was not statistically significant.

Neither of these studies found a reduction in vascular or nonvascular mortality despite a reduction in myocardial infarction occurrence. Discouraging, albeit not statistically significant, trends with respect to stroke were reported. Stroke, should it occur, was more frequently disabling in individuals taking aspirin on a regular basis. In terms of their overall applicability to the general population, care must be taken in extrapolating these results (Hennekens and Buring 1987). The cardiovascular mortality rate among the physicians in the American trial was only 15% of that expected for a general population of white males with a similar age distribution in the USA at that time. It is of importance to note that the Physicians' Health Study involved probands of whom 11% were current cigarette smokers and 70% engaged in regular, vigorous exercise. Studies of prophylactic aspirin administration in a group drawn at random from the general public would avoid such difficulties. A fresh trial could also address the hypothesis of an influence on the clinical severity of strokes, a priori.

As they stand, the current studies do not provide a basis for the administration of aspirin to all men. Due to the selection criteria that were applied, there are no data to determine the risk to benefit ratio for such therapy; indeed, the benefit that was reported in the Physicians' Health Study may have been overestimated as a consequence of the decision to terminate the study prematurely. Similarly, the risk of gastrointestinal side effects as well as stroke is difficult to estimate in a general population. Thus, those volunteers who complained of gastrointestinal side effects or who exhibited evidence of poor compliance during an 18-week run-in period were excluded from the study. However, despite this prerandomization run-in, the incidence of gastrointestinal side effects was greater than for the shorter Veterans' Administration Cooperative study (Lewis et al. 1983) or ISIS-2 (1988) studies. Compliance was 86% for the aspirin group, and gastrointestinal side effects were felt by 26.1% (they were also noted by 25% on placebo).

The Minnesota Heart Survey (Folsom et al. 1988) has provided information on the prevalence of aspirin usage, both overall and for cardiovascular disease prevention. Between 1981–1982 and 1985–1986, use of aspirin increased in men from 8.8% to 11.6%, and from 11.6% to 12.5% in women. The proportion of subjects who admitted to taking aspirin "to avoid a heart attack or stroke" or "because of a previous heart attack or stroke" doubled in men from 1.7% to 3.3% (NS) and quadrupled in women from 0.6% to 2.4% ($P < 0.05$). In 1985, 36.4% of participants who took aspirin had a previous history of hospitalization for myocardial infarction or stroke. This study was performed before the results of the ISIS-2 study were published; it is likely that if repeated, the results would demonstrate a more widespread consumption of aspirin.

As with all areas for which aspirin use has been advocated, there is no consensus as to the optimal regimen of aspirin administration for primary prevention. It is of interest that the Multiple Risk Factor Intervention Trial (MRFIT) collected information on aspirin consumption at each of 7 annual visits among its 12866 participants (GUALLER et al. 1989). For those consuming aspirin on a daily basis, the adjusted relative risk compared with those who did not was 1.63, but in contrast, among those who used aspirin 4–6 days a week, the relative risk was 0.41. None of these trials addressed the issue of primary prevention in women.

IV. Coronary Bypass Grafts

The benefits of surgical therapy for coronary artery disease have been demonstrated by studies performed in the USA (CASS 1983) and in Europe (European Coronary Surgery Study Group 1988). The clinical outcome may be limited, however, by the occurrence of thrombosis or neointimal hyperplasia, events that may involve platelets. The pathological changes occurring in aortocoronary saphenous vein grafts were studied by a number of investigators including UNNI et al. (1974), LAWRIE et al. (1976), and BULKLEY and HUTCHINS (1978). Obviously, the grafts arriving in the histology section, either from reoperation or postmortem specimens, derive from a selected population and may not be truly representative of the changes occurring in such grafts in vivo. UNNI et al. (1974) performed an analysis of the histological changes that arise with increasing time from surgery in saphenous vein grafts from 40 patients. Seven of 13 patients who died less than 24 h after operation had histologically normal grafts; focal absence of endothelial cells was noted in the remainder. BULKLEY and HUTCHINS (1978) found the causes of occlusion to be compression of the vascular lumen in 42%, thrombosis in 31% and dissection of the native coronary artery in 5%–10% in patients who died later. Overall, these investigators found that occlusive thrombi were more common in early graft occlusions, while intimal hyperplasia was more prevalent when occlusion was delayed.

In a canine model of coronary bypass vein grafts (JOSA et al. 1981), aspirin and dipyridamole administration lowered the incidence of thrombosis and in a primate model of a jugular vein bypass to an iliac artery (MCCANN et al. 1980), treatment with aspirin plus dipyridamole reduced intimal hyperplasia. Accordingly, antiplatelet therapy and its ability to prevent graft loss in the clinical setting have been addressed by a number of investigators. The main form of antiplatelet therapy studied has been aspirin, either alone or in combination with dipyridamole.

CHESEBRO et al. examined the influence of antiplatelet therapy commenced in the preoperative period on patency both in the short-term (1982) and over a longer period of follow-up (1984). They studied 407 patients undergoing aortocoronary bypass operations. Patients were randomized to either drug or placebo groups; they did not receive warfarin. The actively treated group commenced dipyridamole 100 mg orally four times daily 2 days prior to surgery and aspirin 7 hours after the operation. Thereafter, they received dipyridamole 75 mg plus aspirin 325 mg three times daily. Within 1 month of operation, 3% of the treatment group had occluded distal anastomoses, in contrast to 10% of the placebo group. These rates were 4% and 15%, respectively, within 6 months. The rates per patient were 8% of the treated group and 21% of the placebo group at 1 month and 10% and 30%, respectively, at 6 months. The later paper by these authors addressed the effect of treatment on the late postoperative occlusion rate. Angiography was performed at a median of 1 year (range 11–18 months) following surgery. The new occlusion rates per graft were 9% for the treated and 14% for the placebo group and per patient, 16% and 27%, respectively.

The Veterans Cooperative study (GOLDMAN et al. 1988) compared placebo, aspirin (325 or 975 mg daily), aspirin 975 mg plus dipyridamole 215 mg, and sulfinpyrazone 801 mg daily with placebo. Treatment was commenced preoperatively. A benefit was recorded for all aspirin-containing regimens over placebo and over sulfinpyrazone on early (60 days) reocclusion rates. The lower dose of aspirin was as effective as the higher dose and the combination of aspirin with dipyridamole. All three aspirin groups had an increase in perioperative blood loss.

BROWN et al. (1985) described an improved outcome for therapy initiated on the 2nd postoperative day. A total of 147 patients were enrolled. Their protocol entailed aspirin 325 mg plus dipyridamole 75 mg three times daily, aspirin 325 mg plus a dipyridamole placebo three times daily, or double placebo three times daily. Patients were recatheterized at 1 year. Some 21% of the placebo group had occluded grafts, 14% of the aspirin and dipyridamole group and 12% of the aspirin group. This difference was statistically significant against placebo for each of the active treatments, but there was no variation between the antiplatelet regimens. They demonstrated that this angiographic benefit translated into clinical benefit: 13% of patients with all grafts patent had persistent pain, 25% of those with one occluded graft and 54% of those with two or more occluded ($P < 0.02$).

Positive results have also been reported for triflusal, a platelet inhibitor which is structurally related to aspirin. GUITERAS et al. (1989) compared aspirin 50 mg plus dipyridamole 75 mg three times daily, triflusal 300 mg plus dipyridamole 75 mg three times daily and placebo in 209 patients.

Treatment was initiated on the morning of surgery and repeated 1 h after surgery. The antiplatelet regimens had no protective effects on occlusion as assessed by angiography 9 days after surgery. However, at 6.5 months postsurgery, there was a benefit of aspirin plus dipyridamole over placebo and of triflusal over aspirin. The occlusion rates for placebo, aspirin-dipyridamole, and triflusal-dipyridamole were 40%, 31%, and 20% in patients, 24%, 15%, and 11% in vein grafts, and 24%, 16%, and 12% in distal anastomoses, respectively. Ticlopidine at a dose of 500 mg daily, commenced on the 2nd postoperative day, resulted in improved graft patency at 10, 180, and 360 days after bypass grafting (Limet et al. 1987). They studied a total of 173 patients. Their data also demonstrated that occlusion occurred mainly in the first 6 months.

Other studies which revealed positive results include that of Mayer et al. (1981), who reported 94% angiographic patency at 3–6 months for patients treated with aspirin 650 mg plus dipyridamole 50 mg daily, in contrast to 82% patency among the control group ($P < 0.02$). The protective effect of antiplatelet therapy was observed for the subgroup of patients who received saphenous vein grafts only; aspirin conferred no additional benefit when internal mammary grafts, which have a high patency rate, were employed. Rajah et al. (1985) reported improved graft patency of 92% for aspirin 330 mg plus dipyridamole 75 mg three times daily commenced on the evening prior to surgery versus a placebo rate of 75% in 125 patients. This benefit was not associated with an increase in intraoperative blood loss.

Aspirin in lower doses has also been demonstrated to be of effect; Lorenz et al. (1984) compared 100 mg daily of aspirin with placebo in 60 patients. This intervention was commenced 24 h postsurgery. At 4 months, 90% of the grafts in the aspirin-treated group were patent compared with 68% in the placebo group ($P = 0.006$). However, the occlusion rate was high in the placebo group and this may have led to an overestimation of the benefits of this regimen of aspirin.

Trials with negative results include the randomized placebo controlled trial of aspirin and dipyridamole carried out by Brooks and his colleagues (1985), in which patients received aspirin 990 mg and dipyridamole 225 mg daily or placebo in addition to routine anticoagulation. In all, 266 patients were studied. It was the intention at the time of study design to commence antiplatelet therapy preoperatively as soon as the patient gave consent. However, an adverse outcome in their fourth patient, who turned out to have been taking active treatment, caused a change to initiation of treatment on the 2nd or 3rd postoperative day. Follow-up angiography was performed at 12 months, but no difference was seen in patency between the two groups, with a placebo patency of 87%.

Pantley et al. (1979) found no benefit for aspirin 325 mg plus dipyridamole 75 mg three times daily or warfarin over placebo among 65 patients. Therapy was initiated on the 3rd postoperative day. Graft patency was 82% in both the control and the aspirin plus dipyridamole group; for those treated with warfarin it was 78%. SHARMA et al. (1983) compared aspirin 325 mg three times daily, aspirin 325 mg plus dipyridamole 75 mg three times daily, and a parallel control group not assigned any therapy who were operated on at the same time and studied prospectively. Study medication was commenced on the 3rd to 5th postoperative day. Angiographic patency at 1 year was 80% for the control group, 79% for the aspirin group, and 83% for the aspirin-dipyridamole group. The patencies were not statistically different either overall or for any individual vessel.

Interpretation of these studies is limited by the variations in dose of aspirin administered, the time of initiation of therapy relative to surgery, and the concomitant use of other agents, in particular warfarin. Another factor that influences the interpretation is the ability to randomize patients but not the individual grafts to the therapy under study; this complicates the statistical analysis of graft patency as an end-point. Another problem is study size; PANTLEY et al. (1979) estimated that 140 patients would be required to give an 80% confidence level of detecting a 15% difference in patency rate between the control group and treatment groups, at the 5% level of significance. Only those studies of CHESEBRO et al. (1984) BROOKS et al. (1985) BROWN et al. (1985) and LIMET et al. (1987) possess this sample size. In conclusion, the outcomes would suggest that antiplatelet therapy is effective in preventing graft occlusion. The optimal dose of aspirin remains to be determined; however, despite a high rate of graft occlusion in the placebo group the trial of LORENZ et al. (1984) provides preliminary evidence that the benefits of a low-dose regimen might be of a similar order to those obtained in other studies involving higher doses of aspirin.

V. Peripheral Arterial Grafts

Bypass grafts performed for peripheral vascular disease are also subject to thrombotic occlusion. Evidence for a potential role of platelets in this process is mainly derived from the demonstration of platelet deposition on these grafts, the modification of such deposition by antiplatelet regimens, and more limited data on the influence of antiplatelet therapy on occlusion rates. These grafts may be performed with veins or with synthetic material, most commonly Dacron and polytetrafluoroethylene (PTFE).

Platelet deposition on these grafts in vivo may be studied utilising homologous ^{111}In-labelled platelets. STRATTON et al. (1982) did not find any abnormal deposition of platelets in 13 healthy volunteers aged 18–37 years. However, in 12 of 15 patients with Dacron grafts placed in the aortofemoral or aortoiliac positions for a mean of 26 months, an abnormal pattern of platelet deposition was present. This pattern was studied over a 96-h period, and in the majority of the patients was irregular, suggesting that this was a dynamic and changing process.

Platelet deposition during the early postoperative period in patients undergoing femoropopliteal bypass surgery was studied by GOLDMAN et al. (1983a). Some 47 patients were randomized to aspirin 300 mg plus dipyridamole 75 mg three times daily, commencing 48 h prior to surgery. Whenever possible, autologous saphenous vein was utilized; otherwise they selected Dacron or PTFE. Indium-labelled platelets were reinjected on the 7th postoperative day. Platelet accumulation was greatest in the placebo patients with Dacron grafts and this was significantly reduced by aspirin/dipyridamole. Platelet deposition was less in patients with PTFE grafts, and this was further reduced by the antiplatelet regimen. Deposition was markedly lower on the saphenous vein grafts; it was unaffected by antiplatelet therapy. In contrast, PUMPHREY et al. (1983) reported that a regimen of dipyridamole 100 mg four times on the day before surgery followed by aspirin 325 mg three times daily postoperatively reduced deposition of platelets on Dacron grafts but not on PTFE grafts. In addition, GOLDMAN et al. (1983b) demonstrated that the "thrombogenicity index" (the mean daily rise in the ratio of radioactivity graft/contralateral thigh) of platelets injected on the postoperative day was the best indicator of the risk of occlusion over the following year. Grafts that occluded had an index of 0.19 ± 0.018 versus an index of 0.07 ± 0.09 for those that remained patent ($P < 0.001$).

GOLDMAN et al. (1982) noted in a group of 9 patients followed over a 12-month period that platelet deposition, despite falling over time, remained demonstrable in the region of the anastomoses. Deposition was also shown in patients with grafts in place for 2, 5, and 9 years. In a series of studies, STRATTON and RITCHIE have reported that platelet deposition is reduced by aspirin plus dipyridamole (1986) but not by ticlopidine (1984) or by sulfinpyrazone (1985) in patients with long-term Dacron grafts.

BLAKELY and POGORILER (1977) studied 169 patients who underwent a variety of peripheral vascular procedures, i.e., endarterectomy, vein graft, or prosthesis, but with randomization stratified for the type of operation and found on benefit of sulfinpyrazone 200 mg three times daily over placebo. DONALDSON et al. (1982) administered aspirin 330 mg three times daily and dipyridamole 75 mg three times daily to 65 patients receiving a total of 73 Dacron grafts for femoropopliteal bypass. Occlusion after a mean follow-up of 10 months was reduced from 38% in the placebo group to 16% in the treatment group ($P < 0.05$).

KOHLER et al. (1984) randomized 100 patients who were scheduled for infrainguinal bypass operations to aspirin 325 mg plus dipyridamole 75 mg three times daily, commencing on the first postoperative day. Patency at 24 months did not differ between the two groups, 67% for control and 57% for the treated group. They did not find a difference between the patency of vein grafts and PTFE grafts. SATIANI (1985) assigned 45 patients, randomly on the basis of age, to receive postoperative aspirin 650 mg daily and 55 patients to no treatment. Aspirin was commenced 1–3 days postoperatively. Patency rates did not differ according to aspirin therapy or the form of graft used.

In conclusion, despite evidence that platelet deposition occurs on peripheral arterial grafts and the potential for platelet products to promote graft occlusion, the trials to date have not been definitive. Many involved too small a study population and compared too many treatment groups. Questions remain as to which form of graft composition, if any, may benefit from prophylactic antiplatelet therapy and also whether the benefit may exist for grafts to some or all sites.

VI. Cerebrovascular Disease

In the interpretation of studies of antiplatelet therapy in cerebrovascular disease, there are two potential responses to inhibition of platelet function, a reduction in the incidence and/or severity of strokes due to thrombotic events and an increase in those resulting from hemorrhagic stroke. Fundoscopic observations such as those of FISHER (1959) lend support to the concept that platelet emboli may be the cause of transient monocular blindness during transient ischemic attacks (TIAs).

Evidence for a direct role of platelets in TIA derives from clinical trials of antiplatelet agents. One of the early trials in this area was the Aspirin in Transient Ischemic Attacks Study (AITIA), reported by FIELDS et al. in 1977 for patients receiving medical therapy alone and in 1978 (FIELDS et al. 1978) for those who underwent surgery prior to antiplatelet therapy. Some 88 patients from the medically treated group were assigned to aspirin 650 mg twice daily and 90 to placebo. Outcome was assessed as favorable or unfavorable on the basis of incidence of death, cerebral or retinal infarction, or failure to reduce the number of TIAs over the first 6 months. There was a statistically significant benefit from aspirin, with an incidence of unfavorable events in the placebo group of 44.2% versus 19.2% in the aspirin-treated group. The surgical group received the same study medications, and these were commenced within 1 week of surgery. A total of 125 patients were studied, and no difference was found between the groups for overall mortality, cerebral infarction, or retinal infarction.

The Canadian Cooperative Study Group (1978) enrolled patients with at least one cerebral or retinal ischemic attack over the previous 3 months. The 585 patients were randomized and assigned to treatment groups of sulfinpyrazone 200 mg plus placebo, acetylsalicyclic acid 325 mg plus placebo, both active agents, and both placebos; each regimen was taken four times daily. End-points analyzed were the incidence of TIAs, stroke, and death. The duration of follow-up averaged 26 months. Aspirin was associated with a risk reduction of 19% ($P < 0.05$), sulfinpyrazone did not lead to risk reduction and its combination with aspirin did not result in any interaction either positive or negative. The researchers found that there was a statistically significant difference in the response to aspirin between male and female patients by post hoc subgroup analysis. For male patients, the risk of stroke or death was reduced by 48% ($P < 0.005$); however, for females this was increased by 42% ($P = 0.35$). Women made up only 25% of the study population. In contrast to the Canadian result, the Danish Cooperative

Study (Sorensen et al. 1983) of 203 patients with either TIA or reversible ischemic neurologic deficit (RIND) was unable to demonstrate any benefit of aspirin 1000 mg daily over placebo.

In the Accidents, Ischemignes Cerebreaux Lies A L'Atheroscelose (AICLA) study, Bousser et al. (1983) compared the effect of aspirin 1 g daily, aspirin 1 g plus dipyridamole 225 mg daily and placebo on fatal and nonfatal cerebral infarction. A total of 604 patients were enrolled and followed up over 3 years. There was a difference between aspirin and placebo ($P < 0.05$), but not between aspirin plus dipyridamole and placebo ($P < 0.06$) or between aspirin alone and aspirin plus dipyridamole. There was also a reduction in myocardial infarction in the two treated groups.

The European Stroke Prevention Study (ESPS Group, 1987) enrolled patients with either TIA, RIND, or stroke. They compared acetylsalicyclic acid 325 mg plus dipyridamole 75 mg three times daily with placebo. Their end-points were stroke and death; over a 24-month follow-up period, they reported significant reductions in total strokes, nonfatal strokes, fatal strokes, and total deaths among their 2500 patients.

The UK-TIA Study Group (1988) enrolled patients with a recent TIA or minor ischemic stroke. They compared aspirin at two doses (300 and 1200 mg daily) and placebo. A total of 1778 men and 657 women were randomized between the three groups. For the end-points of major or disabling stroke and vascular death, there was no difference between the two regimens of aspirin. There was an advantage for aspirin over placebo, but as with the Canadian study they were unable to demonstrate a benefit of aspirin among women in an post hoc analysis. The Dutch TIA Study Group (1988) is evaluating the response to two doses of aspirin (30 and 300 mg) in at least 2500 patients. Preliminary reports suggest comparable efficacy in preventing stroke on both regimens (Patrono C. personal communication).

In the Anturane TIA Italian Study (ATIAIS), Candelise et al. (1982) compared aspirin 500 mg twice daily with sulfinpyrazone 400 mg twice daily among 124 patients with TIA followed up over a mean of 11.2 months did not detect a difference between the two agents. Nor was a difference detected between anticoagulation with warfarin or antiplatelet therapy with aspirin among 241 patients with TIA or slight residual symptoms (Garde et al. 1983). Tohgi (1984) reported a nonsignificant trend in favor of ticlopidine 200 mg daily over aspirin 500 mg daily among 334 patients with TIA. The American-Canadian Co-operative Study Group (1985) did not find any additional benefit of the combination of aspirin plus dipyridamole over aspirin alone among 890 subjects with recent carotid territory TIAs.

The recently reported Ticlopidine Aspirin Stroke Study (TASS, Hass et al. 1989) compared ticlopidine 500 mg daily with aspirin 1300 mg daily. Patients over 40 years of age were enrolled within 3 months of a TIA, amaurosis fugax, reversible ischemic neurologic deficit, or minor stroke. A total of 1987 men and 1082 women were recruited, exclusion criteria included the clinical impression that the patient would be unlikely to survive for 5 years. The primary end-point in this study was death from any cause or stroke. This occurred in 306 patients assigned to ticlopidine and 349 who received aspirin, event rates of 17% and 19%, respectively ($P = 0.048$). The 95% confidence intervals for this effect ranged from −2% to 26%. The groups differed in their incidence of side effects. Diarrhea occurred in 20% of the ticlopidine group and in 10% of those receiving aspirin; rash was also more frequently related to ticlopidine treatment; 12% in comparison with 5%. Severe neutropenia occurred in 13 patients assigned to ticlopidine but in none of the aspirin-treated group. Thus, in this trial, which did not include a placebo group, a slight benefit was observed in response to ticlopidine but at the expense of an increase in side effects, some potentially life-threatening.

In conclusion, antiplatelet therapy has been demonstrated to reduce the incidence of TIAs, strokes and death in many studies. Positive results have been reported in all but one (Sorenson et al. 1983). Aspirin was used at high doses (1000 mg or greater per day) in the majority of these trials. The UK-TIA Study Group (1988) reported no differences between aspirin 300 mg and 1000 mg daily. Where aspirin was compared with other treatment regimens, only the TASS study reported a greater response in the non-aspirin-treated group. However, the TASS group reported increased side effects with ticlopidine as against high-dose aspirin.

Although the results of both the Canadian Cooperative Study Group (1978) and the UK-TIA Study Group (1988) raise the intriguing possibility of a diminished response to aspirin in women with TIAs, the information is far from definitive. In the Canadian study, 41–48 women were assigned to each group, and therefore the numbers were insufficient to address this hypothesis. While there were 203–239 women per group in the UK-TIA study, the numbers of events were small and the confidence intervals correspondingly wide. In both studies, the possibility of a gender-dependent difference in drug response was addressed post hoc rather than as an a priori hypothesis.

VII. Prosthetic Valves

Thromboembolism is a major complication of prosthetic valve replacement, arising with both mechanical and bioprosthetic valves (Fuster et al. 1982; Chesebro et al. 1985). Platelet survival is diminished in patients with prosthetic valves as demonstrated by Dale et al. (1975). Harker and Slichter (1970) performed kinetic studies of platelets in 18 patients with prosthetic valves and found that platelets were selectively consumed in an amount that was proportional to valve area. They also reported that platelet survival was lower with valves in the mitral position than with those in the aortic position. Platelet deposition on the sewing ring of prosthetic valves may be demonstrated utilising indium-labelled platelets infused during the early postoperative phase (DEWANJEE et al. 1984). In an attempt to reduce or eliminate this complication, various anticoagulant and antiplatelet regimens have been examined, both in prospective controlled studies and in retrospective analyses. SULLIVAN et al. (1971) studied 163 patients with prosthetic cardiac valves who were started on warfarin on the 4th postoperative day and randomized to either dipyridamole (400 mg per day) or placebo on day 10. At 12 months, the risk of embolism was significantly reduced by dipyridamole treatment. However, more of the patients treated with both warfarin and dipyridamole were withdrawn from the study. Analysis on an intention-to-treat basis did not demonstrate a difference in the rate of embolic events. A positive effect of aspirin 1000 mg in combination with warfarin versus warfarin alone was observed by DALE (1977). He reported that the incidence of arterial thromboembolic complications was reduced from 9.3 to 1.8 per 100 patients per year. This result led him to study aspirin in the absence of warfarin. This was associated with an unacceptable complication rate of 14.5 thromboembolic episodes per 100 patients per year. A similar negative result was obtained by RIBIERO et al. (1986).

ALTMAN et al. (1976) randomized 122 patients to either anticoagulation alone or anticoagulation plus aspirin 500 mg daily. The rate of thromboembolism was significantly reduced in the aspirin-treated group ($P < 0.005$). Hemorrhagic complications did not differ between them.

A further study by DALE et al. (1977) compared aspirin alone (500 mg twice daily) with placebo among 148 patients, all of whom continued anticoagulant therapy. The incidence of arterial thromboembolism was 9.3 episodes per 100 patient years in the placebo group and 1.8 in the aspirin-treated group ($P < 0.01$).

MOGGIO et al. (1978) in a retrospective analysis reviewed the outcome of their 183 patients who underwent valve replacements with Starr-Edwards valves over an 18-year period. The choice of anticoagulant and/or antiplatelet therapy reflected the individual preferences of the surgeons involved. They concluded that warfarin reduced the rate of thromboembolism compared with that observed when no anticoagulant was administered. Aspirin alone did not lower the incidence of embolic events. NUNEZ et al. (1984) reported a 1.4% incidence of thromboembolic events among 768 patients with mitral valve replacement or aortic plus mitral replacement with bioprosthetic material; none of these events occurred in patients in sinus rhythm. They were treated solely with aspirin, initially 1000 mg daily starting on the 2nd postoperative day and more recently with 500 mg on alternate days commencing on the 1st postoperative day. Among these consecutive groups of patients, the lower dose of aspirin was more effective in reducing the rate of embolism for isolated mitral valve replacement.

BROTT et al. (1981) examined the efficacy of aspirin 20 g administered rectally on the evening of surgery followed by aspirin 1.3 g plus dipyridamole 200 mg daily. They followed up their 50 patients over a 27-month period. The incidence of thromboembolic episodes was 8.7 per 100 patient years.

They compared their results with historical data from patients without therapy and found no difference. They considered the actuarial probability of having an event-free course over 3 years of 81% as being unacceptable. Accordingly, they converted their patients to warfarin therapy, and over the subsequent 4 years, the incidence fell to 1.1 per 100 patient years.

CHESEBRO et al. (1983) carried out a nonblinded trial to compare the combination of warfarin with either aspirin 250 mg twice daily or dipyridamole 100 mg four times daily in patients receiving a mechanical prosthetic heart valve. They did not include a control group of warfarin alone in their original protocol but added this "within a few months of starting randomization." However, this control group was made up of patients who, inadvertently, had not been randomized by the surgical services. Both the anticoagulant and the antiplatelet therapy were commenced 48 h after surgery. They found an excess of gastrointestinal and intracerebral bleeding events in the aspirin-treated group of 6.6 episodes per 100 patient years versus 1.6 for the warfarin plus dipyridamole group and 1.8 for those receiving warfarin alone ($P < 0.001$). The reduced incidence of thromboembolism in the warfarin plus dipyridamole group (0.5 per 100 patient years) did not achieve statistical significance. The rate of thromboembolism in the warfarin group was 1.7 per 100 patient years.

In a comparison of warfarin versus two separate forms of antiplatelet therapy, MOK et al. (1985) concluded that the anticoagulant regime was superior. Their patients, who had mechanical prosthetic valves, received warfarin alone over the first 6 months after surgery and then were randomized to one of three groups, to continue warfarin, to commence a slow-release preparation of aspirin 650 mg plus dipyridamole 150 mg, or to pentoxifylline 400 mg plus aspirin 650 mg daily. After 3 years of the 5-year study the investigators changed the aspirin-dipyridamole group to a combined form of aspirin 330 mg with dipyridamole 75 mg three times daily. The incidence of thromboembolism was 2.2 per 100 patient years in the warfarin group, 8.6 in the aspirin-dipyridamole group and 7.9 in the pentoxifylline group. This difference was significant between the anticoagulant group and each antiplatelet group. Among their 254 patients, there were 5 episodes of bleeding among the warfarin group and 1 in the pentoxifylline group.

In conclusion, patients with prosthetic valves appear to be at increased risk for thromboembolic events. The risk of such events is influenced by the type of valve utilized and the patient's cardiac rhythm. Despite the number of studies in this area, many involved a type of valve different from that used in current surgical practice. Numerous studies have demonstrated warfarin to be effective and superior to antiplatelet therapy in isolation. The addition of antiplatelet to anticoagulant therapy has been found to be more effective than warfarin alone in some, but not all, studies. The combination of aspirin and warfarin may be associated with an excessive risk of hemorrhagic complications (CHESEBRO et al. 1983). DALE et al. (1977) reported augmented gastrointestinal bleeding among their patients receiving both aspirin and warfarin; the majority of all bleeding complications occurred at low thrombotest values. The findings of NUNEZ et al. (1984) suggest that a lower dose of aspirin would be even more effective. This could be expected to reduce the risk of bleeding complications. Many of these studies suffer from being retrospective, including a control population that is less than ideal, or enrolling too small a patient population. There is a need for a prospective comparison of different doses of aspirin, alone and in combination with anticoagulants, in patients subject to current surgical procedures.

VIII. Coronary Angioplasty

Dilatation of coronary artery stenoses is an effective means for the treatment of coronary artery disease (DETRE et al. 1988). Complications that limit the outcome of this procedure include acute occlusion and the recurrence of stenosis (MCBRIDE et al. 1988), both of which may be consequent to platelet activation. In a porcine model of coronary angioplasty, STEELE et al. (1985) examined the deposition of indium-labelled platelets over time on carotid arteries that underwent 5 inflations of 6 atm pressure, each lasting for 30 s. The vessels were examined histologically. Balloon angioplasty completely denuded the dilated area of endothelium; there was partial regrowth after 4 days and by 1 week the endothelium was largely regrown. Marked platelet deposition occurred within 1 h of the procedure. This persisted for over 24 h but was reduced to near normal by 4 days. There was no increase in platelet deposition at 7 days, by which time endothelial regrowth was largely complete. In other studies, the same group (STEELE et al. 1984) demonstrated that low-dose aspirin (40 mg daily) or aspirin 650 mg daily plus dipyridamole 100 mg over 90 min i.v., but not aspirin alone 650 mg daily, could reduce both platelet deposition and mural thrombus formation in this porcine model. In his early writings on the use of this technique, GRUNTZIG et al. (1979) included aspirin 1 g daily for 3 days, commencing on the day prior to the procedure.

THORNTON and her colleagues (1984) compared the ability of anticoagulation with warfarin to prevent the recurrence of stenoses against aspirin 325 mg daily among 248 patients. Both groups received 650 mg of aspirin on the day prior to angioplasty and the warfarin-treated group also received aspirin 325 mg daily at their hospital admission. They defined recurrence as the loss of at least 50% of the gain in luminal diameter accomplished at angioplasty. After 9 months of follow-up, the recurrence rate in the warfarin-treated group was 36% as compared with 27% in the group on aspirin; this difference was not statistically significant. Following a subgroup analysis, they reported that aspirin did reduce reocclusion for patients with at least a 3-month history of angina.

A retrospective analysis was performed by BARNATHAN et al. (1987) to examine the influence of antiplatelet therapy on acute coronary thrombosis complicating coronary angioplasty. Their study involved three groups: The first did not receive aspirin ("control," $n = 121$), the second received aspirin alone or with dipyridamole either before admission or in hospital

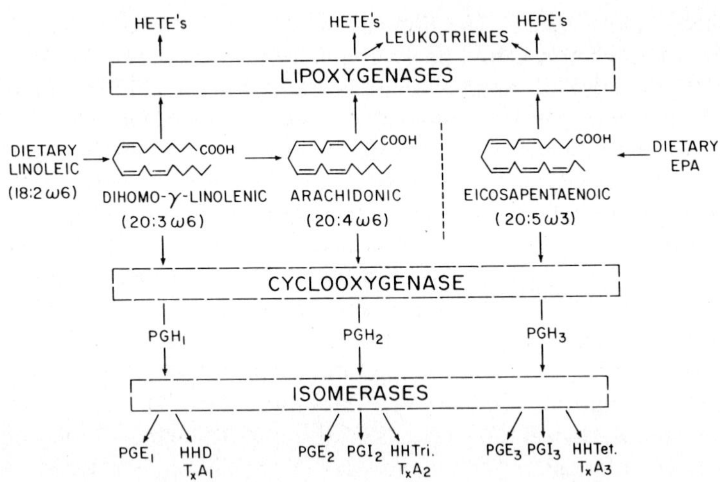

Fig. 6. Formation of the trienoic prostaglandins from eicosapentanoic acid. (From WYNGARDEN and SMITH 1988)

("standard," $n = 110$) and the third received both aspirin and dipyridamole before hospital and in hospital before percutaneous transluminal coronary angioplasty (PTCA) ("maximal," $n = 32$). For the control group the rate of thrombus formation was 21.5%; it was 11.8% in the standard group ($P = 0.07$) and in the maximal group no thrombus formed. Additionally, aspirin reduced clinically significant thrombus formation, as defined by the presence of an acute problem or one requiring intervention.

A randomized, double-blind, placebo-controlled trial in 376 patients was performed by SCHWARTZ et al. (1988) who compared aspirin 330 mg plus dipyridamole 75 mg (with the administration of intravenous dipyridamole to assure adequate blood levels over the time of angioplasty) with placebo. Consistent with the results of BARNATHAN et al. (1987) they reported a reduction in periprocedural events and in particular a reduction in Q-wave infarction from 6.9% to 1.6% ($P = 0.011$). Follow-up angiography was carried out with 249 patients. They did not find any difference in the rate of restenosis between the two groups. The ticlopidine multicenter trial has also demonstrated that antiplatelet therapy with either aspirin 650 mg plus dipyridamole 225 mg daily or ticlopidine 250 mg three times daily reduced the immediate complications of angioplasty (WHITE et al. 1987a; $n = 333$) but did not prevent restenosis (WHITE et al. 1987b; $n = 236$).

KNUDTSON et al. (1986) randomized 280 patients to aspirin plus dipyridamole either alone or in combination with intracoronary prostacyclin (80 ng/kg) before and after dilatation, followed by 5–7 ng/kg min i.v. over 48 h. Acute complications were reduced, but restenosis rates were not. LEMBO et al. (1988) did not detect a difference in the rate of acute complications related to PTCA in patients who received aspirin 325 mg plus dipyridamole 75 mg three times daily compared with those who received aspirin alone.

Administration of ciprostene, a stable analogue of prostacyclin, resulted in a reduction in clinical events, but not in restenosis, over the initial 6 months following PTCA (RAIZNER et al. 1988).

Diets that are rich in marine oils such as eicosapentanoic acid (EPA) lead to the formation of PGI_3 and TXA_3 (Fig. 6). PGI_3 is of similar potency to PGI_2, but TXA_3 is reportedly less effective as an agonist at the thromboxane receptor than TXA_2 (NEEDLEMAN et al. 1979). Epidemiological data suggest that diets rich in fish confer a protection against atherosclerotic disease (KROMANN and GREEN 1980). Various groups have studied the effects of supplementing diets with EPA to determine whether or not they modulate platelet-dependent processes (LEAF and WEBER 1988).

The potential of dietary supplementation with marine oils to modify the complications of coronary angioplasty has been explored by several groups. GRIGG et al. (1989) did not report any protection with max-EPA (10 × 1-g capsules per day) against restenosis; however, they did not commence marine oil until the day before or in some cases the day of angioplasty. This may not have resulted in sufficient incorporation of EPA to modify TXA_3 or PGI_3 formation. The study of REIS et al. (1989) reported an insignificant increase in the relative risk for restenosis of 1.7 (confidence intervals 0.9–3.4) for patients who received 6 g of fish oil daily commencing 5.4 ± 3.2 days before angioplasty. In contrast, DEHMER et al. (1988) commenced marine oil supplementation (3.2 g EPA daily) 7 days before angioplasty and continued it for 6 months. The control group consisted of 39 patients with 53 lesions and the fish oil group, of 43 patients with 50 lesions. Both groups received aspirin 325 mg and dipyridamole 225 mg daily. The proportion of EPA in platelet fatty acids increased from 0.14% ± 0.33% at baseline to 3.7% ± 1.73% by the time of angioplasty. This contrasts with the 8% of platelet fatty acids reported in Eskimo populations (DYERBERG and BANG 1982). They performed follow-up angiography at 3–4 months and in patients with new symptoms repeated follow-up angiography beyond 4 months. Restenosis occurred in 36% of the lesions in the control group and in 16% in the treatment group ($P = 0.026$) and in 46% of patients in the control group but 19% in the treatment group ($P = 0.007$).

Other trials have been reported in a preliminary form; these also differ in outcome. Administration of fish oil, 6–9 capsules per day, resulted in beneficial changes in the lipid profile but in an insignificant trend towards a benefit for single-vessel (16% vs. 33%) over multivessel disease (67% vs. 58%) (SLACK et al. 1987). In contrast, MILNER et al. (1988) reported a reduction from 37% to 20% for clinical restenosis ($P < 0.03$).

In conclusion, antiplatelet therapy appears to reduce the incidence of periprocedural complications among patients undergoing PTCA. Aspirin, either alone or in combination with other antiplatelet agents, with the exception of the results of DEHMER et al. (1988) and SLACK et al. (1987), has not been shown to reduce the incidence of restenosis. However, the studies which have addressed the issue of restenosis have lacked statistical power (Table 3). For example, to demonstrate a reduction in restenosis from 30% to

Table 3. Statistical requirements for trials of fish oil in the setting of percutaneous transluminal coronary angioplasty. Sample size requirements to detect a reduction in restenosis rate from 30% to 15% are $\alpha = 0.05$ and $\beta = 0.05$, for two-arm comparison 172 per group and for three-arm comparison 224 per group (one-tailed) and 260 per group (two-tailed)

	Patient sample sizes in published studies			
	Number of groups	Fish oil	Placebo	Results
SLACK et al. 1987	2	80	82	NS
DEHMER et al. 1988	2	43	39	Fish oil superior
MILNER et al. 1988	3	64	79	Fish oil superior
GRIGG et al. 1989	2	49	55	NS
REIS et al. 1989	2	150	72	NS

15% a two-arm comparison would require 172 patients per group and a three-armed comparison, 224 per group. The studies which have been performed to date are unable to exclude the possibility that the observed positive or negative results could have resulted by chance.

C. Concluding Comments

Unresolved issues in the clinical response to antiplatelet therapy remain to be clarified. In particular, an impression has evolved that a difference in response to prophylactic aspirin exists between men and women in a variety of clinical settings, unstable angina (CAIRNS et al. 1985), TIA (Canadian Cooperative Study Group 1978; UK-TIA Study Group 1988), and post-operative deep venous thrombosis (HARRIS et al. 1977). However, in all these studies the conclusions were on the basis of posthoc subgroup analysis, and the number of women in each study was small.

The results of the various trials of antiplatelet therapy in thrombo-embolic disease demonstrate an important role for platelet activation under these conditions. The majority of these studies utilised aspirin, either alone or in combination with dipyridamole, as the means of inhibiting platelets. There is no evidence to suggest that dipyridamole contributed to the platelet inhibitory effects of aspirin. Despite the widespread use of aspirin, the optimal dose remains uncertain and ongoing investigations need to determine the minimal dose and the means of administration which result in maximal inhibition of thromboxane formation while simultaneously preserving prostacyclin production.

For the present, it has been shown that a daily dosage of aspirin of 160 mg is well tolerated and effective in the secondary prevention of myocardial infarction. However, this regimen was administered over a short term, and the long-term tolerance for this daily dose is unknown. Aspirin

75 mg/day has been shown to reduce the incidence of death and myocardial infarction in patients with unstable angina and preliminary evidence for the efficacy of the same dosage in the prevention of thrombotic stroke has been presented.

References

Aiken JA, Shebuski RJ, Miller OV, Gorman RG (1981) Endogenous prostacyclin contributes to the efficacy of a thromboxane synthetase inhibitor for preventing coronary artery thrombosis. J Pharmacol Exp Ther 219:299–308

Altman R, Boullon F, Rouvier J, de la Fuente L, Favaloro R (1976) Aspirin and prophylaxis of thromboembolic complications in patients with substitute heart valves. J Thorac Cardiovasc Surg 72:127–129

American-Canadian Co-operative Study Group (1985) Persantine aspirin trial in cerebral ischemia part II: endpoint results. Stroke 16:406–415

Antiplatelet Trialists' Collaboration (1988) Secondary prevention of vascular disease by prolonged antiplatelet treatment. Br Med J 1:320–331

Anturane Reinfarction Trial Research Group (1978) Sulfinpyrazone in the prevention of cardiac death after myocardial infarction: the anturane reinfarction trial. N Engl J Med 298:289–295

Anturane Reinfarction Trial Research Group (1980) Sulfinpyrazone in the prevention of sudden cardiac death after myocardial infarction. N Engl J Med 302:250–256

Aspirin Myocardial Infarction Study Research Group (1980) A randomized, controlled trial of aspirin in persons recovered from myocardial infarction. J Am Med Assoc 243:661–669

Bailey JM, Makheja AM, Pash J, Verma M (1988) Corticosteroids suppress cyclooxygenase messenger RNA levels and prostanoid synthesis in cultured vascular cells. Biochem Biophys Res Comm 157:1159–1163

Bakhle YS (1983) Synthesis and catabolism of cyclo-oxygenase products. Br Med Bull 39:214–218

Barnathan ES, Schwartz JS, Taylor L, Laskey WK, Kleaveland JP, Kussmaul WG, Hirshfeld JW (1987) Aspirin and dipyridamole in the prevention of acute coronary thrombosis complicating coronary angioplasty. Circulation 76:125–134

Bhagwat SS, Hamann PR, Still WC, Bunting S, Fitzpatrick FA (1985) Synthesis and structure of the platelet aggregation factor thromboxane A_2. Nature 315: 511–512

Blair IA, Barrow SE, Waddell KA, Lewis PJ, Dollery CT (1982) Prostacyclin is not a circulating hormone in man. Prostaglandins 23:579–589

Blakely JA, Pogoriler G (1977) A prospective trial of sulfinpyrazone after peripheral vascular surgery. Thromb Haemost 38:238 (abstr)

Boston Collaborative Drug Surveillance Group (1974) Regular aspirin intake and myocardial infarction. Br Med J 1:440–443

Bousser MG, Eschwege E, Haguenau M, Lefaucconnier JM, Thibult N, Touboul PJ (1983) "AICLA" controlled trial of aspirin and dipyridamole in the secondary prevention of atherothrombotic cerebral ischemia. Stroke 14:5–14

Brash AR (1985) A review of possible roles of the platelet 12-lipoxygenase. Circulation 72:702–707

Brash AR (1989) 12- and 15-Lipoxygenase products of arachidonic acid at the platelet/vascular interface. In: Patrono C, FitzGerald GA (eds) Platelets and vascular occlusion. Raven Press, New York, pp 141–149

Brash AR, Jackson EK, Saggese CA, Lawson JA, Oates JA, FitzGerald GA (1983) Metabolic disposition of prostacyclin in humans. J Pharmacol Exp Ther 226: 78–87

Breddin K, Loew D, Lechner K, Uberla K, Walter E (1979) Secondary prevention of myocardial infarction comparison of acetylsalicylic acid, phenprocoumon and placebo: a multicenter two-year prospective study. Thromb Heamost 41: 225–236

Brooks N, Wright J, Sturridge M, Pepper J, Magee P, Walesby R, Layton C, Honey M, Balcon R (1985) Randomised placebo controlled trial of aspirin and dipyridamole in the prevention of coronary vein graft occlusion. Br Heart J 53:201–207

Brott WH, Zajtchuk R, Bowen TE, Davia J, Green DC (1981) Dipyridamole-aspirin as thrombembolic prophylaxis in patients with aortic valve prosthesis: prospective study with the model 2320 Starr-Edwards prosthesis. J Thorac Cardiovasc Surg 81:632–635

Brown BG, Cukingnan RA, DeRouen T, Goede LV, Wong M, Fee HJ, Roth JA, Carey JS (1985) Improved graft patency in patients treated with platelet-inhibiting therapy after coronary bypass surgery. Circulation 72:138–146

Bulkley BH, Hutchins GM (1978) Pathology of coronary artery bypass graft surgery. Arch Pathol Lab Med 102:273–280

Bunting S, Gryglewski R, Moncada S, Vane JR (1976) Arterial walls generate from prostaglandin endoperoxides a substance (prostaglandin X) which relaxes strips of mesenteric and coeliac arteries and inhibits platelet aggregation. Prostaglandins 12:897–913

Cairns JA, Gent M, Singer J, Finnie KJ, Froggatt GM, Holder DA, Jablonsky G, Kostuk WJ, Melendez LJ, Myers MG, Sackett DL, Sealey BJ, Tanser PH (1985) Aspirin, sulfinpyrazone, or both in unstable angina: results of a Canadian multicenter trial. N Engl J Med 313:1369–1375

Canadian Cooperative Study Group (1978) A randomized trial of aspirin and sulfinpyrazone in threatened stroke. N Engl J Med 299:53–59

Candelise L, Landi G, Perrone P, Bracchi M, Brambilla G (1982) A randomized trial of aspirin and sulfinpyrazone in patients with TIA. Stroke 13:175–179

Capdevila J, Chacos N, Werringloer J, Prough RA, Estabrook RW (1981) Liver microsomal cytochrome P-450 and the oxidative metabolism of arachidonic acid. Proc Natl Acad Sci USA 78:5362–5366

Capdevila J, Chacos N, Falck JR, Manna S, Negro-Vilar A, Ojeda SR (1983) Novel hypothalamic arachidonate products stimulate somatostatin release from the median eminence. Endocrinology 113:421–423

Carroll MA, Schwartzman M, Capdevila J, Falck JR, McGiff JC (1987) Vasoactivity of arachidonic acid epoxides. Eur J Pharmacol 138:281–283

CASS Principal Investigators and Their Associates (1983) Coronary Artery Surgery Study (CASS): a randomized trial of coronary artery bypass surgery: survival data. Circulation 68:939–950

Catella F, FitzGerald GA (1987) Paired analysis of urinary thromboxane B_2 metabolites in humans. Thromb Res 47:647–656

Catella F, Healy D, Lawson JA, Fitzgerald GA (1986) 11-Dehydrothromboxane B_2: A quantitative index of thromboxane A_2 formation in the human circulation. Proc Natl Acad Sci (USA) 83:5861–5865

Charo IF, Shak S, Karasek MA, Davison PM, Goldstein IM (1984) Prostaglandin I_2 is not a major metabolite of arachidonic acid in cultured endothelial cells from human foreskin microvessels. J Clin Invest 74:914–919

Chesebro JH, Clements IP, Fuster V, Elveback LR, Smith HC, Bardsley WT, Frye RL, Holmes DR, Vlietstra RE, Pluth JR, Wallace RB, Puga FJ, Orszulak TA, Piehler JM, Schaff HV, Danielson GK (1982) A platelet-inhibitor-drug trial in coronary-artery bypass operations: benefit of perioperative dipyridamole and aspirin therapy on early postoperative vein-graft patency. N Engl J Med 307: 73–78

Chesebro JH, Fuster V, Elveback LR, McGoon DC, Pluth JR, Puga FJ, Wallace RB, Danielson GK, Orszulak TA, Piehler JM, Schaff HV (1983) Trial of combined warfarin plus dipyridamole or aspirin therapy in prosthetic heart valve replacement: danger of aspirin compared with dipyridamole. Am J Cardiol 51:1537–1541

Chesebro JH, Fuster V, Elveback LR, Clements IP, Smith HC, Holmes DR, Bardsley WT, Pluth JR, Wallace RB, Puga FJ, Orszulak TA, Piehler JM, Danielson GK, Schaff HV, Frye RL (1984) Effect of dipyridamole and aspirin on late vein-graft patency after coronary bypass operations. N Engl J Med 310:209–214

Chesebro JH, Fuster V, Danielson GK (1985) Time related and chronic risk of thromboembolism after bioprosthetic valve replacement. Circulation 72 (III): 209

Chierchia S, De Caterina R, Crea F, Patrono C, Maseri A (1982) Failure of thromboxane A_2 blockade to prevent attacks of vasospastic angina. Circulation 66:702–705

Ciabattoni G, Maclouf J, Catella C, FitzGerald GA, Patrono C (1987) Radioimmunoassay of 11-dehydrothromboxane B_2 in human plasma and urine. Biochim Biophys Acta 918:293

Coller BS (1985) A new murine monoclonal antibody reports an activation dependent change in the conformation and/or microenvironment of the platelet GpIIb/IIIa complex. J Clin Invest 76:101–108

Coronary Drug Project Research Group (1976) Aspirin in coronary heart disease. J Chron Dis 29:625–642

Craven LL (1956) Prevention of coronary and cerebral thrombosis. Miss Valley Med J 78:213–215

Cunningham FM, Wollard PM (1987) 12(*R*)-hydroxy-5,8,10,14-eicosatetraenoic acid is a chemoattractant for human polymorphonuclear leukocytes in vitro. Prostaglandins 34:71–78

Dale J (1977) Prevention of arterial thromboembolism with acetylsalicyclic acid in patients with prosthetic heart valves. Thromb Haemost 38:66 (abstr)

Dale J, Myhre E, Rootwelt K (1975) Effects of dipyridamole and acetylsalicylic acid on platelet functions in patients with aortic ball-valve prostheses. Am Heart J 89:613–618

Dale J, Myhre E, Storstein O, Stormoken H, Efskind L (1977) Prevention of arterial thromboembolism with acetylsalicylic acid: a controlled clinical study in patients with aortic ball valves. Am Heart J 94:101–111

Davies MJ, Thomas AC, Knapman PA, Hanggartner JR (1986) Intramyocardial platelet aggregation in patients with unstable angina suffering sudden ischemic cardiac death. Circulation 73:418–427

Davis JW, Lewis HD, Phillips PE, Schwegier RA, Yue KT, Hassanein KR (1978) Effect of aspirin on exercise induced angina. Clin Pharmacol Ther 23:505–510

DeClerk F, Beetens J, de Chaffoy de Courcelles D, Freyne E, Janssen PAJ (1989a) R 68 070: thromboxane A_2 synthase inhibition and thromboxane A_2/prostaglandin endoperoxide receptor blockade combined in one molecule-I. Biochemical profile in vitro. Thromb Haemost 61:35–42

DeClerk F, Beetens J, Van de Water A, Vercammen E, Janssen PAJ (1989b) R 68 070; thromboxane A_2 synthetase inhibition and thromboxane A_2/prostaglandin endoperoxide receptor blockade combined in one molecule-II. Pharmacological effects in vivo and ex vivo. Thromb Haemost 61:43–49

Dehmer GJ, Popma JJ, van den Berg EK, Eichorn EJ, Prewitt JB, Campbell WB, Jennings L, Willerson JT, Schmitz JM (1988) Reduction in the rate of early restenosis after coronary angioplasty by a diet supplemented with n-3 fatty acids. N Engl J Med 319:733–740

Detre K, Holubkov R, Kelsey S, Cowley M, Kent K, Williams D, Myler R, Faxon D, Holmes D, Bourassa M, Block P, Gosselin A, Bentivoglio L, Leatherman L, Dorros G, King S, Galichia J, Al-Bassam M, Leon M, Robertson T, Passamani E and the co-investigators of the National Heart, Lung and Blood Institute's Percutaneous Transluminal Coronary Angioplasty Registry (1988) Percutaneous transluminal coronary angioplasty in 1985–1986 and 1977–1981: the National Heart, Lung, and Blood Institute registry. N Engl J Med 318:265–270

Dewanjee MK, Trastek VF, Tago M, Kaye MP (1984) Radioisotopic techniques for noninvasive detection of platelet deposition in bovine-tissue mitral-valve prostheses and in vitro quantification of visceral microembolism in dogs. Invest Radiol 6:535–542

DeWitt DL, El-Harith EA, Smith WL (1989) Prostaglandin endoperoxide G/H synthase as a regulatory enzyme in prostaglandin biosynthesis. In: Patrono C, Fitzgerald GA(eds) Platelets and vascular occlusion. Raven New York, pp 109–118.

DeWitt DL, El-Harith EA, Kraemer SA, Yao EF, Armstrong RL, Smith WL (1990) The aspirin site and heme-binding sites of ovine and murine prostaglandin endoperoxide synthases. J Biol Chem 9:5192–5198

DeWood MA, Spores J, Notske MD, Mouser LT, Burroughs R, Golden MS, Long HT (1980) Prevalence of total coronary occlusion during the early hours of transmural myocardial infarction. N Engl J Med 303:897–902

DiMinno G, Cerbone AM, Mattioli PL, Turco S, Lovine C, Mancini M (1985) Functionally thrombasthenic state in normal platelets following the administration of ticlopidine. J Clin Invest 75:328–338

Donaldson DR, Kester RC, Hall TJ, Rajah SM, Crow MJ, Salter MCP (1982) Do platelet-modifying agents influence the patency of femoropopliteal Dacron bypass grafts? Br J Surg 69:284 (abstr)

Dusting GJ, Moncada S, Vane JR (1977) Disappearance of prostacyclin in the circulation of the dog. Br J Pharmacol 62:414–415P

The Dutch TIA Study Group (1988) The Dutch TIA trial: protective effects of low-dose aspirin and atenolol in patients with transient ischemic attacks or non-disabling stroke. Stroke 19:512–517

Dutta-Roy AK, Sinha AK (1987) Purification and properties of prostaglandin E_1/prostacyclin receptor of human blood platelets. J Biol Chem 262:12685–12691

Dyerberg J, Bang HO (1982) A hypothesis on the development of acute myocardial infarction in Greenlanders. Scand J Clin Lab Invest 161:7–13

Egan JW, Griswold DE, Hillegass LM, Newton JF, Eckardt RD, Slivjak MI, Smith EF (1989) Selective antagonism of peptidoleukotriene responses does not reduce myocardial damage or neutrophil accumulation following coronary artery occlusion with reperfusion. Prostaglandins 37:597–613

Elwood PC, Sweetnam PM (1979) Aspirin and secondary mortality after myocardial infarction. Lancet 2:1313–1315

Elwood PC, Williams WO (1979) A randomised controlled trial of aspirin in the prevention of early mortality in myocardial infarction. J R Coll Gen Pract 29:413–414

Elwood PC, Cochrane AL, Burr ML, Sweetnam PM, Williams G, Welsby E, Hughes SJ, Renton R (1974) A randomized controlled trial of acetyl salicylic acid in the secondary prevention of mortality from myocardial infarction. Br Med J 1:436–440

EPSIM Research Group (1982) A controlled comparison of aspirin and oral anticoagulants in prevention of death after myocardial infarction. N Engl J Med 307:701–708

Erikson LA, Ginsberg MH, Loskutoff DJ (1984) Detection and partial characterization of an inhibitor of plasminogen activator in human platelets. J Clin Invest 74:1465–1472

ESPS Group (1987) The European stroke prevention study (ESPS). Lancet 2: 1351–1354

European Coronary Surgery Study Group (1988) Twelve-year follow-up of survival in the randomized European coronary artery study. N Engl J Med 319:332–337

Falk E (1985) Unstable angina with fatal outcome: dynamic coronary thrombosis leading to infarction and/or sudden death. Circulation 71:699–708

Fields WS, Lemak NA, Frankowski RF, Hardy RJ (1977) Controlled trial of aspirin in cerebral ischemia. Stroke 8:301–314

Fields WS, Lemak NA, Frankowski RF, Hardy RJ (1978) Controlled trial of aspirin in cerebral ischemia. Part II: surgical group. Stroke 9:309–319

Fisher CM (1959) Observations of the fundus oculi in transient monocular blindness. Neurology 9:333–347

Fitzgerald DJ, FitzGerald GA (1989) The role of thrombin and thromboxane A_2 in vascular reocclusion following coronary thrombolysis with tissue type plasminogen activator. Proc Natl Acad Sci USA 86:7585–7589

Fitzgerald DJ, Roy L, Catella C, FitzGerald GA (1986) Platelet activation in unstable angina. N Engl J Med 315:983–989

Fitzgerald DJ, Catella F, Roy L, FitzGerald GA (1988a) Marked platelet activation in vivo after intravenous streptokinase in patients with acute myocardial infarction. Circulation 77:142–150

Fitzgerald DJ, Fragetta J, FitzGerald GA (1988b) Prostaglandin endoperoxides modulate the response to thromboxane synthase inhibition during coronary thrombosis. J Clin Invest 82:1708–1713

Fitzgerald DJ, Wright F, FitzGerald GA (1989) Increased thromboxane biosynthesis during coronary thrombolysis: evidence that TXA_2 modulates the response to tissue-type plasminogen activator in vivo. Circ Res 65:83–94

Fitzgerald GA, Reilly AG, Pedersen AK (1985) The biochemical pharmacology of thromboxane synthase inhibition in man. Circulation 72:1194–1201

FitzGerald GA (1987) Dipyridamole. N Engl J Med 316:1247–1257

FitzGerald GA, Friedman LA, Miyamori I, O'Grady J, Lewis PJ (1979) A double-blind, placebo controlled evaluation of prostacyclin in man. Life Sci 25:665–672

FitzGerald GA, Brash AR, Falardeau P, Oates JA (1981) Estimated rate of prostacyclin secretion into the circulation of normal man. J Clin Invest 68: 1272–1276

Fitzpatrick FA, Wynalda MA (1982) The analytical process for eicosanoid determinations. In: Wu KK, Rossi EC (eds) Prostaglandins in clinical medicine: cardiovascular and thrombotic disorders. Year Book Medical Publishers, Chicago, pp 35–47

Folsom AR, Hiroyasu I, Sprafka JM, Edlavitch SA, Luepker RV (1988) Use of aspirin for prevention of cardiovascular disease-1981-82 to 1985-86: the Minnesota Heart Survey. Am Heart J 116:827–830

Funk C, Furci L, FitzGerald GA (1990) Molecular cloning, primary structure and expression of the human platelet/erythroleukemia cell 12-lipoxygenase. Proc Natl Acad Sci USA 87:5638–5642

Fuster V, Pumphrey CW, McGoon MD, Chesebro JH, Pluth JR, McGoon DC (1982) Systemic thromboembolism in mitral and aortic Starr-Edwards prostheses: a 10–19 year follow up. Circulation 66(I):157–161

Gan Z-R, Gould RJ, Jacobs JW, Friedman PA, Polokoff MA (1988) Echistatin: a potent platelet aggregation inhibitor from the venom of the viper, *Echis carinatus*. J Biol Chem 263:19827–19832.

Garde A, Samuelsson K, Fahlgren H, Hedberg E, Hjerne L-G, Ostman J (1983) Treatment after transient ischemic attacks: a comparison between anticoagulant drug and inhibition of platelet aggregation. Stroke 14:677–681.

Garsky VM, Lumma PK, Friedinger RM, Pitzenberger SM, Randall WC, Veber DF, Gould RJ, Friedman PA (1989) Chemical synthesis of echistatin, a potent inhibitor of platelet aggregation from *Echis carinatus*: synthesis and biological activity of selected analogs. Proc Natl Acad Sci USA 86:4022–4026.

Gerritsen ME, Cheli CD (1983) Arachidonic acid and prostaglandin endoperoxide metabolism in isolated rabbit and coronary microvessels and isolated and cultivated coronary microvessel endothelial cells. J Clin Invest 72:1658–1671

Gerritsen ME, Printz MP (1981) Sites of prostaglandin synthesis in the bovine heart and isolated bovine coronary microvessels. Circ Res 49:1152–1163

GISSI-2 (Gruppo-Italiano per lo Studio della Sopravivienza nell'Infarto Miocardico) (1990) A factorial randomised trial of alteplase versus streptokinase and heparin versus no heparin among 12490 patients with acute myocardial infarction. Lancet 336:65–71

Goetzl EJ, Hill HR, Gorman RR (1980) Unique aspects of the modulation of human neutrophil function by 12-L-hydroperoxy-5,8,10,14-eicosatetraenoic acid. Prostaglandins 19:71–85

Goldman M, Norcott HC, Hawker RJ, Drolc Z, McCollum CN (1982) Platelet deposition on mature Dacron grafts in man. Br J Surg 69:S38–S40

Goldman M, Hall C, Dykes J, Hawker RJ, McCollum CN (1983a) Does ^{111}indium-platelet deposition predict patency in prosthetic arterial grafts? Br J Surg 70: 635–638

Goldman MK, Simpson D, Hawker RJ, Norcott HC, McCollum CN (1983b) Aspirin and dipyridamole reduce platelet deposition on prosthetic femoro-popliteal grafts in man. Ann Surg 198:713–716

Goldman S, Copeland J, Moritz T, Henderson W, Zadina K, Ovitt T, Doherty J, Read R, Chesler E, Sako Y, Lancaster L, Emery R, Sharma GVRK, Josa M, Pacold I, Montoya A, Parikh D, Sethi G, Holt J, Kirklin J, Shabetai D, Moores W, Aldridge J, Masud Z, DeMots H, Floten S, Haakenson C, Harker LA (1988) Improvement in early saphenous vein graft patency after coronary artery bypass surgery with antiplatelet therapy: results of a Veterans Administration Cooperative study. Circulation 77:1324–1332

Golino P, Buja M, Ashton JH, Taylor A, Willerson JT (1988) Effect of thromboxane and serotonin receptor antagonists on intracoronary platelet deposition in dogs with experimentally stenosed coronary arteries. Circulation 78:701–711

Gorman RR, Bunting S, Miller OV (1977) Modulation of human platelet adenylate cyclase by prostaglandin (PGX). Prostaglandins 13:377–388

Gresele P, Arnout J, Deckmyn H, Huybrechts E, Pieters G, Vermylen J (1987) Role of proaggregatory and antiaggregatory prostaglandins in hemostasis: studies with combined thromboxane synthase inhibition and thromboxane receptor antagonism. J Clin Invest 80:1435–1445

Grigg LE, Kay TWH, Manolas EG, Valentine PA, Larkins R, Flower DJ, Manolas EM, O'Dea K, Sinclair AJ, Hopper JL, Hunt D (1989) Determinants of restenosis and lack of effect of dietary supplementation with eicosapentanoic acid on the incidence of coronary artery restenosis after angioplasty. J Am Coll Cardiol 13:665–672

Gruntzig AR, Senning A, Siegenthaler WE (1979) Nonoperative dilatation of coronary-artery stenosis: percutaneous transluminal coronary angioplasty. N Engl J Med 301:61–68

Gualler EM, Neaton JD (1989) An epidemiological study of the impact of different doses of aspirin on cardiovascular disease. Proceedings of the 2nd international conference on preventive cardiology and the 29th annual meeting of the American Heart Association Council on Epidemiology. A43 (abstr)

Guiteras P, Altimiras J, Aris A, Auge JM, Bassons T, Bonal T, Caralps JM, Castellarnau C, Crexells C, Masoti M, Oriol A, Padro JM, Rutllant M (1989) Prevention of aortocoronary vein-graft attrition with low-dose aspirin and triflusal, both associated with dipyridamole: a randomized, double-blind, placebo-controlled trial. Eur Heart J 10:159–167

Hackett D, Davies G, Chierchia S, Maseri A (1987) Intermittent coronary occlusion in acute myocardial infarction: value of combined thrombolytic and vasodilator therapy. N Engl J Med 317:1055–1059

Hamberg M, Hamberg G (1980) On the mechanism of oxygenation of arachidonic acid by human platelet lipoxygenase. Biochem Biophys Res Commun 95: 1090–1097

Hamberg M, Samuelsson B (1974) Prostaglandin endoperoxides. Novel transformations of arachidonic acid in human platelets. Proc Natl Acad Sci 71:3400–3404

Hamberg M, Svensson J, Wakabayashi T, Samuelsson B (1974) Isolation and structure of two prostaglandin endoperoxides that cause platelet aggregation. Proc Natl Acad Sci 71:345–349

Hamberg M, Svensson J, Samuellson B (1975) Thromboxanes: a new group of biologically active compounds derived from prostaglandin endoperoxides. Proc Natl Acad Sci 72:2994–2998

Hamm CW, Lorenz RL, Weber PC, Nober W, Kupper W (1986) Subgroups of patients with unstable angina identified by biochemical evidence of thrombus formation. Circulation 74(II):305 (abstr)

Hammarstrom S, Falardeau P (1977) Resolution of prostaglandin endoperoxide synthase and thromboxane synthase of human platelets. Proc Natl Acad Sci USA 74:3691–3695

Hanson SR, Pareti FI, Ruggeri ZM, Marzec UM, Kunicki TJ, Montgomery RR, Zimmerman TS, Harker LA (1988) Effects of monoclonal antibodies against the platelet glycoprotein IIb/IIIa complex on thrombosis and hemostasis in the baboon. J Clin Invest 81:149–158

Harker LA, Slichter SJ (1970) Studies of platelet and fibrinogen kinetics in patients with prosthetic heart valves. N Engl J Med 283:1302–1305

Harris WH, Salzman EW, Athanasoulis C, Waltman AC, DeSanctis RW (1977) Aspirin prophylaxis of venous thromboembolism after total hip replacement. N Engl J Med 297:1246–1249

Hass WK, Easton JD, Adams HP, Pryse-Phillips W, Molony BA, Anderson S, Kamm B (1989) A randomized trial comparing ticlopidine hydrochloride with aspirin for the prevention of stroke in high-risk patients. N Engl J Med 321: 501–507

Hennekens CH, Buring JE (1987) Epidemiology in medicine. Little, Brown, Boston

Hennekens CH, Karslon LK, Rosner B (1978) A case-control study of regular aspirin use and coronary deaths. Circulation 58:35–38

Henriksson P, Wennmalm A, Edhag O, Vesterqvist O, Green K (1986) In vivo production of prostacyclin and thromboxane in patients with acute myocardial infarction. Br Heart J 55:543–548

Hensby CN, Barnes PJ, Dollery CT, Dargie H (1979) Production of 6-oxo-$PGF_{1\alpha}$ by human lung in vivo. Lancet 2:1162–1163

Hoffmann W, Forster W (1987) Two years follow-up Cottbus reinfarction study with 30 and 60 mg acetylsalicyclic acid. In: Sinzinger M, Schror K (eds) Progress in clinical and biological research, vol 242. Alan R Liss, New York, pp 393–397

Honn KV, Grossi IM, Fitzgerald LA, Umbarger LA, Diglio CA, Taylor JD (1988) Lipoxygenase products regulate IRGpIIb/IIIa receptor mediated adhesion of tumor cells to endothelial cells, subendothelial matrix and fibronectin. Proc Soc Exp Biol Med 189:130–135

Hsia J, Hamilton WP, Kleiman N, Roberts R, Chaitman BR, Ross AM (1990) A comparison between heparin and low-dose aspirin as adjunctive therapy with tissue plasminogen activator for acute myocardial infarction. N Engl J Med 323:1433–1437

Inoue U, Kuwaki K, Ueda K, Shirai T (1987) Angioscopy guided coronary thrombolysis. J Am Coll Cardiol 9:62A (abstr)

International Study Group (1990) In-hospital mortality and clinical course of 20 891 patients with suspected acute myocardial infarction randomised between alteplase and streptokinase with or without heparin. Lancet 336:71–75

ISIS-2 (Second International Study Group of Infarct Survival) Collaborative Group (1988) Randomised trial of intravenous streptokinase, oral aspirin, both, or neither among 17,187 cases of suspected acute myocardial infarction:ISIS-2. Lancet 2:349–360

Joist JH, Niewiarwoski S, Nath N, Mustard JF (1976) Platelet antiplasmin: its extrusion during the release reaction, subcellular localization, characterization and relationship to heparin in pig platelets. J Lab Clin Med 87:659–669

Josa M, Lie JT, Bianco RL, Kaye MP (1981) Reduction of thrombosis in canine coronary bypass vein grafts with dipyridamole and aspirin. Am J Cardiol 47: 1248–1254

Kerins DM, Roy L, FitzGerald GA, Fitzgerald DJ (1989) Platelet and vascular function during coronary thrombolysis with tissue-type plasminogen activator. Circulation 80:1718–1725

Kerins DM, Murray R, FitzGerald GA (1990) Prostacyclin and prostaglandin E_1: molecular mechanisms and therapeutic utility. Prog Hemost 10:307–337

Klimt CR, Knatterud GL, Stamler J, Meier P (1986) Persantine-aspirin reinfarction study. Part II. Secondary coronary prevention with persantine and aspirin. J Am Coll Cardiol 7:251–269

Knudtson ML, Duff HJ, Flintoft VF, Roth DL, Hansen JL (1986) Does short term prostacyclin administration lower the risk of restenosis after PTCA?: a prospective randomized trial. Circulation 74(II):282 (abstr)

Kohler TR, Kaufman JL, Clowes A, Donaldson MC, Kelly E, Skillman J, Couch NP, Whittemore AD, Mannick JA, Salzman EW (1984) Effect of aspirin and dipyridamole on the patency of lower extremity bypass grafts. Surgery 96: 462–466

Kromann N, Green A (1980) Epidemiological studies in the Upernavik district, Greenland: incidence of some chronic diseases, 1950–74. Acta Med Scand 208:401–406

Lawrie GM, Lie JT, Morris GC, Beazley HL (1976) Vein graft and intimal proliferation after aortocoronary bypass: early and long-term angiopathic correlations. Am J Cardiol 38:856–862

Leaf A, Weber PC (1988) Cardiovascular effects of n-3 fatty acids. N Engl J Med 318:549–557

Lembo NJ, Black AJ, Roubin GS, Mufson LH, Wilentz JR, Douglas JS, King SB (1988) Does the addition of dipyridamole to aspirin decrease acute coronary angioplasty complications? The results of a prospective randomized clinical trial. J Am Coll Cardiol 11:237A (abstr)

Lewis HD, Davis JW, Archibald DG, Steinke WE, Smitherman TC, Doherty JE, Schnaper HW, LeWinter MM, Linares E, Pouget JM, Sabharwal SC, Chesler E, DeMots H (1983) Protective effects of aspirin against acute myocardial infarction and death in men with unstable angina: results of a Veterans Administration cooperative study. N Engl J Med 309:396–403

Lewis RA, Austen KH (1984) The biologically active leukotrienes: biosynthesis, metabolism, receptors, functions and pharmacology. J Clin Invest 73:889–897

Limet R, David J-L, Margotteaux P, Larock MP, Rigo P (1987) Prevention of aortocoronary graft occlusion. Beneficial effect on early and late patency rates of venous coronary bypass grafts: a double blind study. J Cardiovasc Surg 94: 773–783

Lorenz RL, von Schacky C, Weber M, Meister W, Kotzur J, Reichardt B, Thiesen K, Weber PC (1984) Improved aortocoronary bypass patency by low-dose aspirin (100 mg daily): effects on platelet aggregation and thromboxane formation. Lancet 1:1262–1264

Lüscher TF, Yang Z, Diederich D, Bühler FR (1989) Endothelium-derived vasoactive substances: potential role in hypertension, atherosclerosis, and vascular occlusion. J Cardiovasc Pharm 14 [Suppl 6]:S63–S69

MacDermot J, Kelsey CR, Waddell KA, Richmond R, Knight RK, Cole PJ, Dollery CT, Blair IA (1984) Synthesis of leukotriene B_4 and prostanoids by human alveolar macrophages: analysis by gas chromatography/mass spectrometry. Prostaglandins 27:163–179

Maclouf J, Fradin A, Vausbinder L, Henson PM, Murphy RC (1989) Development of an ex vivo model to assess transcellular metabolism of arachidonic acid: towards a reappraisal of the biosynthesis of eicosanoids. In: Patrono C,

FitzGerald GA (eds) Platelets and vascular occlusion. Raven, New York, pp 151–159
Mahony C (1989) Effect of aspirin on myocardial ischemia. Am J Cardiol 64: 387–389
Marcus AJ (1984) The eicosanoids in biology and medicine. J Lipid Res 25:1511–1516
Marcus AJ (1990) Thrombosis and inflammation as multicellular processes: pathophysiological significance of transcellular metabolism. Blood 76:1903–1907
Marcus AJ, Weksler BB, Jaffe EA, Broekman MJ (1980) Synthesis of prostacyclin from platelet-derived endoperoxides by cultured human endothelial cells. J Clin Invest 66:979–986
Marcus AJ, Safier LB, Ullman HL, Islam N, Broekman MJ, von Schacky C (1987) Studies on the mechanism of Ω-hydroxylation of platelet 12-hydroxyeicosatetraenoic acid (12-HETE) by unstimulated neutrophils. J Clin Invest 79:179–187
Marder VJ, Sherry S (1988) Thrombolytic therapy: current status. N Engl J Med 318:1512–1520, 1585–1594
Mayer JE, Maj MC, Lindsay WG, Castenada W, Nicoloff DM (1981) Influence of aspirin and dipyridamole on patency of coronary artery bypass grafts. Ann Thorac Surg 31:204–210
Mayeux PR, Morton HE, Gillard J, Lord A, Morinelli TA, Boehm A, Mais DE, Halushka PV (1988) The affinities of prostaglandin H_2 and thromboxane A_2 for their receptor are similar in washed human platelets. Biochem Biophys Res Comm 157:733–739
McBride W, Lange RA, Hillis LD (1988) Restenosis after successful coronary angioplasty: pathophysiology and prevention. N Engl J Med 318:1734–1737
McCann RL, Hagen P-O, Fuchs JCA (1980) Aspirin and dipyridamole decrease intimal hyperplasia in experimental vein grafts. Ann Surg 191:238–243
Mehta P, Mehta J, Lawson D, Krop I, Letts LG (1986) Leukotrienes potentiate the effects of epinephrine and thrombin on human platelet aggregation. Thromb Res 41:731–738
Milner MR, Gallino RA, Leffingwell A, Pichard AD, Brooks-Robinson S, Rosenberg J, Little T, Lindsay J (1989) Usefulness of fish oil supplements in preventing clinical evidence of restenosis after percutaneous transluminal coronary angioplasty. Am J Cardiol 64:294–299
Miwa K, Kambara H, Kawai C (1983) Effect of aspirin in large doses on attacks of variant angina. Am Heart J 105:351–355
Moggio RA, Hammond GL, Stansel HC, Glenn GWL (1978) Incidence of emboli with cloth-covered Starr-Edwards valve without anticoagulation and with varying forms of anticoagulation: analysis of 183 patients followed for 3½ years. J Thorac Cardiovasc Surg 75:296–299
Mok CK, Boey J, Wang R, Chan TK, Cheung KL, Lee PK, Chow J, Ng RP, Tse TF (1985) Warfarin versus dipyridamole-aspirin and pentoxifylline-aspirin for the prevention of prosthetic heart valve thromboembolism: a prospective randomized clinical trial. Circulation 72:1059–1063
Moncada S, Herman AG, Higgs EA, Vane JR (1977) Differential formation of prostacyclin (PGX or PGI_2) by layers of the arterial wall. An explanation for the antithrombotic properties of vascular endothelium. Thromb Res 11:323–344
Moncada S, Korbut R, Bunting S, Vane JR (1978) Prostacyclin is a circulating hormone. Nature 273:767–768
Needleman P, Raz A, Minkes MS, Ferrendeli JA, Sprecher H (1979) Triene prostaglandins: prostacyclin and thromboxane biosynthesis and unique biological properties. Proc Natl Acad Sci USA 314:937–942
Needleman P, Turk J, Jakschik BA, Morrison AR, Lefkowith JB (1986) Arachidonic acid metabolism. Ann Rev Biochem 55:69–102

Siess W, Dray F (1982) Very low levels of 6-keto-prostaglandin $F_{1\alpha}$ in human plasma. J Lab Clin Med 99:388–398
Slack JD, Pinkerton CA, VanTassel J, Orr CM, Scott M, Allen B, Nasser WK (1987) Can oral fish oil supplement minimize re-stenosis after percutaneous transluminal coronary angioplasty? J Am Coll Cardiol 9:64A (abstr)
Smith JB, Dangelmaier C, Mauco G (1985) Quantitation of arachidonate released during the platelet phosphatidylinositol response to thrombin. In: Bailey JM (ed) Prostaglandins, leukotrienes and lipoxins: biochemistry, mechanism of action, and clinical applications. Plenum, New York, pp 205–211
Sorensen PS, Pedersen H, Marquardsen J, Petersson H, Heltberg A, Simonsen N, Munck O, Andersen LA (1983) Acetylsalicyclic acid in the prevention of stroke in patients with reversible cerebral ischemic attacks. A Danish cooperative study. Stroke 14:15–22
Spears JR, Marais J, Serur J, Pomerantzeff O, Geyer RP, Sipzener RS, Weintraub R, Thurer R, Paulin S, Gerstin R, Grossman W (1983) In vivo coronary angioscopy. J Am Coll Cardiol 5:1311–1314
Steele PM, Chesebro JH, Stanson AW, Holmes DR, Badimon L, Fuster V (1984) Balloon angioplasty: effect of platelet-inhibitor drugs on platelet-thrombus deposition in a pig model. J Am Coll Cardiol 3:506 (abstr)
Steele PM, Chesebro JH, Stanson AW, Holmes DR, Dewanjee MK, Badimon L, Fuster V (1985) Balloon angioplasty: natural history of the pathophysiological response to injury in a pig model. Circ Res 57:105–112
Steering committee of the Physicians' Health Study Research Group (1989) Final report on the aspirin component of the ongoing physicians' health study. N Engl J Med 321:129–135
Stratton JR, Ritchie JL (1984) Failure of ticlopidine to inhibit deposition of indium-111-labelled platelets on Dacron prosthetic surfaces in humans. Circulation 69:677–683
Stratton JR, Ritchie JL (1985) The effect of sulfinpyrazone on platelet deposition on Dacron vascular grafts in man. Am Heart J 109:453–457
Stratton JR, Rithie JL (1986) Reduction of indium-111 platelet deposition on Dacron vascular grafts in humans by aspirin plus dipyridamole. Circulation 73:325–330
Stratton JR, Thiele BL, Ritchie JL (1982) Platelet deposition on Dacron aortic bifurcation grafts in man: quantitation with indium-111 platelet imaging. Circulation 66:1287–1293
Sullivan JM, Harken DE, Gorlin R (1971) Pharmacologic control of thromboembolic complications of cardiac-valve replacement. N Engl J Med 25:1391–1394
Tateson JE, Moncada S, Vane JR (1977) Effects of prostacyclin (PGX) on cyclic AMP concentration in human platelets. Prostaglandins 13:389–399
Taylor GW, Morris HR (1983) Lipoxygenase pathways. Br Med Bull 39:219–222
Temple R, Pledger GW (1980) Special report: the FDA's critique of the anturane reinfarction trial. N Engl J Med 303:1488–1492
Theroux P, Ouimet H, McCans J, Latour JG, Joly P, Levy G, Pelletier E, Juneau M, Stasiak J, DeGuise P, Pelletier GB, Rinzler D, Waters D (1988) Aspirin, heparin, or both to treat acute unstable angina. N Engl J Med 319:1105–1111
Thornton MA, Gruntzig AR, Hollman J, Kimg SB, Douglas JS (1984) Coumadin and aspirin in prevention of recurrence after transluminal coronary angioplasty: a randomized study. Circulation 69:721–777
Tohgi H (1984) The effect of ticlopidine on TIA compared with aspirin: a double-blind, twelve-month follow up study. Agents Actions [Suppl]15:279–282
UK-TIA Study Group (1988) United Kingdom transient ischemic attack (UK-TIA) aspirin trial: interim results. Br Med J 296:316–320
Unni KK, Kottke BA, Titus JL, Frye RL, Wallace RB, Brown AL (1974) Pathologic changes in aortocoronary saphenous vein grafts. Am J Cardiol 34:526–532
Vejar M, Lipkin DP, Maseri A, Born GVR, Ciabattoni G, Patrono C (1988) Dissociation of platelet activation and spontaneous myocardial ischemia in unstable angina. Clin Res 36:326A (abstr)

Verheugt FWA, Küpper AJF, Galema TW, Roos JP (1988) Low dose aspirin after early thrombolysis in anterior wall acute myocardial infarction. Am J Cardiol 61:904–906

Weksler BB, Marcus AJ, Jaffe EA (1977) Synthesis of prostaglandin I_2 (prostacyclin) by cultured human and bovine endothelial cells. Proc Natl Acad Sci USA 74:3922–3926

Weksler BB, Pett SB, Alonso D, Richter RC, Stelzer P, Subramanian V, Tack-Goldamn K, Gay WA (1983) Differential inhibition by aspirin of vascular and platelet prostaglandin synthesis in atherosclerotic patients. N Engl J Med 308: 800–805

Weksler BB, Tack-Goldman K, Subramanian VA, Gay WA (1985) Cumulative inhibitory effect of low-dose aspirin on vascular prostacyclin and platelet thromboxane production in patients with atherosclerosis. Circulation 71: 332–340

White CW, Chaitman B, Lassar TA, Marcus ML, Chisholm RJ, Knudson M, Morton B, Khaja F, Vandormael M, Reitman M and the Ticlopidine Study Group (1987a) Antiplatelet agents are effective in reducing the immediate complications of PTCA: results from the ticlopidine multicenter trial. Circulation 76(IV):400 (abstr)

White CW, Knudson M, Schmidt D, Chisholm RJ, Vandormael M, Morton B, Roy L, Khaja F, Reitman M and the Ticlopidine Study Group (1987b) Neither ticlopidine nor aspirin-dipyridamole prevents restenosis post PTCA: results from a randomized placebo-controlled multicenter trial. Circulation 76(IV):213 (abstr)

Wu H, Turner JT, Halenda SP (1991) Activation of phospholipase D by E-series prostaglandins in human erythroleukemia cells. J Pharmacol Exp Ther 258: 607–612

Wyngaarden JB, Smith LH (eds) (1988) Cecil Textbook of Medicine. Saunders, Philadelphia

Xie W, Chipman JG, Robertson DL, Erikson RL, Simmons DL (1991) Expression of a mitogen-responsive gene encoding prostaglandin synthase is regulated by mRNA splicing. Proc Natl Acad Sci USA 88:2692–2696

Yokoyama C, Miyata A, Ihara H, Ulrich V, Tanabe T (1991) Molecular cloning of human platlet thromboxane A synthase. Biochem Biophy Res Comm 178: 1479–1484

Yokoyama C, Tanabe T (1989) Cloning of human gene encoding prostaglandin endoperoxide synthase and primary structure of the enzyme. Biochem Biophy Res Comm 165:888–894

Yoshimoto T, Suzuki H, Yamamoto S, Takai T, Yokoyama C, Tanabe T (1990) Cloning and sequence analysis of the cDNA for arachidonate 12-lipoxygenase of porcine leukocytes. Proc Natl Acad Sci USA 87:2142–2146

CHAPTER 10

Chemical Agents That Inhibit Platelet Aggregation*

J.B. SMITH and D.C.B. MILLS

A. Introduction

The primary importance of platelets in the hemostatic process and their acknowledged involvement in thrombosis have led to an extensive investigation into the mechanisms of platelet adhesion and aggregation. Early studies of the factors which influenced platelet adhesiveness in vitro were made by HELLEM (1960) who measured the removal of platelets from citrated blood passed through a column of glass beads. He showed that erythrocytes contain an acidic, dialyzable, and heat stable factor which causes platelet adhesion to glass and aggregation. This new factor was identified by GAARDER et al. (1961) as ADP. The discovery that a specific, low molecular weight agonist can initiate platelet aggregation led rapidly to the development of a reliable method for its study in vitro. The concept of the optical aggregometer was introduced by BORN (1962) and O'BRIEN (1962). This instrument measures the changes in light transmission during aggregation in platelet-rich plasma by the use of a suitable photometric recording device under controlled conditions of temperature and speed of stirring.

Following the discovery that ADP causes platelet aggregation, a number of widely differing substances, which could have physiological or pathological significance, have been found to have similar actions. They include thrombin (SHERMER et al. 1961), collagen (ZUCKER and BORRELLI 1962), serotonin and epinephrine (MITCHELL and SHARP 1964), vasopressin (HASLAM and ROSSON 1972), thromboxane A_2 (TXA_2) (Hamberg et al. 1975), platelet-activating factor (BENVENISTE et al. 1972), and cathepsin G (SELAK et al. 1988). Occurring simultaneously with the findings that these different substances induce platelet aggregation came the discovery that other agents potently inhibit it. The mechanism of action of these inhibitory agents has been the subject of intensive investigation because of their potential value as antithrombotic drugs. In this chapter, we summarize some of the advances that have been made in classifying inhibitors of platelet aggregation and in understanding how they work.

* Supported in part by grants no. HL37392 and HL36579 from the National Heart, Lung, and Blood Institute, National Institutes of Health.

B. Platelet Physiology

Platelets are released by fragmentation of their mother cells, the megakaryocytes, and circulate in the bloodstream for between 7 and 10 days. The most well-established physiological function of platelets is to participate in hemostasis (i.e., to prevent the loss of blood from ruptured arterial or venous blood vessels), and they do this in two ways: Firstly, by quickly adhering to damaged vessel walls in an injured blood vessel and aggregating to form a hemostatic plug that stems the loss of blood; secondly, by providing a phospholipid-containing surface that greatly accelerates the coagulation of constituents of blood plasma. The initial event in hemostasis involves the adhesion of a relatively few platelets to newly exposed connective tissue (collagen). These adhering platelets secrete ADP and serotonin from storage granules and synthesize TXA_2 from arachidonate in the membrane. The ADP and TXA_2 then act as chemical signals that cause other platelets in the vicinity to become sticky and adhere both to the platelets attached to the vessel wall and to each other to form aggregates.

Injury to blood vessels also triggers the coagulation cascade with the eventual formation of fibrin. In this cascade, a series of coagulation factors in plasma are each converted from an inactive zymogen to an active enzyme with serine protease activity, which is then capable of effecting the proteolytic cleavage of the next zymogen in the sequence. These reactions occur most efficiently on a catalytic surface, and it is now evident that activated platelets provide a suitable surface during normal hemostasis. The early coagulation factors in the cascade are present in plasma in very low concentrations, and since they act as enzymes, they are capable of converting progressively greater quantities of subsequent factors to their active form. For example, Factor XI, an early zymogen in the coagulation cascade, is present in plasma at about 5 μg/ml, whereas fibrinogen, the final substrate for the action of the protease thrombin, is present at 2.5 mg/ml. Thus, the activation of a very small amount of Factor XI in the presence of activated platelets can result in the local generation of a substantial amount of fibrin.

C. Platelet Structure

Human platelets are flat circular disks, 2–3 μm in diameter and about 1 μm thick, with an average volume of 15 fl. They lack nuclei but contain numerous organelles including microfilaments, microtubules, a dense tubular system, glycogen granules, and mitochondria. There are also three types of specific storage granules: the α granules, containing a variety of platelet-specific proteins such as thrombospondin, platelet-derived growth factor, and platelet factor 4; the dense bodies, containing serotonin, nucleotides including ADP, and inorganic ions, pyrophosphate, Ca^{2+}, and Mg^{2+}; and the lysosomes, with an array of acid hydrolases. There are between 150 and 450 million platelets present per milliliter of normal human blood. In patients with thrombocytopenia, due either to a reduced production of platelets or their increased destruction, this figure may fall to as low as 20, with the appearance of spontaneous capillary hemorrhage (purpura). On the other hand, patients with thrombocytosis due to increased production of platelets by the bone marrow may experience peripheral ischemia due to obstruction of capillaries.

D. Platelet Involvement in Thrombosis

That platelets are involved in the initial stages of thrombus formation was realized by the end of the nineteenth century. The early history of research on platelets has been reviewed by Robb-Smith (1967). The first stage in the formation of an intravascular arterial thrombus is the adhesion of platelets to damaged endothelium or exposed collagen fibers. The initial adhesion is followed by the formation of large clumps which then "consolidate" and are often large enough to block the vessel almost completely. In the arterial system, e.g., coronary or carotid arteries, these early changes take place with very little fibrin formation, and only in the later stages is there enough thrombin present to cause clotting. By contrast, in the venous system, e.g., leg veins, thrombus formation is mainly due to the clotting of fibrinogen as a result of the gradual build-up of thrombin in slowly moving blood and may involve platelet activation only to a minor extent. Platelets are also concerned in the reocclusion of coronary arteries that occurs in about 30% of patients who have had arterial stenoses removed by thrombolysis.

Platelets have been implicated in cancer metastasis and are believed to contribute to migraine by the release of serotonin in the brain and to vasospasm by the synthesis and release of TXA_2 in diseased blood vessels. Pulmonary embolism results from the migration to the lungs of thrombi formed in the leg veins via the venous circulation; release of vasoactive agents from platelets in these emboli may contribute to their pathology.

E. Platelet Responses

The most prominent responses of platelets to stimuli are shape change, aggregation, and secretion. Following the adhesion of platelets to a freshly exposed surface such as collagen fibers or the binding of an agonist to its receptor, the discoid platelet rapidly becomes spherical and throws out several long pseudopodia. The shape change occurs in the absence of extracellular Ca^{2+} and is mediated by the mobilization of intracellular calcium as discussed below, whereas the subsequent aggregation response depends on the presence of extracellular Ca^{2+} and fibrinogen. Fibrinogen binds to specific receptors that are not present on the surface of unstimulated platelets but become exposed as a result of agonist-mediated stimulation and allow the platelets to adhere to each other (aggregation). Certain agonists are also able to cause the release of substances from the three different types of platelet

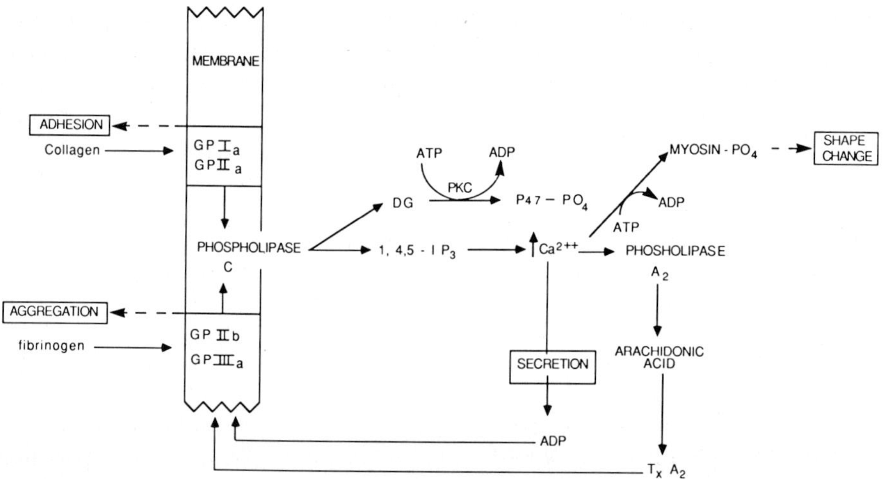

Fig. 1. Some of the mechanisms involved in platelet activation *GPIa*, glycoprotein Ia; *GPIIa*, glycoprotein IIa; *GPIIb*, glycoprotein IIb; *GpIIIa*, glycoprotein IIIa; *DG*, diacylglycerol; *IP3*, inositol trisphosphate; *PKC*, protein kinase C

granules (secretion). A schematic representation of some of the mechanisms involved in platelet activation is shown in Fig. 1.

I. Shape Change

The shape change response greatly enhances the platelets' ability to cling to the vessel wall, to each other, and to fibrin fibrils, and thereby facilitates their role in hemostasis. Adhesion to collagen or stimulation by agonists with the exception of epinephrine leads to platelet shape change. This response consists of a central movement in which platelet granules are pulled towards the center of the cell by a contractile apparatus consisting of myosin, actin, and α-actinin, and a peripheral pseudopodal movement involving actin binding protein, actin, and α-actinin. The arrangement of these cytoskeletal components is so regulated that an increase in the concentration of cytoplasmic free Ca^{2+} causes their activation, while an increase in the concentration of cAMP opposes such changes.

In response to most stimuli, there is a rapid conversion of phosphatidylinositol-4,5-bisphosphate (PIP_2) into two different second messengers, 1,2-diacylglycerol (DAG) and 1,4,5-inositol trisphosphate (IP_3) (see HASLAM 1987; SEISS 1989 for recent reviews). The formation of these second messengers results from the action of phospholipase C which is thought to be controlled through receptor-mediated activation of guanine nucleotide-binding proteins (G-proteins). In platelets, as in other cells, agonist-induced formation of IP_3 precedes the accumulation of inositol monophosphate. This suggests that the primary action of phospholipase C is on PIP_2 and that the decrease in phosphatidylinositol seen in activated platelets may be attributable to replenishment of PIP_2 hydrolysed by phospholipase C rather than to the direct action of the enzyme. The second messenger IP_3 mobilizes Ca^{2+} from the vesicles of the dense tubular system. As mentioned above, intracellular Ca^{2+} is thought to play a very important role in causing platelet shape change as well as in mediating several other platelet functions. The other second messenger, DAG, activates protein kinase C, an enzyme that causes the phosphorylation of several platelet proteins but whose significance is not presently fully understood. Protein kinase C is also activated by phorbol myristate acetate (PMA), which leads to platelet aggregation and secretion (WHITE et al. 1974). It has been suggested that protein kinase C acts synergistically with Ca^{2+} ions in promoting platelet secretion (YAMANISHI et al. 1983).

Analysis of changes in the levels of intracellular free Ca^{2+} in platelets following agonist stimulation was made possible by the introduction of the fluorescent indicator quin 2 (RINK et al. 1982). Quin 2 is a hydrophilic calcium indicator that is introduced into cells as the membrane-permeable acetoxymethyl ester and accumulates in the cells after hydrolysis by cellular esterases. Most agonists cause larger increases in intracellular free Ca^{2+} in the presence of extracellular Ca^{2+}, indicating the calcium enters stimulated platelets from outside, as well as being mobilized from intracellular sources. This is confirmed by the observation that platelets possess receptor-operated calcium channels (ZSCHAUER et al. 1988). Although discrepancies exist in relating measured levels of intracellular free Ca^{2+} and the occurrence of shape change, the weight of evidence indicates that increases in intracellular Ca^{2+} concentration trigger shape change by combining with the calcium binding protein, calmodulin, to activate myosin light chain kinase (DANIEL et al. 1987). This enzyme phosphorylates the light chains of platelet myosin which then interact with actin to cause the central contractile movement associated with shape change. The action of Ca^{2+} is probably assisted by a rapid increase in intracellular protons (from pH 7.15 to 7.35) which results from Na^+/H^+ exchange across the plasma membrane and which can be inhibited by amiloride and its analogues (SIFFERT et al. 1990).

II. Adhesion

Platelet adhesion depends on the presence of a normal platelet membrane and the exposure of subendothelial structures. It is greatly enhanced by the presence, either in the circulating blood or on the vessel wall surface, of the protein called von Willebrand's factor, which is deficient or defective in von Willebrand's disease, a hemorrhagic condition. Newly exposed collagen fibers in the damaged area are the most likely substrate for platelet adhesion, although other microfibrillar structures have been implicated. Platelets can effectively adhere in a Mg^{2+}-dependent manner to either fibrillar or monomeric collagen. Whereas adhesion to the fibrillar substrate is associated with secretion, adhesion to the monomeric substrate does not result in secretion (SANTORO 1986). Von Willebrand factor, which acts as a circulating carrier for the Factor VIII molecule, has an undisputed role in the adhesive process, but its exact mechanism of action is not known. It is most active at high shear rates, such as those found in the arterioles (WEISS et al. 1978).

The platelet surface component that mediates adhesion to collagen was recently identified as a heterodimeric complex of platelet glycoproteins (Gp) Ia and IIa with molecular weights of 160 kDa and 130 kDa, respectively. Platelet GpIa corresponds to the α_2 subunit and platelet GpIIa to the β_1 subunit of the VLA (very late activation) subfamily of the integrin superfamily of cell adhesion molecules (SANTORO et al. 1988). Interestingly, NIEUWENHUIS et al. (1986) described a patient with a bleeding disorder who exhibited impaired collagen-induced platelet aggregation but normal responsiveness to other agonists. This individual was deficient in GpIa.

III. Aggregation

Fibrinogen is believed to bind adjacent platelets together during aggregation, and the platelet receptor for fibrinogen is a Ca^{2+}-dependent, heterodimeric complex of GpIIb and GpIIIa (PARISE and PHILLIPS 1985). Although GpIIb/IIIa is exposed on the surface of unstimulated platelets, it becomes a functional receptor only when platelets are activated. The mechanism by which GpIIb/IIIa is converted to an active receptor is unknown. GpIIb/IIa also binds other plasma proteins including fibronectin and von Willebrand factor, although the role of these proteins in aggregation is unclear. Platelets from patients with the bleeding disorder Glanzmann's thrombasthenia lack GpIIb/IIIa and are unable to bind fibrinogen or aggregate.

GpIIb and GpIIIa are the most abundant proteins on the platelet surface, together forming 10%–20% of the total membrane protein, with 50 000 or more complexes per platelet (JENNINGS and PHILLIPS 1982). GpIIb is the α subunit of the complex (140 kDa) and contains a heavy (115 kDa) and a light (25 kDa) chain linked by a disulfide bridge. GpIIIa, the β subunit, is a single polypeptide with a molecular weight of 105 kDa (PHILLIPS et al. 1988).

F. Inhibition of Platelet Aggregation

I. Cyclic AMP

Platelets have a complex mechanism for regulating their behavior through the control of cAMP levels (Fig. 2). Cyclic AMP is formed from ATP by a membrane-bound enzyme, adenylate cyclase, whose activity is determined by a variety of receptors acting through stimulatory and inhibitory guanine-binding proteins (G_s and G_i). Removal of cAMP is effected by soluble phosphodiesterases, of which the platelet has at least three, differing both in their affinity for cAMP and their relative activity towards cAMP and cGMP

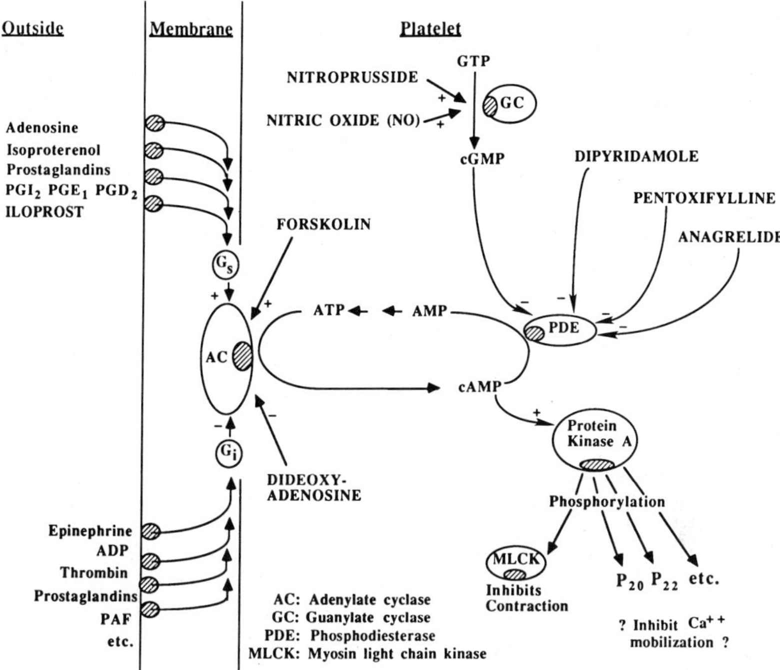

Fig. 2. Regulation of platelet function by agents acting through effects on cAMP or cGMP. *AC*, adenylcyclase; G_S, stimulatory *G* protein; G_i, inhibitory *G* protein; *PDE*, phosphodiesterase; *MLCK*, myosin light chain kinase

(HIDAKA and ASANO 1976). Increased levels of cAMP in platelets, however caused, are associated with inhibition of platelet functions, including aggregation, adhesion, clot promotion, and the secretion of biologically active agents. By contrast, lowering cAMP levels by the use of adenylate cyclase inhibitors has no effect, possibly because the resting level of cAMP in platelets is too low to influence their behavior. The regulation of platelet function by cAMP is thus unidirectional (HASLAM et al. 1978). Mechanisms proposed for the inhibitory effects produced by elevating the cAMP content generally invoke the activation of the cAMP-dependent protein kinase and the associated phosphorylation of several endogenous proteins (HASLAM et al. 1980). Phosphorylation of proteins at 38 and 26 kDa apparent molecular weight (MW_{app}) can be visualized in Fig. 3. These proteins may be involved in the regulation of intracellular calcium ion levels and are different from those that become phosphorylated when platelets are stimulated by aggregating agents.

Platelet adenylate cyclase is stimulated weakly by isoproterenol, by adenosine, and strongly by prostaglandins PGD_2, PGE_1, and PGI_2, all probably acting on specific membrane receptors. It is also inhibited by several agents that cause platelet activation, including epinephrine and ADP, thrombin, platelet activating factor (PAF), and the thromboxane mimetic U44619.

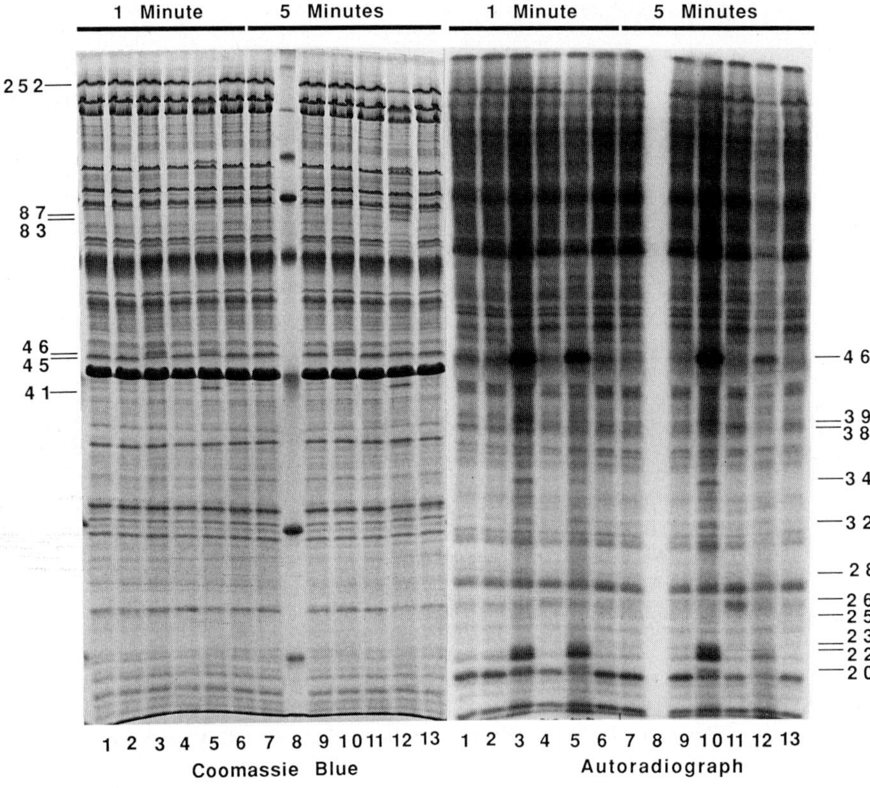

Fig. 3. Phosphorylation of platelet proteins. Washed platelets labeled with ^{32}P were incubated with reagents for 1 or 5 min. They were then dissolved in sodium dodecyl sulfate and mercaptoethanol and subjected to electrophoresis in a discontinuos 12.5% polyacrylamide slab gel (LAEMMLE 1970). The gel was stained, dried, and autoradiographed. Apparent molecular weights (MWapp, in kDa) shown at the sides were derived by interpolation from a polynomial fit to a plot of log MW vs. mobility for the standard proteins in lane 8. *Lanes 1–6*, 1-min incubations; *lanes 7, 9–13*, 5-min incubations. *Lanes 1 & 7*, untreated platelets; *lanes 2 & 9*, 2 m*M* 8-bromo-cGMP (permeant analogue of cGMP); *lanes 3 & 10*, 0.4 μ*M* phorbol myristate acetate (PMA, stimulator of protein kinase C); *lanes 4 & 11*, 2 μ*M* prostaglandin E_1 (adenylate cyclase stimulator) plus 2 m*M* RA_{233} (phosphodiesterase inhibitor similar in structure to dipyridamole); *lanes 5 & 12*, 2 μ*M* A23187 (divalent metal ionophore); *lanes 6 & 13*, 0.1 m*M* sodium nitroprusside (guanylate cyclase stimulator). Note:

1. Appearance of a new protein band at MW_{app} 46 kDa in platelets treated with PMA (*lanes 3 & 10*) or with ionophore (*lane 5*) corresponding to increased phosphorylation of pleckstrin (P47), the principal platelet substrate for protein kinase C (TYERS et al. 1989).
2. Loss of actin binding protein (MW_{app} 252) from platelets treated with ionophore (*lane 12*) and appearance of new bands at 87, 83, and 41 kDa, corresponding to the activation of calcium-dependent neutral protease (calpain) (FOX et al. 1985).
3. Increased phosphorylation of myosin light chains at MW_{app} 22 and 20 kDa with PMA or ionophore (*lanes 3, 5, & 10*).
4. Increased phosphorylation of bands at 39, 34, 32, 28, and 25 kDa with PMA (*lane 10*).

With some other aggregating agents, e.g., serotonin and vasopressin, inhibition of adenylate cyclase is very weak. This may be tentatively attributed to a variable degree of "crosstalk" between receptors and different G-proteins. Recent evidence suggests that the prostaglandins which stimulate adenylate cyclase may also have an inhibitory component to their action mediated by an inhibitory recptor (ASHBY 1986). Other compounds acting directly on the catalytic subunit of adenylate cyclase include the stimulator, forskolin, and the inhibitor, 2′5′-dideoxyadenosine. This latter compound blocks the effects of platelet inhibitors that act by raising cAMP levels and has been useful in determining their mechanism.

The short biological half-life of the naturally occurring prostaglandins and their serious side effects preclude their use as antiplatelet drugs. However, a number of relatively stable synthetic analogues of PGI_2, including iloprost and sulprostone, have been used experimentally to prevent platelet deposition during extracorporeal circulation and in the treatment of obliterative vascular disease.

Inhibition of platelet functions can also be achieved by inhibition of phosphodiesterase and the consequent reduction in the rate of cAMP destruction. Many inhibitors of phosphodiesterases are known, among them papaverine, the methyl xanthines–caffeine, theophylline, and isobutylmethylxanthine (IBMX)–and pyrimidopyrimidine derivatives including dipyridamole. Newer agents which may act at least in part by inhibiting phosphodiesterase are anagrelide (FLEMING et al. 1979) and pentoxifylline (SEIFLAGE and WEITHMANN 1989). Anagrelide, at doses lower than those that inhibit aggregation, causes a fall in the platelet count and has been used to treat patients with primary thrombocythemia (SILVERSTEIN et al. 1988).

II. Cyclic GMP

A second system for regulating platelet responsiveness involves cGMP. This cyclic nucleotide is formed by the action of a soluble enzyme stimulated by oxidizing agents such as sodium nitroprusside and nitric oxide (NO), the principle active component of EDRF, the endothelium-derived relaxing factor (IGNARRO et al. 1987), that causes both vasodilation and platelet inhibition. Nitroprusside and permeant analogues of cGMP weakly stimulate protein phosphorylation in platelets (WALDMANN et al. 1987), although the proteins affected appear to be the same as those phosphorylated with

---

5. Increased phosphorylation of bands at 38 and 26 kDa with elevation of cAMP levels by stimulation of adenylate cyclase in the presence of a phosphodiesterase inhibitor (*lane 11*).
6. General increase in phosphorylation with PMA (*lanes 3 & 10*) and decrease in phosphorylation with ionophore (*lane 12*)

cAMP: The inhibitory action of cGMP may be due to a secondary increase in cAMP, as the phosphodiesterase with low K_m that attacks cAMP is competitively inhibited by cGMP. Phosphorylation of this enzyme in platelets stimulated with forskolin or PGI_2 results in activation, suggesting a negative feedback mechanism for regulating cAMP levels (MACPHEE et al. 1988).

III. Receptor Antagonism

Receptors are components of the cell membrane that specifically and reversibly bind an agonist to form a complex that initiates a sequence of events leading to a cellular response, e.g., shape change, aggregation, or secretion in the case of platelets. The magnitude of the response is proportional to the concentration of the agonist-receptor complex, and the mechanisms by which the response is mediated include the opening of ion channels to permit the passage of cations from the exterior of the cell to the interior or stimulation of the formation of second messengers with effects on intracellular systems.

Receptor antagonists are drugs that selectively inhibit the response elicited by physiologic agonists. They act by competing with the agonist for its binding site on the receptor or by forming a complex with the receptor, inactivating it in a noncompetitive manner. The use of radiolabeled receptor antagonists has made possible the isolation and identification of hormone receptors, and today the complete amino acid sequences of both adrenergic and muscarinic receptors are known. In this section, the specificity of several of the known platelet agonists together with the action of their inhibitors is discussed.

1. Catecholamines

Epinephrine and norephinephrine potentiate platelet aggregation induced by other agonists at concentrations of 10–100 n*M*; at higher concentrations, they bring about aggregation. The naturally occurring L-isomer of norepinephrine is 30 times more effective than the D-isomer, but it is still 4–10 times less potent than epinephrine (BYGDEMAN and JOHNSEN 1969). Aggregation induced by epinephrine differs from that induced by other agonists as it is not preceded by a shape change. It is also slower and less extensive and does not reverse spontaneously (O'BRIEN 1964). High concentrations of epinephrine cause partial aggregation followed after a variable delay by secondary aggregation associated with the release of nucleotides and serotonin and the formation of TXA_2.

O'BRIEN (1964) showed that aggregation induced by epinephrine is inhibited by the α-blocker phentolamine at 10 n*M*, whereas the alkylating α-blocker phenoxybenzamine was active only at 50 μ*M*. Similarly, MILLS and

ROBERTS (1967) found that both potentiation and aggregation induced by the epinephrine were blocked by the α-blocker dihydroergotamine.

Human platelet α-adrenergic receptors were recently purified by REGAN and associates (1986). The receptor is a glycoprotein of 64 kDa containing an essential sulfhydryl residue which can be covalently labeled with tritiated phenoxybenzamine. The binding of several antagonists and agonists showed that this receptor obeyed the characteristic pharmacology of α_2-adrenergic receptors with the potency series for antagonists: yohimbine > phentolamine ≫ prazosin.

Concentrations of epinephrine required to induce platelet aggregation are unphysiological, but catecholamines may contribute to thromboembolic events in stressed individuals by their ability to potentiate platelet aggregation induced by other agonists.

2. Serotonin

RAPPORT et al. (1948) showed that the vasoconstrictor substance present in serum was serotonin, and RAND and REID (1951) demonstrated that it is derived from platelets, from which it is released during clotting. Platelet aggregation induced by serotonin was first observed by MITCHELL and SHARP (1964). In human, citrated, platelet-rich plasma, aggregation is preceded by shape change and is usually weak and reversible. Serotonin induces its maximal response in concentrations between 0.2 and 10 μM, and higher concentrations have less effect (BAUMGARTNER and BORN 1968). Platelet aggregation by serotonin is powerfully and specifically inhibited by methysergide (MITCHELL and SHARP 1964), bromo-LSD, and chlorpromazine (MICHAL and PENGLIS 1969), and by LSD and dibenzyline, but not by morphine or cocaine (MICHAL 1969). BORN et al. (1972) compared the effects of serotonin with structural analogues containing variations in the ring substituents and side chain modifications, including α methylation and alkylation of the amine. Of 17 compounds tested, 16 led to shape change, and 11 produced aggregation, in some cases as powerfully as serotonin. Several compounds were also partial agonists.

DE CLERCK et al. (1982) observed that serotonin-induced human platelet aggregation is inhibited by ketanserin, a selective S_2-receptor antagonist. Platelet responses to serotonin differ widely between species; cat platelets are especially sensitive (TSCHOPP 1970). LEYSEN et al. (1983) showed that radiolabeled ketanserin binds substantially more to cat platelet membranes than it does to preparations from human, cow, horse, pig, rat, and sheep. A total of 21 compounds were tested as inhibitors of ketanserin binding to cat platelets and to rat striatal and prefrontal cortex membranes, in which S_2-receptors had previously been demonstrated. The results indicate that the serotonin receptors on platelets are of the S_2-type.

The secretion of serotonin from platelets does not appear to play a role in human hemostasis as ketanserin has no effect on the bleeding time

(FAITAG et al. 1986), but it may play a role in hemostasis in cats and contribute to human migraine (PEROUTKA 1988) and thromboembolism (THOMAS et al. 1966).

3. ADP

ADP causes aggregation which is preceded by shape change and followed by a second wave of aggregation accompanied by the release of ADP and serotonin (MACMILLAN 1966; MILLS et al. 1968), provided the extracellular calcium concentration is reduced, e.g., by the use of citrate as anticoagulant (MUSTARD et al. 1975). These effects of ADP occur in the concentration range 0.2–5 μM. The only structural analogues of ADP with similar potency as agonists are those which are substituted in the 2-position of the purine ring, such as 2-chloro-ADP, 2-methylthio-ADP (GOUGH et al. 1972) and 2-azido-ADP (MACFARLANE et al. 1982). About 500 ADP receptors per platelet were found using 2-methylthio-[^{32}P] ADP as a radioligand (MACFARLANE et al. 1983). Substituents in other parts of the purine ring or changes in the ribose group cause marked reduction of activity, and the requirement for a pyrophosphate group in the 5′-position is absolute (GAARDER et al. 1961).

Although it was first thought that adenosine and 2-chloroadenosine inhibit ADP-induced aggregation by competing with ADP for its receptor, present evidence indicates that they act by stimulating adenylate cyclase to increase intracellular cAMP. By contrast, ATP is a specific antagonist of the ADP receptor with competitive kinetics ($K_i = 20\,\mu M$) and immediate onset of action (MACFARLANE and MILLS 1975).

As yet no ADP receptor antagonists have been developed that can be used as drugs. The fact that patients with platelet storage pool disease lack ADP in their dense granules and have a mild bleeding tendency (HARDISTY and HUTTON 1967) strongly implicates the release of ADP from platelets in hemostasis and, by analogy, in thrombosis. Thus, ADP receptor antagonists conceivably could be clinically useful tools.

4. Prostaglandin Endoperoxides and Thromboxane A_2

HAMBERG, SAMUELSSON, and their associates (1974) isolated the unstable, intermediate prostaglandin endoperoxides PGG_2 and PGH_2 by incubating arachidonic acid with sheep seminal vesicle microsomes and demonstrated that they induce platelet aggregation. Shortly afterwards (HAMBERG et al. 1975), they detected an even more unstable, intermediate compound, which they named TXA_2, formed when arachidonic acid or PGG_2 was incubated with human platelets. This compound not only aggregated human platelets but also caused contraction of rabbit aorta, and it was suggested that it is identical with "rabbit aorta contracting substance" (RCS) identified by PIPER and VANE (1969). TXA_2 was synthesized chemically in 1985 (BHAGWAT et al. 1985) and shown to have the biological properties expected of it.

It seems probable that PGG_2, PGH_2, and TXA_2 share the same receptor site on platelets. Stable mimetics of these compounds such as 9,11-epoxymethano-PGH_2 (U46619; BUNDY 1975), 9,11-azo-PGH_2 (COREY et al. 1975), and carbocyclic-TXA_2 (LEFER et al. 1980) all act similarly and induce shape change and aggregation which is generally accompanied by the release of constituents of platelet dense granules. On the other hand, stable receptor antagonists such as 9,11-iminoepoxy-PGH_2 (BHAGWAT et al. 1985), SQ-29,548 (OGLETREE et al. 1985), and pinane-TXA_2 (NICOLAOU et al. 1979) inhibit the shape change, aggregation, and secretion induced by prostaglandin endoperoxides, TXA_2, and their stable mimetics but not by other agonists such as ADP and serotonin.

The use of aspirin and other nonsteroidal antiinflammatory drugs that inhibit cyclooxygenase suggests that prostaglandin endoperoxides and TXA_2 contribute to the platelet aggregation that occurs during hemostasis or thromboembolic events. This is discussed in greater detail below.

5. Vasopressin

HASLAM and ROSSON (1972) discovered that vasopressin induces platelet aggregation in heparinized plasma. At a low concentration (1–10 nM) it causes a primary transient aggregation response, while at higher concentrations if brings about secondary irreversible aggregation. It is much less active in citrated, platelet-rich plasma or in other species. Vasopressin acts through V_1-receptors and can be inhibited by selective V_1-receptor antagonists (VANDERWEL et al. 1983). Aggregation is preceded by shape change and requires the presence of extracellular magnesium ions (PLETSCHER et al. 1985).

There is no evidence that vasopressin is involved in either hemostasis or thrombosis. However, infusion of desmopressin (1-deamino-8-D-arginine vasopressin, DDAP), a selective antidiuretic V_2-agonist, reduces bleeding problems in patients with hemophilia and von Willebrand's disease. It may act by increasing plasma levels of Factor VIII-related proteins, including von Willebrand factor.

6. Platelet Activating Factor

BENVENISTE et al. (1972) coined the name PAF for an agent formed during the reaction of leukocytes with antigen which triggered the release of histamine from rabbit platelets. Subsequently, PAF was shown to be a phospholipid, resembling plasmalogens and having the structure 1-*O*-alkyl-2-acetylglycerophosphocholine (HANAHAN et al. 1980). PAF induces shape change, aggregation, and secretion of dense granule constituents in platelets obtained from all species except the rat, in which it is inactive (NAMM et al. 1982). The potency of PAF as a platelet activator varies greatly between species, inducing effects at concentrations as low as 0.1 nM in guinea pig platelet-rich plasma but requiring concentrations of 0.1 μM or higher in human platelet-rich plasma.

Platelet activation by thrombin (discussed below) is not completely inhibited by ADP-scavenging agents nor by inhibitors of cyclooxygenase. Accordingly, a "third pathway" of platelet aggregation, independent of the release of granular ADP and formation of cyclooxygenase metabolites, was postulated (KINLOUGH-RATHBONE et al. 1977). While PAF was initially suggested to account for this "third pathway" (CHIGNARD et al. 1979), this concept has now been disproved by the use of specific PAF antagonists.

A large number of PAF antagonists are now available for experimental use (BRAQUET et al. 1987). They can be classified into three major groups, i.e., compounds structurally related to PAF, natural products such as terpenes, and triazolobenzodiazepines. All of them inhibit PAF-induced aggregation but not that induced by other agonists such as ADP or serotonin. PAF receptor antagonists fail to interfere with thrombin-induced aggregation of aspirin-treated and ADP-depleted platelets (BRAQUET et al. 1987). There is no convincing evidence that PAF participates in either hemostasic or thrombotic events in man.

7. Thrombin

The proteolytic enzyme thrombin, in concentrations of 0.1–1 U/ml, induces shape change, aggregation, and the secretion of granular constituents (THOMAS 1967). However, unlike other aggregating agents, there are no known receptor antagonists for thrombin-induced platelet activation. The effects of thrombin, both as a coagulant and aggregating agent, are inhibited by heparin in the presence of heparin cofactor (CLAYTON and CROSS 1963), and by hirudin, both of which act by combining with and inactivating thrombin.

Thrombin is one of the most important activators of platelets in hemostasis. Since platelets act as the physiological catalyst for thrombin formation, it is possible that sufficient thrombin may be generated at the surface of a platelet aggregate to trigger further aggregation without any fibrin formation. Indeed, lower concentrations of thrombin and shorter exposures are needed to induce platelet activation than to induce coagulation.

8. Collagen

The initial event of hemostasis is the adhesion of platelets to collagen. This is followed by the secretion of constituents from intracellular granules and the formation of TXA_2. While no specific antagonists of the adhesion of platelets to collagen are known, collagen-induced aggregation can be inhibited partly by TXA_2 antagonists or by ADP-removing systems such as creatine phosphate/creatine phosphokinase and almost totally by the combination of both (SMITH and DANGELMAIER, unpublished observations).

IV. Arachidonate Metabolism

1. Source of Arachidonate

The arachidonic acid used for prostaglandin endoperoxide and thromboxane formation is made available by release from platelet membranes by the action of phospholipases. Most studies of the mechanisms involved in the release of arachidonic acid have used thrombin as the stimulus, although some have employed collagen, trypsin, and the divalent cation ionophore A23187. Compared with thrombin, other agonists such as epinephrine, serotonin, ADP, vasopressin, and PAF are poor inducers of arachidonic acid release and eicosanoid formation. BILLS et al. (1977) showed that most of the arachidonic acid is released by the selective action of phospholipase A_2 on 1-acyl-2-arachidonoylphosphatidylcholine. On the other hand, BELL et al. (1979) presented evidence that arachidonic acid is released by the sequential action of phospholipase C and diacylglycerol lipase, phospholipase C acting on phosphatidylinositol to produce 1-steroyl-2-arachidonoylglycerol and diacylglycerol lipase producing free arachidonate. Recently, PURDON et al. (1987) analyzed mass changes in phospholipids of thrombin-sitmulated human platelets and confirmed that platelet phospholipase A_2 is selective for those molecular species of phospholipid containing arachidonic acid. It would therefore appear that the phospholipase A_2 pathway is the major route of arachidonic acid release in human platelets and that the phospholipase C pathway is less significant.

2. Inhibitors of Phospholipase A_2

Prevention of the release of arachidonic acid from platelet phospholipids would abolish thromboxane formation. There is evidence that anti-inflammatory steroids can inhibit phospholipase activity in some cell types by a mechanism that depends on RNA (DANON and ASSOULINE, 1978) and the synthesis of a protein called macrocortin or lipomodulin (BLACKWELL and FLOWER 1983). Steroids do not affect thromboxane formation by platelets, possibly because these cells have a very limited capacity for protein synthesis. Mepacrine and bromophenacylbromide are frequently employed as inhibitors of phospholipase A_2 (VARGAFTIG 1977). However, these highly nonspecific compounds also inhibit phospholipase C (HOFMAN and MAJERUS 1982). Indeed, the most notable observation about the inhibitors of phospholipase A_2 so far studied is their apparent lack of selectivity.

3. Inhibitors of Cyclooxygenase

Aspirin is a relatively potent, selective, and irreversible inhibitor of platelet cyclooxygenase (SMITH and WILLIS 1971); it blocks the formation of prostaglandin endoperoxides and TXA_2 and the associated aggregation. Its effects persist for as long as the platelet remains in circulation (KOCSIS et al. 1973). Aspirin acetylates a serine hydroxyl group near the carboxyl-terminus of cyclooxygenase, an integral membrane homodimer protein of 70 kDa (NUGTEREN et al. 1981). For some time there was concern that the effectiveness of aspirin as an antithrombotic drug might be compromised because it could also inhibit prostacyclin formation by endothelial cells. However, clinical trials have substantiated the effectiveness of aspirin in patients with unstable angina (LEWIS et al. 1983). The main adverse effect of aspirin is gastric intolerance. This may be due to local irritation of the gastric mucosa or to inhibition of the formation of protective prostaglandins. It can be minimized by suitable buffering. Aspirin is contraindicated in patients with hemophilia and is not recommended for pregnant women or for children with viral infections in whom it may give rise to Reye's syndrome. There is no convincing evidence that low doses (300 mg/day) of aspirin are either less or more effective than higher doses. They do, however, produce fewer undesirable side effects (HIRSH et al. 1989).

Several other drugs have been shown to inhibit both cyclooxygenase and platelet aggregation. These are designated nonsteroidal antiinflammatory drugs (NSAID) and include indomethacin, ibuprofen, and naproxen. These drugs have similar side effects to aspirin including gastrointestinal irritation and are more expensive. In contrast to the effect of aspirin, a single dose of indomethacin lasts less than 24 h (KOCSIS et al. 1973). These drugs have not been investigated as antithrombotic agents in clinical trials.

4. Thromboxane Synthase Inhibitors

Platelet thromboxane synthase has a molecular weight of 58.8 kDa and belongs to the group of cytochrome P-450 proteins (HAURRAND and ULLRICH 1985). The first selective inhibitor of thromboxane synthase was imidazole (NEEDLEMAN et al. 1977). Subsequently, 1-carboxyalkyl derivatives of imidazole were found to be more potent inhibitors, and drugs such as dazoxiben (originally called UK-37,248) were developed (TYLER et al. 1981). In the past few years several thromboxane synthase inhibitors have been used in pharmacological studies. These compounds all resemble imidazole in having an aromatic, heterocyclic nucleus linked to a carboxyalkyl or similar side chain.

NEEDLEMAN et al. (1977) studied the effects of imidazole on arachidonic-acid-induced aggregation in vitro. It had very little effect on platelet aggregation even though it inhibited TXA_2 formation as shown by the reduced contraction of rabbit aorta strips. They concluded that TXA_2 was only marginally more effective than prostaglandin endoperoxides in inducing platelet aggregation but was at least 100 times more potent than PGH_2 as a contractor of aortic smooth muscle. Thromboxane synthase inhibitors alone have little inhibitory activity on platelet aggregation, but they may potentiate the inhibitory activity of cAMP phosphodiesterase inhibitors by their ability to divert the metabolism of prostaglandin endoperoxides from TXA_2 to PGD_2, a stimulator of platelet adenylate cyclase (SMITH 1982).

5. Inhibitory Prostaglandins

Three prostaglandins, PGE_1, PGD_2, and PGI_2, are potent inhibitors of platelet aggregation acting through the elevation of cAMP. PGE_2 is less active and in low concentrations stimulates ADP-induced aggregation of rat and pig platelets and enhances the second wave of ADP-induced aggregation of human platelets (SMITH 1980). PGI_2 (prostacyclin), which is 10–20 times as potent an inhibitor as PGE_1 or PGD_2, was discovered by MONCADA et al. (1976), who observed that an unstable factor which inhibits platelet aggregation is formed when PGH_2 or PGG_2 is incubated with microsomes obtained from blood vessels. It is now known that endothelial cells and, to a lesser extent, some smooth muscle cells have the capacity to generate PGI_2 from arachidonate and do so when stimulated with an agonist such as bradykinin.

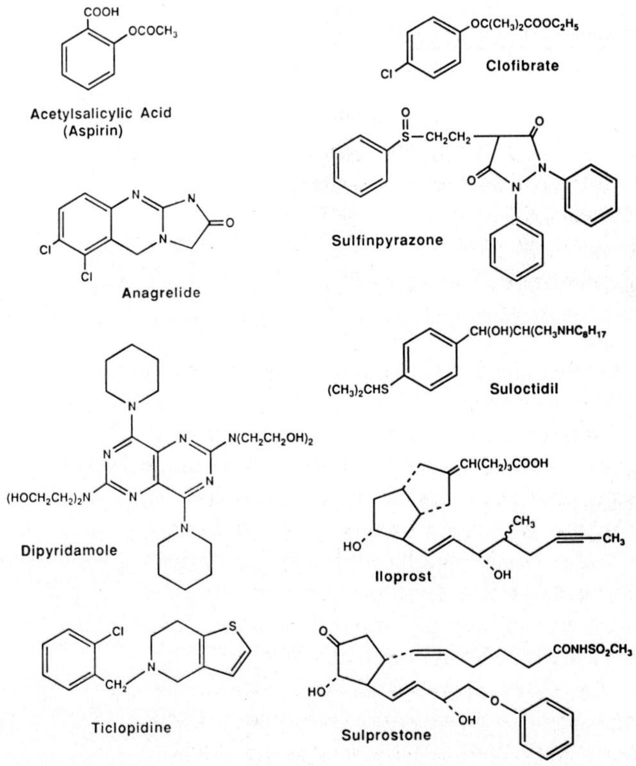

Fig. 4. Chemical structures of some drugs that inhibit platelet activation

V. Experimental Drugs with Unknown Actions

Numerous drugs have been shown to have some degree of antiplatelet activity in one or more of a variety of tests, either in vitro or after administration to experimental animals or human subjects (Fig. 4) (HARKER and GENT 1987). In many cases, these are drugs that had already won acceptance for other properties and were later proved to have activity towards platelets. Among these are:

1. Dipyridamole is the most widely used of the "antiplatelet" drugs besides aspirin. It is a weak inhibitor of platelet phosphodiesterase (HORCH et al. 1970) but more probably acts by inhibiting adenosine transport (BUNAG et al. 1964), thereby enhancing the vasodilator and antiplatelet effects of adenosine released from damaged tissues. It has been used with benefit in combination with aspirin in patients with peripheral vascular disease and with anticoagulants in patients with prosthetic heart valves. In most cases, there is little evidence that aspirin plus dipyridamole is superior to aspirin alone (HIRSH et al. 1989), and its effects on the vessel wall may be more significant than those on platelets.
2. Clofibrate was introduced as an agent for controlling hypercholesterolemia (OLIVER 1963) and has been reported to inhibit platelet function in vitro (CARVALHO et al. 1974).
3. Sulfinpyrazone is an uricosuric agent with very little antiinflammatory activity; it weakly inhibits platelet cyclooxygenase (ALI and McDONALD 1977) and causes some inhibition of platelet function in vitro and in vivo (PACKHAM and MUSTARD 1969). Sulfinpyrazone appears to improve the early survival of patients after a myocardial infarction (SHERRY et al. 1978), but it is not clear that this effect is due to an action on platelets.

There are also a few drugs that have been introduced for experimental use specifically as platelet antagonists. Among these are:

1. Suloctidil, which depletes platelet amine storage granules of serotonin (MILLS and MACFARLANE 1977), is reported to lengthen the platelet survival time in patients with artificial heart valves (COL-DEBEYS et al. 1981) and has been tested in several other in vivo models (ROBA et al. 1983) with variable results.
2. Ticlopidine has essentially no effect on platelets in vitro but causes a marked inhibition of platelet functions in several in vivo and ex vivo models (MAFFRAND et al. 1988). Its mechanism of action is unknown, but it probably acts neither as a cyclooxygenase inhibitor nor through elevation of cAMP (DEFREYN et al. 1989).

G. Conclusions

The participation of platelets in the normal process of hemostasis and in the pathological events that lead to thrombosis pose an exciting challenge to research. On the one hand, it would be helpful to be able to reduce platelet reactivity in situations associated with a high incidence of thrombotic events, as in transient cerebral ischemia and unstable angina pectoris. Although aspirin is effective under these conditions, agents causing a greater degree of inhibition would be, presumably, more effective still. On the other hand, the risks of hemorrhage from too effective a suppression of platelet functions cannot be ignored. One possible solution would stem from the ability to differentiate between the hemostatic and thrombosis-promoting properties of platelets. While this will have to wait for more basic understanding of platelet physiology, the goal of a safe and effective inhibitor, selective for platelets and with a more pronounced activity than the cyclooxygenase inhibitors, remains alluring. In the search for specificity and increased effect several approaches are possible, among them:

1. Aspirin-like drugs with platelet-specific actions, e.g., thromboxane synthase inhibitors and thromboxane receptor antagonists that do not interfere with prostacyclin formation.
2. Antagonists of the platelet-fibrinogen interaction, e.g., antibodies to the GpIIb/IIIa fibrinogen receptor (Coller et al. 1986), and analogues of the fibrinogen domains involved in platelet binding.
3. Antagonists of the interactions of platelets with von Willebrand factor, fibronectin, thrombospondin, and collagen, proteins that are all involved in some way with cell adhesion, aggregation, and hemostasis.
4. Cyclic AMP phosphodiesterase inhibitors or adenylate cyclase stimulators with selective effects for platelets, which would be less prone to cause unacceptable side effects.
5. Antagonists of the ADP receptor. This receptor is apparently unique to platelets and could provide a target for specific inhibitors.

References

Ali M, McDonald JWD (1977) Effect of sulfinpyrazone on platelet prostaglandin synthesis and platelet release of serotonin. J Lab Clin Med 89:868–875

Ashby B (1986) Kinetic evidence indicating separate stimulatory and inhibitory prostaglandin receptors on platelet membranes. J Cyclic Nucleotide Protein Phosphor Res 11:291–300

Baumgartner HR, Born GVR (1968) Effects of 5-hydroxytryptamine on platelet aggregation. Nature 218:137–141

Bell RL, Kennerly DA, Stanford N, Majerus PW (1979) Diglyceride lipase-pathwway for arachidonic acid release from human platelets. Proc Natl Acad Sci USA 76:3238–3241

Benveniste J, Henson PM, Cochrane CG (1972) Leukocyte-dependent histamine release from rabbit platelets: the role of IgE, basophils and a platelet-activating factor. J Exp Med 136:1356–1377

Bhagwat SS, Hamann PR, Still WC, Bunting S, Fitzpatrick FA (1985) Synthesis and structure of the platelet aggregating factor thromboxane A_2. Nature 315: 511–513

Bills TK, Smith JB, Silver MJ (1977) Selective release of arachidonic acid from the phospholipids of human platelets in response to thrombin. J Clin Invest 60:1–6

Blackwell GJ, Flower RJ (1983) Inhibition of phospholipase. Br Med Bull 39: 260–264

Born GVR (1962) Aggregation of blood platelets by adenosine diphosphate and its reversal. Nature 194:927–929

Born GVR, Juengjaroen K, Michal F (1972) Relative activities and uptake by human blood platelets of 5-hydroxytryptamine and several analogues. Br J Pharmacol 44:117–139

Braquet P, Shen TY, Touqui L, Vargaftig BB (1987) Perspectives in platelet-activating factor research. Pharmacol Rev 39:97–145

Bunag RD, Douglas CR, Imai S, Berne RM (1964) Influence of a pyrimido pyrimidine derivative on deamination of adenosine in blood. Circ Res 15:83–88

Bundy GL (1975) The synthesis of prostaglandin endoperoxide analogs. Tetrahedron Lett 24:1957–1960

Bygdeman S, Johnsen O (1969) Studies on the effects of the adrenergic blocking drugs on catecholamine-induced platelet aggregation and uptake of noradrenaline and 5-hydroxytryptamine. Acta Physiol Scand 75:129–138

Carvalho ACA, Colman RW, Lees RS (1974) Clofibrate reversal of platelet hypersensitivity in hyperbetalipoproteinemia. Circulation 50:570–574

Chignard M, Le Couedic JP, Tence M, Vargaftig BB, Beneveniste J (1979) The role of platelet-activating factor in platelet aggregation. Nature 275:799–800

Clayton S, Cross MJ (1963) The aggregation of blood platelets by catecholamines and by thrombin. J Physiol 169:82P

Col-Debeys C, Ferrant A, Moriau M (1981) Effects of suloctidil on platelet survival time following cardiac valve replacement. Thromb Haemost 64:550–553

Coller BS, Folts JD, Scudder LE, Smith SR (1986) Antithrombotic activity of a monovalent antibody to the platelet glycoprotein IIb/IIIa receptor in an experimental animal model. Blood 68:783–786

Corey EJ, Nicolaou KC, Machida Y, Malmsten CL (1975) Synthesis and biological properties of a 9,11-azo-prostanoid: highly active biochemical mimic of prostaglandin endoperoxides. Proc Natl Acad Sci USA 72:3355–3358

Daniel JM, Selak MA, Purdon AD, Salganicoff L (1987) Methods for the study of the role of calcium in platelet function. In: Colman RW, Smith JB (eds) Modern methods in pharmacology, vol 4. Alan R Liss, New York, pp 185–215

Danon A, Assouline G (1978) Inhibition of prostaglandin biosynthesis by corticosteroids requires RNA and protein biosynthesis. Nature 273:552–554

De Clerck F, David JL, Janssen PAJ (1982) Inhibition of 5-hydroxytryptamine-induced and -amplified human platelet aggregation by ketanserin (R 41,468), a selective 5-HT_2 antagonist. Agents Actions 12:388

Defreyn G, Bernay A, Delebassee D, Maffrand JP (1989) Pharmacology of ticlopidine, a review. Semin Thromb Hemost 15:159–166

Faitag B, Bondard I, Duloroy J, Gorin NC (1986) Effect of ketanserin on bleeding time: a comparison with aspirin. Thromb Res 44:261–264

Fleming JS, Buyniski JP (1979) A potent new inhibitor of platelet aggregation and experimental thrombosis anagrelide (BL-4162A). Thrombosis Res 15:373–388

Fox JE, Say AK, Haslam RJ (1979) Effects of collagen, ionophore A23187 and prostaglandin E_1 on the phosphorylation of specific proteins in blood platelets. Biochem J 184:651–661

Fox JEB, Goll EE, Reynolds EC, Phillips DR (1985) Identification of two proteins (actin-binding protein and P235) that are hydrolyzed by endogenous Ca^{2+}-dependent protease during platelet aggregation. J Biol Chem 260: 1062–1066

Gaarder A, Jonsen J, Laland S, Hellem A, Owren PA (1961) Adenosine diphosphate in red cells as a factor in the adhesiveness of human blood platelets. Nature 192:531–532

Gough G, Maguire MH, Penglis F (1972) Analogues of adenosine 5′-diphosphate–new platelet aggregators. Mol Pharmacol 8:170–177

Hamberg M, Svensson J, Wakabayashi T, Samuelsson B (1974) Isolation and structure of two prostaglandin endoperoxides that cause platelet aggregation. Proc Natl Acad Sci USA 71:345–349

Hamberg M, Svensson J, Samuelsson B (1975) Thromboxanes–a new group of biologically active compounds derived from prostaglandin endoperoxides. Proc Natl Acad Sci USA 72:2994–2998

Hanahan DJ, Demopoulos CA, Liehr J, Pinckard RN (1980) Identification of platelet activating factor isolated from rabbit. J Biol Chem 255:5514–5516

Hardisty R, Hutton R (1967) Bleeding tendency associated with a "new" abnormality of platelet behaviour. Lancet 1:983–985

Harker LA, Gent M (1987) The use of agents that modify platelet function in the management of thrombotic disorders. In: Colman RW, Hirsh J, Marder VJ, Salzman EW (eds) Hemostasis and thrombosis. Lippincott, Philadelphia, pp 1438–1456

Haslam RJ (1987) Signal transduction in platelet activation. In: Veratraete M, Vermylen J (eds) Thrombossis and haemostasis. Leuven University Press, Leuven, Netherlands, pp 147–174

Haslam RJ, Rosson GM (1972) Aggregation of human blood platelets by vasopressin. Am J Physiol 223:958–967

Haslam RJ, Davidson MM, Desjardins JV (1978) Inhibition of adenylate cyclase by adenosine analogues in preparations of broken and intact platelets. Evidence for the unidirectional control of platelet function by cyclic AMP. Biochem J 176: 83–95

Haslam RJ, Salama SE, Fox JEB, Lynham JA, Davidson MM (1980) Roles of cyclic nucleotides and of protein phosphorylation in the regulation of platelet function. In: Rotman A, Meyer FA, Gitler C, Silberberg A (eds) Platelets: cellular response mechanisms and their biological significance. Wiley, New York, pp 213–231

Haurand M, Ullrich V (1985) Isolation and characterization of thromboxane synthase from human platelets as a cytochrome-P450 enzyme. J Biol Chem 260: 15059–15067

Hellem AJ (1960) The adhesiveness of human blood platelets in vitro. Scand J Clin Lab Invest 12 [Suppl 51]:1–117

Hidaka H, Asano T (1976) Human blood platelet 3′:5′-cyclic nucleotide phosphodiesterase. Isolation of low K_m and high K_m forms. Biochim Biophys Acta 429:485–497

Hirsh J, Salzman EW, Harker L, Fuster V, Dalen JE, Cairns JA, Collins R (1989) Aspirin and other platelet active drugs. Chest 95:12–18S

Hofman SL, Majerus PW (1982) Modulation of phosphatidylinositol-specific phospholipase C activity by phospholipid interactions, diglycerides and calcium ions. J Biol Chem 257:14359–14364

Horch U, Kadatz R, Kopitar Z, Weisenberger H (1970) Pharmacology of dipyridamole and its derivatives. Thromb Diath Haemorrh 42 [Suppl]:253–266

Ignarro LJ, Buga GM, Wood KS, Byrns RE, Chaudhuri G (1987) Endothelium-derived relaxing factor produced and released from artery and vein is nitric oxide. Proc Natl Acad Sci USA 84:9265–9269

Jennings LK, Phillips DR (1982) Purification of glycoproteins IIb and IIIa from human plasma membranes and characterization of a calcium-dependent IIb-IIIa complex. J Biol Chem 257:10458–10466

Kinlough-Rathbone RL, Packham MA, Reimers HJ Cazenave JJ, Mustard JF (1977) Mechanisms of platelet shape change, aggregation and release induced by collagen, and release induced by collagen, thrombin or A23187. J Lab Clin Med 90:707–719

Kocsis JJ, Hernandovich J, Silver MJ, Smith JB, Ingerman C (1973) Duration of inhibition of platelet prostaglandin formation and aggregation by ingested aspirin or indomethacin. Prostaglandins 3:141–153

Laemmle UK (1970) Cleavage of structural proteins during the assembly of the head of bacteriophage T4. Nature 227:680–685

Lefer AM, Smith EF III, Araki H, Smith JB, Aharony D, Claremon DA, Magolda RL, Nicolaou KC (1980) Dissociation of vasoconstrictor and platelet aggregatory activities of thromboxane by carbocyclic thromboxane A_2, a stable analog of thromboxane A_2. Proc Natl Acad Sci USA 77:1706–1710

Lewis HD, Davis JW, Archibald DG, Steinke WE, Smitherman TC, Doherty JE, Schnaper HW, LeWinter MM, Linares E, Pouget JM, Sabharwal SC, Chesler E, DeMots H (1983) Protective effects of aspirin against acute myocardial infarction and death in men with unstable angina. N Engl J Med 309:396–403

Leysen JE, Gommeren W, De Clerck F (1983) Demonstration of S_2-receptor binding sites on cat blood platelets using [^{3}H]ketanserin. Eur J Pharmacol 88:125–130

Macfarlane DE, Mills DCB (1975) The effects of ATP on platelets: evidence against the central role of released ADP in primary aggregation. Blood 46:309–320

Macfarlane DE, Mills DCB, Srivastava PC (1982) Binding of 2-azidoadenosine [β^{32}P]diphosphate to the receptor on intact human blood platelets which inhibits adenylate cyclase. Biochemistry 21:544–549

Macfarlane DE, Srivastava PC, Mills DCB (1983) 2-Methylthioadenosine [β^{32}P]diphosphate. An agonist and radioligand for the receptor that inhibits the accumulation of cyclic AMP in intact blood platelets. J Clin Invest 71:420–428

Macmillan DC (1966) Secondary clumping effect in human citrated platelet-rich plasma produced by adenosine diphosphate and adrenaline. Nature 211:140–144

Macphee CH, Reifsnyder DH, Moore TA, Lerea KM, Beavo JA (1988) Phosphorylation results in activation of cAMP phosphodiesterase in human platelets. J Biol Chem 263:10353–10358

Maffrand JP, Bernat A, Delabassee D, Defreyn G, Cazenave JP, Gordon JL (1988) ADP plays a key role in thrombogenesis in rats. Thromb Haemost 59:225–230

Michal F (1969) D-receptor for serotonin on blood platelets. Nature 221:1253–1254

Michal F, Penglis F (1969) Inhibition of serotonin-induced platelet aggregation in relation to thrombus production. J Pharm Exp Ther 166:276–284

Mills DCB, Macfarlane DE (1977) Depletion of platelet amine storage granules by the antithrombotic agent, suloctidil. Thromb Haemost 38:1010–1017

Mills DCB, Roberts GCK (1967) Effects of adrenaline on human blood platelets. J Physiol 193:443–453

Mills DCB, Robb IA, Roberts GCK (1968) The release of nucleotides, 5-hydroxytryptamine and enzymes from human blood platelets during aggregation. J Physiol 193:715–729

Mitchell JRA, Sharp AA (1964) Platelet clumping in vitro. Br J Haematol 10:78–93

Moncada S, Gryglewski R, Bunting S, Vane JR (1976) An enzyme isolated from arteries transforms prostaglandin endoperoxides to an unstable substance that inhibits platelet aggregation. Nature 263:663–665

Mustard JF, Perry DW, Kinlough-Rathbone RL, Packham MA (1975) Factors responsible for ADP-induced release reaction of human platelets. Am J Physiol 228:1757–1765

Namm DH, Tadepalli AS, High JA (1982) Species specificity of the platelet responses to 1-O-alkyl-2-acetyl-sn-glycero-3-phosphocholine. Thromb Res 25:341–350

Needleman P, Bryan B, Wyche A, Bronson SD, Eakin E, Ferrendelli JA, Minkes M (1977) Thromboxane synthetase inhibitors as pharmacological tools: differential biochemical and biological effects on platelet suspensions. Prostaglandins 14: 897–907

Nicolaou KC, Magolda RL, Smith JB, Aharony D, Smith EF III, Lefer AM (1979) Synthesis and biological properties of pinane thromboxane A_2, a selective inhibitor of coronary artery constriction, platelet aggregation, and thromboxane formation. Proc Natl Acad Sci USA 70:2566–2570

Nieuwenhuis HK, Akkerman JWN, Houdjik WPN, Sixma JJ (1986) Human blood platelets showing no response to collagen fail to express surface glycoprotein la. Nature 318:470–472

Nugteren DH, Buytenhek M, Crist-Hazelhof E, Moonen P, van der Ouderaa FJ (1981) Enzymes involved in the conversion of endoperoxides. Prog Lipid Res 20:169–172

O'Brien JR (1962) Platelet aggregation. Part I. Some effects of the adenosine phosphates, thrombin, and cocaine upon platelet adhesiveness. Part II. Some results from a new method of study. J Clin Pathol 15:446–455

O'Brien JR (1964) A comparison of platelet aggregation induced by seven compounds and a comparison of their inhibitors. J Clin Pathol 17:275–281

Ogletree ML, Harris DN, Greenberg R, Haslanger MF, Nakane M (1985) Pharmacological actions of SQ-29,548, a novel selective thromboxane receptor antagonist. J Pharm Exp Ther 234:435–441

Oliver MF (1963) Further observations on the effects of atromid and of ethyl chlorophenoxyisobutyrate on serum lipid levels. J Atheroscler Res 8:427–444

Packham MA, Mustard JF (1969) The effect of pyrazole compounds on thrombin-induced platelet aggregation. Proc Soc Exp Biol Med 130:72–75

Parise LV, Phillips DR (1985) Reconstitution of the purified fibrinogen receptor. J Biol Chem 260:10698–10705

Peroutka SJ (1988) 5-Hydroxytryptamine receptor subtypes: molecular, biochemical and physiological characterization. Trends Neurosci 11:496–500

Phillips DR, Caro IF, Parise LV, Fitzgerald LA (1988) The platelet membrane glycoprotein IIb-IIa complex. Blood 71:831–843

Piper PJ, Vane JR (1969) Release of additional factors in anaphylaxis and its antagonism by antiinflammatory drugs. Nature 223:29–35

Pletscher A, Erne P, Burgisser E, Ferracin F (1985) Activation of human blood platelets by arginine-vasopressin. Role of bivalent cations. Mol Pharmacol 28:505–514

Purdon AD, Patelunas D, Smith JB (1987) Evidence for the release of arachidonic acid through the selective action of phospholipase A_2 in thrombin-stimulated human platelets. Biochim Biophys Acta 920:205–214

Rand M, Reid G (1951) Source of 'seretonin' in serum, Nature 168:385

Rapport MM, Green AA, Page IH (1948) Serum vasoconstrictor (serotonin) IV. Isolation and characterization. J Biol Chem 176:1243–1251

Regan JW, Nakata H, Demarinis RM, Caron MC, Lefkowitz RJ (1986) Purification and characterization of the human platelet α_2 adrenergic receptor. J Biol Chem 261:3894–3900

Rink TJ, Smith SW, Tsien RY (1982) Cytoplasmic free calcium in human platelets: Ca^{2+} thresholds and Ca-independent activation for shape change and secretion. FEBS Lett 148:21–26

Roba J, Defreyn G, Biagi G (1983) Anti thrombotic activity of suloctidil. Thromb Res 4:53–58

Robb-Smith AHT (1967) Why the platelets were discovered. Br J Haematol 13: 618–637

Santoro SA (1986) Identification of a 160000 dalton platelet membrane protein that mediates the initial divalent-cation dependent adhesion of platelets to collagen. Cell 46:913–920

Santoro SA, Rajpara SM, Staatz WD, Woods VL (1988) Isolation and characterization of a platelet surface collagen binding complex related to VLA-2. Biochem Biophys Res Commun 153:217–223

Seiflage D, Weithmann KU (1989) Updata on the pharmacology of pentoxifylline and its combination with low dose acetyl salicylic acid (HWA5112). Semin Thromb Hemost 15:1150–1158

Seiss W (1989) Molecular mechanisms of platelet activation. Physiol Rev 69:58–178

Selak MA, Chignard M, Smith JB (1988) Cathepsin G is a strong platelet agonist released by neutrophils. Biochem J 251:293–299

Shermer RW, Mason RG, Wagner RH, Brinkhous KM (1961) Studies on thrombin-induced platelet agglutination. J Exp Med 114:905–920

Sherry S, Gent M, Mustard JF, et al. (1978) Sulfinpyrazone after myocardial infarction. N Engl J Med 298:1257–1259

Siffert W, Siffert G, Scheid P, Akkerman JW (1990) Na^+/H^+ exchange modulates calcium mobilization in human platelets stimulated by ADP and the thromboxane mimetic U46619. J Biol Chem 264:719–725

Silverstein MN, Petitt RM, Solberg LA Jr, Fleming JS, Knight RC, Schacter LP (1988) Anagrelide: a new drug for treating thrombocytosis. N Engl J Med 318:1292–1294

Smith JB (1980) The prostanoids in hemostasis and thrombosis. Am J Pathol 99: 743–804

Smith JB (1982) Effect of thromboxane synthetase inhibitors on platelet function: enhancement by inhibition of phosphodiesterase. Thromb Res 28:477–486

Smith JB, Willis AL (1971) Aspirin selectively inhibits prostaglandin production in human platelets. Nature (New Biology) 231:235–237

Thomas DP (1967) Effect of catecholamines on platelet aggregation caused by thrombin. Nature 215:298–299

Thomas DP, Gurevich V, Ashford TP (1966) Platelet adherence to thromboemboli in relation to the pathogenesis and treatment of pulmonary emboli. N Engl J Med 274:953–956

Tschopp TB (1970) Aggregation of cat platelets in vitro. Thromb Diath Haemorrh 23:601–620

Tyers M, Haslam RJ, Rachubinski RA, Harley CB (1989) Molecular analysis of pleckstrin: the major protein kinase C substrate of platelets. J Cell Biochem 40:133–145

Tyler HM, Saxton CAPD, Parry MJ (1981) Administration to man of UK-37,248-01, as selective inhibitor of thromboxane synthetase. Lancet 1:629–632

Vanderwel M, Lum DS, Haslam RJ (1983) Vasopressin inhibits the adenylate cyclase of human platelet particulate fraction through V_1-receptors. FEBS Lett 164:340–344

Vargaftig BB (1977) Carrageenan and thrombin trigger prostaglandin synthetase-independent aggregation of rabbit platelets: inhibition of phospholipase A_2 inhibitors. J Pharm Pharmacol 29:222–228

Waldmann R, Nieberding M, Walter U (1987) Vasodilator-stimulated protein phosphorylation in platelets is mediated by cAMP- and cGMP-dependent protein kinases. Eur J Biochem 167:441–448

Weiss HJ, Turitto VT, Baumgartner HR (1978) Effect of shear rate on platelet interaction with subendothelium in citrated and native blood. I. Shear dependent decrease of adhesion in von Willebrand's disease and the Bernard Soulier syndrome. J Lab Clin Med 92:750–959

White JG, Rao GHR, Estensen RD (1974) Investigation of the release reaction in platelets exposed to phorbol myristate acetate. Am J Pathol 75:301–304

Yamanishi J, Takai Y, Kaibuchi K, Sano K, Castagna M, Nishizuka Y (1983) Synergistic functions of phorbol ester and calcium in serotonin release from human platelets. Biochem Biophys Res Commun 112:778–786

Zschauer A, van Breemen C, Buhler FR, Nelson MT (1988) Calcium channels in thrombin-activated human platelets. Nature 334:703–706

Zucker MB, Borrelli J (1962) Platelet clumping produced by connective tissue suspensions and by collagen. Proc Soc Exp Biol Med 109:779–787

CHAPTER 11

Anticoagulants, Antithrombotic and Thrombolytic Agents

M. DUGDALE

Thrombi are blood clots that form within the blood stream. Their presence is always pathologic. They can cause disease locally or can break loose (embolize) and lodge downstream, causing major damage distant from their site of origin. Because of the difference in patterns of blood flow in arteries and veins (rapid and high pressure in arteries, slow and low pressure in veins), the thrombi that form in these two sites are structurally different (FREIMAN 1987). Venous clots consist largely of red cells held together by a network of fibrin. They form in areas of stagnant blood, often starting in the pocket of a valve cusp, especially in the legs, where clotting can proceed undisturbed. Once begun, extension of the clot can be remarkably rapid. A thrombus beginning in the deep veins of the calf can extend within a day to the upper thigh, although many will remain localized. These restricted clots may produce local symptoms of pain, tenderness, heat, and swelling or may cause no symptoms at all. The first indication of a clot in the deep veins of legs or pelvis may be the occurrence of pulmonary embolus.

Arterial thrombi develop differently. The initial step is the attachment of platelets to an area of injured endothelium or denuded vessel wall such as occurs with atherosclerosis. Because of the atherosclerotic lesion, there is often narrowing of the vessel lumen, causing local perturbation of the normal laminar flow of blood. The turbulence and eddy currents in the area favor redistribution of platelets to the periphery of the column of blood (they normally flow towards the center, away from the wall) (TURITTO and BAUMGARTNER 1975; TURITTO 1982). The newly arrived platelets react with and stick to the adherent platelets, leading eventually to build-up of a large clump of platelets held together by a fibrin mesh. As flow is further disturbed by the presence of the mass of platelets, clotting can begin, leading to further enlargement of the thrombus. These thrombi can produce symptoms due to ischemia in the area served by the affected artery, or the mass of platelets and fibrin can embolize, causing arterial obstruction in vessels downstream.

Under normal circumstances, blood within blood vessels does not clot. The reasons for this are complex and involve the nature of the interactions between blood platelets and plasma and the endothelial lining of the vessels (WEKSLER 1987). These processes have been the focus of a great deal of investigation in the past decade. Particularly important to our understanding of the initiation of arterial thrombosis is the interaction between platelets and endothelium. This is discussed in detail in other chapters in this volume and, therefore, will not be repeated here. Normal patterns of flow are also important (LEONARD 1987). Disease of the arteries, especially atherosclerosis, causes narrowing and turbulence as described above. In the veins, unidirectional flow depends on the presence of competent valves, especially in the lower extremities. Dilation of veins and incompetence of valves from previous injury or scarring allow for pooling of blood in the veins, which encourages clot formation.

Clot formation is an essential function of the hemostatic mechanism (HIRSH et al. 1987). All necessary proteins are present in inactive form in the blood plasma and are known as factors. Activation occurs at sites of injury, and the resultant fibrin serves both to occlude torn blood vessels (hemostatic plugs) and to hold the tissues together during the process of healing. The fibrin in vessels and tissues is removed by the fibrinolytic system as the tissues heal. Under normal conditions, fibrin forms only in the immediate area of injury. The adjacent, healthy, undamaged endothelium continues to secrete prostacyclin and repels platelets. Thrombin that escapes from the area attaches to thrombomodulin on the endothelial surface, thus activating protein C, which will then inactivate Factors V and VIII. Thrombin and other activated factors escaping into the surroundings will be neutralized by antithrombin III. The pathological clots found in thrombosis are formed via the same mechanisms.

Some knowledge of the coagulation reactions is necessary for understanding the medications used to control thrombotic diseases. Coagulation is triggered by contact of the blood with injured tissue (Fig. 1). Factor XII reacts with this surface and becomes "activated" and in this form reacts with Factor XI, which, in turn, becomes activated. Activated Factor XI (XI_A) now reacts with Factor IX, activating it (IX_A), and in the presence of Factor VIII and phospholipid, activates Factor X (X_A). Simultaneously, phospholipid exposed in the area of injured tissue reacts with Factor VII to form a complex which can also activate Factor X. Both of these pathways are necessary for normal hemostasis and interact at several points. Factor X_A, in the presence of calcium, phospholipid, and Factor V, converts prothrombin to thrombin, which, in turn, converts fibrinogen into fibrin monomers. The monomers spontaneously polymerize and form a clot which subsequently is stabilized by Factor XIII as covalent bonds develop between fibrin polymers. There are at least two inhibitors in the blood plasma that influence activation of coagulation: antithrombin III (AT III) and protein C. AT III reacts with and neutralizes Factors XII_A, XI_A, IX_A, X_A, and thrombin. Protein C, once activated by contact with thrombin, is a potent inhibitor of Factors VIII and V. For expression of its full activity, a co-factor, protein S, is necessary. Deficiency of AT III, protein S, or protein C causes an increased tendency to thromboembolic disease, with thrombi forming mostly in the venous side of the circulation (BROEKMANS et al.

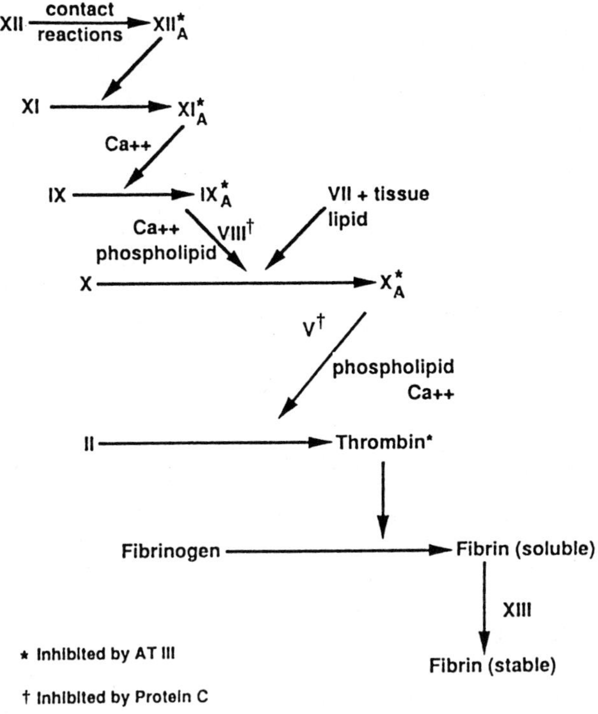

Fig. 1. Coagulation cascade

1983). Vitamin K is necessary for the production of Factors VII, IX, X, and II (prothrombin) and proteins C and S.

The coagulation system is counterbalanced by the fibrinolytic system (HIRSH et al. 1987), the normal function of which is to remove any fibrin that may form intravascularly and from wounds as they heal. The active enzyme is plasmin, which is not found normally in the circulating blood. It exists there in its inactive zymogen form, plasminogen. Plasminogen activators, secreted by injured or ischemic tissue, convert plasminogen to plasmin, which digests fibrin, leaving soluble fragments collectively known as fibrin degradation products. The fibrinolytic system, like the coagulation system, has its specific inhibitors that influence the activity of the plasminogen activators (plasminogen activator inhibitor) and the activity of plasmin (α_2-antiplasmin).

From the above, it can be seen that there are several levels at which the process of thrombosis can be attacked and, hopefully, interrupted. Ideally, the initiating cause should be prevented or eliminated. This would mean, on the arterial side, prevention or reversal of atherosclerosis, at present a still elusive goal, and on the venous side, prevention of venous distension and stasis, which, at least in the legs, is amenable to mechanical and perhaps pharmacologic maneuvers.

Platelet reactivity with vessel walls and with each other can be decreased by certain drugs, especially aspirin. This approach will be most effective in the management of arterial thrombi where selective consumption of platelets occurs which is not corrected by anticoagulation but is stopped by platelet inhibitory drugs (HARKER and SLICHTER 1972). Blood coagulation can be slowed down or prevented directly (e.g., heparin) or indirectly by suppressing production of some of the essential blood factors (e.g., warfarin). This approach has been successful in the management of venous thrombosis where consumption of fibrinogen and platelets occurs, both of which are blocked by anticoagulation (HARKER and SLICHTER 1972). Once the thrombi have formed, removal can be hastened by the application of fibrinolytic drugs. All these approaches can be viewed as antithrombotic measures. Those directed towards prevention or control of the atherosclerotic process are beyond the scope of this chapter. Those directed towards modulation of platelet-vessel wall interaction are presented elsewhere in this volume. This chapter will deal mainly with the anticoagulants and the fibrinolytic agents with a final brief section on other antithrombotics that do not fit into any of the above classes.

A. Anticoagulants

Anticoagulation has been the standard form of treatment of venous thrombosis and pulmonary embolism for more than 40 years. Heparin is usually used for treatment of the acute process and oral anticoagulation for prevention of recurrence and for long-term management. Both forms of therapy are effective.

I. Heparin

Heparin is not a new drug. The history of its discovery in the early years of the twentieth century and its subsequent isolation and identification are nicely summarized by JACQUES (1978, 1979). In 1922 HOWELL produced an extract of dog liver which had anticoagulant properties. He called it heparin because of its organ of origin. Later studies showed it to be a sulfated carbohydrate. Heparin occurs naturally in the tissues of many animals. For clinical use, it is purified from extracts of beef lung or porcine intestinal mucosa. These preparations consist of heparin molecules of widely varying molecular weights, 3000 to greater than 40000 daltons, with an average around 15000 (Fig. 2). Heparin is a highly sulfated glycosaminoglycan consisting of alternating residues of partially sulfated uronic acid and D-glucosamine. The uronic acid residues exist either as L-iduronic acid or D-glucuronic acid. There is variable acetylation of the glucosamine moieties. Polymers may be fairly short or very long, as indicated above. The length of the polymer, the sequence of its components, and the degree of sulfation influence its anticoagulant properties (ROSENBERG 1987).

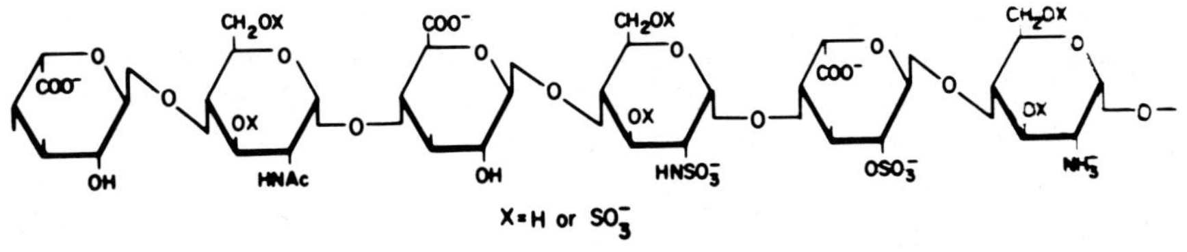

Fig. 2. Structure of a typical heparin molecule

Heparin has no direct anticoagulant activity. It blocks coagulation by greatly accelerating the normal inhibitory reactions of AT III with thrombin, activated Factor X, and other coagulation proteases. At higher concentrations, it stimulates the inhibition of thrombin by heparin cofactor II.

Studies in the past decade have begun to identify the areas of the heparin chain that react with AT III and enhance anticoagulant activity. One specific domain which is eight residues long has been recognized and defined which binds AT III, thereby accelerating the inhibition of X_A. However, this reaction does not alter the rate of inhibition of thrombin and the other proteases. Binding of heparins of longer chain length (16 residues or more) to other domains is necessary for acceleration of these reactions (Rosenberg 1987; Choay 1989). Without heparin, the reactions of AT III with thrombin and the other proteases are very slow. In the presence of heparin, these reactions are almost instantaneous. However, the properties that convey the antithrombotic effect are only partially understood. There are indications that heparin fractions with high anti-X_A activity but little or no antithrombin activity do not restrict thrombosis (Ockelford et al. 1982; Thomas et al. 1982; Buchanan et al. 1985). Therefore, antithrombin activity must be necessary for an effective antithrombotic heparin. Heparin also reacts with platelets. In vitro (Eika 1972; Salzman et al. 1980) and in vivo (Fernandez et al. 1986; Heiden et al. 1977) both aggregation and inhibition of aggregation have been demonstrated. Immediately after a bolus injection of heparin into a human subject, the bleeding time is prolonged, implying interference with platelet adhesion or aggregation. This antiplatelet effect is felt by some to be more important in producing the hemorrhagic complications of heparin therapy than is the anticoagulant effect (Carter et al. 1982; Fernandez et al. 1986).

Commercial heparin preparations contain a large but variable amount of proteoglycan that does not react with AT III or contribute to its antithrombotic properties (Lam et al. 1976). Accordingly, dosages are measured in units of activity rather than in milligrams. Heparin is employed as an anticoagulant in vitro, but its main use is as a therapeutic agent. It can be given as an intravenous infusion (the preferred route), as intermittent intravenous boluses, or subcutaneously. Its main applications are in the treatment of deep vein thrombosis (pelvis and legs) and pulmonary embolism. It is also used extensively for instillation into indwelling arterial and venous catheters and cannulae to maintain patency and is essential for preserving blood fluidity during cardiopulmonary bypass, hemodialysis, or other ex vivo procedures. When administered intravenously in a sufficient dose, anticoagulation occurs immediately. The response of individual patients is not entirely predictable, making it necessary to monitor the effect and adjust the dosage accordingly. An antithrombotic effect depends on the production of adequate anticoagulation (CHIU et al. 1977; HULL et al. 1986). Monitoring is usually done with the activated partial thromboplastin time (APTT), which is quite sensitive to the presence of heparin. Therapeutic levels of heparin are between 0.2 and 0.3 U/ml blood. These levels approximately double the APTT (TRIPLETT et al. 1978). The thrombin time, recalcification time, and whole blood clotting time can also be used as therapeutic monitors (TSAO et al. 1979). With the recent commercial availability of chromogenic substrates, assays for the anti-X_A or antithrombin activity of heparin have become simple enough to be practical for clinical use. They can measure actual heparin levels in the blood (TEIEN et al. 1976; LARSEN et al. 1978). There are animal studies showing that the actual heparin level may be more important that the change in APTT in determining the potential antithrombotic effect (CHIU et al. 1977). This has not yet been demonstrated in the clinical setting.

The variable effect of heparin from patient to patient is due to differences in the rates of heparin clearance, the difference in APTT response to identical levels of heparin, and the disease being treated (HIRSH et al. 1976; CIPOLLE et al. 1981). The half-life of heparin depends on the assay method used, but BJORNSSON et al. (1982) and DE SWART et al. (1982) found, regardless of method, that there is a short 10–15-min period immediately after bolus injection during which heparin rapidly disappears from the blood. This is followed by a much slower, linear decline. In the patient with venous thromboembolism the half-life after the usual initial intravenous therapeutic dose (~75 U/kg) is 80–100 min (HIRSH et al. 1976). In pulmonary embolism it is about half as long for the first 3–4 days of therapy (SIMON et al. 1978). The half-life is dose-dependent, being longer with larger doses because of a decreased rate of clearance (BJORNSSON 1982; MCAVOY 1979). After subcutaneous heparin administration, the peak blood level is reached in 4–6 h and then gradually decreases, with a measurable effect lasting for 10–12 h (PITNEY and DEAN 1976). The duration of effect is dose-dependent, too.

1. Clinical Applications

The value of anticoagulant drugs in the management of pulmonary embolism was demonstrated by BARRITT and JORDON in 1960. The purpose of treatment for pulmonary embolism is to prevent recurrence, which is about 25% if untreated. The patient who survives the initial event will recover if further embolization can be prevented. Heparin does not augment or accelerate the natural thrombolytic capability of the lung. It prevents the growth of clots in the legs or pelvis and hence decreases the likelihood of repeat embolization. The clinical response to initiation of heparin therapy can be seen within a few hours, possibly due to the blocking of humorally mediated pulmonary arteriolar and bronchial constriction as well as to its antithrombotic effect (GUREWICH et al. 1968). The purpose of treatment of deep vein or pelvic thrombosis is primarily to prevent pulmonary embolism. It is not yet clear whether it decreases the incidence of postphlebitic syndrome. There also continues to be some question as to whether patients with thrombosis limited to the deep veins of the calf should be treated with heparin. It has been suggested that if patients with calf-vein thrombosis can be followed by plethysmography or other noninvasive means, they need not be treated unless extension is demonstrated. Untreated, 20% of thrombin will progress up into the thigh; of these patients, up to 27% will develop evidence of pulmonary embolism, and 11%–22% will die of pulmonary embolism (ZILLIACUS 1946). The response to the institution of heparin therapy in the symptomatic patient is rapid and gratifying, with reduction in pain, heat, and swelling usually within the first 24 h.

The preferred course of therapy for pulmonary embolism or deep vein thrombosis is an initial intravenous bolus of approximately 5000 units followed by a continuous intravenous infusion of 1250–1700 U/h. It is imperative that the hourly dose be adjusted to maintain the APTT between 1.5 and 2 times its initial value (HULL et al. 1986). Anything less than this is inadequate and fails to protect from recurrent thrombosis (HULL et al. 1986; BASU et al. 1972). It has been customary to continue heparin for 5–7 days before adding warfarin (or other oral anticoagulant). The two agents are then continued until full anticoagulation with warfarin has been attained (usually 5 days). Heparin can then be discontinued, and anticoagulation maintained orally for at least 3 months (following a first episode of thrombosis) or indefinitely (after recurring deep vein thrombosis or pulmonary embolism). In the less acutely ill patient it may be appropriate to initiate oral anticoagulation simultaneously or the day following the start of heparin therapy. This will reduce the exposure to heparin as well as reduce overall cost by reducing days in the hospital (GORDON-SMITH et al. 1972; KAKKAR et al. 1972).

Intermittent bolus administration of heparin is as effective as the continuous intravenous route for treatment of both pulmonary embolism and deep vein thrombosis (SALZMAN et al. 1975; GLAZIER and CROWELL 1976; WILSON and LAMPMAN 1979). If reliable pumps for intravenous administration that predictably control the rate of infusion are not available, intermittent administration is safer. The appropriate dose (usually 7000–8000 U) is given every 6 h. The incidence of bleeding with intermittent administration was higher in studies in which the 24 h dose of heparin was greater than in those receiving it by infusion (GLAZIER and CROWELL 1976; WILSON and LAMPMAN 1979) but was comparable when the doses were similar (MANT et al. 1977).

With both forms of therapy, there is less than 5% recurrence of thrombosis during the initial 7–10 days of therapy. In the 3 months of continuing anticoagulation, the recurrence rate is about 3%. After anticoagulants are discontinued, 6%–10% will have a recurrence within the next 12 months (SALZMAN et al. 1980; BASU et al. 1972). Bleeding of a significant degree occurs in 5%–10% of patients receiving full-dose heparin either by continuous infusion or in intermittent bolus fashion (BASU et al. 1972; HULL et al. 1986; GLAZIER and CROWELL 1976; WILSON and LAMPMAN 1979; WALKER et al. 1987). The bleeding is often from previously traumatized sites. If accessible, pressure will frequently suffice to control it. If not, heparin should be discontinued until bleeding is controlled, then resumbed cautiously at a lower dose. In extreme cases, anticoagulation can be reversed with protamine sulfate.

Subcutaneous heparin is not dependable for the treatment of acute thrombosis (HULL et al. 1986) unless the dose is adjusted to good antithrombotic levels (HULL et al. 1982). It is best used for prophylaxis in patients at high risk for thrombosis and for the follow-up, long-term treatment of deep venous thrombosis or pulmonary embolism in patients who cannot take oral anticoagulants. One such group involves pregnant women, in whom the coumarin anticoagulants cannot be used because of their teratogenic effect. After initial therapy as described above, subcutaneous heparin is begun at one-third the intravenous dose the patient had required for stable anticoagulation at the correct level. This is usually around 10 000 U and is administered every 12 h. At 6 h after injection, the APTT is checked. This should be 1.5 times the original APTT. If not, the dose is adjusted until this is achieved (RASKOB et al. 1989). This level is then continued indefinitely with occasional monitoring in the pregnant patient whose dose requirements will change during pregnancy (WHITFIELD et al. 1983). In nonpregnant patients, monitoring is not necessary since requirements will remain very stable.

2. Prophylactic (Low-Dose) Heparin

Subcutaneous heparin in low doses ("mini-dose heparin") has been shown to prevent thrombosis in patients at high risk, especially those about to undergo elective hip or pelvic surgery and those recently placed on bed rest because of acute myocardial infarction, stroke, and severe congestive heart failure (HIRSH 1986). Various doses have been tried, commonly 5000 U two or three times daily. It appears to be most effective in patients undergoing elective surgery who receive the first dose 2 h prior to operation. It has proven less effective in patients who have already sustained tissue injury (myocardial infarction, hip fracture). The effectiveness of these low doses of heparin is thought due to the fact that activation of the factors higher in the sequence of clotting reactions can be stopped by much lower doses than is required to block coagulation reactions already under way. YIN (1975) has shown that 1 μg AT III will inhibit 32 U X_A, thus blocking generation of 160 U thrombin. It takes 1000 μg AT III to neutralize this amount of thrombin. This explains its particular effectiveness in the healthy, preoperative patients who is presumable free from clots as opposed to the injured patient in whom clot formation has already begun.

A number of prospective studies (using leg scan, venogram, or Doppler) have demonstrated the effectiveness of mini-dose heparin. These are reveiwed by SALZMAN and HIRSH (1987). In eight trials (GORDON-SMITH et al. 1972; KAKKAR et al. 1972; NICOLAIDES et al. 1972; BALLARD et al. 1973; LAHNBORG et al. 1974; Scottish study 1974; ABERNETHY and HARTSUCK 1974; COVEY et al. 1975) involving a total of 557 elective general surgery patients receiving 5000 U heparin subcutaneously every 12 h, 4% developed thrombosis compared with 27% of the controls (562 patients). In another group of six studies (ROSENBERG et al. 1975; GALLUS et al. 1975; REM et al. 1975; GRUBER et al. 1977; Groote Schurr Hospital Thromboembolus Study Group 1979; International Multicenter Trial 1975) involving 1319 treated (5000 U every 8 h) and 1463 untreated controls, thrombosis developed in 28% of the controls and only 7.6% of the treated patients. Nine studies (MORRIS et al. 1974; HAMPSON et al. 1974; DECHAVANNE et al. 1974; Venous Thrombosis Clinical Study Group 1975; HUME et al. 1973; GALLUS et al. 1973; MANUCCI et al. 1976; MOSKOVITZ 1978; WILSON and LAMPMAN 1979) evaluated mini-dose heparin in elective hip surgery, in which leg vein thrombosis is particularly frequent. Of a total of 289 control patients, 142 (49%) developed thrombosis; of 285 patients receiving heparin, only 21% developed thrombosis.

Mini-dose heparin cannot be used safely in patients at particularly high risk for bleeding (e.g., neurosurgical patients, patients with a preexisting defect in hemostasis). In other patients, the risk of significant bleeding is low (around 2%) (International Multicenter Trial 1975).

3. Complications

The main complication of heparin therapy is bleeding, as discussed above. In the past decade, heparin-induced thrombocytopenia and the arterial thrombosis that in rare instances follows or accompanies it has aroused a lot of interest, although the size of the clinical problem resulting from it remains uncertain. Arterial thrombosis during heparin therapy was first reported in 1958 (WEISMAN and TOBIN 1958), although thrombocytopenia was not mentioned in this report. The problem of thrombocytopenia with or without thrombosis was rarely mentioned again until the late 1970s and through the 1980s, at which time numerous articles appeared describing the laboratory findings, clinical picture, incidence, and suggestions regarding management. The typical clinical picture (KING and KELTON 1984; RICE et al. 1986; CINES et al. 1980) is of thrombocytopenia developing 6–12 days after initial exposure to heparin. The thrombocytopenia may be of reasonable severity with the count falling to 20 000–30 000/mm^3 or less but usually is much milder (80 000–150 000/mm^3). Most patients are clinically asymptomatic, and the platelet count may actually return to normal even though heparin administration is continued (GREEN et al. 1984). Thrombocytopenia can develop regardless of the amount (BELL et al. 1976) or type of heparin the patient is receiving (GREEN et al. 1984). It is more common with heparin of beef lung origin but also occurs with porcine heparin and with low molecular weight heparin. It has been seen in patients whose only exposure to heparin was the small amount used to keep venous cannulae open (BELL et al. 1976). Its occurrence may be higher with certain manufacturers' lots (RICE et al. 1986; STEAD et al. 1984). The incidence has been reported to be between 0% and 24% for patients receiving porcine heparin and between 4% and 30% for those receiving bovine heparin (KING and KELTON 1984; GREEN et al. 1984; POWERS et al. 1979; EIKA et al. 1980). Many of the patients receiving heparin are acutely ill, hence it is not always apparent whether the thrombocytopenia is due to the heparin or is caused by the patient's medical or surgical status or other drugs being concurrently taken. Since the thrombocytopenia itself is often clinically unimportant, the real question relates to the very serious problem of major arterial or venous thrombosis. In almost all reported instances of thrombosis, thrombocytopenia also occurred simultaneously. In one case report, there was a fall in the platelet count, but it remained in the normal range (PHELAN 1983). Some have suggested that the thrombocytopenia precedes the onset of thrombosis (CIMO et al. 1979), but the careful study of KING and KELTON (1984) does not support this (Fig. 3). They demonstrated that they occur simultaneously. Until this question is definitely settled, however, thrombocytopenia must be

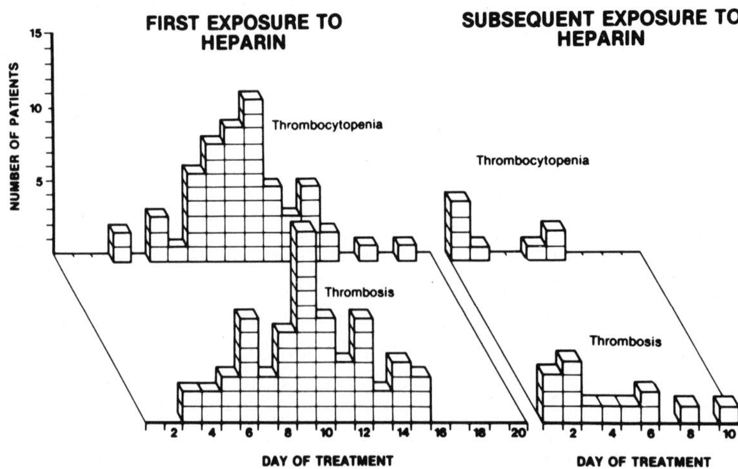

Fig. 3. Heparin induced thrombocytopenia and thrombosis. (Reproduced by permission from KING and KELTON, 1984)

viewed as a possible precursor of major thrombosis. The thrombosis is usually arterial, involves major vessels, and often leads to amputation or death. The incidence of this devastating complication is not known but is clearly much, much less than that of thrombocytopenia. Of the 1456 patients covered by KING and KELTON's (1984) review of prospective and randomized studies, none developed thrombosis, and in reviewing the world's literature they were able to find only 85 reported cases.

The etiology of thrombocytopenia is not fully resolved. In vitro, normal platelets in heparinized blood will aggregate spontaneously (ZUCKER 1977; SALZMAN et al. 1980). These aggregates can be broken up by simple mixing of the blood sample. This type of aggregation is enhanced in the blood of patients who have recently received heparin (SHOJANIA and TURNBULL 1987). Rapid infusion of heparin into experimental animals can produce prompt but transient thrombocytopenia (FIDLER and JACQUES 1948), possibly by this mechanism. These observers also noted the same effect in human subjects; others have not (DAVEY and LANDER 1968). This form of thrombocytopenia is thought not to be immune mediated. The later-developing thrombocytopenia may be antibody mediated as first suggested by WAHL et al. (1978) and subsequently by many other observers. The aggregating activity has been demonstrated in plasma, in the IgG (CHONG et al. 1981) and the IgM fractions (WAHL et al. 1978). There is evidence that heparin attached to the platelet serves as an antigen inducing an antibody that can attack platelets (GREEN et al. 1978), that an IgG-heparin complex forms which activates platelets (KELTON et al. 1988), and that antibodies in the plasma of patients with the heparin-thrombocytopenia syndrome react with heparin which is bound to the endothelium, thus inducing platelets to adhere to the injured endothelium, causing thrombocytopenia and initiating arterial thrombus formation (CINES et al. 1987). Clearly, we do not yet have a full understanding of this clinical syndrome, nor do we have a way of predicting who will develop thrombotic disease. The presence of the heparin-dependent aggregating factor or antibody can be demonstrated in vitro either by its ability to aggregate platelets or by its induction of serotonin release (CINES et al. 1987; SHERIDAN et al. 1986; FRATANTONI et al. 1975).

There is no universal agreement as to the management of heparin-induced thrombocytopenia. Some feel that heparin should always be stopped immediately; others feel that as long as the platelet count remains above $50\,000/mm^3$ and there are pressing reasons for heparin treatment, it should be continued with careful monitoring of the platelet count. If heparin is stopped, the platelet count will return to normal in 3–5 days.

Treatment of heparin-induced thrombosis has been approached in several ways, indicating that the definitive mode of therapy is yet to be found (KING and KELTON 1984). All investigators agree that heparin should be stopped immediately. Dextran (BYGDEMAN 1969), low molecular weight heparin (LEROY et al. 1985), thrombectomy, anticoagulation with warfarin, fibrinolytic therapy, and plasmapheresis (NAND and ROBINSON 1988) have all been used with apparent success in some cases.

Rarely, osteoporosis develops in patients receiving heparin treatment for 3 months or more, in doses exceeding 15000 U per day (GRIFFITH et al. 1965; JAFFE and WILLIS 1965; RUPP et al. 1982; HEIDEN et al. 1977). Fractures of ribs and vertebral bodies have been seen. The incidence is not known but is tiny. Also rare is alopecia and the "blue toe syndrome" in which the toes are discolored and the patient complains of a burning sensation in them. The latter is not a precursor of thrombosis or ischemic gangrene.

II. New Therapies

In the past decade, several new approaches to parenteral anticoagulation have been developed and received a varying extent of clinical evaluation. All these products are designed to increase the safety of anticoagulation while preserving or improving on the antithrombotic value of heparin.

1. Heparin plus Dihydroergotamine

The combination of heparin and dihydroergotamine for clinical use was first described in 1976 (SAGAR et al. 1976). The purpose of the heparin is to provide anticoagulation and of the dihydroergotamine to improve venous tone and, thereby, decrease stasis and increase the rate of blood flow. At the dose used, arterial tone is supposedly not altered. This combination recently became available in the USA as Embolex (Sandoz Pharmaceuticals, East Hanover, NJ). It has been used in several European studies with either general surgical (KOPPENHAGEN et al. 1979) or orthopedic (hip) (KAKKAR et al. 1979) patients and in a recent multicenter trial in the USA (total hip replacement) (BEISAW et al. 1988). Their results suggest that the incidence of deep vein thrombosis is reduced by about 50% in patients receiving both drugs simultaneously. No serious adverse results were reported in these studies. However, there have been several case reports of ergotism with gangrene, amputation, or death in patients receiving this combination (ASHENBURG 1990; CUNNINGHAM et al. 1984). Its role in medical and surgical practice is still to be defined.

2. Low Molecular Weight Heparins

Another approach has been with low molecular weight heparins (LMWH) and nonheparin glycosaminoglycans. LMWH are isolated from normal heparin preparations or, more frequently, are produced by depolymerization of the standard large molecular weight heparin. The method of depolymerization determines the structure and hence the properties of the end-products (CASU 1984; HOLMER 1980). Thus, all LMWH are different chemically and have different anticoagulant and antithrombotic properties. The impetus leading to their development was the observations alluded to

Table 1. The low molecular weight heparins. HARENBERG et al. (1989); SASAHARA et al. (1986)

	MW	APTT (U/mg)	Anti-X_A (U/mg)	USP (U/mg)
Fragmin (Kabi 2165) (Sweden)	4000–6000	40	160	
Enoxaparine (PK 10169) (France)	4000–6000		80	40–60
Fraxiparin (CY 216) (France)	4500	50	200 (Choay units)	

MW, molecular weight; APTT, activated partial thromboplastin time; Anti X_A, inhibition of activated factor X expressed in units/mg (μ/mg); USP, United States Pharmacopoeia.

above that it takes little AT III activity to block X_A and that short heparin molecules (~8 residues) can have high anti-X_A activity with little or no antithrombin activity. By separating these activities, it was hoped to create heparins with higher antithrombotic activity but less tendency to produce bleeding. A large number of LMWH have been produced and studied in vitro and in animals. This review will cover only the four products that have been tried clinically: fragmin, fraxiparin, enoxaparine, and LMWH plus dihydroergotamine (Table 1). All are produced from heparin made from porcine intestinal mucosa, all are given subcutaneously, and all have much longer half-lives than heparin. They are not neutralized as effectively as heparin with protamine sulfate. An important problem is in monitoring their activity in comparison with standard heparin. Most of the LMWH have considerably less effect on the APTT than heparin yet may have a comparable antithrombotic effect (Table 2). Activity is usually described in anti-X_A units or APTT units, but the relevance of these to clinical performance remains unclear. Table 2 summarizes the published clinical data. Most of the studies used [^{125}I]fibrinogen scanning to determine incidence of thrombosis. Effective doses for these agents have been established. In general, they are as protective, perhaps more so in some instances, than standard heparin. Bleeding problems develop with about the same frequency. The major and considerable advantage seems to be the requirement for only one daily subcutaneous dose. None is yet available for clinical use in the USA.

One LMWH, CY222, appears to have an additional and major property of enhancing fibrinolysis. Unfractionated heparin does this to a minor degree, while CY222 is considerably more active. It has been used simultaneously with tissue-plasminogen activator and single-chain urokinase plasminogen activator (JUHAN-VAGUE et al. 1989)

Table 2. Clinical data regarding low molecular weight heparins (LMWH)

	No. of patients (subject/control)	Dose	Freq. DVT % Subject/Control	Bleeding
Fraxiparin (CY 216)				
EUROPEAN FRAXIPARIN STUDY GROUP (1988) General surgery	1896 (960/936)	7500 U preop then daily ×7	2.8/4.5 U	Same
KAKKAR and MURRAY (1985) (double-blind)	395 (196/199)	7500 anti-X_AU preop then daily × 7	2.5/7.5 U	Same
KAKKAR and MURRAY (1985) (open) General surgery	910	7500 anti-X_AU preop then daily × 7	3.4	Most in gynecology patients (12%)
(All controls received 5000 U standard heparin every 8 h; [^{125}I] fibrinogen monitor)				
Fragmin (Kabi 2165)				
CAEN (1988) General surgery (double-blind)	385 (195/190)	2500 U/d preop, then daily ×7 Controls: 5000 U heparin every 12 h	3.1/3.7	Same
ERIKSSON et al. (1988) Orthopedic (hip) surgery	98	2500 U preop then daily ×7 Controls: Dext 70	20/45	Less bleeding with fragmin
BERGQVIST et al. (1986) General surgery (double-blind)	432	5000 U preop then daily ×5–7 days Controls: preop heparin 5000 U then b.i.d. ×5–7 days	6.4/4.3	Bleeding in 11.6% with fragmin and 4.6% with standard heparin

(All used [^{125}I] fibrinogen monitor)				
Enoxaparin (Lovenox R) SAMAMA et al. (1988) General surgery	885 (448/437)	20–60 mg/d preop and daily ×7 Control: heparin 5000 U preop and t.i.d.	20 mg 2.9/3.8 40 mg 2.8/2.7 60 mg 3.8/7.6	Same
TURPIE et al. (1986) Orthopedic (hip) surgery	100 (50/50)	30 mg b.i.d begun postop then ×14 days Control: placebo	12/42	Bleeding in 4% of both groups
PLANES et al. (1987) Orthopedic (hip) surgery	114 (57/57)	Starting preop 40 mg/d vs. 20 mg b.i.d.	6	Same
LEBALC'H et al. (1987) Orthopedic (hip) surgery	237 (124/113)	Preop then every day × 10–15 Control: 5000 U heparin every 8 h	12.5/25	Less bleeding with enoxaparin
LMWH + DHE SASAHARA et al. (1986) General surgery	269 (137/132)	1500 APTTU once daily Control: heparin + DHE b.i.d, DHE + twice daily	10.4/10.3	No thigh or pelvic thrombi with treatment. Both seen in controls

DHE, dihydroergotamine; APTT, activated partial thromboplastin time; Freq. DVT %, percentage of subjects developing deep vein thrombosis; general surgery, type of patient studied; Anti X_AU, units used to express the anticoagulant effect of the heparin; Dext 70, dextran 70.

Several nonheparin sulfated glycosaminoglycans are currently being studied as potential antithrombotic agents. These are constituents of vascular endothelium and are thought to add to the resistance to thrombosis of normal endothelium. Two are receiving particular attention: dermatan sulfate and heparan sulfate (HOPPENSTEADT et al. 1989). In dermatan sulfate, the repeating disaccharide unit consists of D-galactosamine and L-iduronic or D-glucuronic acid. Heparan sulfate is more like heparin with the disaccharide unit consisting of D-glucosamine and D-glucuronic or L-iduronic acid. Dermatan sulfate does not react with AT III and does not inhibit X_A. It does react with heparin cofactor II and accelerates its inhibiting action on thrombin (FERNANDEZ et al. 1986). The action of heparan sulfate is via its reaction with AT III and inhibits both X_A and thrombin (MARCUM and ROSENBERG 1987). Both are much weaker, milligram per milligram, than heparin. Both show antithrombotic properties in experimental animals, possibly with less of a tendency to cause bleeding. Neither is ready yet for clinical trials.

Also undergoing extensive sudy at present is hirudin (MARKWARDT et al. 1989). Originally extracted from the parapharyngeal glands of the medicinal leech, *Hirudo medicinalis*, it is now being produced in large amounts using recombinant methods. The recombinant molecule is identical to the natural product. Hirudin has a high affinity for thrombin and inactivates it by forming a complex with it. The complex blocks all the normal reactions of thrombin at very low concentrations (MARKWARDT 1989). It has been given to human subjects intravenously and subcutaneously for research purposes only (MARKWARDT 1984). Hirudin is not yet ready for clinical trial, although preliminary studies in animals and man are encouraging.

III. Oral Anticoagulants

The oral anticoagulants, because of convenience and long-established effectiveness, are the preferred form of treatment for the patient who requires long-term anticoagulation. There are two groups of compounds that have been used for this purpose: the coumarins and the indanediones (Fig. 4) (O'REILLY 1987). Both are chemically related to vitamin K, and both produce their anticoagulant effect indirectly by blocking the formation, in the liver, of the fully functional Factors VII, IX, X, and prothrombin and the natural inhibitors, proteins C and S. All of these molecules must have, in a posttranslational step, γ-carboxylation of glutamic acid residues. This reaction is mediated by vitamin K_1, which is converted to its epoxide form by the reaction. In a reductase-mediated reaction, the vitamin K_1 epoxide is returned to its functional reduced state (RASKOB et al. 1989). It is this reaction which is probably blocked by the coumarin drugs (Fig. 5). Without γ-carboxylation, Factors II (prothrombin), VII, IX, and X cannot react with the calcium ions that serve to bind them to the phospholipid surfaces (membranes) at which the actual clotting reactions occur. Hence, coagula-

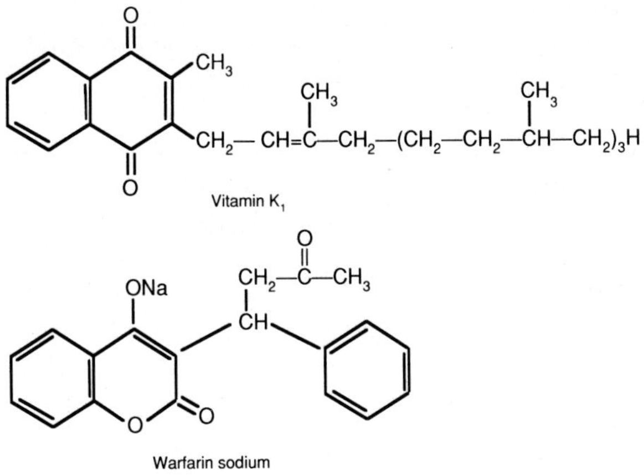

Vitamin K_1

Warfarin sodium

Fig. 4. Structure of vitamin K and warfarin

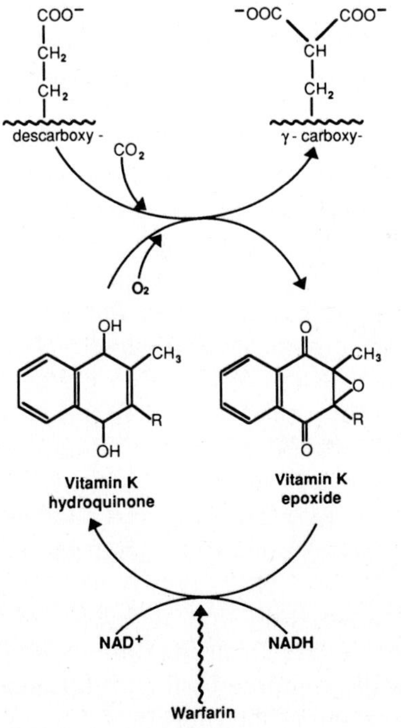

descarboxy-

γ-carboxy-

CO_2

O_2

Vitamin K hydroquinone

Vitamin K epoxide

NAD^+

NADH

Warfarin

Fig. 5. Action of vitamin K in γ-carboxylation of factors II, VII, IX, and X and proteins C and S. Glutamic acid residues on the inactive precursors are converted to γ-carboxyglutamic acid. During this reaction the hydroquinone form of vitamin K is converted to its inactive epoxide form. Under normal circumstances, the epoxide is reduced back to its active hydroquinone form. This reaction is blocked by the coumarin anticoagulants

tion is greatly slowed down. After initiation of warfarin therapy, production of the γ-carboxylated factors stops or is drastically reduced, depending on the dose administered. The rate of disappearance of the factors from the blood is determined entirely by their half-lives since the preformed factors are not affected by the anticoagulant. Factor VII, with a half-life of about 4 h, falls first. By 5–6 days, the activity of all the vitamin-K-dependent factors will be reduced to levels determined by the dose of warfarin given, usually less than 20% with the doses used clinically. However, descarboxylated factors are still present, since the actual synthesis of the proteins is not affected by the anticoagulant (RASKOB et al. 1979). Patients with liver disease and patients with low vitamin K stores will be unusually sensitive to the effect of warfarin. Administration of vitamin K rapidly reverses the anticoagulant effect. Within about 4 h, the production of γ-carboxylated factors resumes, and within 24 h levels of the factors will be back to normal. In the patient with liver disease, recovery may take 2–3 days.

Dicumarol was the first of the oral anticoagulants. It was identified (LINK 1939) as the compound in spoiled sweet-clover silage that caused a hemorrhagic disease in the cattle that ate it. A large number of related coumarins were subsequently identified, and some were tried clinically. Gradually, however, the properties of warfarin (duration of action and ease of anticoagulant control) made it by far the most popular oral anticoagulant used in the USA (more than 95%) (O'REILLY 1987). The indanediones produce effective anticoagulation in a manner similar to the coumarins although they are now rarely used because of their toxic side effects (hypersensitivity reactions in 1%–3% with rash, fever, diarrhea, hepatitis, renal failure, leukopenia) and are no longer available in the USA for clinical use.

Warfarin is administered orally. It is rapidly and almost completely absorbed, with the peak plasma level occurring about 3 h after ingestion. The half-life is about 2.5 days. A loading dose does not cause more rapid achievement of anticoagulation and can lead to serious overdosage (O'REILLY and AGGELER 1968). Warfarin is almost completely bound to albumin (99%), but it is only the free drug that is active in producing the anticoagulant effect (RASKOB 1989). Simultaneous administration of other drugs that displace warfarin from albumin can, therefore, have a marked effect on the degree of anticoagulation. There is sufficient variation from patient to patient in sensitivity to warfarin that the dose must be tailored to the patient's requirements. The usual starting dose in the adult is 7.5–10 mg per day. The effect is usually monitored by the prothrombin time (PT), a global test which is sensitive to diminished levels of Factors VII and X, to some extent to reduction in II but not to the level of Factor IX (POLLER 1986). The antithrombotic effect clearly requires reduction of more than Factor VII alone. The level of Factor VII falls within 36–48 h of institution of warfarin therapy to levels low enough to prolong the PT. However, the patient is not protected against thrombosis until the other factors are also reduced.

Antithrombotic activity is not attained until the patient has taken warfarin for at least 5 days (WESSLER et al. 1978; GITEL and WESSLER 1983). The relationship between anticoagulant level as measured by the PT and the antithrombotic effect to be expected in the patient still remains somewhat controversial (HIRSH and LEVINE 1988; FURIE et al. 1990; SCHULMAN and LOCKNER 1985). This has been in large part due to lack of standardization of the tissue thromboplastins used in the PT, the different between thromboplastins used in Europe and those used in the USA making comparison of trials difficult, and the differences in reactivity of the American thromboplastins used now and those used 20 years ago (HIRSH and LEVINE 1988). Thromboplastin reagents for the PT are made from various animal tissues. In the USA the most commonly used at the present time are derived from rabbit brain and are only weakly sensitive to the changes produced in the blood by warfarin. Thromboplastins used 20–30 years ago were more sensitive to these changes (HIRSH and LEVINE 1988). In the UK, standard reference thromboplastins were developed a decade ago to help standardize anticoagulant therapy. They were made from human brain and are considerably more sensitive to decreasing levels of the vitamin-K-dependent factors (POLLER 1986). Subsequently, the World Health Organization (WHO) adopted one of these British reference thromboplastins as an international reference standard. In order to compare results using local thromboplastins with this international standard, various mathematical approaches were used based on the ratio of normal to patient PT results and the sensitivity (ISI) of the thromboplastin compared with the WHO standard thromboplastin (HULL et al. 1978; KIRKWOOD 1983). The recommendation now is to express the results as the INR (International Normalized Ratio) (LOELIGER et al. 1985). If the ISI of the local thromboplastin is known, the conversion to INR is easily performed by reference to a table. Similar INRs indicate similar degrees of anticoagulation regardless of the actual PTs obtained or the control-to-patient ratios.

Other approaches to monitoring warfarin therapy using chromogenic substrates (FRANCIS et al. 1985) or monospecific antibodies (FURIE et al. 1990) have been suggested. However, the PT, when properly used and understood, is reliable and inexpensive. It is likely to remain the standard at least for the present.

Until recently, proof of the efficacy of anticoagulant therapy (HIRSH 1986) lay entirely on a retrospective study reported by COON et al. in 1969 (DALE et al. 1977) in which they showed that the frequency of recurrence of symptomatic deep vein thrombosis was less in patients who received oral anticoagulants. In 1979, a randomized clinical trial (HULL et al. 1979) using objective documentation of deep vein thrombosis proved that patients treated with warfarin at doses that prolonged the PT 1.5–2 times its original value had no recurrences and that this regimen was superior to low-dose subcutaneous heparin (5000 U every 12 h), with which 25% of patients suffered recurrence. One study done in 1978 (TABERNER et al. 1978) had a

serious is known as coumarin skin necrosis, although it has also been described with indanedione treatment (KOCH-WESER 1968; HORN et al. 1981; HOFFMAN and FRICK 1982). This lesion usually develops after 3–5 days of therapy. Areas of skin overlying abundant subcutaneous fat deposits (breasts, buttocks, thighs) are most frequently affected. After a brief period of localized pain with red or bluish discoloration, large bullae filled with serosanguinous fluid appear followed shortly by formation of a thick black eschar of necrotic skin and subcutaneous fat. Healing occurs over many weeks or months yet may leave remarkably little scar. Many patients, however, have required plastic surgery or mastectomy. Biopsies of the early lesion show thrombi in the dermal venules and capillaries. It has been postulated that thrombosis occurs because of warfarin-induced loss of protein C. It will be recalled that production of protein C is vitamin-K-dependent. The half-life of protein C is quite short, and therefore, the level in the blood falls rapidly after institution of warfarin therapy, before full anticoagulation has been accomplished. This theory is supported by the fact that several cases of coumarin skin necrosis have been described in patients congenitally deficient in protein C (MCGEHEE et al. 1984). However, it fails to explain the peculiar distribution of the lesions to the skin and underlying fat.

No form of treatment has been universally effective; the lesions usually evolve through the typical stages regardless of treatment. It would seem reasonable, considering the pathology, to attempt immediate anticoagulation with heparin, but to be effective, this would have to be started at the very earliest stages of lesion development. Cessation of warfarin and administration of vitamin K is usually recommended, but there are several instances in which warfarin therapy was continued without any new lesions developing and without extension of the initial ones (KOCH-WESER 1968).

Subsequent courses of warfarin may or may not cause skin lesions. The incidence of this complication is not known but is clearly very low. Less than 100 cases had been reported by 1986, when the manufacturer of warfarin estimated that 20 million patients had been treated with this anticoagulant (DUPONT 1986).

Warfarin cannot be used in pregnant women because of its teratogenic effects (HULL et al. 1980; STEVENSON et al. 1980). Taken during the first trimester (6th–12th weeks of gestation) it can produce the "warfarin embryopathy syndrome" with a variety of skeletal abnormalities in the fetus. Taken during the 2nd and 3rd trimesters, it can cause serious developmental anomalies of the central nervous system and eye. The pregnant patient who requires anticoagulation must be treated with heparin.

Allergic reactions, usually minor, have been reported, including fever and skin rashes. A few cases of painful discolored toes have been reported (the purple toe syndrome) (AKLE and JOINER 1981). The cause is not known, but symptoms improve if warfarin is stopped.

B. Thrombolytic Therapy

The feasibility of using fibrinolytic therapy for dissolution of intravascular clots (thrombolysis) is based on the fact that all thrombi contain fibrin, either as a network that holds large numbers of platelets and other cells together or as the major component of the clot (FREIMAN et al. 1987). Removal of this clot would reasonably be the way of restoring tissues to their previous, fully perfused state. Human blood contains an enzyme system capable of digesting fibrin, the fibrinolytic system (ROBBINS 1987). All current thrombolytic therapeutic agents act via this system. As with the coagulation system, the active enzymes of the fibrinolytic system exist in the blood in their inactive zymogen form and become active only under specific conditions. Plasminogen, present in the blood plasma, is the precursor of plasmin, a nonselective serine protease capable of digesting fibrin and a large number of proteins in the plasma and subendothelial structures. There is essentially no free plasmin in the blood since there are potent inhibitors, mainly α_2-antiplasmin, which promptly bind and neutralize it. Under physiological conditions, plasmin is active only in areas of thrombosis with stasis.

The plasminogen molecule has been fully characterized (FRANCIS and MARDER 1990; ROBBINS 1987). It is a single chain molecule with M_r of 88 000 and consists of 790 amino acids. On activation by cleavage at the Arg_{560}-Val_{561} bond, it becomes divided into heavy and light chains held together by a disulfide bond. The heavy chain at the amino-terminal side of the cleavage point contains 5 triple loop "kringle" structures, 4 of which contain lysine-binding sites. It is these sites that bind the plasminogen to fibrin, thereby conferring a degree of substrate specificity. By concentrating the active molecules on the surface of the fibrin, the proteolytic activity is limited to the clot. Any plasmin that escapes from the clot is promptly neutralized by α_2-antiplasmin in the plasma. This inhibitor is much less active against plasmin attached to fibrin. The light chain at the carboxy-terminal side of the cleavage site contains the enzyme center, His_{602}-Asp_{645}-Ser_{740}, which becomes active only after cleavage of the Arg_{560}-Val_{561} bond, which converts plasminogen to plasmin. This occurs when the Arg_{560}-Val_{561} bond is cleaved by very specific serine proteases, the plasminogen activators. Two activators are normally found in human tissues and, in very small amounts, in blood: tissue-type plasminogen activator (t-PA) and urokinase-type plasminogen activator (u-PA). t-PA is secreted locally into the bloodstream from the endothelium in areas of ischemia as in the presence of thrombosis (STALDER et al. 1985; WIMAN et al. 1983; LEVIN et al. 1988). It is a single chain molecule, M_r 60 000, that contains two "kringle" structures very similar to those in plasminogen, one of which confers the ability to bind to fibrin. Additionally, it has a "finger" domain analogous to a similar structure in fibronectin which adds to its affinity for fibrin (ICHINOSE et al. 1986). This affinity for fibrin serves to concentrate t-PA on the surface of a clot,

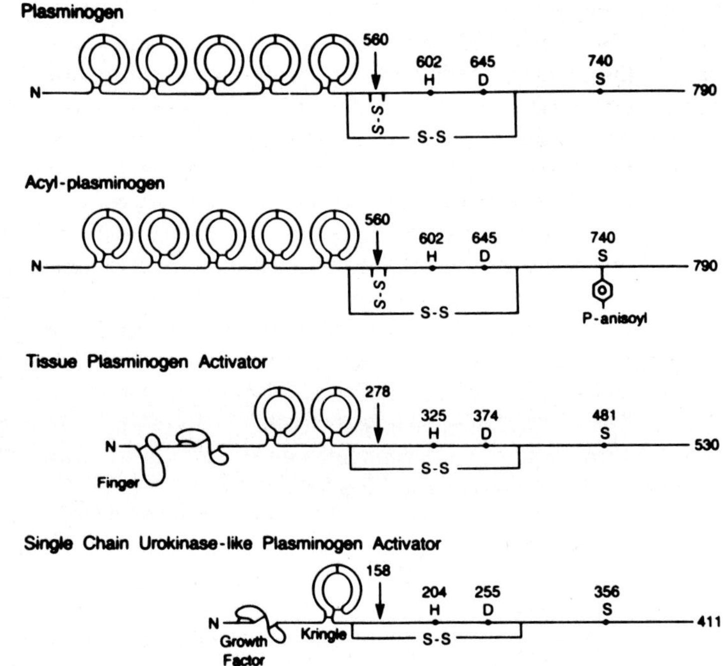

Fig. 6. Structure of plasminogen and its activators. See text for discussion. (Reproduced by permission from FRANCIS and MARDER 1990, p 1315)

thereby enhancing its ability to activate the fibrinolytic system where it is needed with less effect on the proteins that remain in solution. After attachment to fibrin, the molecule undergoes cleavage to a double chain form which is more active in solution. Attached to fibrin, both single- and double-chain t-PA are equally effective in converting plasminogen to plasmin (Fig. 6) (RIJKEN et al. 1982).

Urokinase (WHITE et al. 1966) was originally identified in urine (hence its name) where it exists as a double-chain molecule. It has since been found in human plasma in its single-chain form (scu-PA), $M_r \sim 54000$, which differs from t-PA in having only one "kringle" and no "finger" domain. It does not bind to fibrin. The two-chain form (u-PA, UK) has been the normal type obtained on purification of urine and is the one used therapeutically. u-PA is a serine protease and exits in two forms, S2 ($M_r \sim 54000$) and S1 ($M_r \sim 31000$) which is derived from the higher molecular weight form by proteolytic degradation (LIJNEN et al. 1985). u-PA has a wide range of possible substrates and does not show fibrin selectivity. scu-PA, although it does not bind to fibrin, shows considerable fibrin specificity in an indirect manner. An active competitive inhibitor in plasma abolishes the activity of scu-PA. Fibrin appears to neutralize this inhibition (LIJNEN et al. 1985), allowing expression of its plasminogen-activating function on the fibrin itself.

The era of fibrinolytic therapy began in 1949 when TILLETT and SHERRY administered intrapleural streptokinase to patients and accomplished the dissolution of clotted hemothorax. The preparation they used was too toxic for general intravenous use in humans but was employed successfully in animals for lysis of venous and arterial clots, thus proving the feasibility of this approach to the management of thrombotic disease. Another agent, urokinase, isolated from human urine in 1946 by MACFARLANE and PILLING, was studied within the next decade, but again, matters of purification made it unsuitable for widespread clinical use. Improvement in both products recently have led to increased clinical applications. In the 1978 Handbook for Experimental Pharmacology, urokinase and streptokinase are reviewed in detail, and the reader is referred to these for discussion of the biochemistry, pharmacology, and early clinical work. Since then, enormous advances have continued in the understanding of the thrombolytic process and in the preparation of pure products for clinical use. Urokinase and streptokinase were approved for treatment of deep vein thrombosis and serious pulmonary emboli in the USA around 12 years ago. Concerns about the side effects and especially the dangerous bleeding that could occur during treatment apparently limited their acceptance. Serious and widespread interest in this form of treatment did not begin until it was shown that most cases (~95%) of acute myocardial infarction were due to thrombotic occlusion of a coronary vessel (DEWOOD et al. 1983) and that this thrombus could be digested rapidly with fibrinolytic enzymes, leading to reperfusion of the occluded vessel and considerable clinical gains (RENTROP et al. 1979). An extensive literature has developed in the meantime, dealing with the chemistry, pharmacology, and clinical usage of the two original agents, now highly purified, and newer agents, scu-PA, t-PA, and acylated plasminogen-streptokinase activator complex (APSAC). All of these act to lyse fibrin indirectly through the same mechanism: They are plasminogen activators that, directly or indirectly, cause the conversion of the inactive enzyme plasminogen into its active form, plasmin, which is capable of digesting fibrin and, hence, of dissolving thrombi. They vary, however, in several important properties: affinity for fibrin (as opposed to fibrinogen), antigenicity, half-life, manner of administration, and cost. Each will be reviewed separately, followed by a summary of the main clinical studies which have established their usefulness and compared them with each other and with previous standard therapy (mainly anticoagulation).

I. Streptokinase

Streptokinase is a protein produced by β-hemolytic streptococci, group C, growing in culture. Its potential for dissolving human plasma clots was first recognized in 1933 (TILLETT and GARNER 1933). It was isolated from the culture medium in 1945 and shown to be a single-chain protein with a molecular weight of about 48000 (BACHMANN 1987). During the past 2 decades, a variety of methods have been developed to obtain products of high purity. These are suitable for intravenous and intraarterial use but, being of bacterial origin, are antigenic, can elicit allergic reactions (SHARMA et al. 1982; TOTTY et al. 1982), and can be neutralized by preexisting streptokinase-specific antibodies in the recipient (VERSTRAETE 1978). The activity of streptokinase preparations is measured in international units (IU). A reference standard is available from the WHO. Streptokinase does not convert plasminogen to plasmin directly (WOHL et al. 1978). When added to plasma, it reacts in an equimolar ratio with nonfibrin-bound plasminogen to form a complex. The complex then activates plasminogen to plasmin. Streptokinase has little affinity for fibrin (CAMIOLO et al. 1971). Activation of the fibrinolytic system with streptokinase, therefore, occurs in the plasma, producing the "lytic state" (SHERRY et al. 1959). Fibrin clots are digested, but simultaneously, there is proteolysis of fibrinogen and other components of the coagulation system, leading to considerable impairment in blood coagulability (SHERRY et al. 1959; FLETCHER et al. 1962, 1965). The effects of a bolus infusion of streptokinase are long-lasting (VERSTRAETE et al. 1978). The half-life of the streptokinase plasminogen complex is 23 min, so the fibrinolytic state continues for a few hours after the infusion is completed. Normal levels of fibrinogen and other components of the coagulation system may not be fully restored for 1–2 days. The degree of depletion of these factors is related to the intensity and duration of the infusion. The streptokinase molecule is broken down into several large and small fragments during these reactions, but they remain in complex with fibrin and to varying degrees retain their fibrinolytic activity (SIEFRING and CASTELLINO 1976). The subsequent catabolism and excretion is unknown.

Streptokinase is used in the therapy of myocardial infarction, pulmonary embolism, deep vein thrombosis, arterial thrombosis or embolism, and for the reopening of clotted, implanted cannulae. The dosage, mode of administration and duration of therapy vary with the indication for treatment. A standard dose is usually used, regardless of the patient's size or body weight (VERSTRAETE et al. 1966), which is sufficient to neutralize preexisting streptococcal-specific antibodies in most patients and will initiate an active fibrinolytic state. Since streptokinase is antigenic, a rise in streptococcal-specific antibodies can be expected, and therapeutic reuse within 6 months is likely to be ineffective and associated with more allergic side effects (TOTTY et al. 1982).

The most important indication for thrombolytic therapy is acute myocardial infarction, in which prompt reestablishment of blood flow is necessary to minimize infarction of contractile tissue and preservation of cardiac function. Peripheral thrombotic disease has traditionally been managed with anticoagulants, although thrombolytic therapy may have some advantages (see below). The following dosage regimens have been recommended:

Acute myocardial infarction. Treatment should be as soon as possible after onset of symptoms, preferably within 3 h.

- Intracoronary infusion (ANDERSON et al. 1983; KENNEDY et al. 1983). 140 000 IU administered as a 20 000 IU bolus followed by 2000 IU/min for 60 min. With this approach, 75% of patients had reperfusion of the occluded vessel demonstrated angiographically (vs. 45% in the untreated control patients) within 60 min.
- Intravenous infusion (Gruppo Italiano per lo Studio della Streptochinasi nell' Infarto Miocardico 1987; ISIS-2 1988; RENTROP 1985). Because of the inevitable delay in getting the patient to a center capable of coronary angiography and the further delay in performing the procedure, intravenous administration is now preferred. This should be started as soon as possible after onset of symptoms with best results if given within 1 h and significant benefit up to 6 h. The streptokinase is administered by bolus intravenous infusion in a single dose of 1 500 000 IU given within 1 h. Approximately 50% of patients will achieve patency if it is given within 3 h of onset of symptoms, about 37% if given between 3 and 6 h (VERSTRAETE et al. 1985; CHESEBRO et al. 1987).

Pulmonary embolism (USPET 1974), deep vein thrombosis (GOLDHABER et al. 1984; ARNESEN et al. 1978), arterial embolization (AMERY et al. 1970), and arterial occlusion. More delay between onset of symptoms and initiation of therapy is tolerated in the treatment of all these conditions with the exception of acute, severe pulmonary embolism, for which prompt treatment is necessary. Less intense therapy is used but is given over a protracted period of time, the duration depending on the estimated age of the thrombus (older clots lyse more slowly) and the clinical response. An initial bolus dose of 250 000 IU is given to assure neutralization of preexisting streptococcal-specific antibodies. This is followed by 100 000 IU/h for 24 h or longer. Most pulmonary emboli will clear with 12–24 h of streptokinase treatment. Deep vein thrombosis may require 4–5 days or more. A small percentage of clots will be resistant to lytic therapy.

Implanted cannulae (Physician's Desk Reference 1990; KUDO et al. 1985). The various types of cannulae implanted for venous access in patients requiring long-term intravenous therapy will often become obstructed by clot in spite of careful routine care (i.e., regular flushing followed by instillation of a heparinized solution). Reopening can be accomplished by instilling a concentrated solution of streptokinase (250 000 IU in 2 ml) into each occluded limb, allowing it to remain for 2 h, then aspirating the contents of the cannula followed by flushing with saline.

Streptokinase is available in the USA as Streptase (Hoechst-Roussel) and Kabikinase (Smith Kline & French). Streptase is manufactured by Behringwerke AG, Germany, Kabikinase by Kabivitrum AB, Stockholm, Sweden. Both are supplied in various size vials as a white lyophilized powder. Reconstitution is in either normal saline or 5% dextrose. It is the least expensive of the thrombolytic agents: The cost for intravenous treatment of acute myocardial infarction is between $100 and $200.

II. Urokinase (and Single Chain Urokinase)

Urokinase (BACHMANN 1987) is a serine protease initially isolated from human urine and now produced by recombinant DNA techniques using both bacterial and mammalian cells or from cultures of human embryonic kidney cells and lung adenocarcinoma cells. It occurs mainly in two forms: single chain (M_r ~ 54000; scu-PA) and double chain (u-PA), with the same molecular weight, which is created from the single chain form by cleavage (by plasmin in the presence of fibrin) of a single peptide bond at Lys_{158}-Ile_{159}. Both sorts are direct activators of plasminogen, cleaving the Arg_{560}-Val_{561} bond to produce plasmin. scu-PA is also known as pro-u-PA. The double chain form is considerably more active enzymatically but has no affinity for fibrin. scu-PA has very little fibrinolytic activity, but its rapid conversion to the double-chain form on fibrin immediately renders it fully active. Thus, the proteolytic activity is maximal on the clot (LIJNEN et al. 1985, 1987).

scu-PA is present in plasma in small amounts; u-PA is the main form found in urine. scu-PA infused into human subjects has a half-life of 5 min, while u-PA has a half-life of 10–30 min in the circulation (COLLEN et al. 1984). The fibrinolytic activity of both u-PA and scu-PA is measured in units of activity (IU) (ROBBINS et al. 1987).

Since u-PA has little affinity for fibrin (CAMIOLO et al. 1971), infusion invariably produces a plasma fibrinolytic state with reduction of fibrinogen and Factors V and VIII, as is seen following infusion of streptokinase. With low-dose infusions of scu-PA, there is no reduction in plasma fibrinogen, but at the doses needed for effective thrombolysis, the lytic state is also produced (ZAMARRON et al. 1984). Hence, bleeding is a significant side effect of treatment with both these agents.

Urokinase (u-PA) has been in clinical use for about 20 years. It is available in the USA as Abbokinase (Abbott Laboratories, North Chicago, IL) as a lyophilized powder, 250000 IU/vial. It is administered by slow intravenous injection or by continuous infusion. The approved doses given by the manufacturer (Physician's Desk Reference 1990) are as follows:

- For acute myocardial infarction (TENNANT et al. 1984): 6000IU/min into the occluded coronary artery for up to 2 h. Average total dose for lysis of coronary thrombi is 500000 IU. It is recommended that heparin be given simultaneously and following the infusion to discourage reocclusion.
- For pulmonary embolism (USPET 1974): a priming dose of 4400 IU/kg is given intravenously over 10 min, followed by a continuous infusion of 4400 IU/kg·h for 12 h. Anticoagulation with heparin is begun after the infusion when the thrombin time has fallen to less than twice normal.

- For opening obstructed indwelling venous catheters or devices: u-PA is available for this purpose as a lyophilized powder in 1-ml single-dose vials containing 5000 IU. This is instilled gently in a volume sufficient to fill the device and allowed to remain at least 5 min before attempting aspiration. If it remains occluded, further time, up to 60 min, should be allowed for dissolution of the clot. Once open, blood is aspirated to clear the device of u-PA and fragments of clot, then flushed with saline.
- u-PA has also been recommended for lysis of peripheral arterial and venous clots at various doses as well as intracardiac clots (KREMER et al. 1985).

Urokinase is more expensive than streptokinase. The usual 500 000 IU used in the treatment of acute myocardial infarction costs around $500. It is nonantigenic, and therefore, allergic reactions do not occur during or following its administration.

Relatively little clinical data is yet available on scu-PA. It has proven to be an effective thrombolytic agent in a few cases of acute myocardial infarction (VAN DE WERF et al. 1986). Further studies will undoubtedly be performed. It has a very short half-life of 5 min and, therefore, will have to be given by continuous intravenous infusion with heparin. It is produced by Collaborative Research, Lexington, MA, and by Genentech, San Francisco, CA. The dose used in the above study was 40 mg by continuous intravenous infusion over 60–90 min. Its side effects are not yet fully known, but it does produce the lytic state so that bleeding will not be an unexpected complication. No estimate of cost is yet available, but it is assumed that it will be expensive (similar to t-PA).

III. Tissue Plasminogen Activator

If we consider streptokinase and urokinase the first generation of thrombolytic agents, t-PA is the prominent member of the second generation and has recently become available for clinical use. The second generation products, t-PA, scu-PA, and APSAC, were all developed as agents with increased fibrin specificity that, theoretically, should lyse the thrombus without inducing the plasma lytic state and, therefore, produce less complicating bleeding.

t-PA (LOSCALZO and BRAUNWALD 1988) is the main naturally occurring plasminogen activator of the blood. It has a molecular weight of ~70 000 daltons and occurs in either one- or two-chain forms, the latter being produced from the former by plasmin. Its potency is expressed in international units (IU) of fibrinolytic activity (WHO standard is available), and the half-life is short, 5 min, therefore mandating that it be administered by infusion. For clinical use, it is produced by a human melanoma cell line in culture and by recombinant DNA technology. These are identical in structure and activity to the naturally occurring form. As previously described, t-

PA has a specific affinity for fibrin because of its "kringle" and "finger" domains. Once bound to the clot, it rapidly reacts with the plasminogen already adherent to the clot and converts it to plasmin directly on the desired substrate. Plasmin escaping from the protective environment of the clot is neutralized by α_2-antiplasmin. In animals (AGNELLI et al. 1985), t-PA has been shown to lyse thrombi without producing the plasma lytic state, but in humans the necessary dose and duration of the infusion of t-PA does lead to activation of plasma plasminogen, and decreasing levels of fibrinogen are seen (COLLEN et al. 1986). Bleeding occurs in about the same percentage of patients as with the other thrombolytic agents (CALIFF et al. 1987).

The only approved use for t-PA in the USA is for treatment of coronary thrombosis. As with the older thrombolytic agents, therapy should be started as soon as possible after onset of symptoms. The recommended dose is 100 mg, with 6–10 mg given intravenously as a bolus to initiate therapy, 50–54 mg given by infusion over the 1st h, followed by 20 mg during each of the 2nd and 3rd h. For smaller patients, the dose can be reduced, but the duration of therapy remains at 3 h. Heparin or antiplatelet drugs (aspirin, dipyridamole) can be given simultaneously to reduce the risk of rethrombosis, but this may increase the chances of hemorrhage (see below). The generic term for t-PA is alteplase. It is marketed as Activase by Genentech, San Francisco, CA, and is available in 20-mg and 50-mg vials. Its specific activity is 580 000 IU/mg. It is expensive; the cost for the 100 mg needed for treatment of acute myocardial infarction as described above is about $2750.

IV. Acyl Plasminogen Streptokinase Activation Complex

Several acyl derivatives of streptokinase-plasminogen have been developed with the view of prolonging the effectiveness of the fibrinolytic state induced by streptokinase while increasing its fibrin selectivity by binding to plasminogen.

Serine proteases cleave specific peptide bonds by the formation and subsequent hydrolysis of an unstable acyl bond between the serine residue of the catalytic site on the enzyme and the carbonyl function of the peptide bond of its substrate. By using appropriate lysine or arginine analogues, relatively stable acyl bonds can be formed which block the enzymatic site on the light chain of the plasminogen or plasminogen-streptokinase complex. This renders it resistant to neutralization by α_2-antiplasmin. The complex retains, unaltered, the lysine sites on the heavy chain that react with fibrin and, therefore, will concentrate on the clot. Here it gradually deacylates, exposing the proteolytic site over a period of time (WALKER and DAVIDSON 1987). The acyl derivative that has been most intensively evaluated is the *p*-anisoyl derivative of the plasminogen-streptokinase activator complex (APSAC). In an in vitro system, its deacylation $t_{1/2}$ is 40 min, but it is thought to be slower in human whole blood, approximately 90 min. APSAC has been effective in lysing venous and arterial clots in animal models (DUPE et al. 1983, 1985). Of particular interest is the activity against aged clots that are usually resistant to fibrinolytic therapy.

APSAC has had clinical trials in the UK and Europe which established the dosage at 5–10 mg every 8 h for 24 h for the treatment of pulmonary emboli and up to several days for deep vein thrombosis (WALKER and DAVIDSON 1987). Recent studies have confirmed the effectiveness of APSAC in the management of acute myocardial infarction (AIMS Trial Study Group 1988; MARDER et al. 1986). A 30-mg bolus dose produces reperfusion in most patients. Although the major proteolytic activity of the complex occurs in the thrombi, some degree of systemic fibrinolysis does arise (HOFFMAN et al. 1985; FEARS et al. 1985).

The potential usefulness of APSAC will depend on the clinical validation of its effectiveness, relative fibrin selectivity (reduced risk of bleeding), and its ease of administration (infrequent doses which produce a prolonged effect) in comparison with the other thrombolytic agents.

Since streptokinase is a component of the APSAC complex, allergic reactions may occur, antibodies will be produced, and preexisting streptokinase-specific antibodies may cause resistance to therapy (WALKER et al. 1984). This product has recently become available in the USA as Eminase (Beecham/Upjohn) in 30-U vials at a cost of \$1649/vial (IU $\approx$ 1 mg).

V. Novel Approaches

All the thrombolytic agents currently in clinical use are effective in removing thrombi, but they also carry the risk of producing bleeding. The ideal agent would have very restricted proteolytic activity: The offending clot would be removed, but hemostatic thrombi would be left intact and plasma proteins, platelets, and vessel wall components would not be affected. Attempts towards this goal involve creating hybrid molecules (HABER et al. 1989): One combines the heavy, fibrin-binding chain of plasminogen with the catalytic center of urokinase. Its fibrinolytic activity is double that of urokinase in an in vitro clot assay. Other hybrids combine the heavy chain of plasminogen with the proteolytic chain of t-PA, or the fibrin-binding chain of t-PA and the proteolytic center of low molecular weight scu-PA; neither of these was more active than the parent compounds.

A different approach has been to link fibrin-specific antibodies to plasminogen light chains or plasminogen activator light chains (HABER et al. 1989). Some of these products have promising fibrinolytic activity. This is an active area of research that should produce interesting results in the near future.

1. Defibrotide and Brinase

Two other agents should be mentioned, neither of which is an activator of the plasminogen-plasmin system. Both have been known for a number of years: defibrotide since 1973 (Niada et al. 1981) and brinase since 1963 (Bergkvist 1963), and occasional reports of their clinical use continue to appear in the literature (Coccheri et al. 1982). Defibrotide is a polydesoxyribonucleotide with a chemical structure similar to DNA, which is extracted from mammalian organs. It is described as an antithrombotic agent with fibrinolytic activity which stimulates the production or release of prostacyclin by the endothelium (Niada et al. 1982). Animal studies have shown a dose-response relationship for inhibition of intravascular clot formation without measurable changes in blood coagulation (Niada et al. 1981). Its enhancement of fibrinolysis has also been shown to be dose-dependent (Porta et al. 1984). It appears to increase the physiologic level of activity of the fibrinolytic system while simultaneously reducing the activity of its natural inhibitors. Clinically, it has been used with demonstrated benefit in the treatment of myocardial infarction (Milazzotto et al. 1989; Mattioli et al. 1989). There were absolutely no side effects among the 53 patients receiving it in this study. There have been no studies comparing defibrotide with standard fibrinolytic therapy.

Brinase is a proteinolytic enzyme preparation obtained from the culture medium of *Aspergillus oryzae* growing submerged. It contains a serine protease which provides 98% of the enzymatic activity. The remaining 2% is from a zinc-containing metalloprotease (Frisch 1989). It does not activate the plasmin system (Vanhove et al. 1979). In the circulation, brinase is rapidly complexed to α_2-macroglobulin, which retains part of the enzymatic activity of the uncomplexed molecule. The half-life of the complex in man is 60 min, making brinase one of the longer-acting thrombolytic agents (Bergkvist 1963). Clinically (Verhaeghe et al. 1979), brinase has been used locally by direct instillation into occluded arteries and systemically by intravenous infusion for both arterial and venous thrombosis. When given systemically, it is necessary to measure the inhibitory capacity of the blood. The dose is then adjusted so that this capacity is never exceeded. During treatment there is a modest (15%) fall in the fibrinogen level, but plasminogen values do not change. Tests of paracoagulation often become positive. Brinase is effective via both routes, but there are not sufficient data to make comparisons with either streptokinase or urokinase. Hemorrhages have not been reported, but an allergic reaction was seen in 1 of the 300 patients who have received it. Local reactions at or near the injection site are more frequent: swelling, blister formation, oozing from puncture site.

VI. Side Effects and Complications

By far, the main problem with thrombolytic therapy is the development of a bleeding diathesis which can range from a relatively minor problem to a life-threatening or lethal event. It occurs with all available agents, regardless of fibrin specificity. In the TIMI trial (1985) (t-PA vs. streptokinase in acute myocardial infarction), 15% of patients in both groups developed major bleeding (significant drop in hematocrit) or intracranial bleeding. Minor plus major bleeding occurred in just under 50% of both groups. Intracranial bleeding occurs in about 0.2%–1% of patients and causes serious neurologic damage or death in most (SHERRY et al. 1980). In one major study involving over 5000 patients treated with streptokinase in a 1-h infusion, the incidence of intracranial bleeding, 0.2%, was no greater than in the control group (Gruppo Italiano per lo Studio della Streptochinasi nell' Infarto Miocardico 1987). The higher figure of 1% is likely to be seen in patients receiving more prolonged therapy or the higher dose of t-PA (150 mg for acute myocardial infarction) which is no longer recommended (1.6% incidence) (BRAUNWALD et al. 1987). All agents cause the plasma lytic state which produces a major disruption in all aspects of hemostasis. Fibrinogen is broken down into fragments that not only do not clot but also interfere with the polymerization of fibrin monomers. Factors V and VIII are digested, thus interfering with generation of X_A and, hence, thrombin. These effects are the cause for the prolonged partial thromboplastin (PTT) and thrombin times (ThT) seen in patients receiving fibrinolytic therapy. Platelet function is also disturbed. Surface proteins necessary for aggregation (platelet-platelet interaction) and adhesion (platelet-vessel-wall interaction) are destroyed, thus impeding the development of a hemostatic plug at sites of injury (MARDER and SHERRY 1988; COLLER 1990).

It had been generally accepted that the bleeding diathesis was caused by the disruption of coagulation, but it is likely to be more complex than this. It has been observed clinically that the most frequent site of bleeding is from areas of the invasive procedures which most patients have had shortly before initiation of thrombolytic therapy (surgery, venipunctures, and arterial punctures) (MARDER and FRANCIS 1984). It is also apparent that the longer the thrombolytic state is maintained, the more likely it is the patient will develop clinical bleeding (SHERRY et al. 1980). The newer, more fibrin-selective products are very effective at dissolving thrombi in the coronary arteries, but reocclusion with a fresh clot will occur in a significant percentage of patients unless heparin or antiplatelet therapy is administered simultaneously. These add to the defect in hemostasis and might be expected to increase the possibility of bleeding. Moreover, the incidence of bleeding does not correlate with the intensity of the plasma lytic state as measured by the decrease in circulating fibrinogen and other tests designed to reflect the extent of depletion of coagulation factors (TIMI Study Group 1985; Urokinase Pulmonary Embolism Trial 1973). Fibrinogen falls to very low levels (6%–8% of pretreatment) after the standard 1.5 million IU streptokinase for acute myocardial infarction (TIMI Study Group 1985), whereas with t-PA the fall is a much more modest 40% (VERSTRAETE et al. 1985), but there was the same incidence of bleeding with both of these agents, and the same number of patients required transfusions. Bleeding in both patient groups was largely from previous vessel punctures. These observations imply that the main cause of bleeding is the presence of a recently injured blood vessel. The thrombolytic agents clearly do not distinguish between fibrin in thrombi and fibrin in hemostatic plugs. This type of bleeding can be reduced by minimizing the number of invasive procedures performed in patients who are candidates for fibrinolytic therapy, by drawing blood samples from peripheral veins to which pressure can be applied more effectively if bleeding should supervene, and by selecting the patients for thrombolytic therapy with great caution. As a result of experience, certain patients are considered to have absolute contraindications for thrombolytic therapy: Those with recent (6 months) cerebrovascular event, intracranial tumor, or head injury or surgery, those who have had surgery of the chest or abdomen within the past 10 days, and those with active bleeding, particularly of the gastrointestinal tract, before thrombolytic therapy is begun.

Once therapy with thrombolytic agents is begun, invasive procedures, including blood sampling, must be kept to a minimum. Monitoring of the thrombolytic state is necessary only to establish that it has indeed been accomplished. This can be done with fibrinogen determinations, thrombin times, or prothrombin times. If fibrinogen is falling or the PT or ThT shows prolongation, the plasma lytic state has been achieved, and further monitoring is unnecessary.

If local bleeding occurs, pressure should be applied manually until it is controlled. If bleeding of life-threatening proportions develops, thrombolytic therapy should be stopped, and if necessary, restitution of fibrinogen levels with cryoprecipitate can be done. In extreme cases an antifibrinolytic agent (e.g., epsilon-aminocaproic acid) can also be given.

A concern since the early days of fibrinolytic therapy has been the possibility of producing emboli as the clot is lysed. This probably occurs no more frequently than in the patient receiving heparin therapy alone (MARDER and BELL 1987; BAGLIN et al. 1983).

Rethrombosis after successful lysis of coronary thrombi is a problem with, but not a complication of, thrombolytic therapy. Dissolution of the thrombus does not alter the underlying pathology of the vessel wall that led to the formation of a clot in the first place. Rethrombosis of coronary arteries occurs in 10%–20% of patients regardless of the therapeutic agent used, most commonly within 24 h of initial therapy (BATES et al. 1989). Almost invariably, there is atherosclerotic involvement with narrowing of the vessel and disruption of the endothelium. These are not changed by dissolution of the clot and may need to be addressed mechanically (balloon angioplasty or bypass grafting). The addition of heparin therapy or antiplatelet drugs (ISIS-2 1988) is recommended when the patient is treated with the short-acting, fibrin-favoring agents, but as yet there is no proof that these prevent rethrombosis. Angioplasty soon after completion of thrombolysis is also advocated, but results have not been universally positive (GUERCI et al. 1987; TOPOL 1988; TIMI Study Group 1989).

For central and peripheral arterial thrombi or for pulmonary emboli, local administration of streptokinase or urokinase has been used, hoping to accomplish thrombolysis without systemic activation of the fibrinolytic system. However, when used locally these drugs are given in such a large volume that overflow into patent adjacent vessels and hence into the systemic circulation is inevitable, with consequent activation of the circulating fibrinolytic enzymes. In fact, some observers have noted that dissolution of clots was unlikely unless the lytic state was produced (KOLTS 1985; Gruppo Italiano per lo Studio della Streptochinasi nell' Infarto Miocardico 1987).

The only other complication of note is the occurrence of allergic reactions. Those arising during treatment with streptokinase or APSAC are usually mild (fever, nausea, serum-sickness syndrome), although anaphylaxis can occur (0.1% of patients in a large Italian study). u-PA, scu-PA, and t-PA have not caused allergic reactions to date.

VII. Clinical Considerations

Thrombolytic therapy was first attempted for the treatment of acute myocardial infarction in the late 1950s with streptokinase administered intravenously (FLETCHER et al. 1958) or directly into the coronary artery (BOUCEK and MURPHY 1960). Several larger clinical trials followed, but they failed to prove that thrombolysis improved clinical outcome. Therefore, this form of therapy for acute myocardial infarction did not gain wide acceptance until the late 1980s when several large studies were reported, proving the feasibility of this approach and, more importantly, an impressive improvement in outcome. Other forms of thrombotic disease have received much less attention, presumably reflecting the fact that these affect a much smaller number of people and with lesser morbidity and mortality. Pulmonary embolism was the object of several large clinical trials in the 1960s and 1970s (UPET 1973; USPET 1974), but heparin therapy has proved so safe and effective that thrombolytic therapy to this day is not viewed as the preferred therapeutic approach for most patients. During the same period, the usefulness of thrombolytic therapy for deep vein thrombosis of the leg was examined (KAKKAR et al. 1969). Lesser indications also evaluated have included peripheral arterial embolism (VERSTRAETE et al. 1971) and intraabdominal venous or arterial thrombosis (FLICKINGER et al. 1983), for which it has been found to be effective in some patients.

Several excellent reviews of this very extensive literature have been published recently and are recommended (SHERRY and SOLOMON 1987; VERSTRAETE and COLLEN 1986; MARDER and SHERRY 1988; SAMAMA 1987; KESSLER 1989). The important large studies will be discussed in this review, with reference to particular smaller studies as needed. Each of the major indications will be discussed separately. Some generalizations can be made at the outset. All the fibrinolytic agents currently available can effectively and quickly dissolve thrombi. It is clear that for the older agents streptokinase and urokinase, effectiveness is identical at least for treatment of coronary occlusion. Information comparing t-PA or APSAC with these older agents has been published but only with reference to the treatment of myocardial infarction. Comparative data for scu-PA are only now beginning to appear in the literature. Studies to date have made it clear that fibrinolytic therapy is relatively safe considering the seriousness of the diseases for which it is used. It is also known that the benefits of thrombolytic therapy may be long-lasting and may alter favorably the natural evolution of the disease process.

1. Acute Myocardial Infarction (Coronary Thrombosis)

This is the prime indication for thrombolytic therapy. Considering the very large numbers of patients who develop acute myocardial infarction annually in Europe, the USA, and other industrialized nations, it will clearly continue to be the main reason for using these agents. Thrombolytic therapy for acute coronary thrombosis is not a new idea. In fact, the first clinical trials of streptokinase were in patients with acute myocardial infarction: Fletcher and associates in 1958 used it intravenously; Boucek and Murphy in 1960 tried intracoronary application. Several studies involving large numbers of patients were carried out in the later 1960s and throughout the 1970s, but they generally failed to show improved patient survival and hence generated little enthusiasm. Two were more positive: The European Cooperative Study Group Trial in 1979 showed that mortality at 6 months was 15.6% for those treated with streptokinase within 12 h of onset of pain. For the untreated controls, mortality was 30.6%. The other very important report was that of Rentrop et al. (1979), who demonstrated angiographically that intracoronary infusion of streptokinase rapidly dissolved thrombi. Several other studies were performed around this time, treating only patients fairly early in their disease (i.e., < 12 h). The results were collected and analyzed by Stampfer and coworkers (1982). Their compilation showed that intravenous treatment with streptokinase resulted in a 20% reduction in mortality. Studies using intracoronary administration of streptokinase vs. placebo gave varying results. Three showed mortality differences in favor of the streptokinase-treated group (4%–5% vs. 15%–20%) (Kennedy et al. 1983; Khaja et al. 1983; Anderson et al. 1983). Others failed to demonstrate a mortality difference but did note better preservation of cardiac function (Simoons et al. 1983). Furberg (1984), in an overall comparison of the intracoronary trials reported to that time, concluded that there was no improvement in mortality as a result of streptokinase treatment. Delays in treatment inevitable with the intracoronary approach may partially explain this negative result. However, the intracoronary use of streptokinase did allow reperfusion studies. Marder and Francis (1984), reviewing several such investigations which covered over 700 patients altogether, reported 71% reperfusion. A later review article covering an even larger number of patients gave almost identical results (74% reperfusion) (Rentrop 1985). It should be noted that the dose of streptokinase (and later urokinase) used for intracoronary therapy was large enough to produce systemic effect (i.e., the plasma lytic state).

The question as to the nature of intracoronary clots in myocardial infarction, cause or effect, remained unresolved at the time the earlier studies were done and was not settled until DeWood et al.'s pivotal publication in 1980. They noted that coronary angiography done within 4 h of onset of symptoms demonstrated total occlusion of an artery in 87% of patients with myocardial infarction. If the patients were studied at 6–24 h only 65% were occluded, thus demonstrating that spontaneous thrombolysis does occur. It also explains the incidence of coronary thrombi reported in autopsy series, which may be as low as 20% in patients dying of myocardial infarction (Chandler et al. 1974). His observations stimulated renewed and intense interest in the role of fibrinolytic therapy in the treatment of acute coronary thrombosis.

Several important studies reported in the mid-1980s paved the way for the large clinical trials reported later in the decade. They established the absolute imperative of treatment very early in the course of the disease for maximal benefit and the effectiveness of intravenously administered streptokinase vs. the slower, more cumbersome, and expensive intracoronary route (Schwartz et al. 1982; Mathey et al. 1985; Fine et al. 1986). The importance of early treatment was clearly and dramatically demonstrated by the results of the Italian group (Gissi 1986) that compared intravenously applied streptokinase with placebo: There was a 47% reduction in in-hospital mortality for patients treated within 1 h, 23% for those treated within 3 h, and 17% for those treated within 3–6 h. The findings of a Dutch group (Simoons et al. 1983) support these data using a different end-point. They showed that the magnitude of serum enzyme increments (a measure of the size of the infarction) were directly related to time of treatment after onset of symptoms. Moreover, these beneficial results, as might reasonably be expected, were directly related to achievement of clot lysis with reestablishment of blood flow to the ischemic area. The sooner this was achieved, the greater salvage of contractile tissue and the better the outcome in terms of preservation of cardiac function and survival for the patient (Jennings and Reimer 1983). Intracoronary administration of streptokinase was extensively used in the late 1970s and early 1980s with obvious benefit (4% mortality in patients achieving reperfusion vs. 15% in those who did not) (Marder and Francis 1984; Reimer et al. 1977; Kennedy et al. 1985a,b). But this therapeutic approach required specialized facilities and, most importantly, excessive delay in the initiation of therapy. Inevitably, it was supplanted by the intravenous route after several studies proved both to be equally effective (Taylor et al. 1984; Furberg 1984).

Numerous large and small clinical studies were undertaken during the 1980s and reported in the late 1980s in several European countries, in the USA, and by several transatlantic cooperative trial groups. These produced an enormous and somewhat confusing literature, but all concur on the value of fibrinolytic therapy. Several end-points were used in the different clinical trials: short- and long-term mortality as in the early studies, angiographic reevaluation after completion of therapy for proof of clot dissolution, non-invasive measures of reperfusion such as rises in serum cardiac enzymes (SIMOONS et al. 1986), measurements of left ventricular function (ejection fraction, wall motion) (Multicenter Postinfarction Research Group 1983), and measurement of infarct size (single photon emission tomography and positron emission tomography) (BERGMANN et al. 1982). The major studies all compared streptokinase with placebo using 1.5 million IU over 30 or 60 min. Results are summarized in Table 3.

The results obtained by the GISSI group, already alluded to, are particularly impressive because of both the huge number of patients studied and their results. Not only is short-term mortality greatly improved, the long-term (1 year) is also improved, a point of particular clinical and public health importance. This study has become the "gold standard" for subsequent clinical trials. Reperfusion rates generally with intravenously given streptokinase are about 50%. The Western Washington and New Zealand studies were too small to provide significant results, but the trend is obviously in favor of thrombolytic therapy begun less than 4 h after onset of symptoms. It should be noted that the ISAM study did not demonstrate improvement in survival, but one can imply that the quality of life for post-myocard infarction survivors was better since myocardial function was better preserved in those who received streptokinase.

Follow-up (Table 4) at 1 year continued to show improved survival among the streptokinase-treated patients, especially for those treated within the crucial initial 3 h (GISSI and New Zealand studies). The ISAM results were more disappointing, showing no difference between the treated and placebo groups. The overall conclusion, however, is clear: Streptokinase treatment, administered within 3 h of onset of symptoms and up to 12 h, is effective in preserving myocardial function and in reducing mortality (ISIS Steering Committee 1987).

Urokinase has been used with a much smaller number of patients. MAZEL (1987) demonstrated that an intracoronary infusion would result in reperfusion, but few data have appeared since then. TENNANT et al. (1984) treated 80 patients with either urokinase or streptokinase, given into the occluded coronary artery, and found equal reperfusion rates but more bleeding in the streptokinase-treated group. A Japanese group (YASUNO 1984) reported 94% reperfusion in 10–30 min with large doses (up to 960 000 U) urokinase administered into the occluded coronary artery. A German study (NEUHAUS et al. 1988) comparing u-PA to t-PA given intravenously found them equally effective. The cost of urokinase has undoubtedly been a significant deterrent (about 5 times the cost of streptokinase).

The rate of reinfarction after streptokinase administration is between 10% and 20%. Reocclusion is most likely to occur within the first 24 h

Table 3. Intravenously administered streptokinase (st) vs. placebo in acute myocardial infarction: short-term results

Trial	No. of patients	Length of pain before SK (h)	Mortality			Other
			Control	Treated	*P*	
GISSI (1986)	11 712	<12	13	10.7	0.0002	60′ infusion
		<1	15.4	8.2	0.0001	
		<3	12	9.2	0.0005	
		>3–6	14.1	11.7	0.03	
		>6–9	14.1	12.6	NS	
		>9–12	13.6	15.8	NS	
KENNEDY et al. (1988) (W. WASHINGTON)	368	2–5	9.6	6.3	NS	60′ infusion
		<3	11.5	5.2	NS	
		>3	7.5	7.5	NS	
WHITE et al. (1987) (N. Zealand)	219	<4	12.9	2.3	NS	30′ infusion. Left ventricular function better in SK patients
SCHRÖDER et al. (1987) (ISAM) (W. Germany)	1741	<6	7.1	6.3	NS	60′ infusion. Peak enzymes appear earlier in SK patients. Infarct size smaller in SK patients. Ejection fraction higher in SK patients
		<3	6.5	5.2	NS	
ISIS-2 (1987) (United Kingdom)	4000	<4	12	8.0	Significant	

Table 4. Intravenously administered streptokinase (SK) vs. placebo in acute myocardial infarction: long-term results

Trial	Number of patients (%)	Follow-up at (months)	Mortality			Comments
			Control	Treated	*P*	
GISSI (1987)	11 521 (98.37)	12	19	17.2	0.008	
KENNEDY et al. (1988) (W. WASHINGTON)	338 (91.8) 337 (91.5)	6 12+	(no difference)			Patients treated before 3 h had 17% mortality; controls 30% at 1 year; 19% and 35%, respectively, at 2 years.
SCHRÖDER et al. (1987) (ISAM)	174.1	7 21	11.1 16.1	10.9 14.4	NS NS	More reinfarctions in the SK group (7.2% vs. 4.5%, *P* 0.02)

%, percentage of initial study group available for long-term follow-up.

of successful reperfusion. This demonstrates that thrombolysis does not remove the underlying cause of the initial thrombosis (high-grade stenosis that allows thrombus to form) (HARRISON et al. 1984). In order to evaluate the effect of suppressing one of the factors that cause rethrombosis, the ISIS Study Group (ISIS-2 1988) conducted a very large trial (17 187 patients) comparing four groups: intravenously given streptokinase alone, oral aspirin (160 mg), streptokinase plus aspirin, or neither. The aspirin was administered as soon as possible and continued for 30 days. The results are impressive. Aspirin reduced mortality by 20%, and this was additive to the benefit derived from SK alone. However, there was a slightly higher incidence of stroke in those receiving aspirin.

t-PA at present has become the preferred thrombolytic agent for the treatment of acute coronary occlusion. The dose of 80 mg as a 3-h infusion was established in preliminary studies with concomitant heparin at usual doses. Several large clinical trials have since proven its effectiveness. In most of the trials t-PA is compared with streptokinase, aspirin, or u-PA. The results of these trials are summarized in Table 5. Data on long-time survival after therapy with t-PA are not yet available.

The data summarized in Table 5 represent the administration of t-PA to approximately 3200 patients. It produces a higher reperfusion rate than streptokinase and about the same as urokinase (in one study), but it has a higher reocclusion rate even when heparin therapy is given simultaneously (JOHNS et al. 1988). Heparin plus aspirin alone as was given in the rTTPA (VAN DE WERF and ARNOLD 1988) trial gave excellent reperfusion rates. However, preservation of cardiac function was better and mortality less in those receiving t-PA. There is somewhat more bleeding in patients receiving streptokinase but with t-PA bleeding can be just as severe. t-PA has less effect on the coagulation system, but this may be detrimental. The low fibrinogen levels seen regularly with streptokinase administration impair coagulation and reduce blood viscosity, which improves the rate of blood flow in stenotic areas. Widening the stenosis would seem to be the obvious approach, but angioplasty following t-PA has not substantially affected the end-results (TIMI Study Group 1989; TOPOL 1988).

It summary, until more data are available on the long-term results of t-PA therapy, it is difficult to assign a clear-cut advantage to using this much more expensive product rather than streptokinase. This question is now being addressed in studies currently under way: GISSI-2 (t-PA vs. streptokinase with all patients also receiving aspirin) and ISIS-3 (t-PA vs. streptokinase vs. APSAC with all patients also receiving aspirin).

Clinical data regarding scu-PA are still very preliminary (VAN DE WERF et al. 1986). Because of its short half-life (7 min), it must be given by infusion (intravenous or intracoronary) over 1–3 h. Reperfusion is achieved in about the same percentage of patients as with the other thrombolytic agents. A systemic fibrinolytic state results in most patients, and serious bleeding has occurred. The available data do not suggest that scu-PA offers any particular advantage in the treatment of acute coronary occlusion.

Table 5. Tissue-plasminogen activator (t-PA) in acute myocardial infarction: clinical trials

Trial	No. of patients (study/placebo)	Reperfusion %		Mortality %		Comments
		Control	Study	Control	Study	
GUERCI et al. (1987)	138 72/66 control: placebo	24	66	7.6	5.6	80–100 mg over 3 h. t-PA group had better ejection fraction and less congestive failure
TIMI-I (1985) SHEEHAN et al. (1987) CHESEBRO et al. (1987)	290 143/147 control: SK	30–40	60	8	5	No heparin. Less fall in fibrinogen with t-PA. Bleeding in ~45% both groups. No change in ejection fraction either group overall, only in those treated within 90 min of onset
VAN DE WERF and ARNOLD (1988) (European Cooperative Group)	721 355/366 controls: placebo	77	83	5.7 6.3	2.8 (overall) 1.1 (treated within 3 h of onset)	Heparin and ASA to all patients. t-PA 100 mg over 3 h. 4% reinfarction both groups. t-PA group had better ejection fraction and 20% less infarctions
WILCOX et. al (1988) (ASSET)	5011 2516/2495 control: placebo			9.8	7.2	All patients received heparin. Bleeding in 6.3% t-PA, 0.8% in controls
VERSTRAETE et al. (1985) (European Cooperative Study Group)	129 64/65 control:SK	55	70			Less bleeding with t-PA. Fibrinogen down to 65% for t-PA, 12% for SK

JOHNS et al. (1988) (rTTPA)	68 (no controls)		76			1 mg/kg for 90 min. Those achieving patency randomized to heparin vs. heparin and t-PA for 4 more h. Reocclusion in 19% of the heparin, 0% in t-PA and heparin
MAGNANI (1989) (PAIMS)	171 86/85 control:SK	79	79	8.2	4.6	Better increase in ejection fraction in t-PA group. Fibrinogen <100 mg/dl in 7% t-PA and in 87% SK
NEUHAUS et al. (1988) (GAUS)	238 121/117 control: UK	65.8	69.4	4.0	4.2	Reocclusion early: UK 1.6% t-PA 10.5%. Reocclusion late: UK 13.2% t-PA 8.9%
WHITE et al. (1989) (N. Zealand)	270 135/135 control: SK	75	76	8.9	At 9 months 5.9 (not significant) 5	Ejection fraction, end systolic vol., equal in both groups at 3 weeks. Reinfarction 5% in both groups at 30 days
TIMI-II (1989)	3262					150 mg t-PA and heparin followed by ASA, reduced later in study to 100 mg because of excess intracranial bleeding

SK, Streptokinase; UK, urokinase; ASA, acetylsalicylic acid; rTTPA, recombinant tissue-type plasminogen activator.

Sufficient results have now accumulated to prove that a short, bolus infusion of APSAC is effective therapy in acute coronary occlusion. Its long-lasting effect of 4–6 h is determined by its slow deacylation, which maintains the lytic state for this period of time without need of a long infusion or of adjunctive therapy (heparin or aspirin). Preliminary studies established the effective dose as 30 mg, which is given intravenously over 4–6 min. Published results are summarized in Table 6. All patients received similar doses, i.e., 30 mg, "U", by continuing infusion over 3 h. Although somewhat preliminary, these findings put APSAC well into the group of thrombolytic agents that are effective if used early in the treatment of acute coronary occlusion. Additional data from the ISIS-3 trial and long-term results should help establish its role more firmly. With its ease of administration and effectiveness, this may well become the agent of choice for treatment of acute coronary thrombosis.

2. Arterial Occlusion

In contrast to the vast number of studies done relative to thrombolytic therapy for coronary arteries, peripheral arteries have received little attention. Arterial occlusive disease is generally regarded as a condition requiring a surgical approach (embolectomy with or without reconstructive surgery to the vessel). This has been highly successful, but not all patients are candidates for surgery by virtue of other medical problems or because the occluded vessel is too small to allow a surgical approach (Kartchner and Wilcox 1976). Fibrinolytic therapy is then an acceptable alternative. This has been tried both regionally, with direct infusion of the occluded artery (Hess et al. 1982), or intravenously (Dardik et al. 1984), with systemic activation of the fibrinolytic system. The former is more effective (Marder and Francis 1984) and also permits angiograms during the infusion to evaluate progress in lysis of the thrombus.

Intravenous therapy leads to about 40% patency (complete to partial), but symptoms are at times much improved even if no change in the vessels can be demonstrated by angiography; perhaps collaterals, too small to be visualized, are reopened. Intraarterial therapy gives a somewhat higher reperfusion rate (45%–88%). Rethrombosis can occur with either form of therapy. Intraarterial therapy usually requires a dose which, when given as an infusion for several hours, is sufficient to produce the plasma lytic state. Failure of fibrinolytic therapy or demonstration of high-grade stenosis after successful lysis are indications for surgical intervention. It is more dangerous to attempt fibrinolytic therapy following unsuccessful surgery because of the likelihood of bleeding from the recent surgical wounds. Rarely, embolization from the original site (usually intracardiac) will occur. Streptokinase has been used in the majority of the reported series, but urokinase has also been employed successfully and may be superior to streptokinase (McNamara and Fischer 1985; Belkin et al. 1986). There is a single report of APSAC

Table 6. APSAC in acute myocardial infarction

Trial	No. of patients	Reperfusion %		Mortality %		Comments
		Control	Study	Control	Study	
MARDER et al. (1986)	15	–	60	–	–	Rethrombosis in 1 of 9 at 24 h
BEEN et al. (1985)	32	12	100	–	–	APSAC improved LV function in patients with anterior (37% vs. 23%) but not with inferior infarcts
AIMS (1988)	1004 control: placebo			12.2 (at 30 days)	6.4	Similar results in patients treated within 0–4 h and those treated 4–6 h after onset of symptoms.
				17 (at 1 year)	10	Very low incidence of bleeding
ANDERSON et al. (1988)	240 controls: SK-IC	60	51	<4 h 60 <4.33%		Reperfusion with APSAC in 43 min, with SK in 31 min

APSAC, *p*-anisoyl derivative of plasminogen-streptokinase activator complex; LV, left ventricle; SK, streptokinase; IC, intracoronary.

administered as intravenous boluses every 8 h. Results were similar to those with streptokinase.

Thrombolytic therapy for arterial occlusion has mainly been used for peripheral artery embolization, particularly of the lower extremities (AMERY et al. 1970; MARTIN 1979). In arterial thrombosis, the results are poorer because of the persisting vessel wall disease and stenosis that caused the clot in most of these patients. Surgery is usually required (MARTIN et al. 1970; VERSTRAETE et al. 1971). Thrombolytic therapy has been used successfully in a few cases of renal, hepatic, or superior mesenteric artery thrombosis (MARDER and BELL 1987) and for management of thrombosed prosthetic grafts (DARDIK et al. 1984). It has been effective in lysis of intracardiac clots (prosthetic valves) (ROUDAUT et al. 1987) and left ventricular mural thrombi. There are also some reports of successful thrombolytic therapy for basilar artery thrombosis (DEL ZOPPO et al. 1986; NENCI et al. 1983). The speed with which it can be administered is even more crucial here than in the case of coronary artery thrombosis since brain tissue remains viable only for a very short time once deprived of its arterial blood supply. The use of thrombolysis in stroke remains experimental at this time.

3. Pulmonary Embolism

Thrombolysis for treatment of pulmonary embolism has been approved (FDA 1977) but has never become popular and is rarely viewed as the preferred approach in a particular patient. Heparin therapy is the norm and has been so effective (BARRITT and JORDAN 1960) that any alternative will have to be proved superior. Intuitively, fibrinolytic therapy should be the approach and would also be expected to remove the source of the embolus, usually thrombus in the deep vein of the thigh or pelvis. Heparin stops propagation of the clots in the thigh and lung, while the patient's own fibrinolytic system removes the thrombi. In the lung this is quite effective, and thrombi are resolved spontaneously over several days. One of the main questions, therefore, will be whether the more rapid removal of the clots by thrombolytic agents improves the final outcome sufficiently in terms of preservation of pulmonary tissue and function, cardiac function, and patient survival to warrant the inherent risk of bleeding.

FLETCHER et al. (1959) first showed that streptokinase, intravenously given, produced prompt lysis of pulmonary emboli. Subsequently, a large number of small studies were carried out using streptokinase or urokinase. In two major studies, the UPET (Urokinase Pulmonary Embolism Trial 1970; 1973) and the USPET (Urokinase-Streptokinase Pulmonary Embolism Trial 1974), the effect of urokinase was compared with the effect of heparin alone, and the results of urokinase for 12 h was compared with the results of a 24-h infusion, and streptokinase was compared with urokinase. The doses of SK used were based on those developed for the treatment of acute myocardial infarction: a loading dose of 250 000 IU to neutralize any preexisting streptococcal-specific antibodies followed by 100 000 IU per h for 1–1.5 days. Results (measured by pulmonary angiography) were good, with 28%–60% of patients showing improvement (SERRADIMIGNI et al. 1987; OHAYON et al. 1986; LUOMANMAKI et al. 1983). The dosage of urokinase remains uncertain. The early trials, UPET and USPET, used a loading dose of 4400 IU/kg to establish a lytic state, followed by an infusion of 4400 IU/kg·h to maintain this state for 12 or 24 h. Both regimens were highly effective. Many of the other urokinase trials used different treatment regimens, making comparison of outcome confusing and leaving the question of preferred dose also uncertain. CELLA et al. (1987) have provided an excellent summary of these trials by dividing those with comparable treatment regimens into 4 groups according to the dose of urokinase used. Table 7 is adapted from their study and shows that urokinase is effective therapy, leading to prompt (1–3 days) improvement as demonstrated by angiography or lung scan and produces these results more quickly than heparin. Clinical parameters reported in the UPET and USPET studies improved concomitantly. Streptokinase treatment was equally effective. However, 2 weeks later the patients treated with heparin alone showed improvements on lung scan and arteriograms comparable in all ways to those seen in the urokinase- or streptokinase-treated patients.

More recently, similar clinical trials mostly conducted by GOLDHABER and his group using t-PA have shown that it is as effective as urokinase and streptokinase in obtaining reperfusion of lung tissue and in improving right heart function (GOLDHABER et al. 1988; VERSTRAETE et al. 1988; National Institute of Health Consensus Development Conference 1980). Various regimens were used, but it was finally shown that 100 mg given intravenously

Table 7. Pulmonary embolism urokinase trials, subgroups by dosage

	No. of patients	Dose (IU/kg)		Time	Percentage improvement		
		Loading	Maintenance	(h)	Lung scan	Angiography	Bleeding (%)
Group I	143	4400	4400	12	20–22	41–45	25–31
	125	0	4000–4500	12	–	20–39	0–22
Group II	11	2700	2700	12	–	38	45
	132	0	2000–2750	12–24	–	26–41	0–24
Group III	107	0	1000–1600	24[a]	–	34–51	0–3
Group IV	21	15,000	–	Bolus	–	34	0

[a] One study of 10 patients gave urokinase for 12–72 h

Group I: Urokinase Pulmonary Embolism Trial 1973; USPET 1974; SERRADIMIGNI et al. 1984; Groupe de Recherche Urokinase-Embolie Pulmonaire 1984; OHAYON 1986

Group II: SERRADIMIGNI et al. 1984; Groupe de Recherche Urokinase-Embolie Pulmonaire 1984; BARBARENA 1983; MARINI et al. 1987

Group III: MARINI et al. 1987; GRIGUER et al. 1979; FRANCOIS et al. 1986; BROCHIER et al. 1976

Group IV: DICKIE et al. 1974; DUROUX et al. 1984.

over 2 h produces excellent clot lysis which was not significantly improved by extending the duration of the infusion (Goldhaber et al. 1988). Some 82% of patients who received t-PA at this rate had clot lysis demonstrated by angiography; only 48% of patients receiving standard dose urokinase showed similar improvement after 2 h. Moreover, there was less bleeding with t-PA. In this study, urokinase administration was continued for an additional 22 h (the FDA approved dosage regimen) if lysis was not demonstrated on the angiogram performed after 2 h of treatment. When both groups were reevaluated at 24 h, the angiogram results were identical. The value of t-PA vs. urokinase, therefore, lies in the speed with which dissolution of the clots can be achieved, an important point in a critically ill patient.

Studies in Europe (Verstraete et al. 1988), performed on patients with massive pulmonary embolism, showed that intravenously given t-PA therapy was as effective as t-PA infused into the affected branch of the pulmonary artery. There was no difference in side effects.

All these investigations have demonstrated that thrombolytic therapy rapidly lyses pulmonary emboli in a considerable percentage of patients, with measurable improvement in lung perfusion and right ventricle function. There is a small but significant risk of serious bleeding. Since management with heparin alone is so satisfactory, one of the main remaining questions is who can and should be treated? The NIH Consensus Conference (1980) concluded that thrombolytic therapy should be used in patients with thrombosis of the deep veins of the thigh and pelvis and in those with large pulmonary emboli or significant hemodynamic disturbances from pulmonary emboli. In spite of these recommendations physicians, in general, have not adopted thrombolytic therapy for most of these patients. A recent, large, collaborative, clinical trial, Thrombolysis in Pulmonary Embolism (TIPE) (Terrin et al. 1989), addresses this question from a different perspective. They surveyed the medical records of over 2500 patients with the diagnosis of pulmonary embolism. After disqualifying all those considered to be at risk of bleeding, using very conservative criteria, they found that 53% of the patients would have been acceptable candidates for t-PA treatment. The most pressing question remains unanswered: How many of these patients would have done better with thrombolytic therapy? With the data currently available it seems reasonable to reserve treatment for seriously ill patients in whom the results with thrombolysis are superior to those for thrombectomy. If very rapid improvement is needed, t-PA is probably the preferred agent. Studies underway (Goldhaber et al. 1989) using different dosage regimens for urokinase (5 million U in 2 h) might prove it to be equally efficacious (and less expensive). Results with APSAC would be especially interesting (bolus dose, low cost).

4. Deep Venous Thrombosis

There is general agreement that venous thrombi can be dissolved with thrombolytic therapy and that recently formed thrombi are more readily lysed than old ones (MARDER and BELL 1987). Most cases of venous thrombosis involve the lower extremities. It is a common problem affecting many thousands of patients in the USA yearly. Although known for over 25 years to be effective, thrombolytic therapy has not become the mainstay of treatment; that remains the immediate institution of heparin followed by an extended period of oral anticoagulation. No large clinical trials have ever compared these two forms, although there have been numerous, small, randomized, and controlled studies which, taken in aggregate, provide useful data. Analysis of results ideally requires angiographic evaluation of clots in the veins before and after therapy. The clinical picture is notoriously undependable, with many clots producing no symptoms and similarly many patients with pain and swelling who have no demonstrable clots on angiography. The actual age of clots demonstrated on angiography is, therefore, uncertain. Table 8 summarizes the short-term results of some of these studies in which angiographic documentation was obtained. All compared streptokinase therapy with heparin therapy. Streptokinase was used in the standard dosage of 250000 IU as an initial bolus followed by 100000 IU/h for 3–4 days. Disappearance of the clot, partial or nearly total, was shown in 66% of patients treated with streptokinase but in only 24% of those receiving heparin. Most investigators reported symptomatic improvement corresponding with the angiographic improvement, but in some patients symptoms improved without demonstrable change in the angiogram. Perhaps collaterals too small to be visualized had been reopened.

Short-term reopening of veins, however, does not necessarily indicate long-term benefit for the patient. The postphlebitic syndrome, indicating permanent disruption of normal venous return from the legs, eventually develops in a very large number of patients (90%–94%) treated with heparin (GJÖRES 1956; ELLIOTT et al. 1979). About 15% of these have serious symptoms (claudication or stasis ulcres). Venous insufficiency occurs as a consequence of scarring, failure to recanalize some veins, and incompetent venous valves which were damaged by the thrombi during the acute episode. Preservation of venous valves, therefore, should be an important therapeutic goal. Venographic examinations performed months to years later show impressive differences in most studies: 60% of the venograms in the

Table 8. Streptokinase (SK) vs. heparin for deep vein thrombosis: summary of seven controlled trials. KAKKAR et al. 1969; ROSCH et al. 1976; MARDER et al. 1977; ARNESEN et al. 1982; ELLIOTT et al. 1979; WATZ and SAVIDGE 1979; DUCKERT et al. 1975.

	No. of patients	Degree of lysis		
		Considerable	Some	More
SK	193	89 (46%)	38 (20%)	66 (34%)
Heparin	145	6 (4%)	29 (20%)	110 (76%)

streptokinase-treated patients were normal, whereas only 11% were normal in patients who had received heparin. Persistent changes in the veins predisposes to the postphlebitic syndrome (Immelman and Jeffery 1984). Two reports present a less optimistic outcome (Albrechtsen et al. 1981; Kakkar and Lawrence 1985): Reporting on a total of around 100 streptokinase-treated patients, they found little difference 2 years later in the veins and the patients' functional status between those who had received streptokinase and those treated with heparin.

Employment of urokinase leads to results comparable with those obtained with streptokinase (Trübestein 1984; Van De Loo et al. 1983). Use of t-PA or APSAC has not been described. Thrombolytic therapy has also been successful in the treatment of venous thrombosis in the upper extremities and in the abdomen (Marder and Sherry 1988).

As fibrinolytic therapy is effective in controlling the acute disease and in reducing its serious sequelae, it is remarkable that thrombolysis has not become standard therapy. The answer undoubtedly lies in the fear of inducing serious bleeding with thrombolytic agents. Hemorrhagic complications occur 2.9 times more frequently with streptokinase than with heparin (Samama 1987; Bieger 1976). One might suppose that this is due to the prolonged exposure to streptokinase (usually 3 days). Effective thrombolysis has been demonstrated over 12 h in a small number of patients (Watz and Savidge 1979). A prospective study using a short course of streptokinase or urokinase could be useful in validating the effectiveness. Three days or longer may be unnecessary in many patients. The rate of bleeding complications would probably be less with the shorter duration of thrombolysis. Other than bleeding, there are no complications, embolization occurs no more frequently than in the heparinized patient.

C. Antithrombotic Therapy

Apart from the anticoagulant and fibrinolytic management of thrombosis already described in this chapter and the platelet inhibitory therapy described in other chapters in this volume, there are several further approaches which will be discussed in less detail. Two of these, physical methods and dextran application have been used primarily with surgical patients to reduce postoperative deep vein thrombosis and pulmonary embolism.

I. Dextrans

Dextrans are partially hydrolysed glucose polymers produced by the bacteria *Leuconostoc mesenteroides* which exist in a wide range of molecular sizes. Clinically, two preparations are used, dextran-40 and dextran-70 with average molecular weights of 40000 and 70000 respectively. Both have been shown to have antithrombotic activity which appears to be mainly due to their effect on platelets. Possibly because the dextran molecules are adsorbed to the platelet surface, following exposure, platelet adhesiveness and aggregation are depressed, and the release reaction is impaired (CRONBERG et al. 1966; BYGDEMAN et al. 1966). Clots formed in the presence of dextran have an abnormal structure and lower tensile strength (DHALL et al. 1976).

Several studies were performed during the 1960s and 1970s and are reviewed by KAKKAR (1981) and SALZMAN and HIRSH (1987). Results are not clear cut, and even these reviewers come to different conclusions. In several studies that employed leg scans as the end-point in general or gynecologic surgery patients, dextran appears to reduce the incidence of thrombosis about as much as low-dose heparin prophylaxis. In other studies of similar patients, no benefit was demonstrated. In patients undergoing hip surgery, a considerable reduction (~50%) in the occurrence of deep vein thrombi was found. In a large multicenter trial involving surgical patients in general, dextran was found to have as beneficial an effect as low-dose heparin on the incidence of fatal pulmonary embolism (GRUBER et al. 1980). However, several previous investigations had shown only a non-significant trend in favor of dextran (BRISMAN et al. 1971).

The consensus seems to be that dextran is as effective in the prevention of deep vein thrombosis in the surgical patient as low-dose heparin. Bleeding complications will also occur in about the same percentage of patients (SALZMAN et al. 1971). It, therefore, appears to offer little advantage. Dextran is administered intravenously. A single dose is given at the time of surgery and is not repeated if very early ambulation is expected. The patient who has a considerable period in bed postoperatively is given 500 ml of a 10% w/v solution of dextran-40 daily for 3 days, then every 3rd day until fully ambulatory. Because of its low molecular weight, dextran-40 has a short half-life and, being excreted by the kidneys, can produce a considerable solute diuresis. Dextran-70 is not excreted in this way but is removed slowly by the reticuloendothelial system, making infrequent dosing sufficient to maintain an effective plasma level. Allergic reactions to dextrans are fairly common. Anaphylactic reactions have occurred (RING and MESSMER 1977).

II. Physical Methods

Pulmonary embolism in postoperative patients is a common problem and a major cause of death, especially after hip fracture or surgery. Prevention of pulmonary emboli requires prevention of the thrombi that eventually embolize. The emboli usually come from clots that form in the legs during the periods of immobility associated with surgery (FLANC et al. 1969). It has long been recognized that early ambulation of the postoperative patient reduces the incidence of pulmonary embolism dramatically (SALZMAN et al. 1966). However, not all patients can be mobilized promptly, and various methods designed to decrease venous pooling (thus reducing the opportunity for clot formation) have been devised. Simple elastic stockings, intended to compress superficial veins, thus forcing added flow through the deep veins, did not prove to be effective in preventing thrombosis (ROSENGARTEN et al. 1971). However, stockings designed to exert greater pressure distally (graduated compression stockings) did reduce thrombus formation in general surgical patients (SCURR et al. 1977) and are now widely used with medical and surgical patients. Devices are employed to stimulate electrically the calf muscles intraoperatively (ROSENBERG et al. 1975) or to exert external pneumatic compression (MCMANAMA et al. 1984) on the legs. Both approaches are effective in reducing the incidence of thrombosis to about the same degree as low-dose heparin (SALZMAN and HIRSH 1987). The chief use of these more cumbersome methods would seem to be in those patients who have contraindications to the use of low-dose heparin.

Once thrombosis with pulmonary embolism has occurred, the pharmacologic therapies already described are the preferred approach. Although surgical removal of the embolus from the pulmonary artery seems logical, the mortality associated with this procedure is very high. In the critically ill patient, thrombolysis offers a safer approach (MILLER et al. 1977). In the patient who continues to have proven pulmonary emboli in spite of adequate anticoagulation, surgical interruption of the inferior vena cava may become necessary (STANSEL 1982; GOMEZ et al. 1982). This is now usually accomplished by the placement of a device such as the Greenfield filter (GREENFIELD et al. 1973) which traps emboli but does not totally block blood flow through the vena cava (SCHRÖEDER et al. 1978). It is inserted in its folded shape via the internal jugular vein, then release at the desired site where it opens; the arms hook into the vessel wall, thus holding it in place. These devices are well tolerated by most patients. Should the vena cava become completely occluded, about half of the patients will have leg edema to some degree. Large collateral veins may also develop which can allow passage of emboli.

III. Defibrinogenating Agents

In 1963, REID and associates noted that patients who had been bitten by the Malayan pit viper (*Agkistrodon rhodostoma*) had incoagulable blood yet did not have a hemorrhagic tendency. Since then, extracts from two snake venoms have been developed for clinical use: ancrod from the venom of the Malayan pit viper and batroxobin from the venom of *Bothrops atrox* (South American pit viper). Both of these substances release peptide A from fibrinogen which then undergoes end-to-end polymerization and, in the intact animal, is removed by the reticuloendothelial system. Ancrod further digests peptide A, Batroxobin does not but does activate Factor XIII. Neither acts on any of the other clotting factors. Both are inhibited by α_2-macroglobulin but are not affected by heparin, AT III, or ε-aminocaproic acid. Both are antigenic, although antibody production during treatment is rarely seen. Heterologous antibodies are used to neutralize the action on fibrinogen when it is necessary to reverse the effect of the enzyme. Fibrinogen is then administered, since otherwise hypofibrinogenemia will persist for several days.

Both ancrod and batroxobin have been used clinically in the treatment of both arterial and venous thrombosis. Several reports dealing with small numbers of patients have been published (Kounis and Evans 1979; Kakkar et al. 1969; Olsson et al. 1976) comparing results of treatment or prophylaxis of deep vein thrombosis with defibrinogenating agents with either anticoagulant or fibrinolytic therapy. The consensus is that ancrod is as effective as low-dose heparin for the surgical patient and standard-dose heparin for the patient with venous thrombosis (Pitney 1971; Latallo 1978). Both ancrod and batroxobin are best administered intravenously. An initial slow infusion is given during which the patient's fibrinogen level falls quickly to 50 mg/dl or less. Maintenance of hypofibrinogenemia is accomplished by once or twice daily booster infusions. Therapy is monitored by fibrinogen determinations. In spite of these very low fibrinogen levels, abnormal bleeding is unusual, even in the surgical patient (Olsson et al. 1976). It has been shown that there is a significant decrease in blood viscosity when the fibrinogen level is low and that this should improve blood flow through small or compromised vessels (Lowe 1981).

Very thorough reviews of these enzymes and their uses can be found in the Handbook of Experimental Pharmacology, vol. 46 (Stocker 1978) and by Bell in Colman et al. (1987).

References

Abernethy EA, Hartsuck JM (1974) Postoperative pulmonary embolism: a prospective study utilizing low-dose heparin. Am J Surg 128:739–742

Agnelli G, Buchanan MR, Fernandez I, Boneu B, Van Ryn J, Hirsh J, Collen D (1985) A comparison of thrombolytic and hemorrhagic effects of tissue-type plasminogen activator and streptokinase in rabbits. Circulation 72:178–182

AIMS Trial Study Group (1988) Effect of intravenous APSAC on mortality after acute myocardial infarction: preliminary report of a placebo-controlled clinical trial. Lancet 1:545–549

Akbarian M, Austin WG, Yurchak PM, Scannel JG (1968) Thromboembolic complications of prosthetic cardiac valves. Circulation 37:826–831

Akle CA, Joiner CL (1981) Purple toe syndrome. J R Soc Med 74:219

Albrechtsen V, Anderson J, Einarsson E, Eklof B, Norgren L (1981) Streptokinase treatment of deep-vein thrombosis and the post-thrombotic syndrome. Arch Surg 116:33–37

Amery A, Deloof W, Vermylen J, Verstraete M (1970) Outcome of recent thromboembolic occlusions of limb arteries treated with streptokinase. BMJ 4:639–644

Anderson JH, Rothbard RL, Hockworthy RA, Sorenson SG, Fitzpatrick PG, Dahl CF, Hagan AD, Browne KF, Symkoviak GP, Menlove R, Barry WH, Eckerson HW, Marder VJ for the APSAC Multicenter Investigators (1988) Multicenter reperfusion trial of intravenous anisoylated plasminogen-streptokinase activator complex (APSAC) in acute myocardial infarction: controlled comparison with intracoronary streptokinase. J Am Coll Cardiol 11:1153–1163

Anderson JL, Marshall HW, Bray BE, Lutz JR, Frederick PR, Yanowitz FG, Datz FL, Klausner SC, Hagen AD (1983) A randomized trial of intracoronary streptokinase in the treatment of acute myocardial infarction. NEJM 308:1312–1318

Arnesen H, Heilo A, Jakobsen E, Ly B, Skaga E (1978) A prospective study of streptokinase and heparin in the treatment of deep-vein thrombosis. Acta Med Scand 203:457–463

Arnesen H, Hoiset A, Ly B, Godal HC (1982) Streptokinase or heparin in the treatment of deep-vein thrombosis: follow-up results of a prospective study. Acta Med Scand 211:65–68

Ashenburg RJ (1990) (letter to the editor) J Bone Joint Surg [Am] 72:153

Bachmann F (1987) Plasminogen activators. In: Colman RW, Hirsh J, Marder VJ, Salzman EW (eds) Hemostasis and thrombosis: basic principles and clinical practice, 2nd edn. J B Lippincott, Philadelphia, pp 318–339

Baglin JY, Diebold B, Henin D, Groussard O, Pansard Y, Touche T, Leveque D, Merillon JP, Gourgon R (1983) Thrombose de prothese valvulaire: embolie cerebrale mortelle lors du traitement thrombolytique. Arch Mal Coeur 76: 1077–1080

Ballard RM, Bradley-Watson PJ, Johnstone FD, Kenney A, McCarthy TG, Campbell S, Weston J (1973) Low doses of subcutaneous heparin in the prevention of deep-vein thrombosis after gynecological surgery. J Obstet Gynecol Br Commonw 80:469–472

Barbarena J (1983) Intraarterial infusion of urokinase in the treatment of acute pulmonary thromboembolism: preliminary observations. AJR 140:833–836

Barritt DW, Jordan SC (1960) Anticoagulant drugs in the treatment of pulmonary embolism: a controlled trial. Lancet 1:1309–1312

Basu D, Gallus A, Hirsh J, Cade J (1972) A prospective study of the value of monitoring heparin treatment with the activated PTT. NEJM 287:324–327

Bates ER, Califf RM, Stack RS, Aronson L, George BS, Candela RJ, Kereiakes DJ, Abbottsmith CW, Anderson L, Pitt B, O'Neill WW, Topol EJ, The Thrombolysis and Angioplasty in Myocardial Infarction Study Group (1989) Thrombolysis and angioplasty in myocardial infarction (TAMI-I) trial: influence of infarct location on arterial patency, left ventricular function, and mortality. J Am Coll Cardiol 13:12–18

Been M, de Bono DP, Muir AL, Boulton FE, Hillis WS, Hornung R (1985) Coronary thrombolysis with intravenous anisoylated plasminogen-streptokinase complex BRL 26921. Br Heart J 53:253–259

Beisaw NE, Comerota AJ, Groth HE, Merli GJ, Weitz HH, Zimmerman RC, DiSerio FJ, Sasahara AA (1988) Dihydroergotamine/heparin in the prevention of deep-vein thrombosis after total hip replacement. J Bone Joint Surg [Am] 70:2–10

Belkin M, Belkin B, Bucknam CA, Straut J, Lowe R (1985) Intraarterial fibrinolytic therapy: efficacy of streptokinase vs. urokinase. Arch Surg 121:769–775

Bell WR (1987) Defibrinogenating enzymes. In: Colman RW, Hirsch J, Marder VJ, Salzmann EW (eds) Hemostasis and thrombosis: basic principles and clinical practice, 2nd ed. Lippincott, Philadelphia, pp 886–900

Bell WR, Tomasulo PA, Alving BM, Duffy TP (1976) Thrombocytopenia occurring during the administration of heparin: a prospective study of 52 patients. Ann Int Med 85:155–160

Bergkvist R (1963) The proteolytic enzymes of *Aspergillus oryzae*. III. A comparison of the fibrinolytic and fibrinogenolytic effects of the enzymes. Acta Chem Scand 17:2230–2238

Bergmann SR, Lerch RA, Fox KAA, Ludbrook PA, Welch MJ, Ter-Pogossian MM, Sobel BE (1982) Temporal dependence of beneficial effects of coronary thrombolysis characterized by positron tomography. Am J Med 73:573–581

Bergqvist D, Burmark VS, Frisell J, Hallbook T, Lindblad B, Resberg B, Torngren S, Wallin G (1986) Low molecular weight heparin once daily compared with conventional low-dose heparin twice daily. A prospective double-blind multicenter trial on prevention of postoperative thrombosis. Br J Surg 73:204–208

Bieger R, Bockhout-Mussert RJ, Hohmann F, Loeliger EA (1976) Is streptokinase useful in the treatment of deep-vein thrombosis? Acta Med Scand 199:81–88

Bjerkelund CJ, Orning OM (1969) The efficacy of anticoagulant therapy in preventing embolism related to DC electrical conversion of atrial fibrillation. Am J Cardiol 23:208–216

Bjornsson TD (1982) Dose dependent decrease in heparin elimination. J Pharm Sci 71:1186–1188

Bjornsson TD, Wolfram KM, Kitchell BB (1982) Heparin kinetics determined by 3 assay methods. Clin Pharmacol Ther 31:104–113

Boucek RJ, Murphy WP Jr (1960) Segmental perfusion of the coronary arteries with fibrinolysin in man following a myocardial infarction. J Cardiol 6:525–533

Braunwald E, Knatterud GL, Passamani E, Robertson TL, Solomon R (1987) Update from the thrombolysis in myocardial infarction trial. J Am Coll Cardiol 10:970

Brisman R, Parks L, Haller JA Jr (1971) Dextran prophylaxis in surgery. Ann Surg 174:137–141

Broekmans AW, Veltkamp JJ, Bertina RM (1983) Congenital protein C deficiency and venous thromboembolism: a study of three Dutch families. NEJM 309: 340–344

Buchanan MR, Boneu B, Ofosu F, Hirsh J (1985) The relative importance of thrombin inhibition and factor X_A inhibition to the antithrombotic effect of heparin. Blood 65:198–201

Bygdeman S (1969) Prevention and therapy of thromboembolic complications with dextran. Prog Surg 7:114–139

Bygdeman S, Eliasson R, Gullbring B (1966) Effect of dextran infusion on the adenosine induced adhesiveness and the spreading capacity of human blood platelets. Thromb Diath Haemorrh 15:451–456

Caen JP (1988) A randomized double-blind study between a low molecular weight heparin Kabi 2165 and standard heparin in the prevention of deep-vein thrombosis in general surgery. Thromb Hemost 59:216–220

Califf RM, Stump D, Thornton D, Kereiakes DJ, George BS, Abbottsmith CW, Candela RJ, Boswick JM, Topol EJ, TAMI Study Group (1987) Hemorrhagic complications after tissue plasminogen activator (t-PA) therapy for acute myocardial infarction. Circulation 76:IV–1

Camiolo SM, Thorsen S, Astrup T (1971) Fibrinogenolysis and fibrinolysis with tissue plasminogen activator, urokinase, streptokinase activated human globulin and plasmin. Proc Soc Exp Biol Med 138:277–280

Carter CJ, Kelton JG, Hirsh J, Cerskus AL, Santos AV, Gent M (1982) The relationship between the hemorrhagic versus antithrombotic properties of low molecular weight heparin in rabbits. Blood 59:1239–1245

Casu B (1984) Structure of heparins and their fragments. Nouv Rev Fr Hematol 24:211–219

Cella G, Palla A, Sasahara AA (1987) Controversies of different regimens of thrombolytic therapy in acute pulmonary embolism. Semin Thromb Hemost 13:163–170

Chandler AB, Chapman I, Erhardt LR, Roberts WC, Schwartz CJ, Sinapius D, Spain DM, Sherry S, Ness PM, Simon TL (1974) Coronary thrombosis in myocardial infarction: report of a workshop on the role of coronary thrombosis in the pathogenesis of acute myocardial infarction. Am J Cardiol 34:823–833

Chesebro JH, Knatterud G, Roberts R, Borer J, Cohen LS, Dalen J, Dodge HT, Francis CK, Hillis D, Ludbrook P, Markis JE, Mueller H, Passamani ER, Powers ER, Rao AK, Robertson T, Ross A, Ryan JJ, Sobol BE, Willerson J,

Williams DO, Zaret BL, Braunwald E (1987) Thrombolysis in myocardial infarction (TIMI) trial, phase I: a comparison between intravenous plasminogen activator and intravenous streptokinase. Circulation 76:142–154

Chiu HM, Hirsh J, Yung W, Regoeczi E, Gent M (1977) Relationship between the anticoagulant and antithrombotic effect of heparin in experimental venous thrombosis. Blood 49:171–184

Choay J (1989) Structure and activity of heparin and its fragments: an overview. Semin Thromb Hemost 15:359–364

Chong BH, Grace C, Rozenberg MC (1981) Heparin-induced thrombocytopenia: effect of heparin platelet antibody on platelets. Br J Haematol 49:531–540

Cimo PL, Moake JL, Weinger RS, Ben Menochem Y, Khalil KG (1979) Heparin-induced thrombocytopenia. Association with a platelet aggregating factor and arterial thrombosis. Am J Hematol 6:125–133

Cines DB, Kaywin P, Bina M, Tomaski A, Schreiber AD (1980) Heparin associated thrombocytopenia. NEJM 303:788–795

Cines DB, Tomaski A, Tannenbaum S (1987) Immune endothelial cell injury in heparin-associated thrombocytopenia. NEJM 316:581–589

Cipolle RJ, Seifert RD, Neilan BA, Zaske DE, Haus E (1981) Heparin kinetics: variables related to disposition and dosage. Clin Pharmacol Ther 29:387–393

Coccheri S, De Rosa V, Dettori AG, Ponari O, Bizzi B, Ciavarella N, Isidori A (1982) Effect on fibrinolysis of a new antithrombotic agent: fraction P (defibrotide). A multicenter trial. Int J Clin Pharmacol Res 2:227–245

Collen D, DeCock F, Lijnen HR (1984) Biological and thrombolytic properties of proenzyme and active forms of human urokinase II. Turnover of natural and recombinant urokinase in rabbits and squirrel monkeys. Thromb Haemost 52: 24–26

Collen D, Bounameaux H, De Cock F, Lijnen HR, Verstraete M (1986) Analysis of coagulation and fibrinolysis during intravenous infusion of recombinant human tissue-type plasminogen activator in patients with acute myocardial infarction. Circulation 73:511–517

Coller BS (1990) Platelets and thrombolytic therapy. NEJM 322:33–42

Common HH, Seaman RH, Rosch J, Porter JM, Dotter C (1976) A deep-vein thrombosis treated with streptokinase or heparin: follow-up of randomized study. Angiology 27:645–654

Coon WW, Willie PW III, Symons MJ (1969) Assessment of anticoagulant treatment of venous thromboembolism. Ann Surg 170:559–567

Covey TH, Sherman L, Baue AE (1975) Low dose heparin in postoperative patients. Arch Surg 110:1021–1025

Cronberg S, Robertson B, Nilsson IM, Nilehn JE (1966) Suppressive effect of dextran on platelet adhesiveness. Thromb Diath Haemorrh 16:384–394

Cunningham M, deTorrente A, Ekoe J-M, Ackermann J-P, Humair L (1984) Vascular spasm and gangrene during heparin-dihydro-ergotamine prophylaxis. Br J Surg 71:829–831

Dale J, Myhre JE, Storstein O, Stormorken H, Efskind L (1977) Prevention of arterial thromboembolism with acetylsalicylic acid. A controlled clinical study in patients with aortic ball valves. Am Heart J 94:101–111

Dardik H, Sussman BC, Kahn M, Greweldinger J, Adler J, Mendes D, Svoboda J, Ibrahim IM (1984) Lysis of arterial clot by intravenous or intraarterial administration of streptokinase. Surg Gynecol Obstet 158:137–140

Davey MG, Lander H (1968) Effect of heparin on platelets in vivo. J Clin Pathol 21:55–59

Dechavanne M, Saudin F, Viola JJ, Kher A, Bertrix L, de Mourgues G (1974) Prevention des thromboses veineuses: succes de l'heparine à fortes doses lors des coxarthroses. Nouv Presse Med 3:1317–1319

Del Zoppo GJ, Zeumer H, Harker LA (1986) Thrombolytic therapy in stroke: possibilities and hazards. Stroke 17:595–607 de Swart CAM, Nijmeyer B, Roelofs JMM, Sixma JJ (1982) Kinetics of intravenously administered heparin in normal humans. Blood 60:1251–1258

DeWood MA, Spores J, Notske R, Mouser LT, Burroughs R, Golden MS, Lang HT (1980) Prevalence of total coronary occlusion during the early hours of transmural myocardial infarction. NEJM 303:897–902

DeWood MA, Spores J, Hensley JR, Simpson CS, Eugster GS, Sutherland KI, Grunwald RR, Shields JP (1983) Coronary arteriographic findings in acute transmural MI. Circulation 68[Suppl I]:39–49

Dhall TZ, Bryce WAJ, Dhall DP (1976) Effects of dextran on the molecular structure and tensile behavior of human fibrin. Thromb Haemost 35:737–745

Dickie KJ, de Grott WJ, Cooley RN, Bond TP, Guest MM (1974) Hemodynamic effects of bolus infusion of urokinase in pulmonary embolism. Am Rev Respir Dis 109:48–56

Duckert F, Muller G, Nymen D, Benz A, Prisender S, Madar G, da Silva MA, Widmer LK, Schmitt HE (1975) Treatment of deep-vein thrombosis with streptokinase. BMJ 1:479–481

Dupe RJ, English PD, Smith RAG, Green J (1983) The activity of an acylated streptokinase-plasminogen complex (BR26921) in dog models of thrombosis. In: Davidson JF, Backmann F, Bouvier CA, Kruithof EKO (eds) Progress in fibrinolysis, vol VI. Churchill Livingstone, Edinburgh, pp 240–244.

Dupe RJ, Smith RAG, Green J (1985) Responses of experimental venous clots, aged in vivo in dogs, to acylated and unmodified streptokinase-plasminogen complexes. In: Davidson JF, Donati MD, Coccheri S (eds) Progress in fibrinolysis, vol VIII. Churchill Livingstone, Edinburgh, pp 241–245

DuPont Company (1986) Letter sent to all US physicians. (unpublished)

Duroux P, Simonneau G, Petitpretz P, Herve P (1984) Therapeutic approaches to acute pulmonary embolism. Intensive Care Med 10:99–102

Eika C (1972) The platelet aggregating effect of 8 commercial heparins. Scand J Haematol 9:480–482

Eika C, Godal HC, Loake K, Hamburg T (1980) Low incidence of thrombocytopenia during treatment with hog mucosa and beef lung heparin. Scand J Haematol 25:19–24

Elliott MS, Immelman EJ, Jeffery P, Benatar SR, Funston MR, Smith JA, Shepstone BJ, Ferguson D, Jacobs P, Walker W, Louw JH (1979) A comparative randomized trial of heparin versus streptokinase in the treatment of acute proximal venous thrombosis: an interim report of a prospective trial. Br J Surg 66:828–834

Eriksson BI, Zachrisson BE, Teger-Nilsson A-C, Risberg B (1988) Thrombosis prophylaxis with low molecular weight heparin in total hip replacement. Br J Surg 75:1053–1057

European Cooperative Study Group for streptokinase treatment in acute myocardial infarction (1979) Streptokinase in acute myocardial infarction. NEJM 301: 797–802

European Fraxiparin Study (EFS) Group (1988) Comparison of a low molecular weight heparin and unfractionated heparin in the prevention of deep venous thrombosis in patients undergoing abdominal surgery. Br J Surg 75:1058–1063

Fears R, Green J, Smith RAG, Walker P (1985) Induction of a sustained fibrinolytic response by BRL 26921 in vitro. Thromb Res 38:251–260

Fernandez F, Nguyen P, Van Ryn J, Ofusu FA, Hirsh J, Buchanan MR (1986a) Hemorrhagic doses of heparin and other glycosaminoglycans induce a platelet defect. Thromb Res 43:491–495

Fernandez F, Van Ryn J, Ofosu JA, Hirsh J, Buchanan MR (1986b) The haemorrhagic and antithrombotic effects of dermatan sulfate. Br J Haematol 64:309–317

Fidler E, Jacques LB (1948) The effect of commercial heparin on the platelet count. J Lab Clin Med 33:1410–1423

Fine DG, Weiss AT, Sapoznikov D, Welber S, Applebaum D, Lotan C, Hasin Y, Ben-David Y, Koren G, Gotsman MS (1986) Importance of early initiation of intravenous streptokinase therapy for acute myocardial infarction. Am J Cardiol 58:411–417

Flanc C, Kakkar VV, Clarke MB (1969) Postoperative deep-vein thrombosis: effect of intensive prophylaxis. Lancet 1:477–478

Fletcher AP, Alkjaersig N, Sherry S (1959) The maintenance of a sustained thrombolytic state in man. Induction and effects. JCI 38:1096–1110

Fletcher AP, Alkjaersig N, Sherry S (1962) Fibrinolytic mechanisms and the development of thrombolytic therapy. Am J Med 33:738–752

Fletcher AP, Alkjaersig N, Smyrniotis FE, Sherry S (1958) The treatment of patients suffering from early myocardial infarction with massive and prolonged streptokinase therapy. Trans Assoc Am Physicians 71:287–295

Fletcher AP, Alkjaersig N, Sherry S, Genton E, Hirsh J, Bachmann I (1965) The development of urokinase as a thrombolytic agent. Maintenance of a sustained thrombolytic state in man by its intravenous infusion. J Lab Clin Med 65: 713–731

Flickinger EG, Johnsrude IS, Ogburn NL, Weaver MD, Pories WJ (1983) Local streptokinase infusion for superior mesenteric artery thromboembolism. AJR 140:771–772

Francis CW, Marder VJ (1990) Mechanisms of fibrinolysis. In: Williams WJ, Beutler E, Erslev AF, Lichtman ML (eds) Hematology, 4th edn. McGraw-Hill, New York, pp 1313–1321

Francis CW, Malone JE, Marder VJ (1985) Comparison of chromogenic prothrombin time with clotting prothrombin time in the assessment of clinical coagulation deficiencies. Am J Clin Pathol 84:724–729

Francois G, Charbonnier B, Raynaud P, Garnier LF, Griguer P, Brochier M (1986) Traitement de l'embolie pulmonaire aiguë par urokinase comparée à l'association plasminogène-urokinase. A propos de 67 cas. Arch Mal Coeur 79:435–442

Fratantoni JC, Pollet R, Gralnick HR (1975) Heparin-induced thrombocytopenia: confirmation of diagnosis with in vitro methods. Blood 45:395–401

Freiman G (1987) The structure of thrombi. In: Colman RW, Hirsch J, Marder VJ, Salzman EW (eds) Hemostasis and thrombosis: basic principles and clinical practice, 2nd ed. Lippincott, Philadelphia, pp 1123–1135

Friedli B, Aerichide N, Grondin P, Campeau L (1971) Thromboembolic complications of heart valve prosthesis. Am Heart J 81:702–708

Frisch EP (1989) Clinical pharmacology of the thrombolytic enzyme preparation brinase. Semin Thromb Hemost 15:341–346

Furberg CD (1984) Clinical value of intracoronary streptokinase. Am J Cardiol 53:626–627

Furie B, Diuguid CF, Jacobs M, Diuguid DL, Furie BC (1990) Randomized prospective trial comparing the native prothrombin antigen with the prothrombin time for monitoring oral anticoagulant therapy. Blood 75:344–349

Gallus AS, Hirsh J, Tuttle RJ, Trebilcock R, O'Brien SE, Carrol JJ, Minder JH, Hudecki SM (1973) Small subcutaneous doses of heparin in prevention of venous thrombosis. NEJM 288:545–551

Gallus AS, Hirsh J, O'Brien SE, McBride JA, Tuttle RJ, Gent M (1975) Prevention of venous thrombosis with small subcutaneous doses of heparin. JAMA 235: 1980–1982

GISSI (1986) Effectiveness of intravenous thrombolytic treatment in acute myocardial infarction. Lancet 1:397–402

Gitel SN, Wessler S (1983) Dose-dependent antithrombotic effect of warfarin in rabbits. Blood 61:435–438

Gjores JE (1956) The incidence of venous thrombosis and its sequelae in certain districts of Sweden. Acta Chir Scand [Suppl]206:1–88

Glazier RL, Crowell EB (1976) Randomized prospective trial of continuous versus intermittent heparin therapy. JAMA 236:1365–1367

Goldhaber SZ (1989) Tissue plasminogen activator in acute pulmonary embolism. Chest 95 [Suppl]:282S–289S

Goldhaber SZ, Buring JE, Lipnick RJ, Hennekens CH (1983) Streptokinase versus heparin in acute proximal deep-vein thrombosis: pooled results randomized trials. Circulation 68 (III):III-39 (monogr 101) (abstr 155)

Goldhaber SZ, Buring JE, Lipnick RJ, Hennekens CH (1984) Pooled analyses of randomized trials of streptokinase and heparin in phlebographically documented acute deep-vein thrombosis. Am J Med 76:383–387

Goldhaber SZ, Kessler CM, Heit J, Markis J, Sharma GVRK, Loscalzo J, Dawley D, Nagel JS, Meyerovitz M, Kim D, Vaughan DE, Parker JA, Tumeh SS, Drum D, Reagen K, Selwyn AP, Anderson J, Braunwald E (1988) Randomized controlled trial of recombinant tissue plasminogen activator versus urokinase in the treatment of acute pulmonary embolism. Lancet 2:293–298

Gomez GA, Cutler GS, Wheeler HB (1982) Transvenous interruption of the inferior vena cava. Surgery 93:612–619

Gordon-Smith JC, LeQuesne LP, Grundy DJ, Newcombe JF (1972) Controlled trial of two regimens of subcutaneous heparin in prevention of postoperative deep-vein thrombosis. Lancet 1:1133–1135

Green D, Harris K, Reynolds N, Roberts M, Patterson R (1978) Heparin immune thrombocytopenia: evidence for a heparin-platelet complex as the antigen determinant. J Lab Clin Med 91:167–175

Green D, Martin GJ, Shoichet SH, DeBacker N, Bomalaski JS, Lind RN (1984) Thrombocytopenia: a prospective, randomized, double-blind trial of bovine and porcine heparin. Am J Med Sci 288:60–64

Greenfield FJ, McCurdy JR, Brown PP, Elkins RC (1973) A new intracaval filter promoting continued flow and resolution of emboli. Surgery 73:599–606

Griffith GC, Nicholas G Jr, Asher JD, Flannagan B (1965) Heparin osteoporosis. JAMA 193:85–88

Griguer P, Charbonnier B, Latour F, Fauchier JP, Brochier M (1979) Plasminogen and moderate dose urokinase in the treatment in of acute pulmonary embolism. Angiology 30:1–12

Groote Schurr Hospital Thromboembolus Study Group (1979) Failure of low-dose heparin to prevent significant thromboembolic complications in high-risk surgical patients: interim report of prospective trial. BMJ 1:1447–1450

Groupe de Recherche Urokinase-Embolie Pulmonaire (1984) Rapport préparé par B Charbonnier, Tours: etude multicentrique sur deux protocoles d'urokinase dans l'embolie pulmonaire grave. Arch Mal Coeur 77:773–781

Gruber UF, Duckert F, Fridrich R, Torhorst J, Rem J (1977) Prevention of postoperative thromboembolism by dextran 40, low-doses of heparin or xantinol nicotinate. Lancet 1:207–210

Gruber VD, Seldeen T, Brokop T, Eklof B, Eriksson I, Goldie I, Gran L, Hohl M, Jonsson T, Kristersson S, Ljungstrom KG, Lund T, Maartman Moe H, Svensjo E, Thomson D, Torhorst J Trippestad A, Ulstein M (1980) Incidence of fatal post-operative pulmonary embolism after prophylaxis with dextran-70 and low-dose heparin. BMJ 280:69–72

Gruppo Italiano per lo Studio della Streptochinasa nell' Infarto Miocardico (GISSI) (1987) Long term effects of intravenous thrombolysis in acute myocardial infarction: final report of the GISSI study. Lancet 2:871–874

Guerci AD, Gerstenblith G, Brinker JA, Chandra HC, Gottlieb SO, Bahr RD, Weiss JL, Shapiro EP, Flaherty JT, Bush DE, Chew PH, Gottlieb SH, Halperin HR, Ouyang P, Walford JD, Bell WR, Fatterpaker AK, Llewellyn M, Topal EJ, Healy B, Siu CO, Becker LC, Weisfeldt ML (1987) A randomized trial of intravenous tissue plasminogen activator for acute myocardial infarction with subsequent randomization to elective coronary angioplasty. NEJM 317: 1613–1618

Gurewich V, Cohen M, Thomas DP (1968) Humoral factors in massive pulmonary embolism. Am Heart J 76:784–794

Haber E, Quertermous T, Matsueda JR, Runge MS (1989) Innovative approaches to plasminogen activator therapy. Science 243:51–56

Hampson WGJ, Harris FC, Lucas HK, Roberts PH, McCall IW, Jackson PC, Powell NL, Staddon GE (1974) Failure of low-dose heparin to prevent deep-vein thrombosis after hip replacement arthroplasty. Lancet 2:795–797

Harenberg J, Stehle G, Augustin J, Zimmermann R (1989) Comparative human pharmacology of low molecular weight heparins. Semin Thromb Hemost 15: 414–423

Harker LA, Slichter SJ (1972) Platelet and fibrinogen consumption in man. NEJM 287:999

Harrison DG, Ferguson DW, Collins SM, Skorton DJ, Ericksen EE, Kioschos JM, Marcus ML, White CW (1984) Rethrombosis after reperfusion with streptokinase: importance of geometry of residual lesions. Circulation 69:991–999

Heiden D, Mielke CH Jr, Rodvien R (1977) Impairment by heparin of primary hemostasis and platelet [^{14}C]5-hydroxytryptamine release. Br J Haematol 36: 427–435

Hess H, Ingrisch H, Mietaschk A, Rath H (1982) Local low-dose thrombolytic therapy of peripheral arterial occlusion. NEJM 307:1627–1630

Hirsh J (1986) Effectiveness of anticoagulants. Semin Thromb Hemost 12:21–37

Hirsh J, Levine M (1988) Confusion over the therapeutic range for monitoring therapy in North America. Thromb Hemost 59:129–132

Hirsh J, Van Akin WG, Gallus AS, Dollery CT, Cade JF, Yung WL (1976) Heparin kinetics in venous thrombosis and pulmonary embolism. Circulation 53:691–695

Hirsh J, Deykin D, Poller L (1986) Therapeutic range for oral anticoagulant therapy. Chest 89[Suppl]:11S–15S

Hirsh J, Salzman EW, Marder VJ, Colman RW (1987) Overview of the thrombotic process and its therapy. In: Colman RW, Hirsch J, Marder VJ, Salzman EW (eds) Hemostasis and thrombosis: basic principles and clinical practice, 2nd ed. Lippincott, Philadelphia, pp 1063–1072

Hoffman JJML, Van Rey FJW, Bonnier JJRM (1985) Systemic effects of BR26921 during thrombolytic therapy of acute myocardial infarction. Thromb Res 37: 567–572

Hoffman V, Frick PG (1982) Repeated occurrence of skin necrosis following coumarin intake and subsequently during decrease of vitamin K dependent coagulation factors associated with cholestasis. Thromb Hemost 48:245–246

Holmer E (1980) Anticoagulant properties of heparin and heparin fractions. Scand J Haematol 25:25–39

Hoppensteadt D, Rocanelli A, Walenga JM, Fareed J (1989) Comparative antithrombotic and hemorrhagic effects of dermatan sulfate, heparan sulfate and heparin. Semin Thromb Hemost 15:378–385

Horn JR, Danziger L, Davis RJ (1981) Warfarin-induced skin necrosis: report of 4 cases. Am J Hosp Pharm 38:1763–1768

Howell WH (1922) Heparin, an anticoagulant. Preliminary communication. Am J Physiol 63:434–435

Hull JG, Pauli RM, Wilson KM (1980) Maternal and fetal sequelae of anticoagulation during pregnancy. Am J Med 68:122–140

Hull JH, Murray WJ, Brown HS, Williams BO, Chi SL, Koch GG (1978) Potential anticoagulant drug interactions in ambulatory patients. Clin Pharmacol Ther 24:644–649

Hull R, Delmore T, Genton E, Hirsh J, Gent M, Sackett D, McLaughlin D, Armstrong P (1979) Warfarin sodium versus low-dose heparin in the long-term treatment of venous thrombosis. NEJM 301:855–858

Hull R, Delmore T, Carter C, Hirsh J, Genton E, Gent M, Turpie G, McLaughlin D (1982a) Adjusted subcutaneous heparin versus warfarin sodium in the long-term treatment of venous thrombosis. NEJM 306:189–194

Hull R, Hirsh J, Jay R, Carter C, England C, Gent M, Turpie AGG, McLaughlin D, Dodd P, Thomas M, Roskob J, Ockelford P (1982b) Different intensities of oral anticoagulant therapy in the treatment of proximal-vein thrombosis. NEJM 307:1676–1681

Hull R, Roskob G, Hirsh J, Sackett DG (1984) A cost-effectiveness analysis of alternative approaches for long-term treatment of proximal vein thrombosis. JAMA 252:235–239

Hull R, Roskob GE, Hirsh J, Jay RM, Leclerc JR, Geerts WH, Rosenbloom D, Sackett DL, Anderson C, Harrison L, Gent M (1986) Continuous intravenous heparin compared with intermittent subcutaneous heparin in the initial treatment of proximal-vein thrombosis. NEJM 315:1109–1114

Hume M, Kuriakose TX, Zuch L, Turner RH (1973) ^{125}I-fibrinogen and the prevention of venous thrombosis. Arch Surg 107:803–806

Ichinose A, Takio K, Fujikawa K (1986) Localization of the binding site of tissue-type plasminogen activator to fibrin. J Clin Invest 78:163–169

Immelman EJ, Jeffery PC (1984) The postphlebitic syndrome, pathophysiology, prevention and management. Clin Chest Med 5:537–550

International Multicentre Trial (1975) Prevention of fatal postoperative pulmonary embolism by low-doses of heparin. Lancet 2:45–51

ISAM Study Group (1986) A prospective trial of intravenous streptokinase in acute myocardial infarction (ISAM): mortality, morbidity and infarct size at twenty-one days. NEJM 314:1465–1471

ISIS Steering Committee (1987) Intravenous streptokinase given within 0–4 hours of onset of myocardial infarction reduced mortality in ISIS-2. Lancet 1:502

ISIS-2 (Second International Study of Infarct Survival) Collaborative Group (1988) Randomized trial of intravenous streptokinase, oral aspirin, both or neither among 17187 cases of suspected acute myocardial infarction: ISIS-2. Lancet 2:349–360

Jacques LB (1978) Addendum: the discovery of heparin. Semin Thromb Hemost 4:350–353

Jacques LB (1979) Heparin: an old drug with a new paradigm. Science 206:528–533

Jaffe MD, Willis PW (1965) Multiple fractures associated with long-term sodium heparin therapy. JAMA 193:152–154

Jennings RB, Reimer KA (1983) Factors involved in salvaging ischemic myocardium: effect of reperfusion of arterial blood. Circulation 68[Suppl I]:I25–I36 (AHA monogr 97)

Johanson L, Nylander G, Hedner U, Nilsson IM (1979) Comparison of streptokinase with heparin: late results in the treatment of deep-vein thrombosis. Acta Med Scand 206:93–98

Johns JA, Gold HK, Leinbach RC, Yasuda T, Gimple LW, Werner W, Finkelstein D, Newell J, Ziskind AA, Collen D (1988) Prevention of coronary artery reocclusion and reduction in late coronary artery stenosis after thrombolytic therapy in patients with acute myocardial infarction. A randomized study of maintenance infusion of recombinant tissue-type plasminogen activator. Circulation 78:546–556

Juhan-Vague I, Stassen JM, Alessi MC, Elias A, Aillaud MF, Serradimigni A, Collen D (1989) Potentiation by heparin fragment CY222 (Choay) of thrombolysis induced by human tissue-type plasminogen activator. Semin Thromb Hemost 15:390–394

Kakkar VV (1981) Prevention of venous thromboembolism. Clin Haematol 10:543–582

Kakkar VV, Lawrence D (1985) Hemodynamic and clinical assessment therapy for deep-vein thrombosis: a prospective study. Am J Surg 150:54–63

Kakkar VV, Murray WJG (1985) Efficacy and safety of low molecular weight heparin (CY2116) in preventing postoperative venous thromboembolism: a cooperative study. Br J Surg 72:786–791

Kakkar VV, Flanc C, Howe CT, O'Shea M, Flute PT (1969a) Treatment of deep-vein thrombosis: a trial of heparin, streptokinase and Arvin. BMJ 1:806–810

Kakkar VV, Howe CT, Laws JW, Flanc C (1969b) Late results of treatment of deep-vein thrombosis. BMJ 1:810–811

Kakkar VV, Spindler J, Flute PT, Corrigan T, Fossard DP, Crellin RQ (1972) Efficacy of low-doses of heparin in prevention of deep-vein thrombosis after major surgery: a double-blind randomized trial. Lancet 2:101–106

Kakkar VV, Stamatakis JD, Bentley PG, Lawrence D, De Haas HA, Ward VP (1979) Prophylaxis for postoperative deep-vein thrombosis. Synergistic effect of heparin and dihydroergotamine. JAMA 241:39–42

Kartchner MM, Wilcox WC (1976) Thrombolysis of palmar and digital arterial thrombosis by intraarterial thrombolysis. J Hand Surg [Am] 1:67–74

Kelton JG, Sheridan D, Santos A, Smith J, Sleeves K, Smith C, Brown C, Murphy WG (1988) Heparin-induced thrombocytopenia: laboratory studies. Blood 72:925–930

Kennedy J, Ritchie J, Davis K, Fritz J (1983a) Western Washington randomized trial of intracoronary streptokinase in acute myocardial infarction. NEJM 309: 1477–1482

Kennedy JW, Ritchie JL, Davis KB, Fritz JK (1983b) Western Washington randomized trial of intracoronary streptokinase in acute myocardial infarction. NEJM 309:1477–1482

Kennedy JW, Gensini GG, Timmis GC, Maynard C (1985a) Acute myocardial infarction treated with intracoronary streptokinase: a report of the Society for Cardiac Angiography. Am J Cardiol 55:871–877

Kennedy JW, Ritchie JL, Davis KB, Stadius ML, Maynard C, Fritz J (1985b) The Western Washington randomized trial of intracoronary streptokinase in acute myocardial infarction: a 12-month follow-up report. NEJM 312:1073–1078

Kennedy JW, Martin GV, Davis KB, Maynard C, Stadius M, Sheehan FH, Ritchie JL (1988) The Western Washington intravenous streptokinase in acute myocardial infarction randomized trial. Circulation 77:345–352

Kessler CM (1989) Anticoagulation and thrombolytic therapy: practical considerations. Chest 95[Suppl]:245S–289S

Khaja F, Walton JA Jr, Brymer JF, Lo E, Osterberger L, O'Neill WW, Colfer HT, Weiss R, Tennyson L, Kurian T, Goldberg AD, Pitt B, Goldstein S (1983) Intracoronary fibrinolytic therapy in acute myocardial infarction; report on a prospective randomized trial. NEJM 308:1305–1311

King DJ, Kelton JG (1984) Heparin-associated thrombocytopenia. Ann Int Med 100:535–540

Kirkwood TBL (1983) Calibration of reference thromboplastins and standardization of the prothrombin time rates. Thromb Hemost 49:238–244

Koch-Weser J (1968) Coumarin necrosis. Ann Int Med 68:1365–1367

Kolts RL, Kuehner ME, Swanson MK, Carlson RD, Myers WO, Friedenberg WR (1985) Local intra-arterial streptokinase therapy for acute peripheral arterial occlusions: should thrombolytic therapy replace embolectomy? Am Surg 51: 381–387

Koppenhagen K, Haring R, Zuhlke HV, Wiechmann A, Wenig HG (1979) Efficiency and risk of thromboembolism prophylaxis in surgery. Clinicoexperimental results in 1434 general surgery patients. Thromb Haemost 42:249 (abstr 0589)

Kounis NG, Evans WH (1979) Thromboembolic disease treated with anticoagulants and defibrinating drugs. Practitioner 222:420–422

Kremer P, Fiebig R, Tilsner V, Bleifeld W, Mathey DG (1985) Lysis of left ventricular thrombi with urokinase. Circulation 72:112–118

Kudo S, Chuang VP, Mir S, Bechtel W, Carrasco CH (1985) Transcatheter thrombolysis in cancer patients. Cardiovasc Intervent Radiol 8:1

Lahnborg G, Friman L, Bergstrom K, Lagergren H (1974) Effect of low-dose heparin on incidence of postoperative pulmonary embolism detected by photoscanning. Lancet 1:329–331

Lam LH, Silbert JE, Rosenberg RD (1976) The separation of active and inactive forms of heparin. Biochem Biophys Res Commun 69:570–577

Larsen ML, Abildgaard U, Teien AN, Gjesdahl K (1978) Assay of plasma heparin using thrombin and the chromogenic substrate H-D-Phe-Pip-Arg-pNA (S-2238). Thromb Res 13:285–288

Latallo ZS (1978) Report of the task force on clinical use of snake venom enzymes. Thromb Haemost 39:768–774

LeBalc'h T, Landais A, Butel J, Weill D, Pascariello JC, Planes A (1987) Enoxaparin (Lovenox R) versus standard heparin in prophylaxis of deep-vein thrombosis (DVT) after total hip replacement (THR). Thromb Haemost 58:892 (abstr)

Leonard EF (1987) Rheology of thrombosis. In: Colman RW, Hirsch J, Marder VJ, Salzman EW (eds) Hemostasis and thrombosis: basic principles and clinical practice, 2nd ed. Lippincott, Philadelphia pp 1111–1122

Leroy J, Leclerc MH, Delahousse B, Guerois C, Foloppe J, Gruel Y, Toulemond F (1985) Treatment of heparin-associated thrombocytopenia and thrombosis with low molecular weight heparin. Semin Thromb Haemost 11:326–329

Levin EJ, Marzec U, Anderson J, Harker LA (1984) Thrombin stimulated tissue plasminogen activator release from cultured human endothelial cells. J Clin Invest 74:1988–1995

Lijnen HR, Zamarron C, Collen D (1985) Pro-urokinase kinetics and mechanism of action. Thromb Haemost 54[Suppl 1]:118 (abstr 5698)

Lijnen HR, Stump D, Collen D (1987) Single-chain urokinase-type plasminogen activator: mechanism of action and thrombolytic properties. Semin Thromb Hemost 13:152–159

Link KP (1959) Discovery of dicumoral and its sequels. Circulation 19:97–107

Loeliger EA, Potter L, Samama M, Thomas JM, van der Besselaer AMHP, Vermylen J, Verstraete M (1985) Questions and answers on prothrombin time standardization in oral anticoagulant control. Thromb Haemost 54:515–517

Loscalzo J, Braunwald E (1988) Tissue plasminogen activator. NEJM 319:925–931

Lowe GDO (1981) Defibrinating agents: effects on blood rheology, blood flow and vascular diseases in controlled studies. Bibl Haematologica 47:247–249

Luomanmaki K, Halttunen P, Hekali P, Valle M, Heikila J (1983) Experience with streptokinase treatment of major pulmonary embolism. Ann Clin Res 15:21–25

Macfarlane RG, Pilling J (1946) Observations on fibrinolysis: plasminogen, plasmin and antiplasmin content of human blood. Lancet 2:562–565

Magnani B for the Plasminogen Activator Italian Multicenter Study (PAIMS) Investigators (1989) Comparison of intravenous recombinant single-chain human tissue-type plasminogen activator (rt-PA) with intravenous streptokinase in acute myocardial infarction. J Am Coll Cardiol 13:19–26

Mant MJ, O'Brien BD, Thong KL, Hammond GW, Birtwhistle RV, Grace MG (1977) Hemorrhagic complications of heparin therapy. Lancet 1:1133–1134

Manucci PM, Citteris LA, Panajotopoulos N (1976) Low-dose heparin and deep-vein thrombosis after total hip replacement. Thromb Haemost 36:157–164

Marcum JA, Rosenberg RD (1987) Anticoagulantly active heparan sulfate proteoglycan and the vascular endothelium. Semin Thromb Hemost 13:464–474

Marder VJ, Bell WR (1987) Fibrinolytic therapy. In: Colman RW, Hirsh J, Marder VJ, Salzman EW (eds) Hemostasis and thrombosis: basic principles and clinical practice, 2nd ed. Lippincott, Philadelphia, pp 1393–1437

Marder VJ, Francis CW (1984) An assessment of regional versus systemic thrombolytic treatment of peripheral and coronary artery thrombosis. Prog Hemost Thromb 7:325–356

Marder VJ, Sherry S (1988) Thrombolytic therapy: current status, parts I and II. NEJM 318:1512–1520, 1585–1594

Marder VJ, Soulen RL, Atichartakarn V, Budzinski AZ, Parulekar S, Kim JR, Edward N, Zahavi J, Algazy KM (1977) Quantitative venographic assessment of deep-vein thrombosis in the evaluation of streptokinase and heparin therapy. J Lab Clin Med 89:1018–1029

Marder VJ, Rothbard RL, Fitzpatrick PG, Francisco CW (1986) Rapid lysis of coronary artery thrombi with anisoylated plasminogen-streptokinase activator complex: treatment by bolus intravenous infusion. Ann Int Med 104:304–310

Marini C, DiRicco G, Rossi G, Rindi M, Palla R, Giuntini C (1988) Fibrinolytic effects of urokinase and heparin in acute pulmonary embolism: a randomized clinical trial. Respiration 54:162–173

Markwardt F (1989) Development of hirudin as an antithrombotic agent. Semin Thromb Hemost 15:269–287

Markwardt F, Nowak G, Sturzebecker J, Gresbach V, Walsmann P, Vogel G (1984) Pharmacokinetics and anticoagulant effects of hirudin in man. Thromb Haemost 52:160–163

Markwardt F, Nowak G, Sturzebecker J, Vogel G (1989) Clinicopharmacological studies with recombinant hirudin. Thromb Res 52:393–400

Martin M (1979) Thrombolytic therapy in arterial thromboembolism. Prog Cardiovasc Dis 21:351–374

Martin M, Schoop W, Zietler E (1970) Streptokinase in chronic arterial occlusive disease. JAMA 211:1169–1173

Mathey DG, Sheehan FH, Schofer J, Dodge HT (1985) Time from onset of symptoms to thrombolytic therapy: a major determinant of myocardial salvage in patients with acute transmural infarction. Am Coll Cardiol 6:518–525

Mattioli G, Capello C, Fusaro MT (1989) Treatment of acute myocardial infarction with defibrotide. Semin Thromb Hemost 15:470–473

Mazel MS (1977) Clinical experience with urokinase. In: Paoletti R, Sherry S (eds) Thrombosis and urokinase. Academic, New York, pp 247–252

McAvoy TJ (1979) Pharmacokinetic modeling of heparin and its clinical implications. J Pharmacokinet Biopharm 7:331–354

McGehee WG, Klotz TA, Epstein DJ, Rapaport SI (1984) Coumarin necrosis associated with herditary protein C deficiency. Am Int Med 100:59–60

McManama G, Blume H, Robertson L, Kamm R, Johnson M, Shapiro A, Salzman E (1984) Graded sequential pneumatic calf compression promotes postoperative fibrinolytic activity and prevents venous thrombosis. Circulation 70[Suppl 2] (abstr 1441):360

McNamara TO, Fischer JR (1985) Thrombolysis of peripherial and arterial and graft occlusions: improved results using high-dose urokinase. AJR 144:769–775

Milazotto, F, Carelli M, Citone C, Di Marcotullio G, Giampaolo P, Malinconico V, Polizzi C, Tubaro M, Giovannini E, Boccardi L, Minardi G, Biffani G, De Rubertis C, Nazzari M, Cornelli U (1986) Use of defibrotide in the treatment of acute myocardial infarction. Semim Thromb Hemost 15:464–469

Miller GAH, Hall RJC, Paveth M (1977) Pulmonary embolectomy, heparin, and streptokinase: their place in the treatment of acute massive pulmonary embolism. Am Heart J 93:568–574

Morris GK, Henry APJ, Preston BJ (1974) Prevention of deep-vein thrombosis by low-dose heparin in patients undergoing total hip replacement. Lancet 2: 797–799

Moskovitz PA, Ellenberg S, Feffer HL, Kenmore PI, Neviaser RJ, Rubin BE, Varma VM (1978) Low-dose heparin for prevention of venous thromboembolism in total hip arthroplasty and surgical repair of hip fractures. J Bone Joint Surg [Am] 60:1065–1070

Mueller HS, Rao AK, Forman SA, The TIMI Investigators (1987) Thrombolysis in myocardial infarction (TIMI): comparative studies of coronary reperfusion and systemic fibrinolysis with two forms of recombinant human tissue-type plasminogen activator. J Am Coll Cardiol 10:479–490

Multicenter Postinfarction Research Group (1983) Risk stratification and survival after myocardial infarction. NEJM 309: 331–336

Nand S, Robinson JA (1988) Plasmapheresis in the management of heparin-associated thrombocytopenia with thrombosis. Am J Hematol 28:204–206

National Institute of Health Consensus Development Conference (1980) Thrombolytic therapy in thrombosis. Ann Int Med 93:141–144

Nenci GG, Gresele P, Taramelli M, Agnelli G, Signorini E (1983) Thrombolytic therapy for thromboembolism of vertebrobasilar artery. Angiology 34:561–571

Neuhaus KL, Tebbe U, Gottwik M, Weber MAJ, Feuerer W, Niederer W, Haerer W, Praetorius F, Grosser K-D, Huhman W, Hoepp HW, Alber G, Sheikhzadeh A, Schneider B (1988) Intravenous recombinant tissue plasminogen activator (rt-PA) and urokinase in acute myocardial infarction: results of the German Activator urokinase study (GAUS). J Am Coll Cardiol 12:581–587

Niada R, Mantovani M, Prino G, Pescador R, Berti F, Omini C, Folco GC (1981) Antithrombotic activity of a polydeoxyribonucleotidic substance extracted from mammalian organs: a possible link with prostacyclin. Thromb Res 23:233–246

Niada R, Mantovani M, Prino G, Pescador R, Porta R (1982) PGI 2 generation and antithrombotic activity of orally administered defibrotide. Pharmacol Res Commun 14:949–957

Nicolaides AN, Dupont PA, Desai S, Lewis JD, Douglas JN, Dodsworth H, Fourides G, Luck RJ (1972) Small doses of subcutaneous sodium heparin in preventing deep venous thrombosis after major surgery. Lancet 2:890–893

O'Reilly RA (1987) Vitamin K antagonists. In: Colman RW, Hirsh J, Marder VJ, Salzman EW (eds) Hemostasis and thrombosis: basic principles and clinical practice, 2nd ed. Lippincott, Philadelphia, pp 1367–1372

O'Reilly RA , Aggeler PM (1968) Studies on coumarin anticoagulant drugs: initiation of warfarin therapy without a loading dose. Circulation 38:169–177

Ockelford PA, Carter CJ, Mitchell L, Hirsh J (1982) Discordance between the anti X_A and the antithrombotic activity of an ultra low molecular weight heparin fraction. Thromb Res 28:401–409

Ohayon J, Colle JP, Tauzin-Fin P, Lorient-Roudaut MF, Besse P (1986) Evolution hémodynamique au cours de fibrinolyses de l'émbolie pulmonaire grave. Arch Mal Coeur 79:445–453

Olsson P, Blomback M, Egberg N, Ekestrom S (1976) Experience of extensive vascular surgery on defibrase-defibrinogenated patients. Thromb Res 9:227

Phelan BK (1983) Heparin-associated thrombosis without thrombocytopenia. Ann Int Med 99:637–638

Physician's Desk Reference (1990) Abbokinase (urokinase for injection) and Abbokinase Open-Cath (urokinase for catheter clearance). pp 502–505

Physician's Desk Reference (1990) Steptase (streptokinase). Barnhart, Oradell, NJ, USA, pp 1048–1050

Pitney WR (1971) An appraisal of therapeutic defibrination. Thromb Diath Haemorrh [Suppl]45:43–49

Pitney WR, Dean S (1976) Plasma heparin concentrations during subcutaneous heparin therapy. Aust NZ J Med 6:454–458

Planes A, Vochelle N, Mansat C (1987) Prevention of deep-vein thrombosis (DVT) after total hip replacement (THR) by enoxaparin (Lovenox R): one daily injection of 40 mg versus two daily injections of 20 mg. Thromb Haemost 58:415 (abstr): 117

Poller L (1986) Laboratory control of anticoagulant therapy. Semin Thromb Hemost 12:13–19

Porta R, Pescador R, Mantovani M, Niada R, Prino G, Madonna M (1984) Pharmacokinetics of defibrotide and of its profibrinolytic activity in different animal species. Effects on the levels of fibrinolysis inhibitors and of fibrinogen/fibrin degradation products (FDP). Haemostasis 14:122

Powers PJ, Cuthbert D, Hirsh J (1979) Thrombocytopenia found uncommonly during heparin therapy. JAMA 241:2396–2397

Raskob GE, Carter CJ, Hull RD (1989) Anticoagulant therapy for venous thromboembolism. Prog Hemost Thromb 9:1–27

Reid A, Chan KE, Thean PC (1963) Prolonged coagulation defect (defibrination syndrome) in Malayan viper bite. Lancet 1:621–626

Reimer KA, Lowe JE, Rasmussen MH, Jennings RB (1977) The wavefront phenomenon of ischemic cell death. Myocardial infarct size vs. duration of coronary occlusion in dogs. Circulation 56:786–794

Rem J, Duckert F, Fridrich R, Gruber VF (1975) Subkutane klein Heparindosen zur Thromboseprophylaxe in der allgemeinen Chirurgie und Urologie. Schweiz Med Wochenschr 105:827–835

Rentrop KP (1985) Thrombolytic therapy in patients with acute myocardial infarction. Circulation 71:627–631

Rentrop P, Blanke H, Karsch KR, Kreuger H (1979) Initial experience with transluminal recanalization of the recently occluded infarct-related coronary artery in acute myocardial infarction: comparison with conventionally treated patients. Clin Cardiol 2:92–105

Rice L, Huffman DM, Levine ML, Udden MM, Waddell CC, Luper WE (1986) Heparin-induced thrombocytopenia/thrombosis syndromes: clinical manifestations and insights. Blood 68[Suppl]:339A (abstr 1235)

Rijken DC, Hoylaerts M, Collen D (1982) Fibrinolytic properties of one chain and two chain human extrinsic (tissue-type) plasminogen activator. J Biol Chem 257:2920–2925

Ring J, Messmer K (1977) Incidence and severity of anaphylactoid reactions to colloid volume substitutes. Lancet I:466–469

Robbins KC (1987) The plasminogen-plasmin enzyme system. In: Colman RW, Hirsh J, Marder VJ, Salzman EW (eds) Hemostasis and thrombosis: basic principles and clinical practice, 2nd ed. Lippincott, Philadelphia, pp 340–353

Robbins KC, Barlow GH, Nguyen J, Samama MM (1987) Comparison of plasminogen activators. Semin Thromb Hemost 13:131–138

Rosch J, Dotter CT, Seaman AJ, Porter JM, Common HH (1976) Healing of deep-vein thrombosis: venographic findings in a randomized study comparing streptokinase and heparin. Am J Roentgenol 127:553–558

Rosenberg IL, Evans M, Pollock AV (1975) Prophylaxis of postoperative leg vein thrombosis by low-dose subcutaneous heparin or preoperative calf muscle stimulation: a controlled clinical trial. BMJ 1:649–651

Rosenberg RD (1987) The heparin-antithrombin system: a natural anticoagulant mechanism. In: Colman RW, Hirsh J, Marder VJ, Salzman EW (eds) Hemostasis and thrombosis: basic principles and clinical practice, 2nd ed. Lippincott, Philadelphia, pp 1373–1392

Rosengarten DS, Laird J, Jeyasingh K, Martin P (1971) The failure of compression stocking (Tubigrip) to prevent deep venous thrombosis after operation. Br J Surg 57:296–299

Roudaut M-FL, Ledain L, Roudaut R, Besse P, Boisseau MR (1987) Thrombolytic treatment of acute thrombotic obstruction with disc valve prosthesis: experience with 26 cases. Semin Thromb Hemost 13:201–205

Rupp WM, McCarthy HB, Rohde TD, Blackshear PJ, Goldenberg FJ, Buchwald H (1982) Risk of osteoporosis in patients treated with long term intravenous heparin therapy. Curr Surg 39:419–422

Sagar S, Stamatakis JD, Higgins AF, Nairn D, Maffel FH, Thomas DP, Kakkar VV (1976) Efficacy of low-dose heparin in prevention of extensive deep-vein thrombosis in patients undergoing total hip replacement. Lancet 1:1151–1154

Salzman EW, Hirsh J (1987) Prevention of venous thromboembolism in hemostasis and thrombosis, basic principles and clinical practice. Colman RW, Hirsh J, Marder VJ, Salzman EW (eds) Hemostasis and thrombosis: basic principles and clinical practice, 2nd ed. Lippincott, Philadelphia, pp 1252–1258

Salzman EW, Harris WH, de Sanctis RW (1966) Anticoagulation for prevention of thromboembolism following fractures of the hip. NEJM 275:122–130

Salzman EW, Harris WH, de Sanctis RW (1971) Reduction in venous thrombosis by agents affecting platelet function. NEJM 284:1287–1291

Salzman EW, Deykin D, Shapiro RM, Rosenberg R (1975) Management of heparin therapy: controlled prospective trial. NEJM 292:1046–1050

Salzman EW, Rosenberg RD, Smith MH, Lindon JH, Favreau L (1980) Effect of heparin and heparin fractions on platelet aggregation. J Clin Invest 65:64–73

Samama M, Bernard P, Bonnardot JP, Combe-Tamzali S, Lanson Y, Tissot E on behalf of the participants in the Groupe d'Etude de l'Enoxaparine (GENOX) multicentric trial (1988) Low molecular weight heparin compared with unfractionated heparin in prevention of postoperative thrombosis. Br J Surg 75: 128–131

Samama MM (1987a) Deep vein thrombosis of inferior limbs: are thrombolytic agents superior to heparin? Semin Thromb Hemost 13:178–180

Samama MM (ed) (1987b) Thrombolytic Agents and Treatments. Semin Thromb Hemost 13(2):131–242

Sasahara AA, Koppenhagen K, Haring R, Welzel D. Wolf H (1986) Low molecular weight heparin plus dihydroergotamine for prophylaxis of postoperative deep-vein thrombosis. Br J Surg 73:697–700

Schröder R, Neuhaus K-L, Leizorovicz A, Linderer T, Tebbe U for the ISAM Study Group (1987) A prospective, placebo-controlled, double-blind, multicenter trial of intravenous streptokinase in acute myocardial infarction (ISAM): long-term mortality and morbidity. J Am Coll Cardiol 9:197–203

Schroeder TM, Elkins RC, Greenfield LJ (1978) Entrapment of sized emboli by the KMA-Greenfield intracaval filter. Surgery 83:435–439

Schulman S, Lockner D (1985) Relationship between thromboembolic complications and intensity of treatment during long-term prophylaxis with oral anticoagulants following DVT. Thromb Haemost 53:137–140

Schwartz F, Schuler G, Katus H, Hoffman M, Manthey J, Tillmanns H, Mehmel HC, Kubler W (1982) Intracoronary thrombolysis in acute myocardial infarction: duration of ischemia as a major determinant of late results after recanalization. Am J Cardiol 50:933–937

Scottish Study (1974) A multi-unit controlled trial: heparin versus dextran in the prevention of deep-vein thrombosis. Lancet 2:118–120

Scurr JH, Ibrahim SZ, Faber RG, LeQuesne LP (1977) The efficacy of graduated compression stockings in the prevention of deep-vein thrombosis. Br J Surg 64:371–373

Serradimigni A, Chiche G, Romami A, Philip F (1984) Venous thromboembolism associated with pulmonary embolism. In: Tesi M, Dormandy JA (eds) Superficial and deep venous diseases of the lower limbs. Edizioni Panminerva Medica, Milan, pp 219–222

Sharma G, Cella G, Parisi A, Sasahara A (1982) Thrombolytic therapy. NEJM 306:1268–1276

Sheehan FH, Braunwald E, Conner P, Dodge HT, Gore J, Van Natta P, Passamani ER, Williams DO, Zaret B, Coinvestigators (1987) The effect of intraveneous thrombolytic therapy on left ventricular function: a report on tissue-type plasminogen activator and streptokinase from the Thrombolysis in Myocardial Infarction (TIMI phase I) Trial. Circulation 75:817–829

Sheridan D, Carter C, Kelton JG (1986) A diagnostic test for heparin-induced thrombocytopenia. Blood 67:27–30

Sherry S, Dolomon HA (eds) (1987) Thrombolytic Therapy in cardiovascular diseases. Current practice and future directions. Am J Med 83[Suppl 2A]

Sherry S, Fletcher AP, Alkjaersig N (1959a) Developments in fibrinolytic therapy for thromboembolic disease. Ann Int Med 50:560–570

Sherry S, Fletcher AP, Alkjaersig N (1959b) Fibrinolysis and fibrinolytic activity in man. Physiol Rev 39:343–382

Sherry S, Bell WR, Duckert H, Fletcher AP, Gurewich V, Long DN, Marder VJ, Roberts H, Salzman EW, Sasahara A, Verstraete M (1980) Thrombolytic therapy in thrombosis: an NIH consensus development conference. Ann Int Med 93:141–144

Shojania AM, Turnbull G (1987) Effect of heparin on platelet counts and platelet aggregation. Am J Hematol 26:255–262

Siefring GE, Castellino FJ (1976) Interaction of streptokinase with plasminogen: isolation and characterization of a streptokinase degradation product. J Biol Chem 251:3913–3920

Simon TL, Hyers TM, Gaston JP, Harker LA (1978) Heparin pharmacokinetics: increased requirements in pulmonary embolism. Br J Haematol 39:111–120

Simoons ML, Fioretti P, Van der Brand M, Serruys PW, Krauss XH, Remme P, van der Wall EE, Verheugt F, Res J, Neef KJ (1983) Randomized trial of thrombolysis with streptokinase in acute myocardial infarction. Circulation 68:III-120 (abstr 480)

Simoons ML, Serruys PW, van der Brand M, Res J, Verheugt FWA, Kraus XH, Remme WJ, Bar F, DeZwaan C, van der Laarse A, Vermeer F, Lubsen J (1986) Early thrombolysis in acute myocardial infarction: limitation of infarct size and improved survial. J Am Coll Cardiol 7:717–728

Stalder M, Hauert J, Kruitkof EKO, Bachmann F (1985) Release of vascular plasminogen activator (v-PA) after venous stasis; electrophoretic-zymographic analysis of free and complexed v-PA. Br J Haematol 61:169–176

Stampfer MJ, Goldhaber SZ, Yusuf S, Peto R, Hennekens C (1982) Effect of intravenous streptokinase on acute myocardial infarction; pooled results from randomized trials. NEJM 307:1180–1182

Stansel HC (1982) Vena cava interruption. Contemp Surg 20:43–68

Stead RB, Schafer AI, Rosenberg ID, Handin RI, Josa M, Khuri SF (1984) Heterogeneity of heparin lots associated with thrombocytopenia and thromboembolism. Am J Med 77:185–188

Stevenson RE, Burton OM, Ferlaw GJ, Taylor HA (1980) Hazards of oral anticoagulation during pregnancy. JAMA 243:1549–1551

Stocker K (1978) Defibrinogenation with thrombin-like snake venom enzymes. In: Markwardt F (ed) Fibrinolytics and antifibrinolytics. Seringer, Berlin Heidelberg New York (Handbook of experimental pharmacology, vol 46)

Sullivan JM, Harken DE, Gorlin R (1971) Pharmacologic control of thromboembolic complications of cardiac-valve replacement. NEJM 284:1392–1394

Taberner DA, Poller L, Burslem RW, Jones JB (1978) Oral anticoagulants controlled by the British comparative thromboplastin versus low-dose heparin in prophylaxis of deep venous thrombosis. BMJ 1:272–274

Taylor GJ, Mikell FL, Moses HW, Dove JT, Batchelder JE, Thuall A, Hansen S, Wellons HA, Schneider JA (1984) Intravenous versus intracoronary streptokinase therapy for acute myocardial infarction in community hospitals. Am J Cardiol 54:256–260

Teien AN, Lei M, Abildgaard U (1976) Assay of heparin in plasma using a chromogenic substrate for activated X. Thromb Res 8:413–418

Tennant SN, Dixon J, Venable TC, Page HL, Roach L, Kaiser AB, Frederiksen R, Tacogue L, Kaplan P, Babu NS, Anderson EE, Wooten E, Jennings HS III, Breinig J, Campbell WB (1984) Intracoronary thrombolysis in patients with acute myocardial infarction: comparison of efficacy of urokinase with streptokinase. Circulation 69:756–760

Terrin M, Goldhaber SZ, Thompson B, TIPE Investigators (1989) Selection of patients with acute pulmonary embolism for thrombolytic therapy: thrombolysis in pulmonary embolism (TIPE) patient survey. Chest 95[Suppl]:279S–281S

Thomas DP, Merton RF, Barrowcliffe TW, Thunberg L, Lindahl V (1982) Effects of heparin oligosaccharides with high affinity for antithrombin III in experimental venous thrombosis. Thromb Haemost 47:244–248

Tillett WS, Garner RL (1933) The fibrinolytic activity of hemolytic streptococci. J Exp Med 58:485–502

Tillett WS, Sherry S (1949) The effect in patients of streptococcal fibrinolysin (streptokinase) and streptococcal desoxyribonuclease on fibrinous, purulent and sanguinous pleural exudations. J Clin Invest 28:173–190

TIMI Study Group (1985) The thrombolysis in myocardial infarction (TIMI) trial: Phase I findings. NEJM 312:932–936

TIMI Study Group (1989) Comparison of invasive and conservative strategies after treatment with intravenous tissue plasminogen activator in acute myocardial infarction. Results of the thrombolysis in myocardial infarction (TIMI) phase II trial. NEJM 320:618–627

Topol EJ (1988) Coronary angioplasty for acute myocardial infarction. Ann Int Med 109:970–980

Totty WG, Romano T, Benian GM, Gilula LA, Sherman LA (1982) Serum sickness following streptokinase therapy. Am J Roentgen 138:143–144

Triplett DA, Harms CS, Koepke JA (1978) The effect of heparin on the APTT. Am J Clin Pathol 70:556–559

Trubestein G (1984) Fibrinolytic therapy with streptokinase and urokinase in deep-vein thrombosis. Int Angiol 3:377–382

Tsao CH, Galluzzo TS, Lo R, Peterson KG (1979) Whole-blood clotting, activated PTT and whole blood recalcification time as heparin monitoring tests. Am J Clin Pathol 71:17–21

Turitto VT (1982) Blood viscosity, mass transport and thrombogenesis. Prog Hemost Thromb 6:139–177

Turitto VT, Baumgartner HR (1975) Platelet interaction with subendothelium in a perfusion system: physical role of red blood cells. Microvasc Res 9:335–344

Turpie AGG, Levine MN, Hirsh J, Carter CJ, Joy RM, Powers PJ, Andrew M, Hull RD, Gent M (1986) A randomized controlled trial of a low molecular weight heparin (enoxaparin) to prevent deep-vein thrombosis in patients undergoing elective hip surgery. NEJM 315:925–929

UPET (1970) Urokinase pulmonary embolism trial: phase I results: a cooperative study. JAMA 214:1263–1272

Urokinase Pulmonary Embolism Trial (1973) A national cooperative study. Circulation 47[Suppl II]:II7–II66 (American Heart Association monograph 39)

USPET (1974) Urokinase-streptokinase embolism trial: phase 2 results: a cooperative study. JAMA 229:1606–1613

van de Loo JCW, Kriessman A, Trubestein G, Knoch K, de Swart CAM, Asbeck F, Marbet GA, Schmitt H, Sewell AF, Duckert F, Theiss W, Ritz R (1983) Controlled multicenter pilot study of urokinase-heparin and streptokinase in deep-vein thrombosis. Thromb Haemost 50:660–663

Van de Werf F, Arnold AER for the European Cooperative Study Group for recombinant tissue-type plasminogen activator (1988) Intravenous tissue-plasminogen activator and size of infarct, left ventricular function, and survival in acute myocardial infarction. BMJ 297:1374–1378

Van de Werf F, Nobuhara M, Collen D (1986) Coronary thrombolysis with human single chain urokinase-type plasminogen activator (scu-PA) in patients with acute myocardial infarction. Ann Int Med 104:345–348

Vanhove PH, Donati MB, Claeys H, Verhaeghe R, Vermylen J (1979) Action of brinase on human fibronogen and plasminogen. Thromb Haemost 42:571–581

Venous Thrombosis Clinical Study Group (1975) Small doses of subcutaneous sodium heparin in the prevention of deep-vein thrombosis after elective hip operations. Br J Surg 62:348–350

Verhaeghe R, Verstraete M, Schetz J, Vanhove P, Suy R, Vermylen J (1979) Clinical trial of brinase and anticoagulants as a method of treatment for advanced limb ischemia. Eur J Clin Pharmacol 16:165–170

Verstraete M (1987) Biochemical and clinical aspects of thrombolysis. Semin Hematol 15:35–54

Verstraete M, Collen D (1986) Thrombolytic therapy in the eighties. Blood 67: 1529–1541

Verstraete M, Vermylen J, Amery A, Vermylen C (1966) Thrombolytic therapy with streptokinase using a standard dose scheme. Br Med J 1:454–456

Verstraete M, Vermylen J, Donati MB (1971) The effect of streptokinase infusion on chronic arterial occlusion and stenosis. Ann Int Med 74:377–382

Verstraete M, Vermylen J, Schetz J (1978) Biochemical changes noted during intermittent administration of streptokinase. Thromb Haemost 39:61–68

Verstraete M, Bernard R, Bory M, Brown RW, Collen D, de Bono DP, Erbel R, Huhman W, Lannane RJ, Lubsen J, Mathey D, Meyer J, Michels HR, Rutsch W, Schartt M, Schmidt W, Uebis R, von Eisen R (1985) Randomized trial of intravenous recombinant tissue-type plasminogen activator versus intravenous streptokinase in acute myocardial infarction. Report from the European Cooperative Study Group for recombinant tissue-type plasminogen activator. Lancet 1:842–847

Verstraete M, Miller GAH, Bounameaux H, Charbonnier B, Colle JP, Lecorf G, Marbet GA, Mombaerts P, Olsson CG (1988) Intravenous and intrapulmonary recombinant tissue-type plasminogen activator in the treatment of acute massive pulmonary embolism. Circulation 77:353–360

Wahl TO, Lipschitz DA, Stechschulte DJ (1978) Thrombocytopenia with antiheparin antibody. JAMA 240:2560–2562

Walker ID, Davidson JF (1987) Acylenzymes for Thrombolytic therapy. Semin Thromb Hemost 13:139–145

Walker ID, Davidson JF, Ray AP, Hutton I, Lawrie TDV (1984) Acylated streptokinase plasminogen complex in patients with acute myocardial infarction. Thromb Haemost 57:204–206

Walker MG, Shaw JW, Thomson GJL, Cumming JGR, Lea Thomas M (1987) Subcutaneous calcium heparin versus intravenous sodium heparin in treatment of established deep-vein thrombosis of the legs: a multicentre prospective randomized trial. BMJ 294:1189–1192

Watz R, Savidge GF (1979) Rapid thrombolysis and preservation of valvular venous function in high deep-vein thrombosis. Acta Med Scand 205:293–298

Weisman RE, Tobin RW (1958) Arterial embolism occurring during systemic heparin therapy. Arch Surg 76:219–227

Weksler B (1987) Platelet interactions with the blood vessel wall. In: Colman RW, Hirsh, J, Marder VJ, Salzman EW (eds) Hemostasis and thrombosis: basic principles and clinical practice, 2nd ed. Lippincott, Philadelphia, pp 804–815

Wessler S, Gitel SN, Bank H, Martinowitz U, Stephenson RC (1978) An assay of the antithrombotic action of warfarin: its correlation with the inhibition of stasis thrombosis in rabbits. Thromb Haemost 40:486–498

White HD, Norris RM, Brown MA, Takayama M, Maslowski A, Bass NM, Ormiston JA, Whitlock T (1987) Effect of intravenous streptokinase on left ventricular function and early survival after acute myocardial infarction. NEJM 317:850–855

White HD, Rivers JHT, Maslowski AH, Ormiston JA, Takayama M, Hart HH, Sharpe DN, Whitlock RML, Norris RM (1989) Effect of intravenous streptokinase as compared with that of tissue plasminogen activator on left ventricular function after first myocardial infarction. NEJM 320:817–821

White WF, Barlow GH, Mozen MM (1966) The isolation and characterization of plasminogen activators (urokinase) from human urine. Biochem 5:2160–2169

Whitfield LR, Lele AS, Levy G (1983) Effect of pregnancy on the relationship between concentration and anticoagulant action of heparin. Clin Pharmacol Ther 34:23–28

Wilcox RG, von der Lippe G, Olsson CG, Jensen G, Skene AM, Hampton JR for the ASSET Study Group (1988) Trial of tissue plasminogen activator for mortality reduction in acute myocardial infarction. Anglo-Scandinavian Study of Early Thrombolysis (ASSET). Lancet 2:525–530

Wilson JR, Lampman J (1979) Heparin therapy: a randomized prospective trial. Am Heart J 97:155–158

Wiman B, Mellbring G, Ranby M (1983) Plasminogen activator release during venous stasis and exercise as determined by a new specific assay. Clin Chim Acta 127:279–288

Wohl RC, Summaria L, Arzadon L, Robbins KC (1978) Steady state kinetics of activation of human and bovine plasminogens by streptokinase and its equimolar complexes with various forms of human plasminogen. J Biol Chem 253: 1402–1407

Yasuno M, Saito Y, Ishida M, Suzuki K, Endo S, Takahashi M (1984) Effects of percutaneous transluminal coronary angioplasty: intracoronary thrombolysis with urokinase in acute myocardial infarction. Am J Cardiol 53:1217–1220

Yin ET (1975) Effect of heparin on the neutralization of factor X_A and thrombin by the plasma α-II globulin inhibitor. Thromb Diath Haemorrh 33:43–50

Zamarron C, Lijnen HR, Van Hoef B, Collen D (1984) Biological and thrombolytic properties of proenzyme and active forms of urokinase. I. Fibrinolytic and fibrinogenolytic properties in human plasma in vitro of urokinases obtained from human urine and by recombinant DNA technology. Thromb Haemost 52:19–23

Zilliacus H (1946) On the specific treatment of thrombosis and pulmonary embolism with anticoagulants with particular reference to the postthrombotic sequelae. Acta Med Scand [Suppl]171:1–196

Zucker MB (1977) Biological aspects of heparin action. Fed Proc 36:47–49

CHAPTER 12

Granulocyte-Macrophage Growth Factors

P.J. QUESENBERRY

A. Introduction

Control of granulocyte production can no longer be considered in isolation from control of red blood cell, platelet, or lymphocyte production. This is because there is extensive networking with regard to regulation of these different systems, i.e., regulators and regulator cells which have effects on multiple lineages or which interact to augment effects on different lineages. The classic granulocyte-macrophage (GM) regulators, granulocyte-macrophage or granulocyte-colony stimulating factor (CSF), have major effects on in vitro red blood cell (RBC) and platelet (megakaryocyte) production (METCALF et al. 1986b; SIEFF et al. 1985; ROBINSON et al. 1987; QUESENBERRY et al. 1985) and probably on lymphocyte generation, while interleukin-3 (IL-3) affects megakaryocyte, neutrophil, mast cell, eosinophil, RBC, and monocyte production (IHLE 1983; PRYSTOWSKY et al. 1983). Thus, this chapter, while focusing on GM production, will of necessity touch on and describe elements of all the cell production systems housed in the marrow cavity.

B. Historical Background

A number of early studies suggested the existence of regulators of GM production (HANNA et al. 1967; DELMONTE 1967; ROTHSTEIN et al. 1971; BOGGS et al. 1968; BOGGS et al. 1967; HANKS and AINSWORTH EJ 1964; SAVAGE 1964). These studies demonstrated that fluids or serum from various animal species, when subjected to inflammatory or infectious stresses, would stimulate elevations in the white blood cell and neutrophil counts in vivo, similar to those seen during active bacterial infection. The lipopolysaccharide (LPS) component of the cell wall of gram-negative bacteria produces particularly dramatic effects on granulocyte levels, and its effects on the granulopoietic and hemopoietic systems were studied rather extensively (BOGGS et al. 1967, 1968; HANKS and AINSWORTH 1964; SAVAGE 1964). LPS or endotoxin appeared to have several major effects including stimulation of marrow neutrophil production and release of granulocytes from the bone marrow, the latter apparently mediated via a discrete releasing activity (probably granulocyte-colony stimulating activity, see below). Many earlier studies attempting to demonstrate the existence of granulopoietins specific for stimulating the bone marrow were confounded by the presence of endotoxins or alternatively by the marrow stimulatory influence of foreign proteins. The concept of granulopoietic regulatory hormones remained an unproven hypothesis until the introduction of in vitro culture systems allowing for the final characterization and purification of a number of these regulators.

The introduction of the in vitro clonal agar assay systems by BRADLEY and METCALF (1966) and PLUZNIK and SACHS (1965) laid the base for an explosion of information with regard to the granulopoietic regulatory growth factors. Much of the work preceding this is important in a historical vein, but our current understanding of the regulation of granulocyte and monocyte production has largely evolved since the introduction of clonal hemopoietic cultures and the application of molecular genetic cloning techniques to the study of hemopoiesis. The introduction of these techniques in the early 1960s essentially supplanted earlier approaches for the study of granulopoiesis. Previous studies of the effects of injected substances on neutrophil production were confounded by problems of specificity and in general were either too cumbersome or labor intensive to allow for rigorous purification of bioactive molecules. In the soft agar clonal culture systems, clones of GM derived from single cells grow in the semisolid culture matrix provided by soft agar and culture media. Essential components for this growth are "adequate" lots of pretested fetal calf serum and the presence of stimulatory molecules initially derived from a variety of tissues or bodily fluids (QUESENBERRY and LEVITT 1979). Marrow, spleen, or blood cells from a variety of species, most prominently mouse and man, were found to grow clonally in these systems (QUESENBERRY and LEVITT 1979) and to give rise to colonies consisting of granulocytes and macrophages, granulocytes alone, or macrophages alone. There was marked heterogeneity in colony size and growth factor sensitivity. Classic sigmoid-type dose-response curves were obtained with sources of stimulatory factor initially called colony stimulating activity (CSA). The single cell origin of these type of colonies was formally shown by physical translocation of single cells (MOORE et al. 1972), although in the ordinary situation many of the colonies may not in fact be from single cells. Over the years, since the first descriptions of these assays, modifications of the clonal systems have been reported, including the use of methylcellulose or plasma clot as a semisolid support matrix (AXELRAD et al. 1973; MCLEOD et al. 1974; ISCOVE et al. 1970), the use of different serum supplements or stimuli, and importantly the use of low oxygen tensions, which markedly augment colony formation (BRADLEY et al. 1978). Growth of erythroid colonies, megakaryocyte colonies, and a wide variety of mixed colony types was also obtained in these systems (AXELRAD et al. 1973; MCLEOD et al. 1974; METCALF et al. 1975; NAKAHATA and OGAWA 1982; FAUSER and MESSNER 1978), and various colony forming classes defined by the observed patterns of growth and differentiation (AXELRAD et al. 1973;

McLeod et al. 1974; Gregory 1976; Humphries et al. 1980; Long et al. 1985). Multilineage differentiation was also seen with colonies of 2–5 lineages being described. Ogawa and colleagues classic studies (Suda et al. 1984a,b) assessing the fate of daughter cells from separated doublets have indicated the presence of progenitor cells capable of giving rise to a large number of lineage combinations. In addition, these data indicated that separated daughter cells could produce quite distinct lineages under the same apparent culture conditions. This suggests that within one cell cycle a series of committment decisions can be made for different lineages. Table 1 outlines a number of the described stem/progenitor cells including one of the multipotent cells defined in in vivo systems, i.e., colony forming unit-spleen (CFU-S). It was found that the multilineage colonies appeared to require combinations of growth factors. This was initially studied with crude conditioned media, but with the availability of purified/cloned growth factors it became clear that a number of different combinations can act to stimulate a variety of hemopoietic cell classes in vitro. In fact, a better definition of various progenitor/stem cell classes may be by their growth factor responsiveness rather than by their in vitro phenotype. Thus, colony forming unit (CSF-1, GM-CSF, or GM-CSF + CSF-1), along with the time period of in vitro growth, in fact provides more meaningful information than the older terms of GM-CFU-C, M-CFC, etc. (Fig. 1).

C. Growth Factors

The above-described systems have been utilized to define both the marrow progenitor cells and their regulators. A good deal of initial information was generated with regard to a variety of tissue sources of growth factors. In these studies, bioactive molecules present in conditioned media from different cellular sources were assayed for their effect on colony formation,

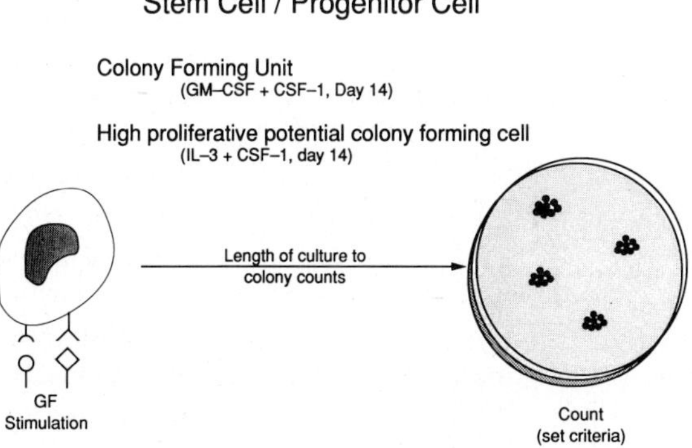

Fig. 1. Model for in vitro progenitor cell characterization

Table 1. Hemopoietic stem/progenitor cells

Stem/progenitor cell	Lineage	Growth factor
Colony forming unit spleen (CFU-S), murine only, day 8–9 and day 10–12	Erythroid, megakaryocyte, granulocyte/ macrophage, and self-renewal	Interleukin-3 (IL-3), probably many others
Granulocyte-macrophage colony forming cell (GM-CFC)	Granulocyte/ macrophage	Granulocyte/ macrophage-colony stimulating factor (GM-CSF) [to some extent granulocyte-colony stimulating factor (G-CSF) and CSF-1]
Macrophage-colony forming cell (M-CFC)	Macrophage/moncyte	CSF-1 (to some extent GM-CSF and IL-3)
Granulocyte-colony forming cell (G-CFC)	Granulocyte	G-CSF (to some extent GM-CSF and IL-3)
High proliferative potential forming cell (HPP-CFC)	Macrophage (potential for granulocyte, megakaryocyte)	CSF-l plus IL-3 and IL-1. Also GM-CSF + CSF-1, IL-3 + G-CSF, G-CSF + CSF-1, G-CSF + GM-CSF
Colony forming unit-erythroid (CFU-E)	Erythroid	Erythropoietin
Burst forming unit-erythroid (BFU-E)	Erythroid	Erythropoietin plus IL-3, GM-CSF, or IL-4
Colony forming unit-megakaryocyte (CFU-M)	Megakaryocyte	IL-3, GM-CSF, G-CSF, IL-6, megakaryocyte and thrombopoietin-like activities
Burst forming unit-megakaryocyte (BFU-M)	Megakaryocyte	IL-3, GM-CSF, thrombopoietin-like activity, plus phorbol myristate acetate (PMA) or cholera toxin
Colony forming unit granulocyte/erythroid/ macrophage and megakaryocyte (CFU-GEMM)	Granulocyte/ megakaryocyte/ macrophage, and possibly T cell	IL-3 and GM-CSF
Blast colony	Blast cell renewal and multilineage differentiation	IL-3, G-CSF, IL-6, possibly GM-CSF
Colony forming unit-diffusion chamber	Granulocyte/ macrophage, some megakaryocyte, erythroid	Not defined
Thy-1^{lo}Lin^{-} ^{s}ca-1^{+}	T, B and myeloid cells	Unknown

largely GM. Monocytes, T lymphocytes, endothelial cells, fibroblasts, and a variety of cell line populations were found to give rise to CSA (Chervenick and LoBuglio 1972; Parker and Metcalf 1974; Song and Quesenberry 1984; Quesenberry et al. 1987; Knudtzon and Mortensen 1975; Bickel et al. 1987; Zucali et al. 1986; Quesenberry and Gimbrone 1980). Vascular smooth muscle (Quesenberry et al. 1981), B lymphocytes (Bickel et al. 1987), keratinocytes (Chodakewitz et al. 1988), and thymic epithelial cells (Le et al. 1988) have also been noted as sources of CSAs. A number of investigations indicated that a variety of manipulations could influence serum levels of CSA in vivo and cellular production in vitro. Radiation, cytotoxic drug administration, viral infection, antigen exposure, and perhaps most dramatically endotoxin injection or bacterial infection caused striking elevations of GM-CSA in a variety of murine species (Shadduck and Nunna 1971; Quesenberry et al. 1975, 1978; Metcalf 1971; Foster et al. 1968; Morley et al. 1971). The common theme here seems to be a functional demand on the monocyte-granulocyte system, leading to increased serum levels of the CSAs. Exposure of different cell populations in vitro to phorbol esters, various mitogens, or endotoxin also resulted in marked increases of CSAs (Alberico et al. 1987; Greenberger et al. 1980; McNeil 1973; Sheriden and Metcalf 1973).

Critical progress in this research has resulted from the biochemical characterization and molecular cloning of a variety of specific polypeptide hormones included under the rubric of CSA. The classic GM-CSAs, granulocyte CSA (G-CSA), macrophage CSA (M-CSA or CSF-1), and GM-CSA were defined by their primary effects on in vitro GM proliferation and differentiation. However, there are a number of growth factors initially defined by their effects on other lineages which have now been shown to influence the granulocyte-macrophage system: These include agents which act early in hemopoietic lineages or synergistically or additively with other growth factors.

I. Colony Stimulating Factor-1

The first of the CSAs to be biochemically defined was M-CSF or CSF-1. Utilizing in vitro agar cloning as an assay and human urine or mouse L cells as a source, Stanley and Guilbert (1981) and Waheed and Shadduck (1979) characterized CSF-1. Murine CSF-1 purified from L-cell-conditioned media was found to be a glycoprotein with a molecular weight of 70000. Previous variations in molecular weight estimates were explained by differing degrees of glycosylation. The core structure of murine CSF-1 consists of a homodimeric protein with a molecular weight of 28000 consisting of two disulfide-bonded, 14000 molecular weight peptide chains. The dimer is transported to cell membranes and proteolytically separated from the membrane-bound segment (Das and Stanley 1982; Rettenmier et al. 1987). Genes for murine CSF-1 have been cloned and expressed (DeLamarter et al. 1987). CSF-1 purified from human urine is a heavily glycosylated homodimer of 45000 molecular weight. Genes for human CSF-1 have also been cloned and expressed (KAWASKI et al. 1985; WONG et al. 1987). The human form is a single gene which encodes several differentially spliced mRNA transcripts ranging in size from 1.5 to 4.5 kilobases (kb). The largest and most abdundant CSF-1 mRNA of 4.5 kb encodes a 61 kDa pre-pro-CSF-1 which is processed to a 21 kDa subunit. Several different sizes of human CSF-1 have been purified from natural sources; the smaller variety is possibly a proteolytic degradation product of the larger 70–90 kDa glycoprotein. CSF-1 has been found to act on early stem cells within the macrophage lineage (STANLEY and GUILBERT 1981; WAHEED and SHADDUCK 1979). Initial observations indicated that human CSF-1 had only marginal CSA for human macrophage progenitors while being an effective stimulator of murine progenitors (KAWASKI et al. 1985; WONG et al. 1987). However, when human marrow progenitors are exposed to "subliminal" (in the picogram range) concentrations of the recombinant human form (rhGM-CSF), their responsiveness to CSF-1 is markedly enhanced (CARACCIOLO et al. 1987).

Macrophage progenitors have been divided into two subpopulations, one responsive to CSF-1 alone and the other requiring two exogenous signals for clonal proliferation (MOORE et al. 1986). The latter cells express Ia antigen and are uniformally in cell cycle. They require CSF-1 and an additional "nonspecific" signal such as endotoxin. The inflammatory neuropeptide substance P and tuftsin could also act as costimulants with CSF-1 (MOORE et al. 1988). CSF-1 interacts with a number of other growth factors to stimulate primitive HPP-CFC-like stem cells (Tables 1, 2) and can augment ongoing division of phenotypically mature macrophages. In addition, both GM-CSF and IL-3 interact additively or synergistically to enhance the proliferative effects of CSF-1 on mature blood monocytes and peritoneal-derived or alveolar macrophages (CHEN and CLARK 1986; LIN et al. 1989). CSF-1 also acts throughout the differentiation sequence, being both a survival and proliferation factor for mature macrophages (TUSHINSKI and STANLEY 1983, 1985). The various functional effects of CSF-1 are described in Table 2.

The CSF-1 gene is found in humans on the long arm of the fifth chromosome in the critical cluster region (5q23–32) which includes genes for GM-CSF, IL-3, IL-4, IL-5 platelet derived growth factor (PDGF) receptor, and endothelial cell growth factor (PETTENATI et al. 1987; ROUSSEL et al. 1983; SHERR et al. 1985; HUEBNER et al. 1985; LEBEAU et al. 1986). The receptor for CSF-1 has now been characterized and found to be the product of the *fms* protooncogene (SHERR et al. 1985). This also codes on the long arm of the fifth chromosome and is deleted in most cases of the $5q^-$ preleukemic syndrome: In 90% there is deletion of all these genes, but in the remaining 10% the CSF-1 and *fms* genes are retained.

Studies characterizing the cellular action of CSF-1 have recently suggested the involvement of G-proteins linking the receptor system to second

Table 2. Biologic actions of colony stimulating factor-1 (CSF-1)

1. Stimulates predominantly macrophage colonies in vitro with some granulocyte component early in culture (STANLEY and GUILBERT 1981; WAHEED and SHADDUCK 1979)
2. Supports survival of differentiated macrophages in vitro; at low doses decreases protein catabolism while at higher concentrations increases protein synthesis and proliferation (TUSHINSKI and STANLEY 1983, 1985)
3. Increases macrophage antitumor activity (WING et al. 1982), the secretion of O_2 reduction products (WING et al. 1985), arachidonic acid (ZIBOH et al. 1982), glucose uptake in murine marrow derived macrophages (HAMILTON et al. 1986), and plasminogen activator (LIN and GORDON 1979)
4. Synergizes with low levels of GM-CSF to give increased human macrophage colony formation and shows other synergistic or additive interactions on various aspects of colony formation with GM-CSF, G-CSF, IL-1, and IL-3 (CARACCIOLO et al. 1987; MCNIECE et al. 1988b,c; MOCHIZUKI et al. 1987)
5. Interacts with receptor which is the c-*fms* protooncogene product (SHERR et al. 1985)
6. Induces synthesis of G-CSF in murine peritoneal cells (METCALF and NICOLA 1985) or in human monocytes (WARREN and RALPH 1986) and enhances production of interferon and TNF by these latter cells after exposure to endotoxin
7. Increases in vitro replication of HIV in blood-derived monocytes (KOYANAQI et al. 1988; GENDELMAN et al. 1988). Induces resistance to viral infection in murine macrophages (LEE and WARREN 1987)
8. Circulatory levels may be regulated by rapid receptor mediated endocytosis and intracellular degradation in macrophages (BARTOCCI et al. 1987)
9. Variable effects when given to cytopenic humans in vivo–some transient increase in neutrophil levels or shortening of duration of leukopenia (KOMIYAMA et al. 1988; MOTOYOSHI et al. 1986)
10. Enhances killing of *Candida albicans* by murine macrophages (KARBASSI et al. 1989)
11. In vivo actions in mice–percentage, in DNA synthesis and absolute number of CFU-GM, CFU-GEMM, BFU-E increased by administration of 20000 U to mice (BROXMEYER et al. 1987a)
12. Action on macrophage colony formation enhanced in humans by subliminal concentrations of GM-CSF (CARACCIOLO et al. 1987)
13. Induces IL-1 from macrophages (MOORE et al. 1980)
14. Induces migration of human monocytes (WANG et al. 1980)

GM, granulocyte/macrophage; IL, Interleukin; HIV, human immunodeficiency virus; CFU, colony forming unit; BFU, blast forming unit; GEMM, granulocyte/erythroid/macrophage/megakaryocyte.

messenger pathways (HE et al. 1988). In addition, it has been found that the CSF-1 receptor autophosphorylates on exposure to CSF-1 and is a tyrosine kinase. Expression of CSF-1 or c-*fms* mRNA or production of the active growth factor has also been demonstrated in some human leukemias or cell lines (HL-60) with a suggestion of possible autocrine mechanisms underlying some of these cases (WAKAMIYA et al. 1987).

In general, the effects of CSF-1 in vivo have been less impressive than that of the other GM growth factors. Effects of cycling of murine stem cells have been demonstrated (BROXMEYER et al. 1987), and CSF-1 administration in an in vivo clinical trial resulted in relatively small, but apparently significant, increases in WBC and neutrophil levels in neutropenic pediatric patients (KOMIYAMA et al. 1988). In this study eight of nine patients responded to a 7-day course of human urinary CSF (equivalent to CSF-1). Repeated cyclical increases were seen in five after therapy had been completed, and three finally remitted completely (i.e., had normal neutrophil counts) after several cycles of fluctuation. In other studies, CSF-1 administration decreased the length of neutrophil nadir in patients treated with cytotoxic chemotherapy (MOTOYOSHI et al. 1986). It seems probable that its major in vivo clinical role may be as part of a synergistic combination with other growth factors. Recently, an enzyme-linked immunosorbent assay (ELISA) for CSF-1 was described and used to measure human serum CSF-1 levels (HANAMURA et al. 1988). This method detected two types of human CSF-1 in both serum and urine, with molecular weights of 85 000 and 45 000. After cancer chemotherapy, serum CSF-1 levels were elevated in one-half of the patients.

II. Granulocyte-Macrophage-Colony Stimulating Factor

GM-CSF was the next hemopoietic growth factor to be characterized biochemically. This was purified from murine lung by BURGESS and colleagues (1977) and subsequently characterized from a human T-cell leukemic line (GASSON et al. 1984). As with CSF-1, GM-CSF was initially defined by its effect on in vitro colony formation, in this instance that of GM colonies. Human GM-CSF was found to be a glycoprotein, with the core protein having a molecular weight of 22 000, while the murine variety is a 23 000 molecular weight glycoprotein. The genes for both murine and human GM-CSF have been cloned. The murine gene was obtained from a murine lung cDNA library (GOUGH et al. 1984) and then from a concanavalin-A-primed T lymphocyte clone. It contains 124 amino acids with a molecular weight of 14 134. The human cDNA was isolated from Mo leukemic cells and from a human T-cell leukemic line (LEE et al. 1985; WONG et al. 1985). It contains 127 amino acids with a molecular weight of approximately 14 000. There is 70% nucleotide homology with the coding region of murine GM-CSF but no cross reactivity. The murine gene is found on chromosome 11 (GOUGH et al. 1984), while the human gene is found in the same cluster region as CSF-1 in the long arm of chromosome 5 (HUEBNER et al. 1985; LEBEAU et al. 1986). Evidence has arisen for the existence of the region upstream of the 5′-end of the GM-CSF gene regulating production of GM-CSF mRNA (CHAN et al. 1986). Further data have suggested the possibility that nucleotide AT sequences 3′ of the gene may influence the stability of the GM-CSF mRNA, and such effects may account for elevated levels of GM-CSF mRNA under certain experimental conditions such as phorbol ester or 1,25-dihydroxyvitamin D_3 stimulation of cells (SHAW and KAMEN 1986; TOBLER et al. 1988). BICKEL et al. (1988) have shown differential inhibition of IL-3 mRNA but not GM-CSF mRNA production by the transcriptional inhibitor 5,6-dichloro-1-β-ribofuranasilbenzamidazole, further indicating posttranscriptional control of GM-CSF production. As with CSF-1, GM-CSF has been found to have actions throughout the GM differentiation pathway (METCALF et al. 1986; SIEFF et al. 1985). It appears to act on relatively early progenitor cells (METCALF et al. 1986; SIEFF et al. 1985; MCNIECE et al. 1988b,c) but also has major effects on end-cell function, influencing phagocytosis, movement, and metabolic activity of mature GM (Table 3) (GASSON et al. 1984; FLEISCHMANN et al. 1986; METCALF et al. 1986b; VADAS et al. 1983; HANDMAN and BURGESS 1979; ARANOUT et al. 1986; WEISBART et al. 1985; DISPERSIO et al. 1987; STANLEY and BURGESS 1983; SILBERSTEIN et al. 1986). CSF-1 has a relatively restricted influence on the macrophage lineage, but GM-CSF has been found to have a wide variety of effects on multiple cellular lineages. It has intrinsic megakaryocyte stimulating effects (ROBINSON et al. 1987; QUESENBERRY et al. 1985), appears to enhance the effect of erythropoietin on in vitro erythroid colony formation, i.e., has burst promoting activity (METCALF et al. 1986; SIEFF et al. 1985), and influences, in concert with other factors, HPP-CFC (MCNIECE et al. 1988b,c) and multipotent progenitor cells in different in vitro systems (SONODA et al. 1988). Other data indicate possible effects on lymphoid systems (T and B cell) (Table 3). Receptors for GM-CSF have been partially characterized on both mature granulocytes and cell lines and the responsiveness of human acute myelogenous leukemia blasts documented (DISPERSIO et al. 1987; WALKER and BURGESS 1985). Constitutive expression of the GM-CSF gene in acute myelobiastic leutemia (AML) blasts has also been noted, suggesting the existence of autocrine mechanisms in some cases of AML (YOUNG et al. 1987). Cells responding to GM-CSF have a low number of high affinity binding receptors with a molecular weight of the cell surface binding protein of approximately 84000 (DISPERSIO et al. 1987). GM-CSF when added to a growth-arrested, factor-dependent cell line induces progression from G_1 into S phase (PLUZNIK et al. 1984). The induction of monocyte tumoricidal toxicity (Table 3) by GM-CSF appears to be mediated by increased release of tumor necrosis factor (CANNISTRA et al. 1988), and enhancement of neutrophil function (F-met-lev-phe-elicited nitroductetrazoliom (NBT) reduction and depolarization) by GM-CSF occurred by increasing the percentage of responsive cells (FLETCHER and GASSON 1988). More recent data suggest the possibility that GM-CSF may have effects on colon adenocarcinoma (BERDEL et al. 1989) or small cell carcinoma (BALDWIN et al. 1987) cell lines. There was a long-standing controversy over whether the in vitro actions of different CSAs (or factors) simply represented in vitro tissue culture artifacts with little in vivo physiologic relevance. This seemed unlikely, given the specificity and potency of action of these growth factors, and recently, with the availability of large amounts of recombinant growth factor for in vivo testing, in vivo activity of the CSFs have been established putting to rest the "relevance question".

Table 3. Biologic actions of granulocyte-macrophage-colony stimulating factor (GM-CSF)

1. Stimulates granulocyte-macrophage, granulocyte, and macrophage colony factor formation in vitro (METCALF et al. 1986c; SIEFF et al. 1985) and proliferation of normal human promyelocytes and myelocytes (BEGLEY et al. 1988)
2. Stimulates megakaryocyte colonies and with erythropoietin acts as erythroid burst promoting activity (METCALF et al. 1986c; SIEFF et al. 1985; ROBINSON et al. 1987; QUESENBERRY et al. 1985)
3. Enhances cytotoxic and phagocytic activity of neutrophils against bacteria, yeast, parasites, and antibody-coated tumor cells. Also enhances ADCC (FLEISCHMANN et al. 1986; METCALF et al. 1986b; VADAS et al. 1983; HANDMAN and BURGESS 1979)
4. Increases cell-cell adhesion and surface expression of adhesion promoting glycoproteins on mature granulocytes (ARANOUT et al. 1986) and administered to humans as a continuous infusion up-regulates the expression of the adhesion glycoprotein cD11 b on granulocytes (SOCINSKI et al. 1988a)
5. Enhances superoxide anion generation in response to f-MLP and increases arachidonic acid release and leukotriene B4 synthesis in neutrophils in response to Ca^{2+} ionophore and chemoattractants (WEISBART et al. 1985; DISPERSIO et al. 1987)
6. Increases synthesis of membrane and nucleoprotein in mature granulocytes (STANLEY and BURGESS 1983)
7. Enhances human eosinophil cytotoxicity and leukotriene synthesis (SILBERSTEIN et al. 1986)
8. Stimulates granulocyte/macrophage and possibly platelet production in vivo in mouse, primates, and man (DONAHUE et al. 1986a,b; VADHAN-RAJ et al. 1987) and expands GM-CFC number in the peripheral blood of treated patients (SOCINSKI et al. 1988b)
9. Stimulates some AML blast progenitors to proliferate in vitro (VALLENGA et al. 1987; MIYAUCHI et al. 1987;) and in vivo (GANSER et al. 1989)
10. Stimulates proliferation of small cell carcinoma cell lines (BALDWIN et al. 1987)
11. Supports in vitro human multipotent progenitor proliferation (SONODA et al. 1988)
12. Enhances PMA and *zymosin*-elicited H_2O_2 release and stimulates Fc-dependent phagocytosis by murine peritoneal macrophages (COLEMAN et al. 1988) and reversibly augments synthesis of 1-A molecules and membrane IL-1 expression in murine marrow macrophages and increases their function as antigen presenting cells (FISCHER et al. 1988)
13. Increases human basophil histamine release (HIRAI et al. 1988)
14. Administration to humans lowers serum cholesterol levels (NIMER et al. 1988)
15. Amplifies IL-2 stimulated T-cell proliferation and acts synergistically with IL-3 in this regard (SANTOLI et al. 1988). Also stimulates one plasmacytoma cell line (VINK et al. 1988)
16. Stimulates guanylate cyclase and decreases adenylate cyclase activity in human blood neutrophils (COFFEY et al. 1988)

ADCC, antibody-dependent cell-mediated cytotoxicity; PMA, phorbol myristale acetate.

Initial research in both mice and primates demonstrated that administration of GM-CSF causes significant increases in granulocytes, monocytes, eosinophils, and to a lesser extent other white cell types in both normal animals or animals subjected to cytotoxic drugs or irradiation-induced marrow suppression (DONAHUE et al. 1986a,b; WELTE et al. 1986; MONRAY et al. 1987; MAYER et al. 1987; BONILLA et al. 1987). Effects on both platelet and reticulocyte counts have been seen in some of these studies.

A number of trials have been carried out assessing the efficacy of GM-CSF under various clinical conditions (VADHAN-RAJ et al. 1987; GROOPMAN et al. 1987; ANTMAN et al. 1988; BRANDT et al. 1988). In general, GM-CSF has been found to augment the total WBC, granulocyte, eosinophil, and questionably lymphocyte count under conditions associated with myelosuppression, i.e., cancer chemotherapy. In one study of 16 adults with metastatic or inoperable sarcoma treated by chemotherapy, rhGM-CSF lessened mean total leukocyte and platelet nadirs (ANTMAN et al. 1988), while in another study in which 19 patients with breast cancer or melanoma were treated by high-dose chemotherapy and autologous marrow transplantation, there was acceleration of recovery of the leukocyte counts, but "no consistent effect" was seen on platelet counts (BRANDT et al. 1988). However, in a separate investigation, infusion of GM-CSF given after treatment with total body irradiation/chemotherapy followed by autologous marrow transplantation accelerated both neutrophil and platelet recovery if the dose was over 60 μg/m^2 daily (NEUMUNAITIS et al. 1988). In primary marrow disorders such as aplastic anemia and myelodysplasia, it is clearly active, although in the former case the effects seem transient, and in the latter case progression of leukemia has been seen especially with patients with elevated blast counts (VADHAN-RAJ et al. 1987; GANSER et al. 1989; BRANDT et al. 1988). GM-CSF also increased WBC and granulocyte counts in AIDS patients, enhanced neutrophil antibody-dependent, cell-mediated toxicity and superoxide generation and in two patients with discrete neutrophil function defects reversed the defects (GROOPMAN et al. 1987; BALDWIN et al. 1988). Since leukemic cells generally respond to GM-CSF with proliferation and in many cases respond synergistically to combinations of the CSFs, great caution needs to be exercised in the use of the factors to treat myelodysplasias or leukemias. Figure 2 presents a scheme for investigating these growth factors in myelodysplastic syndrome (MDS) or acute nonlymphocytic leukemia (ANLL).

An ELISA has been developed for human GM-CSF (CEBON et al. 1988). This assay is quantitative between 100 pg/ml and 2.5 ng/ml for bacterially synthesized hGM-CSF in humans. Following a single intravenous bolus of hGM-CSF in humans there was 2 apparent phases with half-lives of less than 5 min and of 150 min. After subcutaneous administration, detectable serum levels were found within 15–30 min, and serum levels were sustained (at a subcutaneous dose of 10 μg/kg) at >1 ng/ml for over 12 h.

III. Granulocyte-Colony Stimulating Factor

G-CSF was first defined as a relatively selective stimulator of pure granulocyte colonies from normal marrow and as a factor which could induce differentiation of leukemic cell lines (NICOLA et al. 1983, 1985). It

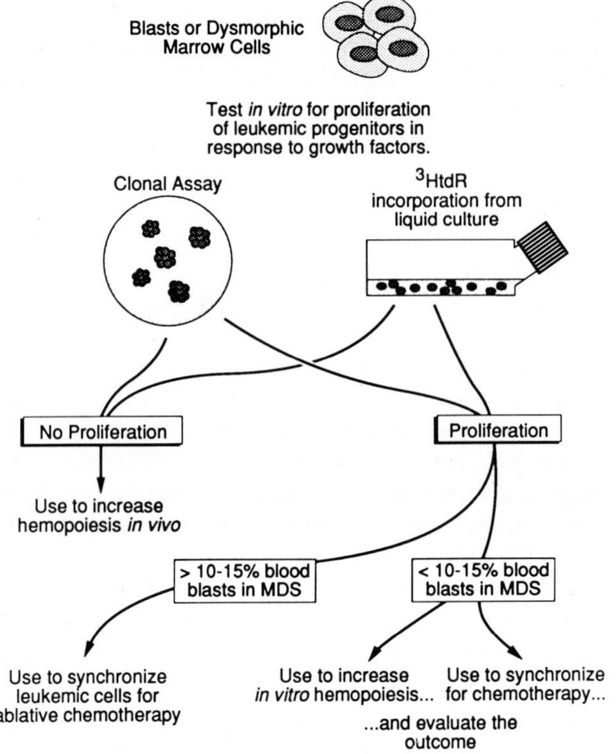

Fig. 2. Growth factor use in leukemic patients

was purified from mouse lung and found to have a molecular weight of 25 000 (NICOLA et al. 1983). hG-CSF was found to have a similar molecular weight and to cross-react on both human and murine marrow cells. The cDNAs for both G-CSFs were cloned (NAGATA et al. 1986; TSUCHIYA et al. 1986), and the human one was found to encode a polypeptide with a 30-amino acid signal sequence followed by a mature G-CSF sequence of 177 amino acids. The calculated molecular weight is 18 987. G-CSF has a significant degree of homology at its amino-terminus with IL-6 (HIRANO et al. 1986). The gene for hG-CSF has been localized on chromosome 17 proximal to the break-point seen in translocation 15:17 which characterizes acute promyelocytic leukemia (SIMMERS et al. 1987). Murine G-CSF along with IL-3 and GM-CSF has been localized to chromosome 11. While G-CSF was first defined as an agent acting to cause differentiation of leukemic cell lines and to stimulate pure granulocyte colonies, its range of actions has been expanded considerably with further testing of the pure and/or recombinant growth factors. G-CSF stimulates some GM progenitors, acts synergistically with IL-3 to stimulate megakaryocyte colonies and blast colonies, and interacts with GM-CSF, IL-3, or CSF-1 to stimulate high proliferation potential colony forming cells (McNIECE et al. 1988a,b; IKEBUCHI et al. 1988). Thus, it appears to have important actions on early marrow stem cells in both mice and humans. As with GM-CSF and CSF-1, G-CSF also has major actions on the differentiated cells of the GM pathway, enhancing phagocytosis, superoxide release, antibody-dependent cellular cytotoxicity, and migration of both neutrophils and monocytes (VADAS et al. 1983; AVALOS et al. 1987; WANG et al. 1988). High-affinity binding sites for G-CSF have been found on neutrophils, and 156 kDa has been estimated as the size of its receptor (AVALOS et al. 1987). In vivo kinetics of hG-CSF-induced neutrophilia was studied in rats and in many aspects mimics the patterns of neutrophil changes seen after endotoxin. There was an initial peripheral neutropenia between 3 and 15 min and a subsequent neutrophilia beginning at 0.5 h, peaking between 12 and 24 h, and returning to normal by 30 h. This initial pattern is probably due to reticuloendothelial sequestration of neutrophils followed by marrow granulocyte release. Hypersegmentation of neutrophil nuclei was seen between 30 and 48 h, and both dexamethasone and γ-interferon inhibited the degree of neutrophilia (ULICH et al. 1988). Treatment with hG-CSF increased numbers of circulating peripheral blood progenitor cells of GM, erythroid, and megakaryocytic lineages up to 100-fold in 30 cancer patients, while in most cases the quantity of marrow progenitor cells was slightly decreased. There was no change in responsiveness of marrow progenitors to G-CSF and GM-CSF in this study (DUHRSEN et al. 1988). Biologic actions of G-CSF are summarized in Table 4.

G-CSF has major effects on leukemic cells, and while defined initially as a differentiation factor it clearly also stimulates proliferation, this effect apparently being more prominent with human cells. It stimulates proliferation of human leukemic cells from patients with acute myelocytic leukemia and in many cases to acts synergistically with IL-3 or GM-CSF in this or in support of proliferation of leukemic cells in liquid culture.

G-CSF has also been established to have in vivo activity in mice, hamsters, primates, and humans, stimulating impressive neutrophil increases with lesser increases in monocytes, "lymphocytes," and at least in one instance platelets (Table 4). G-CSF lessens the extent and/or duration of neutropenia seen after the administration of cytotoxic drugs or irradiation to mice and primates, and in several clinical trials it has now been shown to reduce the neutrophil count depression in patients given aggressive combination chemotherapy (Table 4). In a phase I/II study of G-CSF in cancer patients treated with melphalan, G-CSF administered prior to melphalan caused a transient depression in circulating neutrophils followed by a dose-dependent rise along with increases in lymphocytes and monocytes. G-CSF given after melphalan reduced the period of neutropenia, with bone pain as the only significant side effect. Peripheral blood clearance of G-CSF was studied using a bioassay, and the mean half-life for the second phase was 110 min (MORSTYN et al. 1988). A patient with chronic idiopathic neutropenia was treated with G-CSF and at doses of 3 μg/kg maintained a

Table 4. Biologic action of granulocyte-colony stimulating factor (G-CSF)

1. Stimulates formation of granulocyte colonies in vitro and some GM progenitors, but the latter are not sustained beyond a few days
2. Induces terminal differentiation of WEHI-3B myelomonocytic leukemia cells (NICOLA et al. 1983)
3. Stimulates proliferation and differentiation of some but not all human myeloid leukemic cells (VALLENGA et al. 1987; MIYAUCHI et al. 1987)
4. Acts synergistically with IL-3 to stimulate megakaryocyte colonies and blast colonies (IKEBUCHI et al. 1988; MCNIECE et al. 1988a) and with GM-CSF to stimulate GM colonies and HPP-CFC, and with CSF-1 to stimulate HPP-CFC (MCNIECE et al. 1982, 1988)
5. Increases proliferation of small cell carcinoma H-128 cells, HL-60 and KG1 cells (AVALOS et al. 1987)
6. Primes neutrophils to undergo enhanced oxidative metabolism in response to f-MLP (AVALOS et al. 1987)
7. Increases antibody-dependent, cell-mediated cytotoxicity (ADCC) of human neutrophils and enhances ability to ingest particles (WANG et al. 1988; VADAS et al. 1983)
8. Primes neutrophils for enhanced arachidonic acid release in response to ionophore and chemoattractants (AVALOS et al. 1987)
9. Stimulates leukocytosis predominantly neutrophilic in mouse/primates and man (ULICH et al. 1988; DUHRSEN et al. 1988; OKABE and TAKAKU 1986; GILLIO et al. 1986; GABRILOVE et al. 1987; MORSTYN et al. 1988)
10. Has *chemoactivity* for both neutrophils and monocytes (WANG et al. 1988).

neutrophil level of 1500 per microliter (JAKUBOWSKI et al. 1989). In this patient, G-CSF induced oscillations of neutrophil counts with a frequency of about 40 days. Counts of monocytes, lymphocytes, eosinophils, and platelets also showed oscillation patterns. Preliminary results from one trial of G-CSF in MDS suggests that this treatment may improve hemopoiesis without accelerating the leukemic process (NEGRIN et al. 1988).

IV. Interleukin-3

IL-3 or multi-CSF was first identified as a putative T-cell factor with the capacity to induce the synthesis of 20-α-steroid dehydrogenase in splenic lymphocytes of nude mice. It was subsequently characterized as to its capacity to induce the marker Thy-1 (IHLE 1983). Further work has demonstrated that neither Thy-1 nor 20-α-steroid dehydrogenase are specific T-cell markers as they are seen on myeloid cells at certain stages of differentiation (IHLE 1983; HAPEL et al. 1985). Furthermore, a factor-dependent cell line, FDC-Pl, used for purification turned out to not be selective for IL-3 but also responsive to GM-CSF (ALBERICO et al. 1987). It is remarkable that in spite of these difficulties, IL-3 was characterized and purified successfully; it turned out, however, to have its major biologic effect on myeloid rather than lymphoid cell proliferation and differentiation (IHLE 1983). With the purification and subsequent genetic cloning (IHLE et al. 1982; CLARK-LEWIS et al. 1984; CUTLER et al. 1985; WATSON et al. 1986; FUNG et al. 1984;

YOKOTA et al. 1984), it became apparent that a number of previously described bioactivities including stem cell activation factor inducing CFU-S into cell cycle (SAF), multi-CSF inducing multilineage colonies in in vitro agar culture (CUTLER et al. 1985), burst promoting activity, one of several enhancing the in vitro action of erythropoietin (PRYSTOWSKY et al. 1983), and the mast cell or persisting factor which supported mast cell growth in liquid culture (*P factor*) (CLARK-LEWIS et al. 1984) represented different biologic activities of the 28000-dalton glycoprotein termed IL-3. It also represents one of the synergistic factors acting with CSF-1 to stimulate HPP-CFC (MCNIECE et al. 1982). It enhances in vitro growth of neutrophil, macrophage, eosinophil, and mast cell colonies and is probably the major megakaryocyte stimulator. Its interaction with erythropoietin, CSF-1, GM-CSF, IL-1, or G-CSF to stimulate different classes of in vitro colony forming cells, including BFU-E (PRYSTOWSKY et al. 1983), HPP-CFC (MCNIECE et al. 1982), and blast colony forming units (KOIKE et al. 1985), probably indicates an action on relatively primitive marrow stem cells. However, as with GM-CSF, G-CSF, and CSF-1, it appears to have actions on the more mature progeny of different lineages activating eosinophils (but not neutrophils) (LOPEZ et al. 1987) which respond to rhIL-3 by generating increased levels of leukotriene C4 in response to calcium ionophore, showing increased killing of antibody-coated *Schistosoma mansoni* larvae, and becoming hypodense (ROTHENBERG et al. 1988). It also augments the proliferation of alveolar pulmonary macrophages and in the presence of CSF-1 synergistically acts to stimulate proliferation of blood monocytes and peritoneal macrophages (CHEN and CLARK 1986). Both GM-CSF and IL-3 also cause basophil histamine release (HAAK-FRENDSCHO et al. 1988). Its actions on the lymphoid pathways are less clear. The IL-3-dependent precursor B-cell line, LyD9, differentiates in vitro into mature B cells, producing IgM and IgG when cocultured with bone marrow accessory cells or with dendritic cells and T cells. This is blocked by an IL-4-specific antibody (KINASHI et al. 1988). However, recombinant murine IL-3 failed to stimulate T or B lymphopoiesis in vivo but enhanced the IgM and IgG response to a T-cell-dependent antigen (KIMOTO et al. 1988). IL-3 (and IL-6 also) act synergistically to support proliferation of human and murine multipotential stem cells in G_o and may shorten G_o residence time (YOKOTA et al. 1984; KOIKE et al. 1985). IL-3 interacts with either G-CSF or GM-CSF synergistically to stimulate HPP-CFC (MCNIECE et al. 1988a).

Human IL-3 has been cloned using a gibbon cDNA isolated from a gibbon T-cell line to locate the human gene, and human IL-3 seems to have biologic actions similar to the more extensively studied murine IL-3 (YANG et al. 1986). Recombinant human IL-3 stimulates proliferation and differentiation of erythroid, granulocyte, macrophage, eosinophil, and mixed colonies as well as megakaryocytes from human marrow, but rhGM-CSF provided a stronger stimulus than IL-3 for day 14 myeloid colonies, and rhIL-3 had little stimulatory effect on day 7 colonies. IL-3 had virtually no stimulatory effect on the proliferation of promyelocytes and myelocytes, and there was no influence on several functions of mature neutrophils (ADCC of tumor cells or superoxide anion production after f-met-leu-phe), but mature eosinophils were stimulated by rhIL-3 to kill antibody-coated tumor cells. These data indicated a progressively decreasing effect of rhIL-3 on neutrophil lineages with maturation (LOPEZ et al. 1988). BOT et al. (1988), utilizing purified $CD34^+$ human marrow cells, presented findings indicating that hIL-3 (or multi-CSF) stimulation of CFU-GM, CFU-G, and CFU-M was mediated by accessory monocytes, while effects on early progenitors and CFU-E appeared to be direct. Further work by SONODA et al. (1988) using a serum-free system suggested that hIL-3 or GM-CSF alone or in combination did not effectively support proliferation of progenitor cells but needed the presence of G-CSF or erythropoietin to give neutrophil and erythroid colonies, respectively.

IL-3 is relatively unique amongst the hemolymphopoietic growth factors in that it appears to have a very limited cellular source for production, i.e., T lymphocytes (see below) (IHLE 1983; YANG et al. 1986). Other cell types have not been shown to be sources of IL-3, and this has led to speculation that this growth factor ("hormone") is an emergency-type regulator and not important in baseline regulation. I think it more probable that IL-3 at very low concentrations and in concert with other growth factors is a critical baseline regulator. Again, with the other myeloid growth factors, IL-3 stimulates AML blasts and blast progenitors to proliferate (MIYAUCHI et al. 1987). AML blasts as well as normal murine and human marrow cells have receptors for IL-3 (NICOLA and METCALF 1986; PARK et al. 1986; SORENSON et al. 1986).

Its mechanism of action is as yet unclear. Studies in the IL-3-dependent murine cell line, FDC-Pl, indicated a receptor with a molecular weight of about 67000. Exposure of FDC-Pl cells to IL-3 may lead to the translocation of protein kinase C to the plasma membrane (FARRAR et al. 1985), although there is significant controversy in this area. Phosphorylation of a novel 68 kDa substrate has been reported, and exposure to IL-3 appears to induce tyrosine phosphorylation of a membrane glycoprotein of M_r 150000 in multifactor-dependent myeloid cell lines (KOYASU et al. 1987). IL-3 has been noted to stimulate hexose uptake (WHETTON et al. 1985), enhance arginase activity (SCHNEIDER et al. 1985), and alter calcium mobilization (ROSSIO et al. 1986). Pertussis toxin, which ADP-ribosylates guanine nucleotide binding proteins (G proteins), partially blocks the action of IL-3 on FDC-Pl cells, suggesting that IL-3 may transduce signals from this receptor through G proteins to the inositol phosphate second messenger pathway (HE et al. 1988). The biologic actions of IL-3 are summarized in Table 5.

IL-3 has also been shown to have in vivo activity. When injected into mice it induces a 10-fold increase in blood eosinophils and a three fold increase in granulocytes and monocytes. Splenic hemopoiesis was increased, with prominent effects on mast cells, and many tissues showed increases in

Table 5. Biologic action of interleukin-3 (IL-3)

1. Stimulates formation of granulocyte, macrophage, eosinophil, mast cell, natural killer (NK)-like cell, erythroid and multipotent colonies from murine fetal liver and bone marrow. Similar range of colony formation to human IL-3 (IHLE 1983; LOPEZ et al. 1987) and shows decreasing effects on neutrophil lineages with increasing maturation (LOPEZ et al. 1988)
2. Induces 20α-hydroxy steroid dehydrogenase in splenic lymphocytes from nu/nu mice and also in marrow cells and induces Thy-1 expression in lymphoid and myeloid cells (IHLE 1983)
3. Interacts with erythropoietin to stimulate primitive erythroid stem cells (PRYSTOWSKY et al. 1983) and with CSF-1 to stimulate HPP-CFC (MCNIECE et al. 1982). Also supports proliferation of blast colony forming cells in vitro (KOIKE et al. 1985)
4. Induces CFU-S into cell cycle
5. Induces AML blast progenitors to proliferate (MIYAUCHI et al. 1987)
6. Possibly translocates protein kinase C to plasma membrane of factor dependent cell line cells (FARRAR et al. 1985)
7. Stimulates hexose uptake in WEHI-3B myelomonocytic leukemic cells (WHETTON et al. 1985). Enhances arginase activity (SCHNEIDER et al. 1985) and alters calcium mobilization in factor-dependent murine cell lines (ROSSIO et al. 1986)
8. Stimulates granulocyte, monocyte, eosinophil, and mast cell production in vivo (METCALF et al. 1986) and synergizes with GM-CSF and CSF-1 to induce progenitor cells into cell cycle in mice (BROXMEYER et al. 1987a,b). Sequential treatment of primates with IL-3 followed by GM-CSF acted synergistically to increase blood neutrophil, monocyte, lymphocyte, and eosinophil levels, while alone IL-3 augmented reticulocytes and platelet levels in these primates (DONAHUE et al. 1987)
9. Directly stimulates pulmonary alveolar macrophages to proliferate and acts synergistically with CSF-1 to stimulate proliferation of blood monocytes and peritoneal macrophages (CHEN and CLARK 1986)
10. Stimulates generation of increased levels of leukotriene C4 in response to calcium ionophore and increases killing of *Schistosoma mansoni larvae*. It also induces eosinophils to become hypodense (ROTHENBERG et al. 1988)
11. Induction of basophil histamine release (HAAK-FRENDSCHO et al. 1988)

macrophages or mast cells (METCALF et al. 1986). Single injections of IL-3 induced most types of murine marrow progenitors into cell cycle. In murine species, IL-3, GM-CSF, and CSF-1 in low doses act synergistically to induce progenitor cell cycling (BROXMEYER et al. 1987a,b), and sequential treatment of primates with rhIL-3 followed by low-dose rhGM-CSF increases synergistically blood neutrophil, monocyte, lymphocyte, and eosinophil levels (DONAHUE et al. 1987). In these studies, IL-3 alone augmented reticulocyte and platelet levels.

D. Other Interleukins

The list of growth factors impacting on the GM system continues to grow. The designation of a growth factor as "lymphoid," "myeloid," or "mesenchymal" is clearly arbitrary, and as the growth factors are studied more extensively, less and less lineage specificity is apparent. Growth factors modulating the growth, differentiation, and function of relatively mature lymphoid cells have been termed interleukins (IL-3 is an exception), and IL-1, 2, 4, 5, 6, and 7 have now been described. A relatively large number of biologic effects assessed in a variety of assay systems turned out to be due to a single unique protein. For example, IL-5 was characterized by one group as T-cell replacing factor, by another as B-cell growth factor-2, and by yet another as an eosinophil differentiation factor (KINASHI et al. 1986; SANDERSON et al. 1985; SWAIN and DUTTON 1982). Not surprisingly, with further investigation most of these growth factors have been found to have more general effects on the lymphoid differentiation pathway. Several, including IL-1, 4, 5, and 6, also act on myeloid pathways. General characteristics of both the myeloid growth factors and the interleukins include (a) relative lack of lineage specificity, (b) synergistic or additive interaction with one another, and (c) acting on both progenitor/stem cell and functional mature progeny.

I. Interleukin-1

IL-1 (endogenous pyrogen), along with tumor necrosis factor, is responsible for many of the in vivo effects of endotoxin exposure. It is a major mediator of inflammatory and immune responses and a ubiquitous networking molecule (DINARELLO 1984a). It clearly plays a role in the later steps of T- and B-cell activation, stimulates the proliferation of a variety of mesenchymal cell types, and modulates cartilage and bone metabolism. It has multiple effects on myelopoiesis, inducing early stem cells into cell cycle (possibly by a secondary effect), supporting survival of CFU-GM, and inducing transit of polymorphonuclear granulocytes into the peritoneal cavity. It acts synergistically with other growth factors to promote in vitro generation of blast cell colonies, HPP-CFC, and CFU-Eo, and to support proliferation of AML progenitors (IKEBUCHI et al. 1988; HOANG et al. 1988; ZHOU et al. 1988; ZSEBO et al. 1988; WARREN and MOORE 1988). Many of its actions on the hemopoietic system may be mediated by its capacity to induce GM-CSF, G-CSF, or CSF-1 from a variety of tissues including fibroblasts, endothelial cells, monocytes, keratinocytes, and thymic nonlymphoid cells (KUPPER et al. 1988; SEELENTAG et al. 1987; HERRMANN et al. 1988; FIBBE et al. 1986, 1988; ZUCALI et al. 1987; RENNICK et al. 1987). It also modulates T cell GM-CSF and IL-3 production. IL-1 is derived from a wide variety of tissues, perhaps the most widely studied being the monocyte-macrophage (LEMAIRE 1988). Other sources include glial retinal cells, T cells, polymorphonuclear neutrophil leulcocytes (PMNs), astrocytes, epidermal cells, and endothelial cells (ROBERGE et al. 1988; TARTAKOVSKY et al. 1988; LINDEMANN et al. 1988; DINARELLO 1988).

The biologic activity termed IL-1 is mediated by two separate polypeptides of 17.5 kDa, coded for in humans by separate genes on the long arm of chromosome 2 and with only 20% homology but interacting with the same receptor and having virtual identical biologic activities (DINARELLO 1988). The cDNA for both forms has been cloned, and control of genomic production in monocytes was noted to involve both transcriptional (endotoxin induction) and posttranscriptional (phorbol ester induction) mechanisms (FENTON et al. 1988). The mRNA for IL-1 β predominates, and this is the major secreted form. IL-1 α is mostly membrane bound. A recent report suggests that there is decreased IL-1 production in aplastic anemia (GASCON and SCALA 1988). The biologic actions of IL-1 are summarized in Table 6.

II. Interleukin-2

The effects of IL-2 are predominantly as a T cell growth factor (SMITH 1988). B cells have also been shown to have IL-2 receptors, and IL-2 may also

Table 6. Biologic actions of interleukin-1 (IL-1)

1. Endogenous pyrogen (DINARELLO 1984a, 1988)
2. Neutrophilia induction (DINARELLO 1984a, 1988)
3. Chemotactic for monocytes and neutrophils (SAYERS et al. 1988)
4. Induces hypoferremia in vivo (GORDEUK et al. 1988)
5. Induces cartilage degradation and chondrocyte prostanoid production. Increased bone resorption (LORENZO et al. 1988; CHIN and LIN 1988; IKEBE et al. 1988; HUBBARD et al. 1988; HOM et al. 1988)
6. Stimulates proliferation of many cell, types, including fibroblasts, glial, mesangial, and synovial cells and osteoblast cell lines (DINARELLO 1984a, 1988; HOANG et al. 1988; IKEDA et al. 1988)
7. Augments B cell response and proliferation of thymocytes and potentiates proliferation of T cells stimulated by lectins or alloantigens (LARSSON et al. 1980; SIMTH et al. 1980; PIKE and NOSSAL 1985)
8. Stimulates prostaglandins in multiple cell types (DAYER et al. 1986; AKAHOSHI et al. 1988)
9. Synergizes with IL-3, CSF-1, G-CSF, CM-CSF to stimulate different stem cell classes including blast colony forming cells, HPP-CFC, and AML progenitors. Also induces CFU-S into cell cycle (IKEBUCHI et al. 1988; HOANG et al. 1988; ZHOU et al. 1988; ZSEBO et al. 1988; WARREN and MOORE 1988)
10. Variably induces G-CSF, GM-CSF, and CSF-1 from a variety of tissues including fibroblasts, endothelial cells, monocytes, keratinocytes, marrow stromal cells, and human thymic nonlymphoid cells. It also induces T cell, GM-CSF, and IL-3 production. Also induces IL-2, IFNr and IFNB2 (IL-6) (ZUCALI et al. 1986, 1987; KUPPER et al. 1988; SEELENTAG et al. 1987; HERRMANN et al. 1988; FIBBE et al. 1986, 1988; RENNICK et al. 1987; BAGBY et al. 1986)
11. Induces IL-2 receptors and gene expression (SMITH et al. 1980)
12. Radioprotective effect in mice (NETA and OPPENHEIM 1988)
13. Induces thymic hypoplasia (MORRISSEY et al. 1988)
14. IL-1 β decreases rat thyroid hormone and thyroid stimulating hormone (TSH) levels in vivo and in vitro, releases adrenocorticotrophic hormone, luteinizing hormone, TSH, growth hormone, and prolactin from cultured rat pituitary cells (DUBUIS et al. 1988; BEACH et al. 1989; BENDTZEN et al. 1987)
15. Inhibits Leydig cell testosterone production (CALKINS et al. 1988)
16. Histamine release from human basophils (HAAK-FRENDSCHO et al. 1988)
17. Induces synthesis of acute phase proteins by hepatocytes (DINARELLO 1984b)

play a role in B-cell differentiation (WALDMAN et al. 1984). Monocytes or monocyte cell lines treated with gamma interferon (IEN-γ) also express IL-2 receptors (HERRMANN et al. 1985), and GM or mast cell lines have high levels of IL-2 surface receptors (BIRCHENALL-SPARKS et al. 1986), while the major impact of IL-2 on myelopoiesis is a secondary one. However, IL-2 has been shown recently to inhibit murine GM-CFU-C directly (NALDINI et al. 1987). The source of IL-2 is antigen-stimulated T cells (SMITH 1988).

III. Interleukin-4

IL-4 is the designation of a previously described B cell growth factor variously termed B cell stimulatory factor-1 (BSF-1), B cell differentiation factor (BCDF1), and IgG induction factor (HOWARD et al. 1982; VITETTA et al. 1984; NOMA et al. 1986; COFFMAN et al. 1986). IL-4 has been found to be a 20-kDa glycoprotein (GRABSTEIN et al. 1986; OHARA et al. 1987). It has been cloned by several groups (LEE et al. 1986; YOKOTA et al. 1986; OTSUKA et al. 1987) and its receptors characterized (OHARA and PAUL 1987; PARK et al. 1987). It is produced by T cells and marrow stromal cells. Studies by several groups have now shown that IL-4, while not having intrinsic direct activity on hemopoietic lineages, interacts with G-CSF to stimulate G and GM colony formation in vitro, with erythropoietin (Ep) to stimulate

Table 7. Biologic actions of interleukin-4 (IL-4)

1. Costimulant with IgM-specific antibodies for entry of resting B cells into DNA synthesis (HOWARD et al. 1982)
2. Increases expression of class II MHC molecules on resting B cells (NOELLE et al. 1984)
3. Promotes secretion by B lymphocytes of IgG and IgE (VITETTA et al. 1984; NOMA et al. 1986)
4. Stimulates growth of activated T cells (LEE et al. 1986; HU-LI et al. 1987)
5. Enhances growth of mast cell lines in response to IL-3 (LEE et al. 1986)
6. Interacts with rG-CSF to enhance proliferation of granulocyte or GM-CFC (BROXMEYER et al. 1988)
7. Increases proliferation of CFU-E in presence of erythropoietin (Ep) and with Ep stimulates colony formation by primitive erythroid (BFU-E) and multipotent (CFU-MIX) progenitor cells. In combination with rIL-1, rEp or supernatant of T cell hybridoma FS7-206.18 stimulates megakaryocyte colony formation (PESCHEL et al. 1987)
8. Induces pre-B cell in liquid culture (WOODWARD et al. 1990)
9. Inhibits Il-2-mediated B cell CLL proliferation and inhibits LAK cell induction (DEFRANCE et al. 1988)
10. Induces class I and class II MHC antigen expression on murine bone marrow derived macrophages and modulates human blood monocytes, causing changes suggesting differentiation to macrophages (STUART et al. 1988; TE VELDE et al. 1988)
11. Induces activated killer cells (PEACE et al. 1988)
12. Induces cultured monocytes-macrophages to form giant multinucleated cells (MCINNES and RENNICK 1988)

early and late erythroid progenitors and multipotent progenitors, and with IL-1, Ep, and a T-cell hybridoma supernatant to stimulate megakaryocyte colonies. The biologic actions of IL-4 are summarized in Table 7.

IV. Interleukin-5

IL-5 is a heavily glycosylated, 23-kDa protein (Tominaga et al. 1988; Takatsu et al. 1985) produced by a gene at band 31 q5 on the long arm of human chromosome 5 (Sutherland et al. 1988). It was initially studied by a number of groups as either a B cell growth factor termed T-cell replacing factor (TCRF) (Schimpl and Wecker 1972; Takatsu et al. 1980), B cell growth factor-2 (BCGF-2 or BSF-2) (Swain and Dutton 1982), or as an eosinophil differentiation factor (EDF) (Campbell et al. 1987). IL-5 has been shown to support eosinophil colony formation by human marrow cells and to interact with both IL-3 and GM-CSF to induce eosinophils in liquid culture (Clutterbuck and Sanderson 1988). IL-5 is produced by T cells or T-cell lines (Schimpl and Wecker 1972; Sanderson et al. 1986). Its biologic activities are summarized in Table 8.

V. Interleukin-6

IL-6, a 21-28-kDa protein, was also studied in a number of assay systems prior to its definitive characterization (Hirano et al. 1986; Van Damme et al. 1987; Sehgal et al. 1987; Gauldie et al. 1987). This protein enhances Ig secretion and induces differentiation of B lymphocytes (B cell stimulatory factor-2, BSF-2) and is the hybridoma plasmacytoma growth factor (HPGF) and hepatocyte stimulating factor (HSF). Both high- and low-affinity receptors have been characterized and found on transformed B-cell lines, myeloma lines, myeloid leukemia lines, a rat pheochromocytoma cell line, resting and activated B cells, and resting T cells. Both human and murine genes have been isolated and have a similar structure with 5 exons and 4 introns (Tanabe et al. 1988; Yasukawa et al. 1987). These genes show 60% sequence similarity, and the 3′ untranslated and first 300-bp sequence of the 5′ flanking region are highly conserved (>80%). The gene codes for a protein of 468 amino acids including the 19-amino acid signal peptides.

Table 8. Biologic actions of interleukin-5 (IL-5)

1. Promotes IgM secretion and proliferation by BCL1 B cell line, induces hapten-specific IgG secretion in vitro by in vivo antigen-primed B cells, and promotes differentiation of normal B cells (Schimpl and Wecker 1972; Takatsu et al. 1980; Swain and Dutton 1982)
2. Stimulates eosinophil colony formation and differentiation in liquid culture and synergizes with GM-CSF and IL-3 in eosinophil induction in liquid culture (Campbell et al. 1987; Clutterbuck and Sanderson 1988)

There are 5 molecular weight forms secreted by monocytes (21–28 kDa) (BAUER et al. 1988). IL-6 is produced by a wide variety of cell types including monocytes, fibroblasts, activated T and B cells, endothelial cells, smooth muscle cells, marrow stromal cells, and glial, T cell, *myoma*, osteosarcoma, glioblastoma, bladder carcinoma, and cervical carcinoma cells (HIRANO et al. 1986, 1987; ZILBERSTEIN et al. 1986; NORDAN et al. 1987; HAEGEMAN et al. 1986).

IL-6 acts synergistically with IL-3 to support proliferation of murine multipotent progenitors in culture and hasten the appearance of blast cell colonies (WONG et al. 1988; IKEBUCHI et al. 1987). It indirectly stimulates a number of different hemopoietic colonies and appears to stimulate directly proliferation and differentiation of GM and megakaryocytic progenitors (WONG et al. 1988; IKEBUCHI et al. 1987; CHIU et al. 1988; MCGRATH et al. 1989, unpublished data). There is extensive sequence homology between the amino-terminus of IL-6 and G-CSF (HIRANO et al. 1986). IL-6 also acts synergistically with IL-3 to support CFU-meg (MCGRATH et al. 1989, unpublished data) and is a growth factor for multiple myeloma plasma cells (KAWANO et al. 1988). Its actions are summarized in Table 9.

Table 9. Biologic actions of interleukin-6 (IL-6)

1. Ability to enhance Ig secretion by B lymphocytes and induce differentiation of B cells (HIRANO et al. 1986; VAN DAMME et al. 1987b; BILLIAU 1987)
2. Synergism with Il-3 on murine multipotent hemopoietic progenitors (WONG et al. 1988; IKEBUCHI et al. 1987)
3. Supports murine neutrophil-macrophage, eosinophil, mast cell and megakaryocyte colonies (WONG et al. 1988; IKEBUCHI et al. 1987; CHIU et al. 1988; MCGRATH et al. 1989)
4. Promotes growth of EBV-infected B cells (TOSATO et al. 1988)
5. Inducer of acute phase proteins in hepatocytes (GAULDIE et al. 1987)
6. Serves as a second signal in murine T cell activation (GARMAN et al. 1987)
7. Ability to induce an antiviral state in fibroblasts (VAN DAMME et al. 1987b)
8. Growth inhibitor for human fibroblasts (KOHASE et al. 1986)
9. Growth factor for certain mouse-rat hybridomas and mouse plasmacytomas (SANDERSON et al. 1986; VAN DAMME et al. 1987b)

VI. Interleukin-7

IL-7 is a 25-kDa protein which stimulates pre-*pre*-B cell proliferation (NAMEN et al. 1988a,b). It was isolated from adherent marrow stromal cells transfected with the plasmid pSV3 noncontaining transforming sequences of SV40. Its role in GM production remains to be defined.

E. Inhibitors

Inhibitors of GM production have been difficult to study because of the issue of specificity of in vitro inhibition. Studies on inhibitors were particularly awkward to interpret when nondefined (conditioned media, for example) sources of stimulators were used and tested against mixed populations of marrow cells. The availability of characterized GFs, serum-free systems, and purified stem cells suggests that the point has been reached at which biologically meaningful inhibitors of GM (or "myeloid") cell production can now be defined. Despite the above noted problems, a number of inhibitors of in vitro GM production have been fairly well characterized. Lactoferrin appears to block production of CSF by a subset of monocytes (BROXMEYER and PLATZER 1984), while acidic isoferritin directly inhibits cycling progenitors (BROXMEYER et al. 1986a). Leukemic inhibition factors also appear to act on normal progenitors (QUESENBERRY et al. 1978), and prostaglandins directly inhibit stem cell proliferation (PELUS et al. 1981). Tumor necrosis factor (TNF) and IFN both inhibit various stages of GM colony formation, and TNF is a potent inhibitor of CFU-GEMM, BFU-E, and CFU-E (RAEFSKY et al. 1985; BROXMEYER et al. 1986; PEETRE et al. 1986). TNF and IFN act synergistically to inhibit CFU-GM day 14 or day 7. Transforming growth factor-β (TGF-β) appears to be a relatively selective inhibitor of early as opposed to more differentiated stem cell classes (ISHIBASHI et al. 1987; KELLER et al. 1989). TGF-β is a highly conserved polypeptide which has been shown to inhibit epithelial cell growth while having either inhibitory of stimulatory effects on mesenchymal cell growth. It is produced by a variety of cells, including platelets, bone cells, and T lymphocytes, and by histochemical staining has been localized to areas of active hemopoiesis in bone marrow or fetal liver. Recent work has indicated that TGF-β inhibits a variety of primitive and/or multilineage stem cells including CFU-GEMM, CFU-GM, and several classes of HPP-CFC (HPP-CFC-1, HPP-CFC-2, and HPP-CFC-HLGF-1), while not affecting more differentiated, unilineage,GM progenitors, i.e., formation of pure granulocyte or pure macrophage CFU-C (ISHIBASHI et al. 1987; KELLER et al. 1989).

F. Cellular Production and Networking

The variety of cellular sources, the number of different interacting growth factors with overlapping activities, and the presence of various inhibitor molecules all contribute to the almost bewildering potential complexity of growth factor regulation. Recent observations also suggest the presence of holocrine, paracrine, and autocrine growth factor loops in which one growth factor may induce either itself or another growth factor. Thus, there is a great capacity for extensive networking and modulation. Given this complexity, it is extraordinary that the biologic effects seen when growth factors are administered in vivo so closely parallel their effect in in vitro culture systems.

As noted above, cellular sources include monocytes-macrophages, B-cell lines, T cells, fibroblasts and stromal fibroblasts, endothelial and vascular smooth muscle cells, dendritic cells, keratinocytes, and a variety of cell lines and malignant tissues. In general, these various cell types produce GM-CSF, G-CSF, and CSF-1, or various combinations, but not IL-3, which appears to be restricted to a T-lymphocyte origin (NIEMAYER et al. 1989). Production of these growth factors has been detected by selective bioassay with cell lines and/or differential antibody blocking or Northern blot analysis of mRNA. GF production may be detected only after exposure of cells to various inducers such as IL-1, TNF, IFN, phorbol esters, endotoxin, lectins, or other cytokines like GM-CSF or IL-3, or may be seen without such induction. This last has been termed constitutive production. It is not clear whether this is truly a meaningful distinction since mRNA assays may be negative when bioactivity is detectable by sensitive cell line assays. It seems likely that in many cases a failure to detect "constitutive" production of a GF relates to the sensitivity of detection of its mRNA and that small but biologically meaningful levels of GF may be produced in the uninduced state. Application of polymerase chain reaction techniques (MULLIS and FALLONA 1987) to this type of mRNA analysis should clarify these issues. In vivo biologic models for studying the effects of endotoxin, bacterial infection, or antigen exposure suggest a common theme for GF control. Exposure of peripheral "producer cells" such as monocytes, endothelial cells, or fibroblasts to noxious foreign substances probably results in the release of marrow active GFs and of networkers such as IL-1, which then amplifies the system. These released bioactivities may also modulate local marrow stromal cell GF production to augment further the overall response. Clearing the foreign substance with decrease in GF release may then shut the response off along with possible augmented inhibitor production. Actions of G-CSF and GM-CSF suggest that G-CSF may act to induce immediate release of marrow granulocytes with transit to sites of infection/inflammation, while GM-CSF may focus their activity in one location by preventing further migration. This type of scenario may hold for emergency responses but does not necessarily explain baseline marrow GM production.

G. Microenvironment

Early studies on the influence of the marrow or splenic microenvironment on cell differentiation pathways suggested that local marrow stromal cells exert potent regulatory influences (CURRY et al. 1967; CURRY and TRENTIN 1967; WOLF and TRENTIN 1968; BERNSTEIN 1970). The introduction of the murine, Dexter, long-term, marrow cultures has opened this area for detailed study (DEXTER et al. 1977). In Dexter cultures, murine marrow cells are suspended in media with horse serum and hydrocortisone supplement and kept at 33°C with various feeding schedules. Long-term production (months) of granulocytes, macrophages, megakaryocytes, and most stem cells, including CSF-S day 9, CFU-D, HPP-CFC, GM-CFC, and CFU-meg, occurs, but this active hemopoiesis is critically dependent upon the formation of an adherent stromal cell layer (DEXTER et al. 1977; TESTA and DEXTER 1977; WILLIAMS et al. 1978; DOUKAS et al. 1985; MCGRATH et al. 1987). While neither erythropoiesis nor production of T or B lymphocytes happens in this system (JONES-VILLENEUVE and PHILLIPS 1980; SCHRADER et al. 1984), progenitor/stem cells for these lineages are demonstrable by in vivo transplantation (lymphoid) (SCHRADER and SCHRADER 1978) or in vitro addition of erythropoietin and mechanical agitation of the cultures (erythroid) (DEXTER et al. 1984). Initially, investigators had difficulty demonstrating the presence of myeloid growth factors in this system, leading some to suggest that this indicated the irrelevance of these GFs (DEXTER 1979; WILLIAMS et al. 1978; DEXTER and SHADDUCK 1980). However, the failure to detect bioactivity probably related to the binding, utilization, and/or degradation of GFs in the system (GUALTIERI et al. 1984), and manipulations such as irradiation or irradiation with lectin exposure revealed that the isolated stromal cells were rich sources of multilineage GFs including CSF-1, GM-CSF, and G-CSF (ALBERICO et al. 1987; MCGRATH et al. 1987; GUALTIERI et al. 1984). Furthermore, stromal cell lines have now been found to make IL-4, IL-6, IL-7, and a pre-B GF which synergizes with CSF-1 and IL-3 in vitro for myeloid colony formation (LEE et al. 1986; WOODWARD et al. 1989; CHIU et al. 1988; NAMEN et al. 1988a,b).

Initial characterization of the murine Dexter stromal layers suggested the presence of macrophages, endothelial cells, fat cells, and blanket cells (ALLEN and DEXTER 1976), while other studies indicated that two cell types, the macrophage and an alkaline-phosphatase-positive preadipocyte fibroblast, were sufficient for stromal support in this culture system (SONG and QUESENBERRY 1984; GUALTIERI et al. 1984; TAVASSOLI and TAKAHASHI 1982). Myeloid, predominantly granulocytic, cells form "cobblestone"-appearing areas, and this growth seems to occur directly on top of the preadipocytic cells. The extracellular matrix appears to play an important role in the stromal support of myeloid cell growth (ZUCKERMAN and WICHA 1983). Some researchers have specifically implicated proteoglycans by suggesting that GFs may bind to them and that this may be how the GFs are presented to their target cells (GORDON et al. 1987). Given the potential for very low levels of GFs acting synergistically, it seems plausible that an important mode of local regulation may relate to the presentation to the target stem cell of packets of GFs, in either the right mixture of the right configuration, attached to matrix or cell surface proteoglycans.

The Whitlock-Witte culture system representing a modification of the Dexter cultures from which hydrocortisone is omitted, preselected fetal calf sera substituted for horse sera, the temperature raised to 37°C, and 2-mercaptoethanol added allows for the prolonged growth of pre-B and B cells, again dependent upon the formation of an adequate adherent stromal layer (WHITLOCK and WITTE 1987; KINCADE et al. 1986). If established Dexter cultures are switched to Whitlock-Witte conditions, myelopoiesis will switch to lymphopoiesis, after a short lag period (Johnson and Dorshkind 1986). With this change there is a major shift to large epithelial preadipocytes with a concomitant decrease in the percentage of macrophages in the stromal layer (Ruland et al. 1990). These observations suggest that alterations in the stromal cell phenotype, possibly in turn related to differential growth factor production, direct primitive stem cells into separate differentiation pathways.

H. Conclusions

The stage is set for exploration of the true nature of myeloid regulation. Identification of growth factors, their receptors, genetic modes of regulation, and the regulatory cell networks with their autocrine/paracrine loops begins to give us the essential features of the system. Other general characteristics include GF cross-lineage effects, synergies by low levels of GFs, and the potential for spatial restriction of GF presentation. The myeloid system would appear to have many redundancies and a tremendous capacity for modulation and, in the end, to be essentially deterministic.

Acknowledgement. I would like to thank Ms. Wendy Burton for the excellent typing and editing of this chapter.

References

Akahoshi T, Oppenheim JJ, Matsushima K (1988) Interleukin-1 stimulates its own receptor expression on human fibroblasts through the endogenous production of prostaglandin(s). J Clin Invest 82:1219–1224

Alberico T, Ihle JN, Quesenberry P (1987) Stromal growth factor production in irradiated lectin exposed long-term murine bone marrow cultures. Blood 69: 1120–1127

Allen TD, Dexter TM (1976) Cellular interrelationships during in vitro granulopoiesis. Differentiation 6:191

Antman KS, Griffin JD, Elias A, SOcinski MA, Ryan L, Cannistra SA, Oette D, Whitley M, Frei E, Schnipper LE (1988) Effect of recombinant human granulocyte-macrophage colony stimulating factor on chemotherapy-induced myelosuppression. N Engl J Med 319:593–598

Aranout MA, Wang EA, Clark SC, Sieff CA (1986) Human recombinant granulocyte-macrophage colony stimulating factor increases cell-to-cell adhesion and surface expression of adhesion-promoting surface glycoproteins on mature granulocytes. J Clin Invest 78:597–601

Avalos BR, Hedzat C, Baldwin GC Golde DW, Gasson JC, DiPersio JF (1987) Biological activities of human G-CSF and characterization of the human G-CSF receptor. Blood 70:165a (abstr)

Axelrad AA, McLeod DL, Shreeve MM, Health DS (1973) Properties of cells that produce erythrocytic colonies in vitro. In: Robinson WA (ed.) Hemopoiesis in culture: second international workshop. HEW Publication, NIH Government Printing Office, Washington, p 226

Bagby GC, Dinarello CA, Wallace P, Wagner C, Hefeneider S, McCall E (1986) Interleukin-1 stimulates granulocyte-macrophage colony stimulating activity release by vascular endothelial cells. J Clin Invest 78:1316–1323

Baldwin GC, DePersio J, Kaufman SE, Quan SG, Golde DW, Gasson JC (1987) Characterization of human GM-CSF receptors on non-hematopoietic cells. Blood 70:166a (abstr)

Baldwin GC, Gasson JC, Quan SG, Fleischmann J, Weisbart R, Oette D, Mitsuyasu RT, Golde DW (1988) Granulocyte-macrophage colony stimulating factor enhances neutrophil function in acquired immunodeficiency syndrome patients Proc Natl Acad Sci USA 85:2763–2766

Bartocci A, Mastrogiannis DS, Migliorati G, Stockert RJ, Wolkoff AW, Stanley ER (1987) Macrophages specifically regulate the concentration of their own growth factor in the circulation. Proc Natl Acad Sci USA 84:6179–6183

Bauer J, Ganter U, Geiger T, Jacobshagen U, Hirano T, Mastsuda T, Kishimoto T, Andus T, Acs G, Gerok W, Cilberto G (1988) Regulation of interleukin-6 expression in cultured human blood monocytes and monocyte derived macrophages. Blood 72:1134–1140

Beach JE, Smallridge RC, Kinzer CA, Berinton EW, Holaday JW, Fein HG (1989) Rapid release of multiple hormones from rat pituitaries perfused with recombinant interleukin-1. Life Sci 44:1–7

Begley CG, Nicola NA, Metcalf D (1988) Proliferation of normal human promyelocytes and myelocytes after a single pulse stimulation by purified GM-CSF or G-CSF. Blood 71:640–645

Bendtzen K, Rasmusen AK, Beck K, Feldt-Rasmussen V, Egeberg J (1987) Cytokines in autoimmunity. Immunol Today 8:203–204

Berdel WE, Danhauser-Riedel S, Steinhauser G, Winton EF (1989) Various human hematopoietic growth factors (interleukin-3, GM-CSF, G-CSF) stimulate clonal growth of nonhematopoietic tumor cells. Blood 73:80–83

Bernstein SE (1970) Tissue transplantation as an analytic and therapeutic tool in hereditary anemias. Am J Surg 119:448

Bickel M, Amstad P, Tsuda H, Sulis C, Asofsky R, Mergenhagen SE, Pluznik DH (1987) Induction of granulocyte-macrophage colony stimulating factor by lipopolysaccharide and antiimmunoglobulin M-stimulated murine B cell lines. J Immunol 139:2984–2988

Bickel M, Mergenhagen SE, Pluznik DH (1988) Posttranscriptional control of murine granulocyte/macrophage colony stimulating factor (GM-CSF). Exp Hematol 16:414(abstr)

Billiau A (1987) Interferon beta 2 as a promoter of growth and differentiation of B cells. J Immunol Today 8:84–87

Birchenall-Sparks MC, Farrar WL, Rennick D, Kilian PL, Ruscetti FW (1986) Regulation of expression of the interleukin 2 receptor on hematopoietic cells by interleukin-3. Science 233:455–458

Boggs DR et al. (1967) Mechanisms controlling homeostasis of neutrophilic leukocytes. Haematol Lett 10:43

Boggs DR et al. (1968) Neutrophil releasing activity in plasma of normal human subjects injected with endotoxin. Proc Soc Exp Biol Med 127:689

Bonilla MA, Gillio AP, Potter GK, D' Reilly RS, Souza LM, Weltak (1987) Effects of recombinant human G-CSF and GM-CSF on cytopenia associated with repeated cycles of chemotherapy in primates. Blood 70:130a

Bot FJ, Dorssers L, Wagemaker G, Lowenberg B (1988) Stimulating spectrum of human recombinant multi-CSF (IL-3) on human marrow precursors; importance of accessory cells. Blood 71:1609–1614

Bradley TR, Metcalf D (1966) The growth of mouse bone marrow cells in vitro. Aust J Exp Biol Med Sci 44:287

Bradley TR, Hodgson GS, Rosendaal M (1978) The effect of oxygen tension on haemopoietic and fibroblast cell proliferation in vitro. J Cell Physiol 97:517–522

Brandt SJ, Peters WP, Atwater SK, Kurtzberg J, Borowitz MJ, Jones RB, Shpall EJ, Bast RC Jr, Gilbert CJ, Oette DH (1988) Effect of recombinant human granulocyte macrophage colony stimulating factor on hematopoietic reconstitution after high dose chemotherapy and autologous bone marrow transplantation. N Engl J Med 318:869–876

Broxmeyer HE, Platzer E (1984) Lactoferrin acts in I-A and I-E/C antigen subpopulations of mouse peritoneal macrophages in the absence of T lymphocytes and other cell types to inhibit production of granulocyte-macrophage colony stimulating factors in vitro. J Immunol 133:306

Broxmeyer HE, Lu L, Bicknell DC et al. (1986a) The influence of purified recombinant human H-subunit and L-subunit ferritins on colony formation in vitro by granulocyte-macrophage and erythroid progenitor cells. Blood 68:1257

Broxmeyer HE, Williams DE, Lu L (1986b) Cooper S, Anderson SL, Beyer GS, Hoffman R, Rubin By The suppressive influences of human tumor necrosis factors on bone marrow hematopoietic progenitor cells from normal donors and patients with leukemia: synergism of tumor necrosis factor and interferon-γ. J Immunol 136:4487

Broxmeyer HE, Williams DE, Cooper S, Shadduck RK, Gillis S, Waheed A, Urdal DL, Bicknell DC (1987a) Comparative effects in vivo of recombinant murine interleukin-3, natural murine colony-stimulating factor-1, and recombinant murine granulocyte-macrophage colony stimulating factors on myelopoiesis in mice. J Clin Invest 79:721–730

Broxmeyer HE, Williams DE, Hangoc G, Cooper S, Gillis S, Shedduck RK, Bicknell DC (1987b) Synergistic myelopoietic actions in vivo after administration to mice of combinations of purified natural murine colony stimulating factor-1, recombinant murine interleukin-3 and recombinant murine granulocyte/macrophage colony stimulating factor. Proc Natl Acad Sci USA 84:3871

Broxmeyer HE, Lu L, Cooper S, Tushinski R, Mochizuki D, Rubin BY, Gillis S, Williams DE (1988) Synergistic effects of purified recombinant human and murine B cell growth factor-1/interleukin-4 on colony formation in vitro by hematopoietic progenitor cells. J Immunol 141:3852–3856

Burgess AW, Camakaris J, Metcalf D (1977) Purification and properties of colony stimulating factor from mouse lung-conditioned medium. J Biol Chem 252: 1998–2003

Calkins JH, Sigel MM, Nankin HR, Lin T (1988) Interleukin-1 inhibits Leydig cell steroidogenesis in primary culture. Endocrinology 123:1605–1610

Campbell HD, Tucker WQJ, Hort Y, Martinson ME, Mayo G, Clutterbuck EJ, Sanderson CJ, Young IG (1987) Molecular cloning and expression of the gene encoding human eosinophil differentiation factor (interleukin-5). Proc Natl Acad Sci USa 84:6629

Cannistra SA, Vellenga E, Groshek P, Rambaldi A, Griffin JD (1988) Granulocyte-monocyte colony stimulating factor and interleukin-3 stimulate monocyte cytotoxicity through a tumor necrosis factor-dependent mechanism. Blood 71: 672–676

Caracciolo D, Shirsat N, Wong GG, Lange B, Clark S, Rovera G (1987) Recombinant human macrophage colony stimulating factor (M-CSF) requires subliminal concentrations of granulocyte/macrophage (GM)-CSF for optimal stimulation of human macrophage colony formation in vitro. J Exp Med 166: 1851–1860

Cebon J, Dempsey P, Fox R, Kannourakis G, Bonnem E, Burgess AW, Morstyn G (1988) Pharmacokinetics of human granulocyte macrophage colony stimulating factor using a sensitive immunoassay. Blood 72:1340–1347

Chan JY, Slamon DF, Nimer SD, Golde DW, Gasson JC (1986) Regulation of expression of human granulocyte/macrophage colony stimulating factor. Proc Natl Acad Sci USA 83:8669

Chen BD, Clark CR (1986) Interleukin-3 regulates the in vitro proliferation of both blood monocytes and peritoneal exudate macrophages: synergism between a macrophage lineage-specific colony stimulating factor and IL-3. J Immunol 137:563–570

Chervenick PA, LoBuglio AF (1972) Human blood monocytes: stimulators of granulocyte and mononuclear colony formation in vitro. Science 178:164–166

Chin JE, Lin YA (1988) Effects of recombinant human inter-leukin-1 beta on rabbit articular chondrocytes. Stimulation of prostanoid release and inhibition of cell growth. Arthritis Rheum 31:1290–1296

Chiu CP, Moulds C, Coffman RL, Rennick D, Lee F (1988) Multiple biological activities are expressed by a mouse interleukin-6 cDNA clone isolated from bone marrow stromal cells. Proc Natl Acad Sci USA 85:7099–7103

Chodakewitz JA, Kupper TS, Coleman DL (1988) Keratinocyte-derived granulocyte/macrophage colony stimulating factor induces DNA synthesis by peritoneal macrophages. J Immunol 140:832–836

Clark-Lewis I, Kent SBH, Schrader JW (1984) Purification to apparent homogeneity of a factor stimulating the growth of multiple lineages of hemopoietic cells. J Biol Chem 259:7488

Clutterbuck EJ, Sanderson CJ (1988) Human eosinophil hematopoiesis studied in vitro by means of murine eosinophil differentiation factor (IL-5): production of functionally active eosinophils from normal human bone marrow. Blood 71: 646–651

Coffey RG, Davis JS, Djeu JY (1988) Stimulation of guanylate cyclase activity and reduction of adenylate cyclase activity by granulocyte-macrophage colony stimulating factor in human blood neutrophils. J Immunol 140:2695–2701

Coffman RL, Ohara J, Bond MW, Carty J, Zlotnik A, Paul WE (1986) B cell stimulatory factor-1 enhances the IgE response of lipopolysaccharide-activated B cells. J Immunol 136:4538–4541

Coleman DL, Chudakewitz JA, Bartiss AH, Mellors JW (1988) Granulocyte-macrophage colony stimulating factor enhances selective effect on functions of tissue-derived macrophages. Blood 72:573–578

Curry JL, Trentin JJ (1967) Hemopoietic spleen colony studies. I. Growth and differentiation. Dev Biol 15:395

Curry JL, Trentin JJ, Wolf N (1967) Hemopoietic spleen colony studies. II. Erythropoiesis. J Exp Med 125:703

Cutler RL, Metcalf D, Nicola NA, Johnson GR (1985) Purification of a multipotential colony stimulating factor from pokeweed mitogen-stimulated mouse spleen cell conditioned medium. J Biol Chem 260:6579–6587

Das SK, Stanley ER (1982) Structure-function studies of a colony stimulating factor (CSF-1). J Biol Chem 257:13679–13684

Dayer JM, Rochemonteix B, Burrus B, Demczuk S, Dinarello CA (1986) Human recombinant interleukin-1 stimulates collagenase and prostaglandin E2 production by human synovial cells. J Clin Invest 77:645–648

Defrance T, Vanbervliet B, Banchereau J (1988) Interleukin-4 inhibits proliferation but not the differentiation of activated human B cells in response to interleukin-2. International Society of Experimental Hematology meeting, Houston, abstr 358

DeLamarter JF, Hession C, Semon D, Gough NM, Rothenbuhler R, Mermod J-J (1987) Mucleotide sequence of a cDNA encoding murine CSF-1 (macrophage-CSF). Nucleic Acids Res 15:2389–2390

Delmonte L (1967) Time- and dose-dependent stimulation of hemopoietic colony forming potential with granulocytosis-promoting factor (GPF) in inbred mice. Exp Hematol 12:57

Dexter RM, Shadduck RK (1980) The regulation of haemopoiesis in long-term bone marrow cultures. I. Role of L-cell colony stimulating factor. J Cell Physiol 102:279–286

Dexter TM (1979) Cell interactions invitro Clin Haematol 8:453–468

Dexter TM, Allen TD, Lajtha LG (1977) Conditions controlling the proliferation of haemopoietic stem cells in vitro. J Cell Physiol 91:335

Dexter TM, Spooncer E, Simmons P, Allen TD (1984) In: Wright DC, Greenberger

JS (eds) Long term marrow cultures. Alan R Liss, New York, pp 57–96
Dinarello CA (1984a) Interleukin-1. Rev Infect Dis 6:51
Dinarello CA (1984b) Interleukin 1 and the pathogenesis of the acute phase response. N Engl J Med 311:1413–1418
Dinarello CA (1988) Biology of interleukin-1. FASEB J 2:108–115
Dispersio J, Billing P, Kaufman S et al. (1987) The human GM-CSF receptor: mechanisms of transmembrane signalling and neutrophil priming. Blood 70:170a (abstr)
Donaheu R, Wang E, Stone D, Kaman R, Wong G, Sehgal P, Nathan D, Clark S (1986b) Stimulation of haematopoiesis in primates by continuous infusion of recombinant human GM-CSF. Nature 321:872
Donahue RE, Karlsson S, Clark S, Anderson WF, Nienhuis AW (1986a) Recombinant human GM-CSF accelerates neutrophil and platelet recovery following autologous bone marrow transplantation. Blood 68:281a (abstr)
Donahue RE, Seehra J, Norton C et al. (1987) Stimulation of hematopoiesis in primates with human interleukin-3 and granulocyte-macrophage colony stimulating factor. Blood 70:133a (abstr)
Doukas MA, Niskanen E, Quesenberry PJ (1985) Lithium stimulation of granulopoiesis in diffusion chambers–a model of humoral, indirect stimulation of stem cell proliferation. Blood 65:163–168
Dubuis J-M, Dayer J-M, Siegrist-Kaiser CA, Burger AG (1988) Human recombinant interleukin-1 beta decreases plasma thyroid hormone and thyroid stimulating hormone levels in rats. Endocrinology 123:2175–2181
Duhrsen U, Villeval JL, Boyd J, Kannovrakis G, Morstyn G, Metcalf D (1988) Effects of recombinant human granulocyte colony stimulating factor on hematopoietic progenitor cells in cancer patients. Blood 72:2074–2081
Farrar W, Thomas TP, Anderson WB (1985) Altered cytosol/membrane enzyme redistribution on IL-3 activation of protein kinase C. Nature 315:235
Fauser AA, Messner HA (1978) Granuloerythropoietic colonies in human bone marrow, peripheral blood and cord blood. Blood 52:1243–1248
Fenton MJ, Vermeulen MW, Clark BD, Webb AC, Auron PE (1988) Human pro-IL-1 beta gene expression in monocytic cells is regulated by two distinct pathways. J Immunol 140:2267–2273
Fibbe WE, Van Damme J, Billiou A, Vooglt PJ, Duinker Ken N, Kluck PMC, Falkenburg JHF (1986) Interleukin-1 (22-K factor) induces release of granulocyte-macrophage colony stimulating activity from human mononuclear phagocytes. Blood 68:1316–1323
Fibbe WE, Van Damme J, Billiau A, Duinkerken N, Lurvink E, Ralph P, Altrock BW, Kaushansky K, Willemze R, Falkenburg JHF (1988) Human fibroblasts produce granulocyte-colony stimulating factor, macrophage-colony stimulating factor and granulocyte-macrophage colony stimulating factor following stimulation by interleukin-1 and poly (rI). poly (rC). Blood 72:860–866
Fischer HG, Frosch S, Reske K, Reske-Kunz AB (1988) Granulocyte-macrophage colony stimulating factor activates macrophages derived from bone marrow cultures to synthesis of MHC class II molecules and to augmented antigen presentation function. J Immunol 141:3882–3888
Fleischmann J, Golde DW, Weisbart RH, Gasson JC (1986) Granulocyte macrophage colony stimulating factor enhances phagocytosis of bacteria by human neutrophils. Blood 68:708–711
Fletcher MP, Gasson JC (1988) Enhancement of neutrophil function by granulocyte-macrophage colony stimulating factor involves recruitment of a less responsive subpopulation. Blood 71:652–658
Foster R, Metcalf D, Kirchmyer R (1968) Induction of bone marrow colony stimulating activity by a filterable agent in leukemic and mouse serum. J Exp Med 127:853–855
Fung MC, Hapel AJ, Ymer S, Cohen DR, Johnson RM, Campbell HD, Young IG

(1984) Molecular cloning of cDNA for murine interleukin-3. Nature 307: 233–237

Gabrilove J, Jakubowski A, Fain K, Sher H, Grovs S, Sternberg C, Yagoda A, Clarkson, B (1987) A phase I/II study of rhG-CSF in cancer patients at risk for chemotherapy induced neutropenia. Blood 70:135a (abstr)

Ganser A, Volkers B, Greher J, Ottmann OG, Walther F, Becher R, Bergman L, Schulz G, Hoelzer D (1989) Recombinant human granulocyte-macrophage colony stimulating factor in patients with myelodysplastic syndromes – a phase I/II trial. Blood 73:31–37

Garman RD, Jacobs KA, Clark SC, Raulet DH (1987) B cell stimulatory factor 2 (B2 interferon) functions as a second signal for interleukin-2 production by mature murine T cells. Proc Natl Acad Sci USA 84:7629

Gascon P, Scala G (1988) Decreased interleukin-1 production in aplastic anemia. Am J Med 85:668–674

Gasson JC, Weisbart RH, Kaufman SE, Clark SC, Hewick RM, Wong GG, Golde DW (1984) Purified human granulocyte-macrophage colony stimulating factor: direct action on neutrophils. Science 226:1339–1342

Gauldie J, Richards C, Harnish D, Lansdorp P, Baumann H (1987) Interferon beta 2/B-cell stimulatory factor type 2 shares identity with monocyte-derived hepatocyte-stimulating factor and regulates the major acute phase protein response in liver cells. Proc Natl Acad Sci USA 84:7251–7255

Gendelman HE, Orenstein JM, Martin MA, Ferrua C, Mitra R, Phipps T, Wahl LA, Lane HC, Fauci AS, Burke DS, Skillman D, Meltzer MS (1988) Efficient isolation and propagation of human immunodeficiency virus on recombinant colony stimulating factor 1-treated monocytes. J Exp Med 167:1428–1441

Gillio AP, Bonilla MA, O'Reilly RJ, Potter GK, Boone T, Souza L, Weltek (1986) Effect of recombinant human G-CSF on hematopoietic reconstitution following autologous bone marrow transplantation in primates. Blood 68:283a (abstr)

Gordeuk VR, Prithviraj P, Dolinar T, Brittenham GM (1988) Interleukin-1 administration in mice produces hypoferremia despite neutropenia. J Clin Invest 82:1934–1938

Gordon MY, Riley GP, Watt SM, Geaves MF (1987) Compartmentalization of a haematopoietic growth factor (GM-CSF) by glycosaminoglycans in the bone marrow microenvironment. Nature 326:403

Gough NM, Gough J, Metcalf D, Kelso A, Grail D, Nicola NA, Burgess AW, Dunn AR (1984) Molecular cloning of cDNA encoding a murine haematopoietic growth regulator, granulocyte-macrophage colony stimulating factor. Nature 309:763–767

Grabstein K, Eisenman J, Mochizuki D, Shanebeck K, Conlon P, Hopp T, March C, Gillis S (1986) Purification to homogeneity of B cell stimulating factor. A molecule that stimulates proliferation of multiple lymphokine-dependent cell lines. J Exp Med 163:1405

Greenberger JS, Newberger PE, Sakakeeny M (1980) Phorbol myristate acetate stimulates macrophage differentiation and replication and alters granulopoiesis and leukemogenesis in long term bone marrow cultures. Blood 56:368–379

Gregory CJ (1976) Erythropoietin sensitivity as a differentiation marker in the hemopoietic system: studies of three erythropoietic colony responses in culture. J Cell Physiol 89:289–302

Croopman JE, Mitsuyasu RT, Deleo MJ, Oette DH, Golde DW (1987) Effect of recombinant human granulocyte-macrophage colony stimulating factor of myelopoiesis in the acquired immunodeficiency syndrome. N Engl J Med 317:593–598

Gualtieri RJ, Shadduck R, Baker DG, Quesenberry PJ (1984) Hematopoietic regulatory factors produced in long term bone marrow cultures and the effect of in vitro irradiation. Blood 64:516–525

Haak-Frendscho M, Arai N, Arai K, Baeza ML, Finn A, Kaplan AP (1988) Human recombinant granulocyte-macrophage colony stimulating factor and interleukin-3 cause basophil histamine release. J Clin Invest 82:17–20

Haegeman G, Content J, Volckaert G, Eerynck R, Tavernier J, Fiers W (1986) Structural analysis of the sequence encoding for an inducible 26-kDa protein in human fibroblasts. Eur J Biochem 159:625

Hamilton JA, Vairo G, Lingelbach SR (1986) CSF-1 stimulates glucose uptake in murine bone marrow-derived macrophages. Biochem Biophys Res Commun 138:445–454

Hanamura T, Motoyoshi K, Yoshida K, Saito M, Miura Y, Kawashima T, Nishida M, Takaku F (1988) Quantitation and identification of human monocytic colony stimulating factor in human serum by enzyme-linked immunosorbent assay. Blood 72:886–892

Handman E, Burgess AW (1979) Stimulation by granulocyte-macrophage colony stimulating factor of *Leishmania tropica* killing by macrophages. J Immunol 122:1134–1137

Hanks GE, Ainsworth EJ (1964) Endotoxin protection and colony forming units. Radiat Res 32:367–382

Hanna MG Jr, Nettesheim P, Fisher WD, Peters LC, Francis MW (1967) Serum alpha globulin fraction: survival-and-recovery effect in irradiated mice. Science 157:1458–1461

Hapel AJ, Osborne JM, Fung MC, Young I, Allan W, Hume D (1985) Expression of 20-α-hydroxysteroid dehydrogenase in mouse macrophages, hemopoietic cells and cell lines and its induction by colony stimulating factors. J Immunol 134: 2492

He Y, Hewlett E, Temeles D, Quesenberry P (1988) Inhibition of interleukin-3 and colony stimulating factor-I-stimulated hemopoietic stem cell proliferation by pertussis toxin. Blood 71:1187–1195

Herrmann F, Cannistra SA, Levine H, Griffin JD (1985) Expression of interleukin-2 receptors and binding of interleukin-2 by gamma-interferon induced human leukemia and normal monocytes. J Exp Med 162:1111–1116

Herrmann F, Oster W, Meuer SC, Lindemann A, Mertelsmann RH (1988) Interleukin-1 stimulates T lymphocytes to produce granulocyte-monocyte colony stimulating factor. J Clin Invest 81:1415–1418

Hirai K, Morita Y, Misaki Y, Ohta K, Takaishi T, Suzuki S, Motoyoshi K, Miyamoto T (1988) Modulation of human basophil histamine release by hemopoietic growth factors. J Immunol 141:3958–3964

Hirano T, Yasukawa K, Harada H, Taga T, Watanabe Y, Matsuda T, Kashiwamura S, Nakajima K, Koyama K, Iwamatsu A, Tsunasawa S, Sakiyama F, Matsui H, Takahara Y, Taniguchi T, Kishimoto T (1986) Complementary DNA for a novel human interleukin (BSF-2) that induces B lymphocytes to produce immunoglobulin. Nature 324:73–76

Hirano T, Taga T, Yasukawa K, Nakajima K, Nakano N, Takatsuki F, Shimizu M, Murashima A, Tsunasawa S, Sakiyama F, Kishimoto T (1987) Human B cell differentiation factor defined by an anti-peptide antibody and its possible role in autoantibody production. Proc Natl Acad Sci USA 84:228

Hoang T, Haman A, Goncalves O, Letendre F, Mathieu M, Wong GG, Clark SC (1988) Interleukin-1 enhances growth factor-dependent proliferation of the clonogenic cells in acute myeloblastic leukemia and of normal human primitive hemopoietic precursors. J Exp Med 168:463–474

Hom JT, Bendele AM, Carlson DG (1988) In vivo administration with interleukin-1 accelerates the development of collagen-induced arthritis in mice. J Immunol 141:834–841

Howard M, Farrar J, Hilfiker M, Johnson B, Takatsu K, Hamaoka T, Paul WE (1982) Identification of a T cell derived B cell growth factor distinct from interleukin-2. J Exp Med 155:914–923

Hubbard JR, Steinberg JJ, Bednar MS, Sledge CB (1988) Effect of purified human interleukin-1 on cartilage degradation. J Orthop Res 6:180–187

Huebner K, Isobe M, Croce CM, Golde DW, Kaufman SE, Gasson JC (1985) The human gene encoding GM-CSF in a 5q21-q32, the chromosome region deleted in the 5q-anomaly. Science 230:1282–1285

Hu-Li J, Sheuach EM, Mizuguchi J, Ohara J, Mosmann T, Paul WE (1987) B cell stimulatory factor 1 (interleukin 4) is a potent costimulant for normal resting T lymphocytes. J Exp Med 165:157

Humphries RJ, Eaves AC, Eaves CJ (1980) Expression of stem cell behavior during macroscopic burst formation in vitro. In: Baum SJ, Ledney GD, Van Bekkum DW (eds) Experimental hematology today. Karger, Basel, p 39

Ihle JN (1983) Biochemical and biological properties of interleukin-3: a lymphokine mediating the differentiation of a lineage of cells which includes prothymocytes and mast-like cells. J Immunol 131:282

Ihle JN, Keller J, Henderson L et al. (1982) Procedures for the purification of IL-3 to homogeneity. J Immunol 129:2431

Ikebe T, Hirata M, Koga T (1988) Effects of human recombinant tumor necrosis factor-alpha and interleukin-1 on the synthesis of glycosaminoglycan and DNA in cultured rat costal chrondrocytes. J Immunol 140:827–831

Ikebuchi K, Wong GG, Clark SC, Ihle JN, Hirai Y, Ogawa M (1987) Interleukin-6 enhancement of interleukin-3-dependent proliferation of multipotential hemopoietic progenitors. Proc Natl Acad Sci USA 84:9035–9039

Ikebuchi K, Ihle JN, Hirai Y, Wong GG, Clark SC, Ogawa M (1988) Synergistic factors for stem cell proliferation: further studies of the target stem cells and the meahanism of stimulation by interleukin-1, interleukin-6 and granulocyte colony stimulating factor. Blood 72:2007–2014

Ikeda E, Kusaka M, Hakeda Y, Yokota K, Kumegawa M, Yamamoto S (1988) Effect of interleukin-1 beta on osteoblastic clone MC3T3-E1 cells. Calcif Tissue Int 43:162–166

Iscove NN, Till JE, McCulloch EA (1970) The proliferative states of mouse granulopoietic progenitor cells. Proc Soc Exp Biol Med 134:33–36

Ishibashi T, Miller SL, Burstein SA (1987) Type B transforming growth factor is a potent inhibitor of murine megakaryocytopoiesis in vitro. Blood 69:1737

Jakubowski AA, Souza L, Kelly F, Fain K, Budman D, Clarkson B, Bonilla MA, Moore MAS, Gabrilove J (1989) Effects of human granulocyte colony stimulating factor in a patient with idiopathic neutropenia. N Engl J Med 320:38–42

Johnson A, Dorshkind K (1986) Stromal cells in myeloid and lymphoid long term bone marrow cultures can support multiple hemopoietic lineages and modulate their production of hemopoietic growth factors. Blood 68:1348

Jones-Villeneuve E, Phillips RA (1980) Potentials for lymphoid differentiation by cells from long-term cultures of bone marrow. Exp Hematol 8:65–76

Karbassi A, Becker JM, Foster JS, Moore RN (1989) Enhanced killing of *Candida albicans* by murine macrophages treated with macrophage colony stimulating factor: evidence for augmented expression of mannose receptors. J Immunol 39:417–421

Kawano M, Hirano T, Matsuda T, Taga T, Horii Y, Iwato K, Asaoku H, Tang B, Tanabe O, Tanaka H, Kuramoto A, Kishimoto T (1988) Autocrine generation and essential requirement of BSF-2/IL-6 for human multiple myeloma. Nature 332:83–85

Kawaski ES, Ladner MB, Wang AM, Van Arsdell J, Warren MK, Coyne MY, Schweickart VL, Lee M-T, Wilson KJ, Boosman A, Stanley ER, Ralph P, Mark DF (1985) Molecular cloning of a complementary DNA encoding human macrophage-specific colony stimulating factor (CSF-1). Science 230:291–296

Keller JR, McNiece IK, Sill KP, Ellingsworth LR, Quesenberry PJ, Sing DK, Ruscetti FW (1990) Transforming growth factor beta directly regulates primitive murine hematopoietic cell proliferation. Blood 75:596–602

Kimoto M, Kindler V, Higaki M, Ody C, Izui S, Vassalli P (1988) Recombinant murine IL-3 fails to stimulate T or B lymphopoiesis in vivo but enhances immune responses to T cell dependent antigens. J Immunol 140:1889–1894

Kinashi T, Harada N, Severinson E, Tanabe T, Sideras P, Konishi M, Azuma C, Tominaga A, Bergstedt-Lindquist S, Takahashi M (1986) Cloning of complementary DNA encoding T cell replacing factor and identity with B cell growth factor II. Nature 324:70–73

Kinashi T, Inaba K, Tsubata T, Tashiro K, Palacios R, Honjo T (1988) Differentiation of an interleukin-3-dependent precursor B cell clone into immunoglobulin-producing cells in vitro. Proc Natl Acad Sci USA 85:4473–4477

Kincade PW, Witte PL, Landreth KS (1987) Stromal cell and factor dependent B lymphopoiesis in culture. In: Paige CJ, Gisler RH (eds) Differentiation of B lymphocytes. Springer, Berlin Heidelberg, New York (Current topics in microbiology and immunology, vol 135)

Knudtzon S, Mortensen BI (1975) Growth stimulation of human bone marrow cells in agar culture by vascular cells. Blood 46:937–943

Kohase M, Henriksen-DeStefano D, May LT, Vilcek J, Sehgal PB (1986) Induction of B2-interferon by tumor necrosis factor: a homeostatic mechanism in the control of cell proliferation. Cell 45:659–666

Koike K, Ihle JN, Ogawa M (1985) Selective culture of murine hemopoietic blast cell colonies based on cell cycle dormancy and requirement for low concentrations of interleukin-3. Blood 66:168a

Komiyama A, Ishiguro A, Kubo T, Matsuoka T, Tasukohchi S, Yasui K, Yangisawa M, Yamada S, Yamazaki M, Akabane T (1988) Increases in neutrophil counts by purified human urinary colony stimulating factor in chronic neutropenia of childhood. Blood 71:41–45

Koyanaqi Y, O'Brien WA, Zhao JQ, Golde DW, Gasson JC, Chen SY (1988) Cytokines alter production of HIV-1 from primary mononuclear phagocytes. Science 241:1673–1675

Koyasu S, Tojo A, Miyajima A, Akiyama T, Kasuga M, Urabe A, Schreurs J, Arai K, Takaku F, Yahara I (1987) Interleukin-3-specific tyrosine phosphorylation of a membrane glycoprotein of M_r 150000 in multifactor-dependent myeloid cell lines. EMBO J 6:3979–3984

Kupper TS, Lee F, Birchall N, Clark S, Dower S (1988) Interleukin-1 binds to specific receptors on human keratinocytes and induces granulocyte-macrophage colony stimulating factor mRNA and protein. J Clin Invest 82:1787–1792

Larsson EL, Iscove NN, Coutinho A (1980) Two distinct factors are required for induction of T cell growth. Nature 283:664

Le PT, Kurtzberg J, Brandt SJ, Niedel JE, Haynes BF, Singer KH (1988) Human thymic epithelial cells produce granulocyte and macrophage colony stimulating factors. J Immunol 141:1211–1217

Le Beau MM, Westbrook CA, Diaz MO, Larson RA, Rowley JD, Gasson JC, Golde DW, Sherr CJ (1986) Evidence for the involvement of GM-CSF and fms in the deletion (5q) in myeloid disorders. Science 231:984–987

Lee F, Yokota T, Otsuka T, Meyerson P, Villaret D, Coffman R, Mosmann T, Rennick D, Roehm N, Smith G, Zlotnik A, Arai KI (1986) Isolation and characterization of a mouse interleukin cDNA clone that expresses B cell stimulatory factor 1 activities and T cell and mast-cell stimulating activities. Proc Natl Acad Sci USA 83:2061

Lee F, Yokota T, Otsuka T et al. (1985) Isolation of cDNA for a human granuloctye-macrophage colony stimulating factor by functional expression in mammalian cells. Proc Natl Acad Sci USA 82:4360

Lee M-T, Warren MK (1987) CSF-1-induced resistance to viral infection in murine macrophages. J Immunol 138:3019–3022

LeMaire I (1988) Neurotensin enhances IL-1 production by activated alveolar macrophages. J Immunol 140:2983–2988

Lin HS, Gordon S (1979) Secretion of plasminogen activator by bone marrow derived mononuclear phagocytes and its enhancement by colony stimulating factor. J Exp Med 150:231–245

Lin H-S, Lokeshwar BL, Hsu S (1989) Both granulocyte-macrophage CSF and macrophage CSF control the proliferation and survival of the same subset of alveolar macrophages. J Immunol 142:515–519

Lindemann A, Riedel D, Oster W, Meuer SC, Blohm D, Mertelsmann RH, Hermann F (1988) Granulocyte-macrophage colony stimulating factor induces interleukin 1 production by human polymorphonuclear neutrophils. J Immunol 140:837–839

Long MW, Gragowski LL, Heffner CH, Boxer LA (1985) Phorbol diesters stimulate the development of an early murine progenitor cell. J Clin Invest 76:431–438

Lopez AF, To LB, Yang Y-C, Gamble JR, Shannon MF, Burns GF, Dyson PG, Juttner CA, Clark S, Vadas MA (1987) Stimulation of proliferation, differentiation and function of human cells by primate interleukin-3. Proc Natl Acad Sci USA 84:2761

Lopez AF, Dyson PG, Bik To L, Elliott MJ, Milton SE, Russell JA, Juttner CA, Yang Y-C, Clark SC, Vadas MA (1988) Recombinant human interleukin-3 stimulation of hematopoiesis in humans: loss of responsiveness with differentiation in the neutrophilic myeloid series. Blood 72:1797–1804

Lorenzo JA, Sousa SL, Centrella M (1988) Interleukin-1 in combination with transforming growth factor-alpha produces enhanced bone resorption in vitro. Endocrinology 123:2194–2200

Mayer P, Lam C, Obenaus H, Liehl E, Besemer J (1987) Recombinant human GM-CSF induces leukocytosis and activates peripheral blood polymorphonuclear neutrophils in nonhuman primates. Blood 70:206–213

McGrath HE, Liang C, Alberico T, Quesenberry PJ (1987) The effect of lithium on growth factor production in long term bone marrow cultures. Blood 70: 1136–1140

McInnes A, Rennick DM (1988) Interleukin 4 induces cultured monocytes/macrophages to form giant multinucleated cells. J Exp Med 167:598–611

McLeod DL, Shreeve MM, Axelrad AA (1974) Improved plasma culture system for production of erythrocytic colonies in vitro: quantitative assay method for CFU-E. Blood 44:517–534

McNeil TA (1973) Release of bone marrow colony stimulating activity during immunological reactions in vitro. Nature 244:175–176

McNiece IK, Bradley TR, Kriegler AB, Hodgson GS (1982) A growth factor produced by WEHI-3 cells for murine high proliferative potential GM-progenitor colony forming cells. Cell Biol Int Rep 6:243

McNiece IK, McGrath HE, Quesenberry PJ (1988a) Granulocyte colony stimulating factor augments in vitro megakaryocyte colony formation by interleukin-3. Exp Hematol 16:807–810

McNiece IK, Stewart FM, Deacon DH, Quesenberry PJ (1988b) Synergistic interactions between hematopoietic factors as detected by in vitro murine bone marrow colony formation. Exp Hematol 16:383–388

McNiece IK, Robinson BE, Quesenberry PJ (1988c) Stimulation of murine colony forming cells with high proliferative potential by the combination of GM-CSF and CSF-1. Blood 72:191–195

Metcalf D (1971) Acute antigen induced elevation of serum colony stimulating factor (CSF) levels. Immunology 21:427–436

Metcalf D, Nicola NA (1985) Synthesis by mouse peritoneal cells of granulocyte-colony stimulating factor, the differentiation inducer for myeloid leukemia cells: stimulation by endotoxin, macrophage colony stimulating factor and multi-colony stimulating factor. Leuk Res 9:35–50

Metcalf D, McDonald HR, Odartchenko N, Surdat B (1975) Growth of mouse megakaryocyte colonies in vitro. Proc Natl Acad Sci USA 72:1744–1748

Metcalf D, Bagby CG, Johnson GR, Nicola NA, Lopez AF, Williamson DJ (1986a) Effects of purified bacterially synthesized murinemulti-colony stimulating factor (interleukin-3) on hematopoiesis in normal adult mice. Blood 68:46

Metcalf D, Begley CG, Johnson GR, Nicola NA, Vadas MA, Lopez AF, Williamson DJ, Wong GG, Clark SC, Wang EA (1986b) Biologic properties in vitro of a recombinant human granulocyte-macrophage colony stimulating factor. Blood 67:37–45

Metcalf D, Burgess AW, Johnson GR, Nicola NA, Nice EC, DeLamarter J, Thatcher DR, Mermod J-J (1986c) In vitro actions on hemopoietic cells of recombinant murine GM-CSF purified after production in *Escherichia coli*. Comparison with purified native GM-CSF. J Cell Physiol 128:421–431

Miyauchi J, Kelleher CA, Yang Y-C, Wong GG, Clark SC, Minden MD, Minkin S, McCulloch EA (1987) The effects of three recombinant growth factors IL-3, GM-CSF and G-CSF on the blast cells of acute myeloblastic leukemia maintained in short term suspension culture. Blood 70:657–663

Mochizuki DY, Eisenman JR, Conlon PJ, Larson AD, Tushinski RS (1987) Interleukin-1 regulates hematopoietic activity, a role previously ascribed to hemopoietin 1. Proc Natl Acad Sci USA 84:5267–5271

Monray RL, Skelly RR, MacVittie TJ, Davis TA, Sauber JJ, Clark SC, Donahue RE (1987) The effect of recombinant GM-CSF on the recovery of monkeys transplanted with autologous bone marrow. Blood 70:1696–1699

Moore MAS, Williams N, Metcalf D (1972) Purification and characterization of the in vitro colony forming cells in monkey hemopoietic tissue. J Cell Physiol 79:283–292

Moore RN, Oppenheim JJ, Farrar JJ, Carter CS Jr, Waheed A, Shadduck RK (1980) Production of lymphocyte-activating factor (interleukin-1) by macrophages activated with colony stimulating factors. J Immunol 125:1302

Moore RN, Joshi JG, Deana DG, Pitruzzello FJ, Horohov DW, Rouse BT (1986) Characterization of a two-signal dependent Ia^+ mononuclear phagocyte progenitor subpopulation that is sensitive to inhibition by ferritin. J Immunol 136:1605–1611

Moore RN, Osmand AP, Dunn JA, Doshi JG, Rouse BT (1988) Substance augmentation of CSF-1 stimulated in vitro myelopoiesis: a two-signal progenitor restricted, tuftsin-like effect. J Immunol 141:2699–2703

Morley A, Rickard KA, Howard D, Stohlman F Jr (1971) Studies on the regulation of granulopoiesis. IV. Possible humoral regulation. Blood 37:14–22

Morrissey PJ, Charrier K, Alpert A, Bressler L (1988) In vivo administration of interleukin-1 induces thymic hypoplasia and increased levels of serum corticosterone. J Immunol 141:1456–1463

Morstyn G, Campbell L, Souza LM, Alton NK, Keech J, Green M, Sheridan W, Metcalf D, Fox R (1988) Effect of granulocyte colony stimulating factor on neutropenia induced by cytotoxic chemotherapy. Lancet 1:667–672

Motoyoshi K, Takaku F, Maekawa T, Miura Y, Kimura K, Furusawa S, Hattori M, Nomura T, Mizoguchi H, Ogawa M (1986) Protective effect of partially purified human urinary colony stimulating factor on granulocytopenia after antitumor chemotherapy. Exp Hematol 14:1069–1075

Mullis KB, Fallona FA (1987) Specific synthesis of DNA in vitro via a polymerase-catalyzed chain reaction. Methods Enzymol 155:335–350

Nagata S, Tsuchiya M, Asano S, Yamamoto O, Hirata Y, Kubota N, Oheda M, Nomura H, Yamazaki T (1986) The chromosomal gene structure and two mRNAs for human granulocyte colony stimulating factor. EMBO J 5:575–581

Nakahata T, Ogawa M (1982) Identification in culture of a new class of hemopoietic colony forming units with extensive capability to self-renew and generate multipotential colonies. Proc Natl Acad Sci USA 79:3843–3847

Naldini A, Fleischmann WR, Ballas ZK, Klimpel KD, Klimpel GR (1987) Interleukin-2 inhibits in vitro granulocyte macrophage colony formation. J Immunol 139:1880–1884

Namen AE, Lupton S, Hjerrild K, Wignall J, Mochizuki DY, Schmierer A, Mosley B, March CJ, Urdal D, Gillis S (1988a) Stimulation of B cell progenitors by cloned murine interleukin-7. Nature 333:571–573

Namen AE, Schmierer AE, March CJ, Overell RW, Park LS, Urdal DL, Mochizuki DY (1988b) B cell precursor growth-promoting activity. Purification and characterization of a growth factor active on lymphocyte precursors. J Exp Med 167:988–1002

Negrin RS, Haeuber DH, Nagler A, Souza LM, Greenberg PL (1988) Treatment of myelodysplastic syndromes with recombinant human granulocyte-colony-stimulating factor. Exp Hematol 16:519 (abstr)

Neta R, Oppenheim JJ (1988) Cytokines in therapy of radiation injury. Blood 72:1093–1097

Neumunaitis J, Singer JW, Buckner CD, Hill R, Storb R, Thomas ED, Applebaum FR (1988) Use of recombinant human granulocyte-macrophage colony stimulating factor in autologous marrow transplantation for lymphoid malignancies. Blood 72:834–836

Nicola NA, Metcalf D (1986) Binding of iodinated multipotential colony stimulating factor (interleukin-3) to murine bone marrow cells. J Cell Physiol 128:180–188

Nicola NA, Metcalf D, Matsumoto M, Johnson GR (1983) Purification of a factor inducing differentiation in murine myelomonocytic leukemia cells. Identification as granulocyte colony stimulating factor. J Biol Chem 258:9017–9023

Nicola NA, Begley CG, Metcalf D (1985) Identification of the human analogue of a regulator that induces differentiation in murine leukaemic cells. Nature 314: 625–628

Niemayer CM, Sieff CA, Mathey-Preuot B, Wimperer JZ, Bierer BE, Clark SC, Nathan DG (1989) Expression of human interleukin-3 (multi-CSF) is restricted to human lymphocytes and T cell tumor lines. Blood 73:945–951

Nimer SD, Champlin RE, Golde DW (1988) Serum cholesterol-lowering activity of granulocyte-macrophage colony stimulating factor. JAMA 260:3297–3300

Noelle R, Krammer PH, Ohara J, Uhr JW, Vitetta ES (1984) Increased expression of Ia antigens on resting B cells: an additional role for B cell growth factor. Proc Natl Acad Sci USA 81:6149–6153

Noma Y, Sideras P, Naito T, Bergstedt-Lindquist S, Azuma C, Severinson E, Tanabe T, Kinashi T, Matsudfa F, Yaoita Y (1986) Cloning of cDNA encoding the murine IgGl induction factor by a novel strategy using SP6 promoter. Nature 319:640–646

Nordan RP, Pumphrey JG, Rudikoff S (1987) Purification and NH_2-terminal sequence of a plasmacytoma growth factor derived from the murine macrophage cell line, P388D1. J Immunol 139:813

Ohara J, Paul WE (1987) Receptors for B cell stimulatory factor-1 expressed on cells of haematopoietic lineage. Nature 325:537

Ohara J, Coligen JE, Zoon K, Meloy WL, Paul WE (1987) High efficiency purification and chemical characterization of B cell stimulatory factor-1/interleukin-4. J Immunol 139:1127

Okabe T, Takaku F (1986) In vivo granulocytopoietic activities of human recombinant granulocyte colony stimulating factor. Exp Hematol 14:475

Otsuka T, Villaret D, Yokota T, Takabe Y, Lee F, Arai N, Arai KI (1987) Structure analysis of the mouse chromosomal gene encoding interleukin-4 which expresses B cell, T cell and mast cell stimulating activities. Nucleic Acids Res 15:333

Parker JW, Metcalf D (1974) Production of colony stimulating factor in mitogen stimulated lymphocyte cultures. J Immunol 112:502–510

Park LS, Friend D, Gillis S, Urdal DL (1986) Characterization of the cell surface receptor for a multi-lineage colony stimulating factor (CSF-2). J Biol Chem 261:205–210

Park L, Friend D, Sarsenfeld HM, Urdal DL (1987) Characterization of the human B cell stimulatory factor 1 receptor. J Exp Med 166:476

Peace DJ, Kern DE, Schultz KR, Greenberg PD, Cheever MA (1988) IL-4-induced lymphokine activated killer cells. Lytic activity is mediated by phenotypically distinct natural killer-like and T cell-like large granular lymphocytes. J Immunol 140:3679–3685

Peetre C, Gulberg U, Nilsson E, Olsson I (1986) Effects of recombinant tumor necrosis factor on proliferation and differentiation of leukemia and normal hemopoietic cells in vitro. Relationship to cell surface receptor. J Clin Invest 78:1694

Pelus LM, Broxmeyer HE, Moore MAS (1981) Regulation of human myelopoiesis by prostaglandin E and lactoferrin. Cell Tissue Kinet 14:515

Peschel C, Paul WE, Ohara J, Green I (1987) Effects of B cell stimulatory factor-1 (interleukin-4) on hematopoietic progenitor cells. Blood 70:254

Pettenati MJ, Le Beau LL, Lemons RS, Shima EA, Kawasaki ES, Larson RA, Sherr CJ, Diaz MO, Rowley JD (1987) Assignment of CSF-1 to 5q33.1: evidence for clustering of genes regulating hematopoiesis and for their involvement in the deletion of the long arm of chromosome 5 in myeloid disorders. Proc Natl Acad Sci USA 84:2970

Pike BL, Nossal GJV (1985) Interleukin-1 can act as a B cell growth and differentiation factor. Proc Natl Acad Sci USA 82:8153

Pluznik DH, Sachs L (1965) The cloning of normal "mast" cells in tissue culture. J Cell Comp Physiol 66:319–324

Pluznik DH, Cunningham RE, Noguchi PD (1984) Colony stimulating factor controls proliferation of CSF-dependent cells by acting during G1 phase of the cell cycle. Proc Natl Acad Sci USA 81:7451–7455

Prystowsky MB, Ihle JN, Rich I, Keller J, Offen G, Naujokos M, Coken M, Goldwasser E, Fitch FW (1983) Two biologically distinct colony stimulating factors are secreted by a T lymphocyte clone. J Cell Biochem 6:37

Quesenberry P, Gimbrone M (1980) Vascular endothleium as a regulator or granulopoiesis: production of colony stimulating activity by cultured human endothelial cells. Blood 56:1060–1067

Quesenberry P, Levitt L (1979) Hematopoietic stem cells. N Engl J Med 301:755, 819, 868

Quesenberry P, Halperin J, Ryan M, Stohlman F Jr (1975) Tolerance to the granulocyte-releasing and colony stimulating factor elevating effects of endotoxin. Blood 45:789

Quesenberry PJ, Rappeport JM, Fountebuoni A, Sullivan R, Zuckerman K, Ryan M (1978a) Inhibition of normal murine hematopoiesis by leukemic cells. N Engl J Med 299:71–75

Quesenberry P, Cohen H, Levin J, Sullivan R, Bealmear P, Ryan M (1978b) Effects of bacterial infection and irradiation on serum colony stimulating factor levels in tolerant and nontolerant CF1 mice. Blood 51:229

Quesenberry PJ, Gimbrone MA, Doukas MA, Goldwasser E (1981) Vascular derived tissues as a source of colony stimulating activity (CSA). Clin Res 29:830a (abstr)

Quesenberry PJ, Ihle JN, McGrath E (1985) The effect of interleukin-3 and GM-CSA-2 on megakaryocyte and myeloid clonal colony formation. Blood 65:214

Quesenberry P, Song Z, McGrath H et al. (1987) Multilineage synergistic activity produced by a murine adherent marrow cell line. Blood 69:827

Raefsky EL, Platanias LC, Zoumbos NC, Young NS (1985) Studies of interferon as a regulator of hematopoietic cell proliferation. J Immunol 135:2507

Rennick D, Yang G, Gemmell L, Lee F (1987) Control of hemopoiesis by a bone marrow stromal cell clone: lipopolysaccharide and interleukin-1 inducible production of colony stimulating factors. Blood 69:682

Rettenmier CW, Roussel MF, Ashmun RA, Ralph P, Price K, Sherr CJ (1987) Synthesis of membrane bound colony stimulating factor-1 (CSF-1) and down modulation of CSF-1 receptors in NIH 3T3 cells transformed by cotransfection of the human CSF-1 and c-*fms* (CSF-1 receptor) genes. Mol Cell Biol 7: 2378–2387

Roberge FG, Caspi RR, Nussenblatt RB (1988) Glial retinal Muller cells produce IL-1 activity and have a dual effect on autoimmune T helper lymphocytes.

Antigen presentation manifested after removal of suppressive activity. J Immunol 140:2193–2196

Robinson BE, McGrath HE, Quesenberry PJ (1987) Recombinant murine granulocyte macrophage colony stimulating factor has megakaryocyte colony stimulating activity and augments megakaryocyte colony stimulation by interleukin-3. J Clin Invest 79:1648

Rossio JL, Ruscetti FW, Farrar WL (1986) Ligand-specific calcium mobilization in IL2 and IL3 dependent cell lines. Lymphokine Res 5:163–172

Rothenberg ME, Owen WF, Silberstein DS, Woods J, Soberman RJ, Austen KF, Stevens RL (1988) Human eosinophils have prolonged survival, enhanced functional properties and become hypodense when exposed to human interleukin-3. J Clin Invest 81:1986–1992

Rothstein G, Hugl EH, Bishop CR, Athens JW, Ashenbrucker HE (1971) Stimulation of granulocytopoiesis by a diffusible factor in vivo. J Clin Invest 50: 2004–2007

Roussel MF, Sherr CJ, Baker PE, Ruddle FH (1983) Molecular cloning of the c-*fms* locus and its assignment to human chromosome 5. J Virol 48:770–773

Ruland LJ, Quesenberry PJ, Balian G (1990) A 17 kilodalton polypeptide, sensitive to bacterial collagenase, is synthesized by bone marrow macrophages in myeloid and lymphoid cultures. Exp Hematol 18:969–973

Sanderson CF, O'Garra A, Warren DJ, Klaus GGB (1986) Eosinophil differentiation factor also has B cell growth factor activity: proposed name interleukin-4. Proc Natl Acad Sci USA 83:437

Sanderson CJ, Warren DJ, Strath M (1985) Identification of a lymphokine that stimulates differentiation in vitro. Its relationship to interleukin-3 and functional properties of the eosinophils produced in cultures. J Exp Med 162:60

Santoli D, Clark SC, Kreider BL, Maslin PA, Rovera G (1988) Amplification of IL-2-driven T cell proliferation by recombinant human IL-3 and granulocyte-macrophage colony stimulating factor. J Immunol 141:519–526

Savage AM (1964) Hematopoietic recovery in endotoxin treated lethally X-irradiated BUB mice. Radiat Res 23:180–191

Sayers TJ, Wiltrout TA, Bull CA, Denn AC, Dilano AM, Lokesh B (1988) Effect of cytokines on polymorphonuclear neutrophil infiltration in the mouse. J Immunol 141:1670–1677

Schimpl A, Wecker E (1972) Replacement of T cell function by a T cell product. Nature 237:15

Schneider E, Ihle JN, Dy M (1985) Homogeneous interleukin-3 enhances arginase activity in murine hematopoietic cells. Lymphokine Res 4:95–102

Schrader JW, Schrader S (1978) In vitro studies on lymphocyte differentiation. I. Long term in vitro culture of cells giving rise to functional lymphocytes in irradiated mice. J Exp Med 148:823–828

Schrader JW, Schrader S, Clark-Lewis I, Crapper R (1984) In: Wright DG, Greenberger JS (eds) Long term bone marrow culture. Alan R Liss, New York, pp 293–307

Seelentag WK, Mermod J-J, Montesano R, Vassalli P (1987) Additive effects of interleukin-1 and tumor necrosis factor-alpha on the accumulation of the three granulocytes and macrophage colony stimulating factor mRNAs in human endothelial cells. EMBO J 6:2261–2265

Sehgal PB, May LT, Tamm I, Vilcek J (1987) Human B_2 interferon and B cell differentiation factor BSF-2 are identical. Science 235:731–732

Shadduck RK, Nunna NG (1971) Granulocyte colony stimulating factor. III. Effect of alkylating agent induced granulocytopenia. Proc Soc Exp Biol Med USA 137:1479–1482

Shaw G, Kamen R (1986) A conserved AU sequence from the 3′ untranslated region of GM-CSF mRNA mediates selective mRNA degradation. Cell 46:659–667

Sheriden JW, Metcalf D (1973) CSF production and release following endotoxin. In:

Robinson WA (ed) Hemopoiesis in culture. DHEW Publication No (NIH) 74–205, Washington, pp 135–143

Sherr CJ, Rettenmier CW, Sacca R, Roussel MF, Look AT, Stanley ER (1985) The c-*fms* proto-oncogene product is related to the receptor for the mononuclear phagocyte growth factor, CSF-1. Cell 41:665–676

Sieff CA, Emerson SG, Donahue RE, Nathan DG (1985) Human recombinant granulocyte-macrophage colony stimulating factor: a multilineage hematopoietin. Science 230:1171–1173

Silberstein DS, Owen WF, Gasson JC, DiPersio JF, Golde DW, Bina JC, Soberman R, Austen KF, David JR (1986) Enhancement of human eosinophil cytotoxicty and leukotriene synthesis by biosynthetic (recombinant) granulocyte-macrophage colony stimulating factor. J Immunol 137:3290–3294

Simmers RN, Webber LM, Shannon MF, Garson OM, Wong G, Vadas MA, Sutherland GR (1987) Localization of the G-CSF gene on chromosome 17 proximal to the breakpoint in the t (15:17) in acute promyelocytic leukemia. Blood 70:330–332

Smith KA (1988) Interleukin-2: inception, impact and implications. Science 240: 1169–1176

Smith KA, Lachman LB, Oppenheim JJ, Favata MF (1980) The functional relationship of the interleukins. J Exp Med 151:1551

Socinski MA, Cannistra SA, Sullivan R, Elias A, Antman K, Schnipper L, Griffin JD (1988a) Granulocyte macrophage colony stimulating factor induces the expression of the CDllb surface adhesion molecule on human granulocytes in vivo. Blood 72:691–697

Socinski MA, Elias A, Schnipper L, Cannistra SA, Antman KH, Griffin JD (1988b) Granulocyte-macrophage colony stimulating factor expands the circulating haemopoietic progenitor cell compartment in man. Lancet 1:1194–1198

Song ZX, Quesenberry PJ (1984) Radioresistant murine marrow stromal cells: a morphologic and functional characterization. Exp Hematol 12:523

Sonoda Y, Yang Y-C, Wong GG, Clark SC, Ogawa M (1988) Analysis in serum-free culture of the targets of recombinant human hemopoietic growth factors: interleukin-3 and granulocyte-macrophage colony stimulating factor are specific for early developmental stages. Proc Natl Acad Sci USA 85:4360–4364

Sorenson P, Farber NM, Krystal G (1986) Identification of the interleukin-3 receptor using an iodinatable, cleavable, photoreactive cross-linking agent. J Biol Chem 261:9094

Stanley ER, Guilbert LF (1981) Methods of purification, assay, characterization and target cell binding of a colony-stimulating factor (CSF-1). J Immunol Methods 42:253–284

Stanley IJ, Burgess AW (1983) Granulocyte-macrophage colony stimulating factor stimulates the synthesis of membrane and nuclear proteins in murine neutrophils. J Cell Biochem 23:241–258

Stuart PM, Zlotnik A, Woodward JG (1988) Induction of class I and class II MHC antigen expression on murine bone marrow-derived macrophages by IL-4 (B cell stimulatory factor 1). J Immunol 140:1542–1547

Suda J, Suda T, Ogawa M (1984a) Analysis of differentiation of mouse hemopoietic stem cells in cultures by sequential replating of paired progenitors. Blood 64: 393–399

Suda T, Suda J, Ogawa M (1984b) Diseparate differentiation in mouse hemoopietic colonies derived from paired progenitors. Proc Natl Acad Sci USA 81: 2520–2524

Sutherland GR, Baker E, Callen DF, Campbell HD, Young IG, Sanderson CJ, Garson OM, Lopez AF, Vadas MA (1988) Interleukin-5 is at 5q3l and is deleted in the 5q- syndrome. Blood 71:1150–1152

Swain SL, Dutton RW (1982) Production of a B cell growth-promoting activity, (DL) BCGF, from a cloned T cell line and its assay on the BCLl B cell tumor. J Exp Med 156:1821

Takatsu K, Tominaga A, Mamaoka T (1980) Antigen induced T cell replacing factor (TRF). I. Functional characterization of TRF-producing helper T cell subset and genetic studies on TRF production. J Immunol 124:2414

Takatsu K, Harada N, Hara Y, Yamada G, Takahama Y, Dobashi K, Hamaoka T (1985) Purification and physico-chemical characterization of murine T cell replacing factor (TRF). J Immunol 134:382

Tanabe O, Akira S, Kamiya T, Wong GG, Hirano T, Kishimoto T (1988) Genomic structure of the murine IL-6 gene. J Immunol 141:3875–3881

Tartakovsky B, Finnegan A, Muegge K, Brody DT, Kovacs EJ, Smith MR, Berzofsky JA, Young HA, Durum SK (1988) IL-1 is an autocrine growth factor for T cell clones. J Immunol 141:3863–3867

Tatakis DN, Schneeberger G, Dziak R (1988) Recombinant interleukin-1 stimulates prostaglandin E2 production by osteoblastic cells: synergy with parathyroid hormone. Calcif Tissue Int 42:358–362

Tavassoli M, Takahashi K (1982) Morphological studies on long term culture of marrow cells: characterization of the adherent stromal cells and their interactions in maintaining the proliferation of hemopoietic stem cells. Am J Anat 164:91

Testa NG, Dexter TM (1977) Long term production of erythroid precursor cells (BFU) in bone marrow cultures. Differentiation 9:193

te Velde AA, Klomp JP, Yard BA, de Vries JE, Figdor CG (1988) Modulation of phenotypic and functional properties of human peripheral blood monocytes by IL-4. J Immunol 140:1548–1554

Tobler A, Miller CW, Norman AW, Koeffler HP (1988) 1,25-Dihydroxyvitamin D_3 modulates the expression of a lymphokine (GM-CSF) posttranscriptionally. J Clin Invest 81:1819

Tominaga A, Matsumoto M, Hjarada N, Takahashi T, Kikuchi Y, Takatsu K (1988) Molecular properties and regulation of mRNA expression for murine T cell-replacing factor/IL-5. J Immunol 140:1175–1181

Tosato G, Seamon KB, Goldman ND, Sehgal PB, May LT, Washington GC, Jones KD, Pike SE (1988) Monocyte-derived human B cell growth factor identified as interferon-beta-2 (BSF-2, IL-6). Science 239:502–504

Tsuchiya M, Asano S, Kaziro Y, Nagata S (1986) Isolation and characterization of the cDNA for murine granulocyte colony stimulating factor. Proc Natl Acad Sci USA 83:7633–7637

Tushinski RJ, Stanley ER (1983) The regulation of macrophage protein turnover by a colony stimulating factor (CSF-1). J Cell Physiol 116:67–75

Tushinski RJ, Stanley ER (1985) The regulation of mononuclear phagocyte entry into S phase by the colony stimulating factor, CSF-1. J Cell Physiol 122:221–228

Ulich TR, del Castillo J, Souza L (1988) Kinetics and mechanisms of recombinant human granulocyte-colony stimulating factor-induced neutrophilia. Am J Pathol 133:630–638

Vadas MA, Nicola NA, Metcalf D (1983) Activation of antibody dependent cell mediated cytotoxicity of the human neutrophils and eosinophils by separate colony stimulating factors. J Immunol 130:795–799

Vadhan-Raj S, Keating M, LeMaistre A, Hittelman WN, McCredie K, Trujillo JM, Broxmeyer HE, Henney C, Gutterman JU (1987) Stimulation of hematopoiesis in patients with myelodysplastic syndrome by recombinant granulocyte-macrophage colony stimulating factor. Blood 70:144a (abstr)

Vallenga E, Young DC, Wagner K, Wiper D, Ostapovicz D, Griffin JD (1987) The effects of GM-CSF and G-CSF in promoting growth of clonogenic cells in acute myeloblastic leukemia. Blood 69:1771–1776

Van Damme J, DeLey M, Van Snick J, Dinarello CA, Billou A (1987a) The role of interferon-B1 and the 26-kDa protein (interferon-B2) as mediators of the antiviral effect of interleukin-1 and tumor necrosis factor. J Immunol 139:1867

Van Damme J, Openakker G, Simpson RJ, Rubira MR, Cayphas S, Vink A, Billior A, Van Snick J (1987b) Identification of the human 26-kd protein, interferon B2

(IFN-B2) as a B cell hybridoma/plasmacytoma growth factor induced by interleukin-1 and tumor necrosis factor. J Exp Med 165:914

Vink A, Vandenabeele P, Uyttenhove C, Cayphas S, Van-Snick J (1988) Plasmacytoma growth factor activity of murine granulocyte-macrophage colony stimulating factor. J Immunol 141:1996–1999

Vitetta ES, Brooks K, Chen YW, Isakson P, Jones S, Layton J, Mishra GC, Pure E, Weiss E, Word C (1984) T cell derived lymphokines that induce IgM and IgG secretion in activated murine B cells. Immunol Rev 78:137–157

Waheed A, Shadduck RF (1979) Purification and properties of L cell-derived colony-stimulating factor. J Lab Clin Med 94:180–194

Wakamiya N, Horiguchi J, Kufe D (1987) Detection of c-*fms* and CSF-1 RNA by in situ hybridization. Leukemia 1:518–520

Waldman TA, Goldman CK, Robb RJ, Depper JM, Leonard WJ, Sharrow SU, Bongiouanni KF, Korsmeyer SJ, Greene WC (1984) Expression of interleukin 2 receptors on activated human B cell. J Exp Med 160:1450–1466

Walker F, Burgess AW (1985) Specific binding of radioiodinated granulocyte-macrophage colony stimulating factor to hemopoietic cells. EMBO J 4:933–939

Wang JW, Griffin JD, Rambaldi A, Chen ZG, Mantovani A (1980) Induction of monocyte migration by recombinant macrophage colony stimulating factor. J Immunol 141:575–579

Wang JW, Chen ZG, Colella S, Bonilla MA, Welte K, Bordignon C, Mantovani A (1988) Chemotactic activity of recombinant human granulocyte colony-stimulating factor. Blood 72:1456–1460

Warren DJ, Moore MAS (1988) Synergism among interleukin-1, interleukin-3 and interleukin-5 in the production of eosinophils from primitive hemopoietic stem cells. J Immunol 140:94–99

Warren MK, Ralph P (1986) Macrophage growth factor CSF-1 stimulates human monocyte production of interferon, tumor necrosis factor and colony stimulating activity. J Immunol 137:2281–2285

Watson JD, Crosier PS, March CJ, Conlon PJ, Mochizuki DY, Gillis S, Urdal DL (1986) Purification to homogeneity of a human hematopoietic growth factor that stimulates the growth of a murine IL-3-dependent cell line. J Immunol 137: 854–857

Weisbart RH, Golde DW, Clark SC, Wong G-G, Jasson JC (1985) Human granulocyte-macrophage colony stimulating factor is a neutrophil activator. Nature 314:361–363

Welte K, Bonilla MA, Gillio AP, Boone T, Gabrilove JL, Potter G, O'Reilly RJ, Souza LM (1986) In vivo effects of combined recombinant human G-CSF and GM-CSF on hematopoiesis in primates. Blood 68:183a

Whetton AD, Bazill GW, Dexter TM (1985) Stimulation of hexose uptake by haemopoietic cell growth factor occurs in WEHI-3B myelomonocytic leukaemia cells: a possible mechanism for loss of growth control. J Cell Physiol 123:73–78

Whitlock CA, Witte ON (1987) Long term culture of B lymphocytes and their precursors from murine bone marrow. Proc Natl Acad Sci USA 79:3608

Williams N, Jackson H, Sheridan APC, Murphy MJ, Elste A, Moore MAS (1978) Regulation of megakaryopoiesis in long-term murine bone marrow cultures. Blood 51:245–255

Wing EJ, Waheed A, Shadduck RK, Nagle LS, Stephenson K (1982) Effect of colony stimulating factor on murine macrophages. J Clin Invest 69:270–276

Wing EJ, Ampel NM, Waheed A, Shadduck RK (1985) Macrophage CSF (M-CSF) enhances the capacity of murine macrophages to secrete oxygen reduction products. J Immunol 135:2052–2056

Wolf NS, Trentin JJ (1968) Hemopoietic colony studies. V. Effect of hemopoietic organ stroma on differentiation of pluripotent stem cells. J Exp Med 127:205

Wong GG, Witek JS, Temple PA, Wilkens KM, Leary AC, Luxemburg DP, Jones SS, Brown EL, Kan RM, ORREC (1985) Human GM-CSF: molecular cloning of the complementary DNA and purification of the natural and recombinant proteins. Science 228:810

Wong GG, Temple PA, Leary AC, Witek-Gianatti JS, Yang Y-C, Ciarletta DB, Chung M, Murtha P, Kriz R, Kaufman RJ, Ferenz CR, Sibley BS, Turner KJ, Hewick RM, Clark SC, Yanai N, Yokota H, Yamada M, Saito M, Motoyoshi K, Takaku F (1987) Human CSF-1: molecular cloning and expression of 4-kb cDNA encoding the human urinary protein. Science 235:1504–1508

Wong GG, Witck-Giannotti JS, Temple PA, Kriz R, Ferenz C, Hewick RM, Clark SC, Ikebuchi K, Ogawa M (1988) Stimulation of murine hemopoietic colony formation by human IL-6. J Immunol 140:3040–3044

Woodward TA, Baber GB, McNiece IK, Robinson BE, Quesenberry PJ (1990) Induction of early B lineage cells by hemopoietic growth factors. Blood 75: 2130–2136

Yang Y-C, Ciarletta AB, Temple PA, Chung MP, Kovacic S, Witek-Giannotti SS, leary AC, Kriz R, Donahoe RE, Wong GG, Clark SC (1986) Human interleukin-3 (multi-CSF): identification by expression cloning of a novel hematopoietic growth factor related to murine interleukin-3. Cell 47:3

Yasukawa K, Hirano T, Watanabe Y, Muratani K, Matsuda T, Nakai S, Kishimoto T (1987) Structure and expression of human B cell stimulatory factor 2 (BSF-2) gene. EMBO J 6:2939–2945

Yokota T, Lee F, Rennick D, Hall C, Arai N, Mosmann T, Nabel G, Cantor H, Arai K (1984) Isolation and characterization of a mouse cDNA clone that expresses mast cell growth factor activity in monkey cells. Proc Natl Acad Sci USA 81:1070–1074

Yokota T, Otsuka T, Mosmann T, Banchereau J, DeFrance T, Blanchard D, DeVries JE, Lee F, Arai K (1986) Isolation and characterization of a human interleukin cDNA clone, homologous to mouse B cell stimulatory factor 1, that expresses B cell and T cell stimulating activities. Proc Natl Acad Sci USA 83:5894–5898

Young DC, Wagner K, Griffin JD (1987) Constitutive expression of the granulocyte-macrophage colony stimulating factor gene in acute myeloblastic leukemia. J Clin Invest 79:100–106

Zhou Y-Q, Stanley ER, Clark SC, Hatzfeld JA, Levesque J-P, Federici C, Watt SM, Hatzfeld A (1988) Interleukin-3 and interleukin-1-alpha allow earlier bone marrow progenitors to respond to human colony stimulating factor-1. Blood 72:1870–1874

Ziboh VA, Miller AM, Wu M-C, Yunis AA, Jimenez J, Wong G (1982) Induced release and metabolism of arachidonic acid from myeloid cells by purified colony stimulating factor. J Cell Physiol 113:67–72

Zilberstein A, Ruggieri R, Korn JH, Revel M (1986) Structure and expression of cDNA and genes for human interferon-B-2, a distinct species inducible by growth stimulatory cytokines. EMBO J 5:2529–2537

Zsebo KM, Wypych J, Yuschenkoff VN, Lu H, Hunt P, Dukes PP, Langley KE (1988) Effects of hematopoietin-1 and interleukin-1 activities on early hematopoietic cells of the bone marrow. Blood 71:962–968

Zucali JR, Dinarello CA, Oblon DF, Gross MA, Anderson L, Weiner RS (1986) Interleukin 1 stimulates fibroblasts to produce granulocyte-macrophage colony stimulating activity and prostaglandin E2. J Clin Invest 77:1857–1863

Zucali JR, Broxmeyer HE, Dinarello CA, Gross MA, Weiner RS (1987) Regulation of early human hematopoietic (BFU-E, and CFU-GEMM) progenitor cells in vitro by interleukin-1-induced fibroblasts-conditioned medium. Blood 69:33

Zuckerman KS, Wicha MS (1983) Extracellular matrix production by the adherent cells of long term murine bone marrow cultures. Blood 61:540

CHAPTER 13

Chemical Agents Which Suppress Myelopoiesis: Agranulocytosis and Leukemia

R.A. JOYCE

A. Introduction

The blood system represents a conduit by which cells travel from sites of production, maturation, and storage in the bone marrow to reach a milieu in which they are functionally active. Quantitative neutrophil deficiencies in the blood are referred to as neutropenia or granulocytopenia (blood neutrophils <1500/μl) (ZACHARSKI et al. 1971). Agranulocytosis is the virtual absence of mature neutrophils (band forms and mature polymorphonuclear leukocytes) on a blood smear. In this chapter, the term myelopoiesis refers to the proliferation and differentiation of marrow cells into mature neutrophils.

It is worth noting that agranulocytosis is a relatively modern disorder (SCHULTZ 1922), first mentioned in association with a clinical syndrome of fever, sore throat, sepsis, and death. During the subsequent 10 years, similar cases of agranulocytosis were reported, many in association with the use of aminopyrine, an analgesic and antipyretic agent of the time (MADISON et al. 1934; RAWLS 1936). Despite this recognized association, the syndrome reappeared when dipyrine, a derivative of aminopyrine, came into clinical use 3 decades later (HUGULEY 1964).

The marrow-suppressive effects of some chemical agents are recognized, dose-related, and reproducible in animal studies and human clinical trials. Other drug-induced neutropenias are idiosyncratic and unpredictable. Neutropenia, in the absence of infection, may be asymptomatic for extended periods, and so, it may be difficult to identify the etiologic agent and the mechanism responsible for the neutropenia.

The syndrome of agranulocytosis may have one pathophysiologic mechanism or many overlapping causes. Chemical agents are capable of suppressing marrow productioin, resulting in neutropenia. Still other agents may directly alter mature cell distribution in the blood or mature cell lifespan, resulting in similarly deficient blood neutrophil concentrations. Thus, neutropenia can result from any one of three mechanisms or by combinations of them: (a) decreased production with reduced outflow of cells from the marrow; (b) increased destruction of neutrophils beyond the replacement capabilities of the marrow production pool; (c) shift of blood neutrophils out of the circulating pool of blood cells.

B. Normal Marrow Cell Kinetics

Some understanding of marrow cell kinetics is essential for the interpretation of how chemical agents suppress myelopoiesis and when or whether normal myelopoiesis is expected to return following withdrawal of the responsible agent. Blood cells are constantly being lost and must be replaced. These mature cells depend on a replacement system of myelopoietic tissue which must have two distinguishing capabilities, self-replication and differentiation into more mature cells. The cellular organization of the hematopoietic system has four general classes of cells: (a) stem cells, (b) multilineage and lineage-specific progenitor cells, (c) marrow cells of the production and maturation pools, and (d) functional end-products, which include mature circulating blood cells (Fig. 1).

The stem cell has no special morphologic feature to identify it. It has been defined by its ability for self-renewal and differentiation (Abramson et al. 1977). Normally, it does neither, as cells in this pool are cycle inactive, leaving mature cell supplies to more differentiated marrow elements. However, primitive stem cells have the capacity to regenerate the entire hematopoietic system (Boggs et al. 1982). Following marrow ablation, self-renewal precedes differentiation, a step which ultimately preserves the system but leaves a critical time during which the host must survive without a supply of functioning mature cells (Chervenick et al. 1969). Using the hematopoietic system of the mouse, Till and McCulloch (1961) first described microscopic nodules present on the spleen surface 10 days following lethal irradiation and injection with syngeneic bone marrow (Till and McCoulloch 1961). Examination of these nodules revealed them to be composed of erythrocytic, neutrophilic, or megakaryocytic tissue or combinations of all three. Later studies from their laboratory clearly demonstrated that the nodules began from a single cell (or CFU-S) and that these colonies were manifestations of clonal evolution (Becker et al. 1963). More recently, this population of cells has been further dissected and charac-

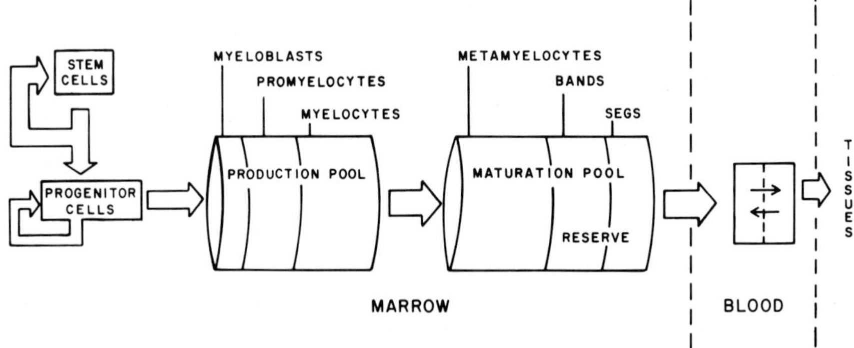

Fig. 1. Model of neutrophil production, maturation, and distribution. (Adapted from Boggs and Winkelstein 1990) SEGS, Segmented neutrophils

terized. Not every spleen colony is representative of stem cell clonal evolution. Initially, they were separated into early (more mature) and later appearing (day 12–14) CFU-S (MAGLI et al. 1982; HARRIS et al. 1984; BERTONCELLO et al. 1985). Based on their ability to survive 5-fluorouracil treatment, it is now estimated that only 10% or less of the CFU-S day 12 represent pluripotent stem cells (VAN ZANT 1984).

Evidence for the existence of a stem cell pool in man comes from chromosome studies in patients with chronic myelocytic leukemia. Here, the typical form of this disease is manifested by chromosome defects with a translocation of a portion of chromosome 22, most often to chromosome 9 (ROWLEY et al. 1973). WHANG and associates (1963) found this chromosome defect not only in neutrophils but also in erythrocyte and megakaryocyte precursors. The presence of this defect in these three distinctive cell lines of bone marrow origin suggested that the defect in chronic myelocytic leukemia arises from a cell which is a common stem cell for these three precursors. Similar common stem cell defects have been described in patients with paroxysmal nocturnal hemoglobinuria where common cytochemical defects have been identified in neutrophils, platelets, and erythrocytes (BURROUGHS et al. 1988). Demonstrations of single glucose-6-phosphate dehydrogease gene expression in granulocytes, red cells, and megakaryocytes of heterozygotes with chronic myelocytic leukemia (FIALKOW et al. 1969), idiopathic myelofibrosis (JACOBSON et al. 1976), and polycythemia vera (ADAMSON et al. 1976) have provided additional evidence for the existence of pluripotential stem cells.

Stem cells are either in a state of G_0 generative cycle or in a prolonged generative cycle. In support of this, BECKER and coworkers (1965) exposed murine cells to suicidal doses of tritiated thymidine prior to cell transplantation and produced little difference in the number of colony forming units (CFUs) in recipients. Efforts continue to further isolate and characterize these cells based on their biochemical or physical properties, response or lack of it to hematopoietic growth factors in vitro, and their surface antigenicity. The discovery of the CD34 antigen on 2%–3% of human bone marrow cells, including the stem cells, has aided greatly in efforts to isolate these cells using fluorescence-activated cell sorting (BERENSON et al. 1988). Using a CD34-specific antibody and a panel of antibodies directed at more mature cells, SUTHERLAND and coworkers (1989) have been able to assay cells that initiate sustained hematopoiesis in vitro in stromal layers of long-term marrow cell cultures.

Chemical agents can alter this primitive stem cell pool to cause suppression of hematopoiesis and pancytopenia. It has long been recognized that there is an association between drug-induced marrow suppression and the eventual evolution of leukemia. This association has been noted with occupational benzene exposure and following therapeutic administration of cytotoxic chemotherapy, most notably the alkylating agents (see below). The precise mechanism responsible for the evolution of a leukemic clonal proliferation of cells, often with expression of chromosomal abnormalities, is as yet not well defined.

Progenitor cells also have no identifying morphologic features but do have membrane receptors for cytokines which permit the formation of clones or colonies of cells in semisolid media in the presence of appropriate colony stimulating factors (CSFs). These cells are named based on the cell type of their progeny, such as CFU-neutrophil, -monocytes/macrophage, -eosinophil, -megakaryocyte, and -erythrocyte. Their ability to expand and mature serves to protect the more primitive stem cell compartment. The technique of in vitro growth of colonies of granulocytes in semisolid media was first described using cells collected from mouse marrow and spleen (PLUZNIK et al. 1965; BRADLEY et al. 1966). These assay systems have been useful in more clearly identifying the pathophysiologic mechanisms for human neutropenia and marrow suppression following exposure to various chemical agents (YOUNG et al. 1987).

Morphologically identifiable cells of the neutrophil series are found in the peripheral blood and bone marrow. In a normal steady state, the blood neutrophil compartment is maintained by inflow from the bone marrow balancing the outflow to tissues. The average neutrophil spends only several hours in the blood (ATHENS et al. 1961a; DRESCH et al. 1975). Loss from the blood is a random function. That is, the neutrophil that has just entered the blood from the marrow is as likely to leave in its first circulatory circuit as is one which has been around for many hours. The rapid rate of turnover indicates that, on the average, the mass of blood neutrophils is replaced 2.5 times each day (BOGGS 1967). It is this rapid turnover that marks a drop in blood neutrophil concentration as a primary indicator of disrupted marrow cell production and maturation.

The determination of the concentration of neutrophils in venous blood samples can be misleading. Under normal circumstances, approximately one-half of blood neutrophils are marginated on the walls of capillaries or postcapillary venules and are not represented by the circulating neutrophil concentration measurements of collected blood samples (ATHENS et al. 1961b). Thus, one may underestimate the number of blood neutrophils by such a concentration determination (Fig. 1). This underestimation is greater when neutropenia is present. Maximal blood neutrophil increment following epinephrine infusion, used as a measure of the marginal neutrophil pool, is raised in neutropenic subjects. Although absolute neutrophil increments are greater in subjects who are less severely neutropenic, there is a significant enhancement of the percentage of neutrophil increment in neutropenic patients as compared with normal subjects. Furthermore, there is an inverse correlation between the blood neutrophil concentration and the percentage increment following epinephrine, indicating an inverse relationship between the sizes of the circulating and marginal neutrophil pools as the neutropenia becomes more profound (JOYCE et al. 1976). This distribution favoring neutrophil margination may play a protective role in chronically neutropenic patients and may serve to explain the lack of symptoms of infection in some patients with long-standing neutropenia. One of the more useful determinations in explaining the change in neutrophil concentration in the blood is a ratio of band forms to segmented neutrophils. With a sudden inflow of neutrophils from the bone marrow, the band to segmented cell ratio will increase. Thus, if neutropenia is accompanied by little or no increase in the band to segmented neutrophil ratio, it is not considered as functionally severe as neutropenia in which all neutrophils in the blood are bands (JOYCE et al. 1978). Such circumstances exist following administration of agents which increase neutrophil adherence (see pseudoneutropenia below).

Morphologic examination of the bone marrow reveals a continuum of neutrophil maturation in which, for functionally descriptive purposes, three subcompartments may be distinguished (Fig. 1). The production pool consists of cells capable of undergoing mitosis: myeloblasts, promyelocytes, and myelocytes. The postmitotic maturation pool consists of metamyelocytes, band and segmented neutrophils. Further subdivision of the maturation pool separates the effective storage pool or marrow granulocyte reserve of band and segmented neutrophils from the metamyelocytes, which are not readily released into the blood (CRADDOCK et al. 1960; JOYCE et al. 1979).

In the normal subject, there are at least 15 times as many band and segmented neutrophils in the marrow granulocyte reserve of the bone marrow as there are in the blood. This reserve can be released to the blood upon demand. Such demand is probably controlled by circulating humoral factors, some of which are described elsewhere in this volume. Therefore, this storage pool constitutes an effective means of rapidly delivering a large number of neutrophils to a site of infection and can supply the blood with extra cells until production has time to catch up with the increased need. With a normal marrow structure, and even with extreme neutropenia, it is unusual for cells less mature than a band to be released to the blood. Thus, with neutropenia due to increased peripheral cell loss, we see a preserved production pool as well as metamyelocytes but very few band and segmented neutrophil forms in the marrow. This is the circumstance often termed "maturation arrest," used to describe the bone marrow following exposure to agents causing rapid peripheral neutrophil destruction. An explanation for this morphologic picture that seems more reasonable than arrest is the following. With the increased demand for cells in the blood, as is assumed to occur with most instances of neutropenia, the marrow neutrophil is released to the blood as soon as it matures to the band stage, and the marrow storage pool becomes depleted (JOYCE et al. 1976).

In the average normal subject, a period of approximately 11 days is required for a myelocyte to divide, mature into a segmented neutrophil, and enter and then leave the blood. It must be realized, however, that much of this time is spent within the storage pool (BISHOP et al. 1970). If there is increased demand for cells, or if the storage pool is attenuated, then the time required for a myelocyte to mature and enter the blood can be markedly reduced. The generation time for the normal myelocyte is about 2 days (BISHOP et al. 1970). Increased production is probably accomplished by a combination of decreased generation time, skipped division, and increased feed-in from the stem cell compartment.

The normal site of replenishment for blood neutrophils is the production pool of the marrow. After the last mitosis of the myelocyte stage, a further period of maturation occurs. Normally, the mature cells spend a significant length of time in the storage pool of the bone marrow. From this, they are released to the blood for a brief transit and then migrate out of the blood vessels into tissues and body cavities. Here, they presumably provide a cleansing function by phagocytic activity. The "functional home" of the neutrophil is clearly beyond the blood in tissues, body cavities, and beginning exudates. In the absence of a normal number of neutrophils available for migration into such sites, infections are more frequent and abnormally severe, since they cannot be contained and localized by the rapid entrance of neutrophils into exudates.

C. Pathophysiologic Mechanisms for Drug-Induced Neutropenia

Laboratory investigations of the pathophysiology of drug-induced neutropenia have produced confusing and, at times, conflicting results. An immune basis for aminopyrine-associated neutropenia is generally accepted and fits with the clinical observations. For example, rechallenge of a patient who has recovered from aminopyrine agranulocytosis with small doses of the drug is followed within 6–10 h by recurrent neutropenia (DAMESHEK et al. 1936). Further studies have described a serum factor from an aminopyrine-sensitive patient capable of producing neutropenia in normal subjects and inducing in vitro lysis of granulocytes in the presence of the drug (MOESCHLIN et al. 1952). However, reproduction of in vitro granulocyte lysis has been inconsistent (PAYNE 1961). Other studies of drug-induced neutropenia have demonstrated leukoagglutins, but the significance of in vitro leukoagglutination has been questioned (HARTL 1965). Drug-dependent leukocyte antibodies must be distinguished from leukocyte isoantibodies, such as occur following pregnancy, transfusion of blood products, and various other circumstances (PAYNE 1961). Furthermore, the abnormal sequestration of immunologically injured cells may escape detection by available in vitro tests.

It has been suggested that certain drugs, most notably the penicillins and other β-lactam antibiotics, alter leukocyte membranes or complex with them as a haptene, causing a cell-specific antibody response and immune destruction of "sensitized" cells (LEVIN et al. 1971; HOMAYOUNI et al. 1989). HARTL (1965) suggested that drug-protein conjugates, drug-specific antibodies, and complement all interact to alter neutrophil adherence, aggregation, and metabolism, with consequent cell destruction.

The ability to establish short-term clonogenic assays of granulocyte and monocyte/macrophage progenitor cells (CFU-GM) in vitro from marrow cell samples of neutropenic patients has added to the pathophysiologic investigation of drug-induced neutropenia. The findings of reduced progenitor cells associated with peripheral neutropenia and marrow myeloid hypoplasia have implicated drug-induced marrow toxicity as a cause of neutropenia in some instances. Such findings offer an explanation for a delay in blood neutrophil recovery following withdrawal of certain chemical agents. Reduction of CFU-GM colony formation in vitro with addition of the chemical agent or its metabolites, with or without autologous serum, has supported the implication of direct marrow toxicity of the agent in question in some cases and of immune-mediated toxicity in others (KELTON et al. 1979). However, the large scale use of these assays has produced conflicting data. This has led to the hypothesis that some chemical agents associated with neutropenia may cause this effect by immune-mediated peripheral cell destruction with or without a similar immune-mediated marrow suppression in some cases and by direct marrow suppression in others. Marrow precursor cells bear certain unique surface markers that are no longer expressed as the cell matures. Examples include the HLA antigens, which are present on early neutrophil precursor cells but not in mature neutrophils (CLINE et al. 1977). Other membrane antigens are more fully expressed in mature cells. It is possible, and has been reported, that certain immune-mediated neutropenias represent antibody formation directed against early neutrophil precursor cells, appearing as marrow production defects, antibodies directed at mature cells only, or combinations of the two (KELTON et al. 1979).

The neutropenias observed in association with certain chemical agents appear to be more clearly associated with marrow myeloid toxicity. Such is the case in instances of neutropenia associated with exposure to phenothiazines or hydantoins. Neutropenia in these instances is preceded by a variable period of latency and is often dose-dependent. The agranulocytosis is usually associated with reduced marrow cellularity (PISCIOTTA et al. 1958, 1964). In studies reported by PISCIOTTA and associates (1962), chlorpromazine inhibited tritiated thymidine incorporation into DNA. Later observations by this group, that a similar inhibition of DNA synthesis can be detected in subjects not sensitized to chlorpromazine, led to the conclusion that certain drug-induced neutropenias, in particular, chlorpromazine-induced neutropenia, is observed only in patients with a coincident defective marrow cell proliferative potential. These patients are capable of compensating for such defects in the absence of exposure to the drug (PISCIOTTA 1965; PISCIOTTA et al. 1965).

As a generalization, studies of immune-mediated mechanisms of neutropenia associated with exposure to chemical agents and evaluation of marrow cellularity and in vitro progenitor cell assays support the clinical impression that there are two types of drug-induced neutropenia: Those following short drug exposure with a rapid onset of neutropenia suggesting rapid mature cell destruction and those associated with suppression of marrow myeloid production and more prolonged drug exposure, often in high doses.

Any classification of drug-induced neutropenia seems to lead to extensive lists of exceptions and reports of different etiologies in individual cases. What follows is a hematopoietic-based categorization compiled with the following assumptions. Not all idiosyncratic neutropenias have identifiable immune mechanisms, nor are they necessarily limited to increased peripheral destruction of neutrophils without concomitant suppression of marrow production. Furthermore, chemical agents which are recognized to alter marrow suppression may, instead, cause enhanced mature cell destruction under other circumstances.

D. Neutropenia Associated with Cytotoxic Chemotherapeutic Agents

A few cancer chemotherapeutic agents have selective effects on neoplastic cell proliferation. These include asparaginase and bleomycin, both of which have minimal effects upon normal hematopoietic cells (BOGGS et al. 1974). The majority of chemotherapeutic agents have a straight dose-related hematopoietic toxicity with marrow suppression and subsequent peripheral pancytopenia including neutropenia. A schematic outline of their mechanisms and sites of action is shown in Fig. 2.

To understand the effects of chemotherapeutic agents on hematopoietic cells, it is useful to know whether they are cycle active or not. The cycle active drug affects only cells that are in active generative cycle. Most of these are inhibitors of DNA synthesis, such as hydroxyurea (CARTER 1972), or act as mitotic inhibitors, such as the vinca alkaloids (JOHNSON et al. 1963). Noncycle active agents such as the alkylating drugs will damage cells in active mitotic cycle but will also influence potentially dividing cells (WHEELER 1962). Still other agents, such as 6-mercaptopurine and cyclophosphamide (HILL et al. 1975), have effects which are intermediate between the two but are probably more active upon cells in generative cycle (BRUCE et al. 1966). In general, however, most chemotherapeutic agents are active more or less at specific stages of the cell cycle (GILL et al. 1975).

As noted previously, the normal stem cell compartment is not in generative cycle. Thus, exposure to a cycle active drug such as vinblastine results in quite different alterations to blood neutrophil concentrations compared with changes following agents such as cyclophosphamide. The neutrophil levels following single doses of vinblastine sulfate or cyclophosphamide administered to normal mice are shown in Fig. 3. Both of these agents lead to the absence of blood neutrophils. However, the duration of neutropenia following cyclophosphamide is more prolonged and recovery of blood neutrophils is delayed when compared with the neutrophil changes following administration of vinblastine. As a cycle active agent, a single dose

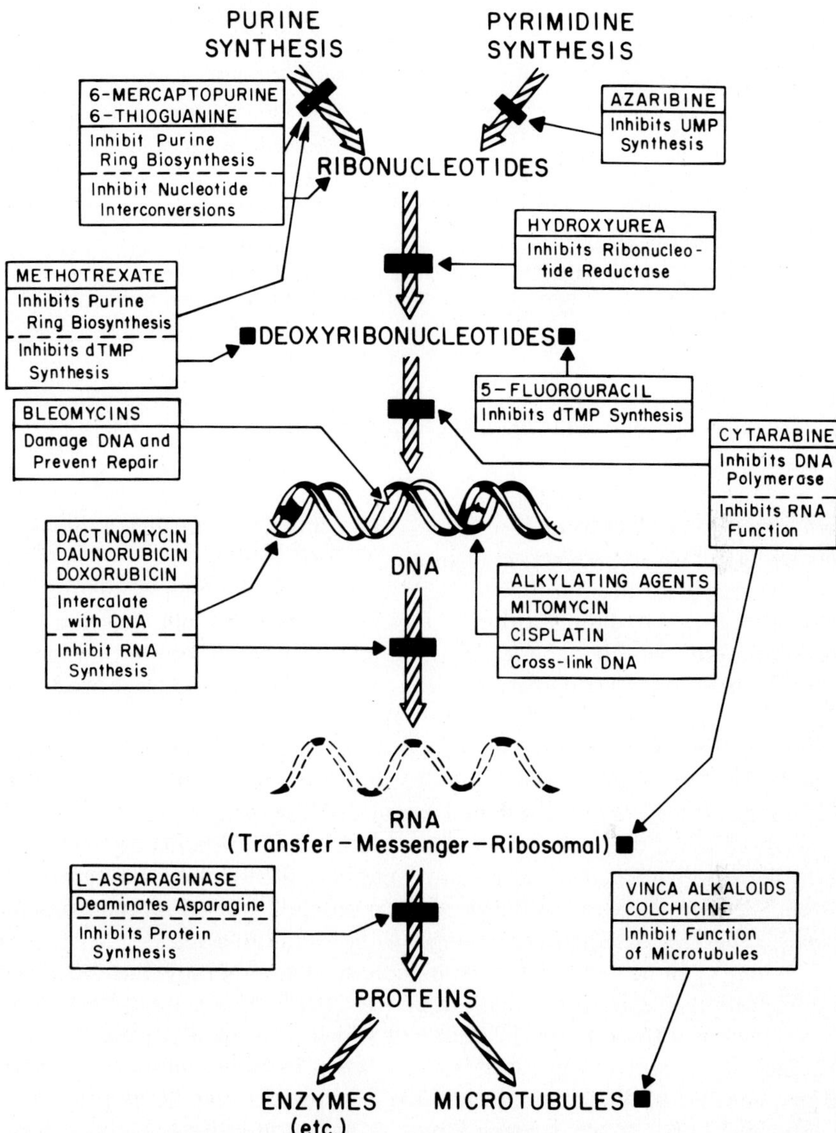

Fig. 2. Summary of the mechanisms and sites of action of chemotherapeutic agents useful in the treatment of neoplastic disorders. (Adapted from GILMAN et al. 1980)

of vinblastine would be expected to spare the stem cell compartment, leading to more rapid regeneration of mature neutrophils. This was the case when marrow progenitor cells from these animals were quantitated. Conversely, cyclophosphamide-induced neutropenia is associated with a more prolonged period of neutropenia during which time the cells of the stem cell

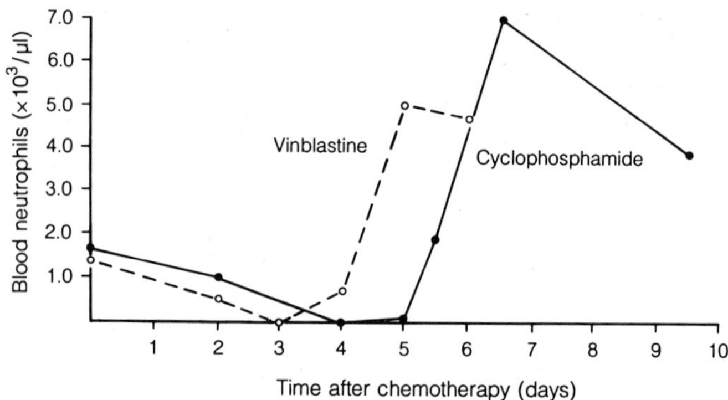

Fig. 3. Blood neutrophil concentrations from mice following single administration of cyclophosphamide, 200 mg/kg, or vinblastine, 4.0 mg/kg (Joyce et al. 1980)

pool undergo self-replication prior to differentiation, causing a delay in marrow granulocyte production (Joyce et al. 1977, 1980).

Differences in the duration of neutropenia and the rate of mature cell recovery following administration of these two drugs in single doses to mice are supported by the experience of administration of chemotherapeutic agents in man. Vinblastine can be given every 7–10 days without producing progressive toxicity in most patients, suggesting that any damage in marrow cell production can be repaired during this time period. Conversely, a longer period of time is required following exposure to cyclophosphamide or other alkylating agents administered in comparable doses. An alkylating agent administered at a dose that will induce a level of neutropenia equivalent to that following vinblastine and given repetitively will deplete the neutrophil system. Under these circumstances, a prolonged period of neutropenia ensues, reflective of repetitive damage to the stem cell pool.

A major clinical basis for combination chemotherapy has been the demonstration that agents which are active when employed alone against a given category of neoplastic disease and which have qualitatively different toxicities will result in increased activity when used in combination. Such agents, because of differing dose-limiting host toxicity, can be used together at the same doses as when given alone. A variation in this approach could involve two agents in combination, both of which affect the same normal organ but at different times. As an example, cytosine arabinoside produces myelosuppression with maximum depression occurring at approximately 1–2 weeks, whereas the nitrosoureas take 4–6 weeks to produce myelosuppression. Thus, these agents could be given in combination at nearly full doses, which would result in a more prolonged myelosuppression but without and increase in its degree at any one time.

The use of cytotoxic agents, even at low doses, may deplete the stem cell pool over time (Finch 1967). Clinically, this is manifested by a period of latency during which the agent is continued in the absence of severe neutropenia while the stem cell pool is reduced. Under such circumstances, severe and prolonged neutropenia follows, and recovery is delayed until the stem cell compartment is regenerated. This point serves to emphasize that the blood neutrophil concentration is an insensitive, albeit convenient barometer of chemotherapeutic marrow toxicity.

Allopurinol is a xanthine oxidase inhibitor used to reduce serum and urinary uric acid concentrations. It is rarely associated with idiosyncratic neutropenia. However, because it inhibits the enzymatic oxidation of mercaptopurine to 6-thiouric acid, its concomitant use with mercaptopurine or azathioprine, which is cleaved in vivo to mercaptopurine, requires a reduction in the dosage of these cytotoxic agents to prevent untoward marrow suppression.

As noted in another chapter in this volume, the administration of colony stimulating factors (CSFs) in association with cytotoxic chemotherapeutic agents has been demonstrated to shorten the period of time required for progenitor cell recovery and return of mature functioning cells to the circulation. It remains to be seen whether the repetitive use of these agents in association with cytotoxic chemotherapy will outstrip the capacity of the stem cell pool to regenerate itself and result in a compromised marrow stem cell pool.

E. Drug-Induced Myeloid Suppression

Many drugs with distinct therapeutic benefits not due to their cytotoxic activity have a recognized association with hypoproliferative neutropenia and, in severe cases, marrow aplasia. Often, the reported instances of neutropenia are more frequent than those associated with idiosyncratic or immune-mediated neutropenia. In general, they comprise the majority of the cases of neutropenia recorded in tabulations of drug-associated blood dysplasias (Table 1). Such listings have been published by the American Medical Society Council on Drugs (Wintrobe 1968). As described below, most are due to drug-induced suppression of neutrophil production in the marrow. Similar findings have been reported from Stockholm, gathered from computerized data of hospital records (Arneborn et al. 1982). These tabulations are useful in identifying potential marrow toxic side effects of chemical agents but are incomplete and based on voluntary reporting with the former and exclude widespread out-of-hospital drug administration with the latter.

As discussed earlier, the durations of neutropenia due to agents which affect marrow neutrophil production tend to be more prolonged after removal of the causative agent when compared with those in which peripheral destruction of mature cells is the principle reason for neutropenia. In this regard, the clinical course and risk of infection from drug-associated

Table 1. Number of cases of drug-associated leukopenia

Drug	Etiologic mechanisms	
	Impaired production	Idiosyncratic
Analgesics		
Aminopyrine		15
Dipyrone		22
Phenylbutazone	44	
Acetylsalicylic acid	87	
Antibiotics		
Sulfonamides		26
Chloramphenicol	18	
Penicillin		7
Sulfonamides		
Nonbacteriocidal		21
Anticonvulsants		15
Phenothiazines	143	
Antithyroid		23
Totals	292	129

Classification of mechanisms of leukopenia based on most commonly reported defect. Data reported by: The Panel on Hematology (1965/1967) Registry on adverse reactions. Council on Drugs, AMA, Chicago. See WINTROBE (1968).

myeloid suppression are similar to instances of marrow toxicity following cytotoxic chemotherapy. Although immune-mediated peripheral destruction of neutrophils can also be seen with some of the following agents, marrow proliferative defects are more commonly noted. Their use warrants routine measurement of blood cell concentrations, especially with circumstances under which drug excretion and metabolism are altered by coincident renal and/or hepatic dysfunction.

I. Ethanol

Multiple factors contribute to the increased susceptibility to bacterial infections in the alcoholic patient. These patients often have associated anemia and thrombocytopenia, splenomegaly with blood cell sequestration, and nutritional folate deficiency. Ethanol, however, contributes to suppression of marrow cell proliferation as well. When ethanol is added in physiologic concentrations (100–600 mg/100 ml) to marrow cell cultures, there is a dose-related suppression of marrow granulocyte colony formation (TISMAN et al. 1973). The clinical findings of reduced marrow granulocyte production in acutely intoxicated patients in the absence of splenomegaly, infection, and megaloblastic anemia support the impression that ethanol suppresses granulocyte production in some patients (LIU 1980). Later studies confirmed the suppressive effects of ethanol on marrow cell production and demonstrated that acetaldehyde also inhibited myeloid and erythroid growth in vitro (MEAGHER et al. 1982).

II. Phenothiazines

This group of agents includes chlorpromazine, thioridazine, and prochlorperazine. These are sulfur-containing tricyclic compounds effective as sedatives and antiemetics. Agranulocytosis may occur after a 3–6 week latent period of drug administration (KORST 1959) and often can be avoided when the drug is readministered in smaller amounts to patients who had been previously neutropenic (PISCIOTTA et al. 1958). In an 8-year study of 6000 patients at the Milwaukee County Mental Health Clinic treated with chlorpromazine, leukopenia was noted with an incidence of 10%. However, agranulocytosis developed in only 5 patients (PISCIOTTA 1973). A more generalized marrow aplasia affecting the erythroid marrow and platelet production may be present in affected patients and is reversible with discontinuation of the drug. Such patients have been reported to have a proliferative defect as measured by diminished mitotic and tritiated thymidine labeling indices (PISCIOTTA et al. 1962). A preexisting, compensated, marrow proliferative defect exposed by treatment with tricyclic agents is believed to be the explanation for the agranulocytosis in sensitive patients (PISCIOTTA 1965; PISCIOTTA et al. 1965). The observation of the more frequent incidence of phenothiazine-induced neutropenia in female subjects over the age of 50 years remains unclear (PISCIOTTA 1958).

III. Anticonvulsants

The use of these agents has been associated with a relatively high incidence of neutropenia and, in more severe cases, even marrow aplasia. No common mechanism has been identified. Most of the cases are noted after prolonged use of the agent and may be seen in association with fever, skin rash, and detection of leukoagglutinins (ABBOTT et al. 1950). The marrow may show suppressed myeloid precursors in some (ABBOTT et al. 1950; PISCIOTTA 1971) or noncomplement-dependent antibody suppression of myeloid production in vitro in others (TAETLE et al. 1979). An incidence as high as 6% has been reported with the use of methyloxazolidine (DAVIS et al. 1947). The most common serious reaction associated with the use of trimethadione involves depression of marrow cell production (ABBOTT et al. 1950). This drug is recommended for use only in controlling petit mal seizure disorders refractory to treatment with other antiepileptic drugs. Less commonly, diphenylhydantoin administration results in leukopenia in 2% of cases (SPARBERG 1963) and may produce effects similar to those observed with phenothiazines since decreased [^{3}H]uridine uptake by marrow cells has been reported in affected patients (PISCIOTTA 1971). Such cases must be distinguished from the neutropenias associated with megaloblastic marrow changes and low folate concentrations.

IV. Antiinflammatory Agents

The mechanisms responsible for hematopoietic toxicity observed with the use of these agents vary, as does the severity of the defect, ranging from isolated neutropenia in some to severe aplastic anemia in others. Phenylbutazone is chemically similar to aminopyrine, though cross-reactivity of phenylbutazone has not been demonstrated in vivo in aminopyrine-sensitive patients (Von Rechenberg 1953). Blood cell changes may be seen early or after prolonged exposure to the drug (Mauer 1955). Evidence for phenylbutazone suppression of marrow granulocyte precursor cells has been demonstrated in sensitive patients recovering from hematopoietic toxicity (Smith et al. 1977). The incidence of neutropenia associated with phenylbutazone has been as high as 0.6% (Leonard 1953). Oxyphenbutazone is reported to be less toxic than phenylbutazone, though it can be more toxic when added to marrow cell cultures (Smith et al. 1977). Acetylsalicylic acid has rarely been implicated as a cause of leukopenia, although in vitro studies of both murine and human marrow cultures have demonstrated a dose-dependent inhibition of granulocyte/macrophage colony formation with the addition of acetylsalicylic acid (Gabourel et al. 1977). Use of gold salts has been effective in reducing the severity of chronic debilitating inflammatory diseases such as rheumatoid arthritis. However, these agents are suspected to be a cause of the neutropenia in some patients with Felty's syndrome (rheumatoid arthritis, splenomegaly, and neutropenia) (Joyce et al. 1980). In vitro suppression of granulocyte progenitor cells has been reported with the addition of gold salts to marrow cell cultures (Howell et al. 1975).

V. Antiviral Agents

The interferons are a diverse group of glycoproteins secreted from various cells in response to viral infections and other stimuli. Although they were initially recognized for their antiviral activity, they have been useful clinically as cytotoxic agents and modulators of the immune system (Merigan 1983). Alpha interferon (IFN-α) is a product of leukocytes. Its use has been associated with selective neutropenia as well as overall marrow suppression. When added to marrow cell cultures, it has a concentration- and time-related suppressive effect on granulocyte progenitor cells. Similar toxicity is noted for normal as well as leukemic cells (Greenberg et al. 1977). It appears to decrease DNA synthesis of granulocyte progenitor cells but is not cell cycle stage-specific in its effects. There are over 13 different IFN-α species, 2 distinct forms of fibroblast-derived IFN-β, and IFN-γ, a product of stimulated T lymphocytes (FRIEDMAN et al. 1983). Similar effects on circulating blood cells have been observed with both IFN-β and IFN-γ and appear to be the result of impaired marrow cell production (KURZROCK et al. 1986).

Ganciclovir is an acyclic analogue of thymidine which is active against all human herpes viruses. It is a potent inhibitor of viral DNA polymerase in its triphosphate form. It has been demonstrated to halt the progression of cytomegalovirus retinitis and gastrointestinal disease in immunocompromised hosts, such as patients with AIDS (JACKSON 1988). Its most common adverse reaction is neutropenia, which appears to be dose-related (LASKIN et al. 1987). Lower doses of the drug can be reinstituted in patients previously neutropenic while being treated with ganciclovir, suggesting that the neutropenia is due to inhibition of marrow production (JACKSON 1988).

Azidothymidine is a thymidine analogue used in the treatment of patients with AIDS. Dose-limiting toxicities of the agent include progressive neutropenia and anemia (RICHMAN et al. 1987). Neither human nor murine toxicity studies have demonstrated thrombocytopenia associated with use of this agent. We have studied the hematopoietic effects of azidothymidine in mice (JOYCE et al. 1988). There was a dose-dependent reduction in blood neutrophil concentrations and hematocrits during chronic (18 day) administration. No significant change in marrow cellularity or platelet levels was detected. The numbers of granulocyte and erythrocyte progenitor cells in the marrow were reduced without significant alterations of the less mature, multipotential progenitor cells. T-lymphocyte release of CSF in vitro was lowered in these mice. Both neutropenia and anemia were corrected while azidothymidine administration was continued by simultaneous administration of GM-CSF. It appears that the hematopoietic toxicity of azidothymidine results from impaired release of growth factors necessary for granulocyte as well as erythrocyte progenitor cell growth and maturation.

VI. H_2 Receptor Antagonists

Cimetidine is an H_2 receptor antagonist which has rarely been associated with agranulocytosis and, in some cases, suppression of marrow cell production (FRESTON 1979). A dose-related toxicity of cimetidine has been reported (GROSS et al. 1984). Although the precise mechanism has not been defined, it may involve inhibition of the histamine-induced initiation of marrow progenitor cell DNA synthesis (GROSS et al. 1984). Recent evidence has been provided in mice that IL-3-induced cycling of more mature stem cells (CFU-S day 8) is abrogated by specific H_2 receptor blockade and that disruption of histamine synthesis abolishes entry of stem cells into S phase in response to IL-3 (SCHNEIDER et al. 1990). Neutropenia has also been noted with the other H_2-receptor antagonists, metiamide (FELDMAN et al. 1976) and ranitidine (LIST et al. 1988).

VII. Miscellaneous Agents

Suppression of marrow granulocyte production with associated neutropenia has been reported with a variety of other drugs, including phenindione (Wintrobe 1968; Wright 1970), procainamide (Bluming et al. 1976; Ellrodt et al. 1984), and arsenicals (Loveman 1932; Kasich 1944). Of particular note is the neutropenia associated with the antibiotic combination of trimethoprim and sulphamethoxazole, both inhibitors of folic acid metabolism. Their effects can be corrected by simultaneous administration of folinic acid (Golde et al. 1978).

F. Idiosyncratic Neutropenias

These neutropenias which develop in response to drug administration are usually sudden and may be accompanied be fever, skin rash, eosinophilia, and monocytosis. Nuclear-specific antibodies and other serum factors may be detected, but their significance pertaining to the neutropenia is not clear. These clinical and laboratory changes fit with the reports of transient serum leukoagglutinins and leukocytotoxic antibodies in many cases. The bone marrow of patients with idiosyncratic neutropenia is usually cellular or hypercellular, with an abundance of cells in the neutrophil production and maturation pools up to and including the metamyelocyte stage of development. Blood neutrophil recovery is usually prompt, and neutrophil concentrations usually return to normal or above normal levels within several days of withdrawal of the causative agent. A longer duration of neutropenia may be encountered with agents or their metabolites which concentrate in extravascular tissue, such as procainamide or its slow-reacting analogue (Ellrodt et al. 1984). Readministration of agents associated with idiosyncratic neutropenia, even at very low doses, will usually result in prompt return of the neutropenia and is not recommended. Furthermore, there is considerable overlap in the immune reaction with drugs of similar composition, as is the case with the various β-lactam antibiotics (Rouveix et al. 1983).

The incidence of neutropenia with drugs in this category is low. Conversely, the list of agents reported to cause idiosyncratic neutropenia is extensive. An encyclopedic tabulation of each drug reported to be associated with idiosyncratic neutropenia is beyond the scope of this text. Rather, an attempt has been made to identify categories of drugs which either are well described as causing rapid peripheral destruction of neutrophils or are more commonly associated with the clinical findings of idiosyncratic neutropenia. The major categories are analgesics, antibiotics, cardiovascular agents, thyrostatics, and sulfonamides.

I. Analgesics

Aminopyrine is the benchmark agent which led to the clinical recognition of agranulocytosis. Like aminopyrine, dipyrine is a phenylprazoline derivative.

The association of agranulocytosis with these two agents has resulted in their withdrawal from clinical use. Antipyrine, another phenylprazoline derivative, remains available as a topical otic preparation. Although phenylbutazone is structurally similar to aminopyrine, its hematopoietic toxicity is more often directed to the early stages of marrow neutrophil production. Idiosyncratic immune-mediated neutropenia from phenylbutazone is rare (WEISSMAN et al. 1959). Various other nonsteroidal antiinflammatory agents and analgesics have been associated with idiosyncratic neutropenia, including ibuprofen (GRYFE et al. 1976), but the incidence is generally reported to be less than 1%. Indomethacin and other inhibitors of prostaglandin synthesis may actually enhance neutrophil production by opposing the negative effect of prostaglandin E in neutrophil progenitor cell growth and differentiation (KURLAND et al. 1978; BOORMAN et al. 1982).

II. Antibiotics

It is fortunate that the incidence of idiosyncratic neutropenia with the use of these agents is low, given the significance of such a development in subjects with active infection. Penicillin has rarely been implicated as a causative agent of agranulocytosis (NOORABECHI et al. 1973). Neutropenia has been reported with various semisynthetic penicillins, including ampicillin (GRAF et al. 1968), methicillin (LEVIN et al. 1970), piperacillin and mezlocillin (KIRKWOOD et al. 1985), ticarcillin (GASTINEAU et al. 1981), amoxicillin (DESGRANDCHAMPS et al. 1987), nafcillin (ZAKHIRCH et al. 1978), oxacillin (CHU et al. 1977), and carbenicillin. With the exception of carbenicillin, the neutropenias associated with these antibiotics have been of the idiosyncratic type (KAMMER 1984). Carbenicillin, in high doses, has been reported to be toxic to marrow granulocyte precursor cells (REYES et al. 1973). The cephalosporins represent a large category of β-lactam antibiotics whose classification is generally made according to their overall antimicrobial activity (MANDELL et al. 1985). The incidence of idiosyncratic neutropenia with such agents is similar to that of the other β-lactam antibiotics (ROUVEIX et al. 1983). The frequency of neutropenia increases when these drugs are used in large doses or for prolonged periods of time (NEFTEL et al. 1985). Under these circumstances, neutropenia has been reported in incidences of as high as 15%.

Other structurally dissimilar antibiotic drugs have been associated with idiosyncratic neutropenia and include the aminoglycosides (CHANG 1975), metronidazole (LEFEBVRE et al. 1965), nitrofurantoin (PALVA et al. 1973), rifampin (LIEDERMAN et al. 1970), and ristocetin (NEWTON et al. 1958). The latter two drugs are more commonly associated with thrombocytopenia. Chloramphenicol suppresses marrow production in a dose-related fashion. Idiosyncratic neutropenia has been noted (HUGULEY et al. 1966), although instances of aplastic anemia are more common. The antibacterial sulfonamides will be considered separately. Rare instances of idiosyncratic neutropenia due to isoniazid have been reported (HANSON 1961). Finally, the anthelmintic agent, levamisole, was initially developed for its activity against intestinal nematodes. It also has immunostimulatory effects and has been used in the treatment of patients with chronic inflammatory arthritis, including rheumatoid arthritis. It has recently been found to be efficacious when used in conjunction with 5-fluorouracil in patients with colorectal carcinoma. The incidence of idiosyncratic agranulocytosis in patients treated with levamisole is as high as 10% (TEERENHOVI et al. 1978). An interesting association of agranulocytosis with HLA-B27 in patients with rheumatoid arthritis has been noted (VEYES et al. 1978) but has not been observed in the agranulocytosis of levamisole for noninflammatory diseases (TEERENHOVI et al. 1978).

III. Cardiovascular Drugs and Diuretics

A number of antiarrhythmic drugs have been associated with idiosyncratic neutropenia, including propranolol (NAWABI et al. 1973) and quinidine. Reports of marrow aplasia in association with quinidine have shown transient immune-mediated inhibition of granulocyte and erythrocyte precursor cells in the presence of autologous serum and drug. There was no evidence of drug-mediated peripheral blood cell destruction (KELTON et al. 1979; ASCENSAO 1984). Although lidocaine has not been associated with idiosyncratic neutropenia, tocainide, a primary amino analogue of lidocaine has been reported in association with a lupus-like illness and neutropenia (OLIPHANT et al. 1988).

Various antihypertensive agents and diuretics have been connected with idiosyncratic neutropenia, including ethacryinic acid (WALKER 1966) and chlorthalidone (TURNER et al. 1964). Neutropenia has been more commonly associated with the use of methyldopa (CLOSS et al. 1984). This latter drug is also associated with a Coombs positive reaction and autoimmune hemolytic anemia (WORLLEDGE et al. 1966).

Agranulocytosis has also been reported with the use of carbonic anhydrase inhibitors, acetazolamide and methazolamide (FRAUNFELDER 1979), and with the acetylcholinesterase inhibitor, captopril (COOPER et al. 1983). Neutropenia in association with captopril treatment has been seen in approximately 0.3% of patients (VIDT 1982). These agents appear to influence marrow production (EDWARDS et al. 1981) in a way described, in severe cases, as aplastic anemia rather than idiosyncratic neutropenia (UNDERWOOD 1956; WERBLIN et al. 1979). Yet, the low incidence of neutropenia considering the wide use of these agents favors their designation as idiosyncratic.

Procainamide is an effective antiarrhythmic agent that induces formation of nuclear-specific antibodies in most patients who take the drug for an extended period of time (WOOSLEY et al. 1978). Severe neutropenia or agranulocytosis is a relatively infrequent complication. The use of sustained-release procainamide has been associated with a higher incidence of agranulocytosis (MEYERS et al. 1985). Procainamide-induced neutropenias have been associated with both marrow hyperplasia and, in other reports, hypoplastic marrow changes. Flecainide has been used to treat severe ventricular arrhythmias. It is a local anesthetic that decreases intracardiac conduction. This agent also binds to neutrophil surfaces and has been noted to cause a haptene-mediated neutropenia similar to that associated with the cephalosporins (SAMLOWSKI et al. 1987).

IV. Thyrostatic Agents

Neutropenia is a frequent side effect observed with the use of drugs in this category. Both immune destruction of mature neutrophils and suppression of marrow cell production have been reported. Although neutropenia may be detected in as many as 10% of patients treated with propylthiouracil or methimazole, the more severe toxicity of agranulocytosis is much less frequent, affecting 0.3%–0.6% of subjects (TROTTER 1962; ROSOVE 1977). Onset of neutropenia is usually delayed, from 2–10 weeks of drug exposure, and may be associated with a fever, skin rash, and arthralgias (COOPER et al. 1983). Patients retreated with thiouracil develop neutropenia more rapidly. Serum antibodies have been reported in patients neutropenic from either propylthiouracil or methimazole (AMRHEIN et al. 1970; SATO et al. 1985). Neutropenia is more common in patients over the age of 40 years. The risk of neutropenia with methimazole appears to be dose-related, occurring less frequently in patients treated with less than 30 mg per day (COOPER 1983).

V. Sulfonamides

This category of drugs includes a wide variety of agents such as antibacterial drugs, diuretics like chlorothiazide (SCHOTLAND et al. 1963), chlorthalidone, and acetazolamide, as well as the oral hypoglycemic agents, tolbutamide (BEST 1963) and chlorpropamide (STEIN et al. 1964). Considering the widespread use of these agents, neutropenia arises infrequently, with a reported incidence of 1% or less (HUGULEY 1966). An immune basis for neutropenia has been suggested in view of its association with skin rash, fever, and arthralgias.

G. Pseudoneutropenia

Several physical and biological agents are associated with brief periods of neutropenia following their exposure to blood cells. Initial reports of this reaction were based on observations of acute changes in blood neutrophil concentrations within the fist 30 min of administration of endotoxin, the lipopolysaccharide component of bacterial cell walls. These acute changes in blood neutrophil concentrations were shown to represent a shift from the circulating pool into the marginal pool (ATHENS et al. 1961). Other agents have been demonstrated to induce increased neutrophil margination by means of raised expression of various cell membrane components responsible for the adherence properties of the mature neutrophil.

I. Complement Activation

The acute neutropenia which occurs during the 1st h of hemodialysis (BRUBAKER et al. 1971) or during cardiopulmonary bypass (CHENOWETH et al. 1981) or blood pheresis (SCHIFFER et al. 1975) has been shown to be due to complement activation with resulting neutrophil aggregation and shift into the marginal pool (CRADDOCK et al. 1977a). Exposure of blood to cellophane membranes, used as filters in these procedures, results in activation of the plasma complement system and release of C5a, the complement component which has been shown to enhance neutrophil adherence (CRADDOCK et al. 1977b).

II. Expression of Membrane Adhesion Molecules

Transient neutropenia is observed during the first 1–2 h of infusion of human recombinant CSFs. These growth factors promote proliferation and differentiation of hematopoietic progenitor cells and enhance mature neutrophil chemotaxis and bacteriocidal activity associated with up-regulation of the expression of the neutrophil membrane surface antigen CD11b (SOCINSKI et al. 1988; KAPLAN et al. 1988). This is an adhesion molecule involved with neutrophil adherence. These data suggest that this transient neutropenia represents a shift of cells from the circulating neutrophil pool into the marginal pool. Similar transient episodes of neutropenia have been observed with infusion of tumor necrosis factor (TNF), which also has been shown to up-regulate CD11b (LOGAN et al. 1990). Returning to the initial shifts in blood neutrophils seen with endotoxins, it is of interest that endotoxin induces the release of a variety of different cytokines including TNF and IL-1 as well as the growth factors G-CSF and GM-CSF.

H. Secondary Leukemia

Secondary leukemia has been recognized as a distinct clinical entity since 1964. It was first described in reports of the hematopoietic toxicity in workers chemically exposed to benzine (ENRICO et al. 1964). It is an acute myelogenous leukemia (AML) usually preceded by several months of anemia, neutropenia, and/or thrombocytopenia. This preleukemic phase is associated with marrow changes of ineffective cell production and myelodysplastic changes. Chromosomal defects are common. A high incidence of AML has also been reported in adults with occupational exposure to petroleum products, solvents, and insecticides (MITELMAN et al. 1978).

Other agents used for the treatment of noncancerous conditions have been considered potentially leukemogenic. Their common feature is suppression of marrow production and, in some cases, aplastic anemia. They include chloramphenicol (COHEN et al. 1967), hexachlorcylohexane (JEDLICKA 1958), and phenylbutazone (JENSON et al. 1965), among others. Statistical analyses of the relative risks are difficult to interpret and are generally unsatisfactory or nonexistent.

More recently, drug-related acute leukemia in patients following treatment of primary malignancy has been the object of statistical analysis. The incidence of leukemia is increased in patients treated with cytotoxic chemotherapy for Hodgkin's disease (KALDOR et al. 1990a), multiple myeloma (BERGSAGEL et al. 1979), ovarian carcinoma (KALDOR et al. 1990b) breast cancer (FISHER et al. 1985), and lung cancer (PEDERSON-BJERGAARD et al. 1985).

Of the cytotoxic chemotherapeutic agents, the alkylating ones have been most frequently noted for their leukemogenic potential. Of these, chlorambucil and melphalan are believed to be the most leukemogenic in patients treated for ovarian carcinoma (KALDOR 1990b). Chlorambucil administration to patients with polycythemia vera is associated with a significantly higher incidence of evolution to AML as reported by the Polycythemia Vera Study Group (BERK et al. 1981). The leukemic potential of these agents also seems to be a factor of dose and duration of therapy. Other cytotoxic agents which alter DNA synthesis are known for their leukemic potential, including cisplatin and the anthracycline antibiotics (KALDOR et al. 1990a). A notable exception is actinomycin D, which is a potent carcinogen in the rat but is not thought to be leukemogenic in man (KALDOR et al. 1988).

A common denominator in the background of patients with this highly refractory form of AML is exposure to agents which directly or indirectly alter the stem cell pool. This is especially the case with ones that interfere with DNA synthesis (Fig. 1). The delay in recognition of the leukemogenic potential of many of these drugs has undoubtedly been due to the long latency period prior to the onset of the clinical manifestations of leukemia, usually 4–6 years (KALDOR et al. 1990b). Three factors have aided in the recognition of drug-associated leukemias: improved treatment schemes allowing prolonged survival and cure of patients with primary malignancy, recognition of a chronic prodromal syndrome of "preleukemia" characterized by refractory anemia and myelodysplastic marrow changes, and identification of nonrandom clonal chromosomal changes associated with these secondary leukemias, especially defects of chromosomes 5 and 7 (ROWLEY et al. 1977).

Over 75% of patients with secondary AML have chromosomal defects involving chromosome 5 and/or 7 (ROWLEY et al. 1977, 1981; NOWELL et al. 1981; ALBAIN et al. 1983). The relative consistency of the deletion of the long arm of chromosome 5 (−5q) and 7 (−7q) in the secondary leukemias with prior exposure to various chemical agents suggests a close or causal association. It is not yet understood whether the relative resistance of these secondary leukemias to remission induction therapy is in some way due to these chromosomal changes. However, there is certainly a proposed association. The genes which code for the growth factors M-CSF, GM-CSF, IL-3, 4, and 5, platelet-derived growth factor, and myelomonocytic differentiation antigen, CD14, are all located on 5q while the erythropoietin gene is located on chromosome 7 (COLTMAN et al. 1990).

J. Conclusions

Various mechanisms have been implicated and, in some instances, acknowledged to explain chemically induced neutropenia. An understanding of the normal kinetics of marrow neutrophil production and distribution is helpful in defining the severity, duration, and ultimate outcome of the neutropenia. The proliferation of pharmacologic agents that are and will be useful in the treatment of both malignant and nonmalignant disorders suggests that a compendium of drugs associated with neutropenia or other toxic side effects has become less valuable. Progress in the further understanding of the biochemistry of cell metabolism and the structure of the surface membranes of both mature and immature myeloid elements will no doubt be valuable in defining the myelosuppressive and peripherally destructive mechanisms of chemically induced neutropenia and ways to avoid or treat such conditions.

Acknowledgement. I wishes to thank Ms. Nell Kelly for her efforts in contributing to the preparation and editing of this chapter.

References

Abbott JA, Schwals RS (1950) The serious side effects of the newer antiepileptic drugs: their control and prevention. N Engl J Med 242:943–949

Abramson S, Miller RG, Phillips RA (1977) The identification in adult bone marrow of pluripotent and restricted stem cells of the myeloid and lymphoid systems. J Exp Med 145:1567–1579

Adamson JW, Fialkow PJ, Murphy S (1976) Polycythemia vera: stem-cell and probable clonal origin of the disease. N Engl J Med 295:913–916

Albain KS, Le Beau MM, Vardiman JW, Golomb HM, Rowley J (1983) Development of dysmyelopoietic syndrome in a hairy cell leukemia patient treated with chlorambucil: cytogenetic and morphologic evaluation. Cancer Genet Cytogenet 8:107–115

Amrhein JA, Kenny FM, Ross D (1970) Granulocytopenia, lupus-like syndrome, and other complications of propylthiouracil therapy. J Pediatr 76:54–63

Arneborn P, Palmblad J (1982) Drug-induced neutropenia – a survey for Stockholm 1973–1978. Acta Med Scan 212:289–292

Ascensao JL, Flynn PJ, Slungaard A, Wachsman W, Zanjani ED, Jacob HS (1984) Quinidine-induced neutropenia: report of a case with drug-dependent inhibition of granulocyte colony generation. Acta Haematol 72:349–354

Athens JW, Haab OP, Raab SO, Mauer AM, Ashenbrucker H, Cartwright GE,

Wintrobe MM (1961a) Leukocyte studies. IV. The total blood circulating and marginal granulocyte pools and the granulocyte turnover rate in normal subjects. J Clin Invest 40:989–995

Athens JW, Raab SO, Haab OP, Mauer AM, Ashenbrucker H, Cartwright GE, Wintrobe MM (1961b) Leukokinetic studies III. The distribution of granulocytes in the blood of normal subjects. J Clin Invest 40:159–164

Becker AJ, McCulloch EA, Till JE (1963) Cytological demonstration of the clonal nature of spleen colonies derived from transplanted mouse marrow cells. Nature 197:452–454

Becker AJ, McCulloch EA, Siminovitch L, Till JE (1965) The effect of differing demands for blood cell production on DNA synthesis by hematopoietic colony-forming cells of mice. Blood 26:296–308

Berenson RJ, Andrews RG, Bensinger WI, Kalamasy D, Knitter G, Buckner CD, Bernstein ID (1988) Antigen CD34+ marrow cells engraft lethally irradiated baboons. J Clin Invest 81:951–955

Bergsagel DE, Barley AJ, Langley GR, MacDonald RN, White DF, Miller AB (1979) The chemotherapy of plasma-cell myeloma and the incidence of acute leukemia. N Engl J Med 301:743–748

Berk PD, Goldberg JD, Silverstein NM, Weinfeld A, Donovan PB, Ellis JT, Landow SP, Laszlo J, Najean Y, Pisciotta AV, Wasserman LR (1981) Increased incidence of acute leukemia in polycythemia vera associated with chlorambucil therapy. N Engl J Med 304:441–447

Bertoncello I, Hodgson GS, Bradley TR (1985) Multiparameter analysis of transplantable hemopoietic stem cells: I. The separation and enrichment of stem cells homing to marrow and spleen on the basis of rhodamine-123 fluorescence. Exp Hematol 13:999–1006

Best WR (1963) Drug-associated blood dyscrasias. JAMA 185:286–290

Bishop CR, Athens JW (1970) Studies of granulocytopoiesis in abnormal conditions. In: Stohlman F Jr (ed) Hematopoietic cellular proliferation. Grune and Stratton, New York, p 229

Bluming AZ, Plotkin D, Rosen P, Theissen R (1976) Severe transient pancytopenia associated with procainamide ingestion. JAMA 236:2520–2521

Boggs DR (1967) The kinetics of neutrophilic leukocytes in health and in disease. Semin Hematol 4:359–386

Boggs DR, Winkelstein A (1990) White cell manual, 5th edn. Davis, Philadelphia

Boggs DR, Boggs SS, Saxe DF, Grass LA, Canfield DR (1982) Hematopoietic stem cells with high proliferative potential: assay of their concentration in marrow by the frequency and duration of cure of w/w^v mice. J Clin Invest 70:242–253

Boggs SS, Sartiano GP, DeMessa A (1974) Minimal bone marrow damage in mice given bleomycin. Cancer Res 34:1938–1942

Boorman GA, Luster ML, Dean JH, Luebke RW (1982) Effect of indomethacin on the bone marrow and immune system of the mouse. J Clin Lab Immunol 7:119–126

Bradley TR, Metcalf D (1966) The growth of mouse bone marrow cells in vitro. Aust J Exp Biol Med Sci 44:287–299

Brubaker LH, Nolph KD (1971) Mechanisms of recovery from neutropenia induced by hemodialysis. Blood 38:623–631

Bruce WR, Meeker BE, Valeriote FA (1966) Comparison of the sensitivity of normal hematopoietic and transplanted lymphoma colony-forming cells to chemotherapeutic agents administered in vivo. J Natl Cancer Inst 37:233–245

Burroughs SF, Devine DV, Browne G, Kaplan ME (1988) The population of paroxysmal nocturnal hemoglobinuria neutrophils deficient in decay-accelerating factor is also deficient in alkaline phosphatase. Blood 71:1086–1089

Carter SK (1972) Current status of new agents. Cancer Chemother Rep 3:33–47

Chang JC (1975) Agranulocytosis associated with gentamicin. JAMA 232:1154–1155

Chenoweth DE, Cooper SW, Hugli TE (1981) Complement activation during

cardiopulmonary bypass: evidence for generation of C3a and C5a anaphylatoxins. N Engl J Med 304:497–503
Chu J, O'Connor DM, Schmidt RR (1977) The mechanism of oxacillin-induced neutropenia. J Pediatr 90:668–669
Cline MJ, Billing R (1977) Antigens expressed on human B lymphocytes and myeloid stem cells. J Exp Med 146:1143–1145
Closs SP, Cummins D, Contreras M, Armitage SE (1984) Neutropenia due to methyldopa antibodies. Lancet 1:1479
Cohen T, Creger WB (1967) Acute myeloid leukemia following seven years of aplastic anemia induced by chloramphenicol. Am J Med 43:762–770
Coltman CA Jr, Dahlberg S (1990) Treatment-related leukemia. N Engl J Med 322:32–33
Cooper DS, Goldminz D, Levin AA, Ladenson PW, Daniels GH, Molitch ME, Ridgway EC (1983) Agranulocytosis associated with antithyroid drugs. Ann Intern Med 98:26–29
Cooper RA (1983) Captopril-associated neutropenia. Who is at risk? Arch Intern Med 143:659–660
Craddock CG, Perry S, Lawrence JS (1960) The dynamics of neutropenia and leukocytosis. Ann Intern Med 52:281–294
Craddock PR, Fehr J, Brigham KL, Kronenberg RS, Jacob HS (1977a) Complement and leukocyte-mediated pulmonary dysfunction in hemodialysis. N Engl J Med 296:769–774
Craddock PR, Hammerschmidt D, White JG, Dalmasso AP, Jacob HS (1977b) Complement (C5a)-induced granulocyte aggregation in vitro: a possible mechanism of complement-mediated leukostasis and leukopenia. J Clin Invest 60:260–264
Dameshek W, Colmes A (1936) The effect of drugs in the production of agranulocytosis with particular reference to amidopyrine hypersensitivity. J Clin Invest 15:85–97
Davis JP, Lennox WG (1947) The effect of trimethyl oxazolidine deine (tridione) in the blood. J Pediatr 31:24–33
Desgrandchamps D, Schnyder C (1987) Severe neutropenia in prolonged treatment with orally administered augmentin (amoxicillin/clavulanic acid). Infection 15:260–261
Dresch C, Najean Y, Bauchet J (1975) Kinetic studies of ^{51}Cr and DF^{32}P labelled granulocytes. Br J Haematol 29:67–80
Edwards CR, Drury P, Penketh A, Damluji SA (1981) Successful reintroduction of captopril following neutropenia. Lancet 1:723
Ellrodt AG, Murata GH, Riedinger MS, Steward ME, Mochizuki C, Gray R (1984) Severe neutropenia associated with sustained-release procainamide. Ann Intern Med 100:197–201
Enrico C, Vigliali EC, Saita G (1964) Benzene and leukemia. N Engl J Med 221:872–876
Failkow PJ, Lisker R, Detter J (1969) Hemizygous manifestation in a patient with leukemia. Science 163:194–195
Feldman EJ, Isenberg JL (1976) Effects of metiamide in gastric acid hypersecretion, secretion, steatorrhea and bone marrow function in a patient with systemic mastocytosis. N Engl J Med 295:1178–1179
Finch SC (1967) Recognition of radiation-induced late bone marrow changes. Ann NY Acad Sci 145:748–751
Fisher B, Rockette H, Fisher ER, Wickerham L, Redmond C, Brown D (1985) Leukemia in breast cancer patients following adjuvant chemotherapy or postoperative radiation: the NSABP experience. J Clin Oncol 3:1640–1658
Fraunfelder FT (1979) Interim report: national registry of possible drug-induced ocular side effects. Ophthalmology 86:126–130
Freston JW (1979) Cimetidine and granulocytopenia. Ann Intern Med 90:264–265

Friedman RM, Vogel SN (1983) Interferons with special emphasis on the immune system. Adv Immunol 34:97–140

Gabourel JD, Moore MAS, Bagby GC Jr, Davies GH (1977) Effect of sodium salicylate on human and mouse granulopoiesis in vitro. Arthritis Rheum 19:59–64

Gastineau D, Spector R, Philips D (1981) Severe neutropenia associated with ticarcillin therapy. Ann Intern Med 94:711–712

Gilman AG, Goodman LS, Gilman A (1980) The pharmacologic basis of therapeutics, 6th edn. Macmillan, New York, p 1255

Golde DW, Bersch N, Quan SG (1978) Trimethoprim and sulfamethoxazole inhibition of hematopoiesis in vitro. Br J Haematol 40:363–367

Graf M, Tarlov A (1968) Agranulocytosis with monohistiocytosis associated with ampicillin therapy. Ann Intern Med 69:91–95

Greenberg PL, Mosny SA (1977) Cytotoxic effects of interferon in vitro on granulocyte progenitor cells. Cancer Res 37:1794–1799

Gross S, Worthington-White DA (1984) Cimetidine suppression of CFU-C in males. Am J Hematol 17:279–286

Gryfe CI, Rubenzahl S (1976) Agranulocytosis and aplastic anemia possibly due to ibuprofen. Can Med Assoc J 114:877

Hanson JE (1961) Hypersensitivity to isoniazid with neutropenia and thrombocytopenia. Ann Rev Respir Dis 83:744–748

Harris RA, Hogarth PM, Wadeson LJ, Collins P, McKenzie IFC, Penington DG (1984) An antigenic difference between cells forming early and late hematopoietic spleen colonies (CFU-S). Nature 307:638–643

Hartl W (1965) Drug allergic agranulocytosis (Schultz's disease). Semin Hematol 2:313–337

Hill BT, Boserga R (1975) The cell cycle and its significance for cancer treatment. Cancer Treat Rev 2:159–175

Hodinka L, Geher P, Meretey K, Gyodi EK, Petranyi GG, Bozsoky S (1981) Levamisole-induced neutropenia and agranulocytosis; association with HLA B27 leukocyte agglutinating and lymphocytotoxic antibodies. Int Arch Allergy Appl Immunol 65:460–464

Homayouni H, Gross PA, Setia U, Lynch TJ (1979) Leukopenia due to penicillin and cephalosporin homologues. Arch Intern Med 139:827–828

Howell A, Gumpel JM, Watts RWE (1975) Depression of bone marrow colony formation in gold-induced neutropenia. Br Med J 22:432–434

Huguley CM Jr (1964) Agranulocytosis induced by dipyrine, a hazardous antipyretic and analgesic. JAMA 189:938–941

Huguley CM Jr (1966) Hematological reactions. JAMA 196:408–410

Huguley CM, Lea JW Jr, Butts JA (1966) Adverse hematologic reactions to drugs. Prog Hematol 5:105–123

Jackson MA, Mills J (1988) Serious cytomegalovirus disease in the acquired immunodeficiency syndrome (AIDS). Ann Intern Med 108:585–594

Jacobson R, Fialkow PJ (1976) Idiopathic myelofibrosis: stem cell abnormality and probable neoplastic origin. Clin Res 24:439

Jedlicka V (1958) Paramyeloblastic leukemia appearing simultaneously in two blood cousins after simultaneous contact with gammexane (hexachlorocyclohexane). Acta Med Scand 81:445–460

Jenson MK, Roll K (1965) Phenylbutazone and leukemia. Acta Med Scand 178:505–513

Johnson IS, Armstrong JG, Gorman M, Burnett JP (1963) The vinca alkaloids: a new class of oncolytic agents. Cancer Res 23:1390–1427

Joyce RA, Boggs DR (1978) Chemotherapy and leukokinetics. In: Brodsky I, Kahn SB, Conroy JF (eds) Cancer chemotherapy III. Grune & Stratton, New York, p 303

Joyce RA, Boggs DR (1979) Visualizing the marrow granulocyte reserve. J Lab Clin Med 93:101–110

Joyce RA, Chervenick PA (1977) Corticosteroid effect on granulopoiesis in mice following cyclophosphamide. J Clin Invest 60:277–283

Joyce RA, Chervenick PA (1980) Lithium effect on granulopoiesis in mice following cytotoxic chemotherapy. Adv Exp Med Biol 127:145–154

Joyce RA, Boggs DR, Chervenick PA (1976a) Neutrophil kinetics in hereditary and congenital neutropenias. N Engl J Med 295:1385–1390

Joyce RA, Boggs DR, Hasiba U, Srodes CH (1976b) Marginal neutrophil pool size in normal subjects and neutropenic patients as measured by epinephrine infusion. J Lab Clin Med 88:614–620

Joyce RA, Boggs DR, Chervenick PA, Lalezari P (1980) Neutrophil kinetics in Felty's syndrome. Am J Med 69:695–702

Joyce RA, Chervenick PA, Kang MY (1988) Azidothymidine induced marrow toxicity. Blood 72[Suppl 1]:122

Kaldor JM, Day NE, Hemminki K (1988) Quantifying the carcinogenicity of antineoplastic drugs. Eur J Cancer Clin Oncol 24:703–711

Kaldor JM, Day NE, Clarke EA, Van Leeuwen FE, Henry-Amar M, Fiorentino MV, Bell J, Pedersen D, Band P, Assouline D, Koch M, Choi W, Prior P, Blair V, Langmark F, Kirn VP, Neal F, Peters D, Pfeiffer R, Karjalainen S, Cuzick J, Sutcliffe SB, Somers R, Pellae-Cosset B, Pappagallo GL, Fraser P, Storm H, Stovall M (1990a) Leukemia following Hodgkin's disease. N Engl J Med 322:7–13

Kaldor JM, Day NE, Pettersson F, Clarke EA, Pedersen D, Mehnert W, Bell J, Host H, Prior P, Karjalainen S, Neal F, Koch M, Band P, Choi W, Kirn VP, Arslan A, Zaren B, Belch AR, Storm H, Kittelmann B, Fraser P, Stovall M (1990b) Leukemia following chemotherapy for ovarian cancer. N Engl J Med 322:1–6

Kammer RB (1984) Host effects of beta lactam antibiotics. In: Root RK, Sande MA (eds) New dimensions in antimicrobial therapy. Churchill Livingstone, New York, pp 101–119

Kaplan SS, Basford RE, Wing EJ, Shadduck RK (1988) The effect of recombinant human granulocyte macrophage colony-stimulating factor on neutrophil activation in patients with refractory carcinoma. Blood 73:636–638

Kasich M (1944) Agranulocytosis following mapharsen therapy. Arch Dermatol Syphil 50:302–305

Kelton JG, Huang AJ, Mold N, Logue G, Rosse WF (1979) The use of in vitro techniques to study drug-induced pancytopenia. N Engl J Med 301:621–624

Kirkwood CF, Lasezkay GM (1985) Neutropenia associated with mezlocillin and piperacillin. Drug Intell Clin Pharm 19:112–114

Korst DR (1959) Agranulocytosis caused by phenothiazine derivatives. JAMA 170:2076–2081

Kurland JI, Bockman RS, Broxmeyer HE, Moore MAS (1978) Limitation of excessive myelopoiesis by the intensive modulation of macrophage-derived prostaglandin E. Science 199:552–555

Kurzrock R, Quesada JR, Rosenblum MG, Sherwin SA, Gutterman JU (1986) Phase I study of I.V. administered recombinant gamma interferon in cancer patients. Cancer Treat Rep 70:1357–1364

Laskin OL, Stahl-Bayliss CM, Kalman CM, Rosecan LR (1987) Use of ganciclovir to treat serious cytomegalovirus infections in patients with AIDS. J Infect Dis 115:323–327

Lefebvre Y, Hesseltine HC (1965) The peripheral white blood cells and metronidazole. JAMA 194:15

Leonard JC (1953) Toxic effects of phenylbutazone with special reference to disorders of the blood. Br Med J 1:1311–1313

Levin AS, Winer RS, Fudenberg HH (1971) Granulocytopenia caused by anticephalothin antibodies. Clin Res 19:424

Levitt BH, Gottlieb AJ, Rosenberg IR, Klein JJ (1964) Bone marrow depression due to methicillin, a semisynthetic penicillin. Clin Pharmacol Ther 5:301–306
Liederman E, Mogabgab WJ (1970) Rifampin in beta-hemolytic streptococcal pharyngitis and occurrence of leukopenia. Clin Med 77:36
List AF, Beaird DH, Kummet T (1988) Ranitidine-induced granulocytopenia: recurrence with cimetidine administration. Ann Intern Med 108:566–567
Liu YK (1980) Effects of alcohol on granulocytes and lymphocytes. Semin Hematol 17:130–136
Logan TF, Kaplan SS, Bryant JL, Ernstoff MS, Krause JR, Kirkwood JM (1991) Granulocytopenia in cancer patients treated in a Phase I trial with recombinant tumor necrosis factor (TNF). J Immunotherapy 10:84–95
Loveman AB (1932) Toxic granulocytopenia, purpura hemorrhagica and aplastic anemia following the arsphenamines. Ann Intern Med 5:1238–1256
Madison FW, Squier TL (1934) Etiology of primary granulocytopenia (agranulocytic angina). JAMA 102:755–759
Magli MC, Iscove NN, Odartchenko N (1982) Transient nature of early hematopoietic spleen colonies. Nature 295:527–529
Mandell GL (1985) Cephalosporins. In: Mandell GL, Douglas RG Jr, Bennett JE (eds) Principles and practice of infectious diseases, 2nd edn. Wiley, New York, pp 180–187
Mauer EF (1955) The toxic effects of phenylbutazone (butazolidin). N Engl J Med 253:404–410
Meagher RC, Sieber F, Spivak JL (1982) Suppression of hematopoietic – progenitor-cell proliferation by ethanol and acetaldehyde. N Engl J Med 307:845–849
Merigan TC (1983) Human interferon as a therapeutic agent – current status. N Engl J Med 308:1530–1531
Meyers DG, Gonzalez ER, Peters LL, Davis RB, Feagler JR, Egan JD, Nair CK (1985) Severe neutropenia associated with procainamide: comparison of sustained release and conventional preparations. Am Heart J 109:1393–1395
Mitelman F, Brandt L, Nilsson PG (1978) Relation among occupational exposure to potential mutagenic/carcinogenic agents, clinical findings, and bone marrow chromosomes in acute nonlymphocyte leukemia. Blood 52:1229–1237
Moeschlin S, Wagner K (1952) Agranulocytosis due to the occurrence of leukocytic-agglutinins. Acta Haematol 8:29–35
Nawabi IU, Ritz ND (1973) Agranulocytosis due to propranolol. JAMA 223:1376–1377
Neftel KA, Hauser SP, Muller MR (1985) Inhibition of granulopoiesis in vivo and in vitro by beta lactam antibiotics. J Infect Dis 152:90–97
Newton RM, Ward VG (1958) Leukopenia associated with ristocetin administration. JAMA 166:1956–1959
Noorabechi B, Kohout E (1973) Apparent penicillin-induced arrest of mature bone marrow elements. Br Med J 2:26–27
Nowell P, Glick JH, Bucolo A, Finan J, Creech R (1981) Cytogenetic studies of bone marrow in breast cancer patients after adjuvant chemotherapy. Cancer 48:667–673
Oliphant LD, Goddard M (1988) Tocainide-associated neutropenia and lupus-like syndrome. Chest 94:427–428
Palva IP, Lehmola U (1973) Agranulocytosis caused by nitrofurantoin. Acta Med Scand 194:575–576
Payne R (1961) Leukocyte agglutinins in human sera. Am J Hum Genet 13:306–319
Pedersen-Bjargaard J, Osterlind K, Hansen M, Philip P, Pedersen AG, Hansen HH (1985) Acute nonlymphocytic leukemia, preleukemia, and solid tumors following intensive chemotherapy of small cell carcinoma of the lung. Blood 66:1393–1397
Pisciotta AV (1965) Studies on agranulocytosis, VII. Limited proliferative potential of chlorpromazine sensitive patients. J Lab Clin Med 65:240–247

Pisciotta AV (1971) Drug-induced leukopenia and aplastic anemia. Clin Pharm Ther 12:13–43
Pisciotta AV (1973) Immune and toxic mechanisms in drug-induced agranulocytosis. Semin Hematol 10:279–310
Pisciotta AV, Kaldhl J (1962) Studies on agranulocytosis. IV. Effects of chlorpromazine on nucleic acid synthesis of bone marrow cells in vitro. Blood 20:364–376
Pisciotta AV, Santos AS (1965) Studies in agranulocytosis. VI. The effect of clinical treatment with chlorpromazine on nucleic acid synthesis of granulocyte precursors in normal persons. J Lab Clin Med 65:228–239
Pisciotta AV, Ebbe SN, Lennon ES, Metsger GO, Madison FW (1958) Agranulocytosis following administration of phenothiazine derivatives. Am J Med 15:210–223
Pisciotta AV, Santos AS, Keller C (1964) Studies on agranulocytosis.V. Patterns of recovery from drug-induced bone marrow damage. J Lab Clin Med 63:445–458
Pluznik DH, Sachs L (1965) The cloning of normal "mast" cells in tissue culture. J Cell Comp Physiol 66:319–324
Rawls WB (1936) The effects of amidopyrine upon the red, white, and polymorphonuclear blood cells of a series of 100 patients. Am J Med Sci 192:175–179
Reyes MP, Palutke M, Lerner AM (1973) Granulocytopenia associated with carbenicillin: five episodes in 2 patients. Am J Med 54:413–418
Richman DD, Fischl MA, Grieco MH, Gottlieb MS, Volberding PA, Laskin OL, Leedom JM, Groopmen JE, Mildvan D, Hirsch MS, Jackson GG, Durack DT, Nusinoff-Lehrman S and the AZT Collaborative Working Group (1987) The toxicity of azidothymidine (AZT) in the treatment of patients with AIDS and AIDS-related complex. N Engl J Med 317:192–197
Rosove MH (1977) Agranulocytosis and antithyroid drugs. West J Med 126:339–343
Rouveix B, Lassoued K, Vittecoq D, Regnier B (1983) Neutropenia due to beta lactamine antibiotics. Br Med J 287:1832–1834
Rowley J (1973) A new consistent chromosomal abnormality in chronic myelogenous leukaemia identified by quinacrine fluorescence and Giemsa staining. Nature 243:290–293
Rowley JD, Golomb HM, Vardiman JW (1977) Non-random chromosomal abnormalities in acute non-lymphocytic leukemia in patients treated for Hodgkin disease and non-Hodgkin lymphomas. Blood 50:759–770
Rowley JD, Golomb HM, Vardiman JW (1981) Non-random chromosome abnormalities in acute leukemia and dysmyelopoietic syndromes in patients with previously treated malignant disease. Blood 58:759–767
Samlowski WE, Frame RN, Logue GL (1987) Flecanide-induced immune neutropenia. Documentation of a haptene-mediated mechanism of cell destruction. Arch Intern Med 147:383–384
Sato K, Miyakawa M, Han DL, Kato S (1985) Graves' disease with neutropenia and marked splenomegaly: autoimmune neutropenia due to propylthiouracil. J Endocrinol 8:551–555
Schiffer CA, Aisner J, Wiernik PH (1975) Transient neutropenia induced by transfusion of blood exposed to nylon fiber filters. Blood 45:141–146
Schneider E, Piquet-Pellorce C, Dy M (1990) New role for histamine in interleukin-3-induced proliferation of hematopoietic cells. J Cell Physiol 143:337–343
Schotland MG, Grumbach MM (1963) Neutropenia in an infant secondary to hydrochlorothiazide therapy. Pediatrics 31:754–757
Schultz W (1922) Über eigenartige Halserkrankungen. Dtsch Med Wochensch 48:1495
Smith CS, Chinn S, Watts RWE (1977) The sensitivity of human bone marrow granulocyte/monocyte precursor cells to phenylbutazone, oxyphenbutazone and gamma-hydroxphenylbutazone in vitro, with observations on the bone marrow

colony formation in phenylbutazone-induced granulocytopenia. Biochem Pharmacol 26:847–852

Socinski MA, Cannistra SA, Sullivan R, Elias A, Antman K, Schnipper L, Griffin JD (1988) Granulocyte-macrophage colony-stimulating factor induces the expression of the DC11b surface adhesion molecule in human granulocytes in vivo. Blood 72:691–697

Sparberg M (1963) Diagnostically confusing complications of diphenylhydantoin therapy. Ann Intern Med 59:914–930

Stein JH, Hamilton HE, Sheets RF (1964) Agranulocytosis caused by chlorpropamide. Arch Intern Med 113:186–190

Sutherland HJ, Eaves CJ, Eaves AC, Dragowska W, Lansdorp PM (1989) Characterization and partial purification of human marrow cells capable of initiating long-term hematopoiesis in vitro. Blood 74:1563–1570

Taetle R, Lane TA, Mendelsohn J (1979) Drug-induced agranulocytosis: in vitro evidence for immune suppression of granulocytosis and a cross-reacting lymphocyte antibody. Blood 54:501–512

Teerenhovi L, Heinonen E, Grohn P, Klefstrom P, Mehtonen M, Tiilikainen A (1978) High frequency of agranulocytosis in breast-cancer patients treated with levamisole. Lancet 2:151–152

Till JE, McCulloch EA (1961) A direct measurement of the radiation sensitivity of normal mouse bone marrow cells. Radiat Res 14:213–222

Tisman G, Herbert V (1973) In vitro myelosuppression and immunosuppression by ethanol. J Clin Invest 52:1410–1414

Trotter WR (1962) The relative toxicity of antithyroid drugs. J New Drugs 2:333–343

Turner NA, Woodliff HJ (1964) Neutropenia associated with chlorthalidone therapy. Med J Aust 1:361–363

Underwood LC (1956) Fatal bone marrow depression after treatment with acetazolamide (Diamox). JAMA 161:1477–1478

Van Zant G (1984) Studies of hematopoietic stem cells spared by 5-fluorouracil. J Exp Med 159:679–690

Veys EM, Mielants H, Verbruggen G (1978) Levamisole-induced adverse reactions in HLA B27-positive rheumatoid arthritis. Lancet 1:148

Vidt DG, Bravo EL, Fouad FM (1982) Drug therapy: captopril. N Engl J Med 306:214–219

Von Rechenberg HK (1953) Untersuchungen über Butazolidin und Irgapyrin in ihren Beziehungen zur Agranulozytose. Acta Haematol 9:353–370

Walker JG (1966) Fatal agranulocytosis complicating treatment with ethacrynic acid. Ann Intern Med 64:1303–1305

Weissman G, Xefteris ED (1959) Phenylbutazone leukopenia. Arch Int Med 103:957–961

Werblin TP, Pollack IP, Liss RA (1979) Aplastic anemia and agranulocytosis in patients using methazolamide for glaucoma. JAMA 241:2817–2818

Whang J, Frei E III, Tjio JH (1963) The distribution of the Philadelphia chromosome in patients with chronic myelogenous leukemia. Blood 22:664–673

Wheeler GP (1962) Studies related to the mechanisms of action of cytotoxic alkylating agents: a review. Cancer Res 22:651–688

Wintrobe MM (1968) The therapeutic millennium and its price: a view from the hematopoietic system. J R Coll Physicians Lond 3:99–119

Woolsey RL, Drayer DE, Reigenberg MM, Nies AS, Carr K, Dates JA (1978) Effect of acetylator phenotype on the rate at which procainamide induces antinuclear antibodies and the lupus syndrome. N Engl J Med 298:1157–1159

Worlledge SM, Carstairs KC, Dacie JV (1966) Autoimmune haemolytic anaemia associated with alpha-methyldopa therapy. Lancet 2:135–139

Wright JS (1970) Phenindione sensitivity with leukaemoid reaction and hepato-renal damage. Postgrad Med J 46:452–455

Young GA, Croaker G, Vincent PC, Forrest P, Morris TC (1987) The CFU-C assay in patients with neutropenia, and in particular, drug-associated neutropenia. Clin Lab Haematol 9:245–253

Zacharski LR, Elveback LR, Linman JW (1971) Leukocyte counts in healthy adults. Am J Clin Pathol 56:148–150

Zakhirch B, Rout RK (1978) Unusually high occurrence of drug reactions to nafcillin. Yale J Biol Med 51:449–455

CHAPTER 14

Drugs Useful in the Chemotherapy of the Acute Leukemias

R.L. CAPIZZI and K. AGRAWAL

A. Introduction

Traditionally, the only curative measures for neoplastic diseases have been surgery and/or radiation therapy. These modalities cure only localized forms. Since they are disseminated malignancies, the leukemias require systemic therapy. Collaborative research efforts between clinicians and pharmacologists over the past 30 years have enabled the development of regimens that are curative for several subsets of patients with acute leukemia.

Overall, the leukemias are the ninth most prevalent form of cancer in the USA, constituting 5%–6% of all cancers. National statistics, which group the acute and chronic leukemias together, indicate an incidence of 5–10 cases per 100000 population (ELLISON 1982). Although the incidence of leukemia appears to be on the rise, this probably reflects more frequent diagnosis of the chronic leukemias as a result of increased medical surveillance of an aging population. Approximately 60% of leukemia patients have one of the chronic variants, and 60% of all leukemia patients are over age 50 (Table 1).

The designation of acute or chronic leukemia is based on natural history and morphology. The acute leukemias are commonly fulminating diseases. Patients characteristically have a short period of illness, and their presenting medical complaints reflect the symptoms and signs of bone marrow failure due to the replacement of its normal elements with leukemia cells. These signs and symptoms involve anemia, neutropenia, and thrombocytopenia. While the patients may have marked leukocytosis, the predominant cell in the peripheral blood, as in the bone marrow, is an immature blast with or without some morphologic features of differentiation indicating the lineage of origin. In contrast, many patients with either of the chronic leukemias, chronic lymphocytic leukemia (CLL) or chronic granulocytic leukemia (CGL), may be initially diagnosed at the time of a routine physical examination. The patient may be totally asymptomatic, and the only clue to the diagnosis of chronic leukemia may be leukocytosis composed of lymphocytosis or neutrophilia for CLL and CGL, respectively. Aside from an absolute increase in number, one would be hard pressed to make a diagnosis of CLL or CGL on morphological criteria only. The lymphocytes

Table 1. Overall percentage of leukemias at different ages. From GUNZ and HENDERSON (1983)

Type	Patients in age groups (years)		
	0–14	15–19	50+
All leukemias	20%	20%	60%
Acute	35%	23%	42%
Chronic	4%	15%	81%

of CLL and the neutrophils of CGL are morphologically indistinguishable from their normal counterparts. Thus, additional laboratory features are important to recognize these entities. Two other features distinguish the acute from the chronic leukemias. Without therapy, the median lifespan of patients with chronic leukemias is measured in years, whereas that for patients with acute leukemiais is measured in weeks or months (GUNZ and HENDERSON 1983). However, the most notable feature differentiating acute from chronic leukemias is their response to therapy: Acute leukemias are examples of disseminated malignancies that can be cured with available drugs, while virtually none of the chronic leukemias, as yet, fall into this category. Cure rates (percentage disease-free for more than 10 years) for acute lymphocytic (lymphoblastic) leukemia (ALL) in children average 50%, with a range of 10%–80% depending on the cytoimmunologic subtype and other prognostic features. The cure rate for ALL in adults is between 10% and 30%. Cure rates for acute myeloid (myeloblastic) leukemia (AML) range between 15% and 30%, the lower figure for adults and the higher one for children.

This overview will focus on drugs useful in the treatment of the acute leukemias. The acute leukemias are divided into two broad types, ALL and AML. As noted in Table 1, they have a bimodal distribution as a function of age, 0–14 years and in those over age 50. This distribution reflects the preponderance of ALL or AML as a function of age (Table 2). ALL is more commonly a disease of childhood and AML, a disease of older adults. Age is also one of the most important prognostic indicators for response to therapy, duration of response, and presumed curability for both ALL and AML patients. These variations obviously correspond to the intrinsic

Table 2. Age distribution of the acute leukemias

	Children	Adults
ALL	81%	25%
AML	19%	75%

ALL, acute lymphocytic leukemia; AML, acute myeloid leukemia.

chemosensitivity of the leukemias and also important host factors in the ability of the patient to tolerate and survive the toxic effects of chemotherapy, especially the period of virtually complete bone marrow ablation during which the patient is extremely susceptible to serious infections and bleeding. Comorbid diseases related to common adult problems such as atherosclerosis, hypertension, substance abuse, etc. frequently alter organ function, which in turn, may affect drug metabolism, pharmacokinetics, and organ reserve. Thus, the care of the older adult with acute leukemia not infrequently involves all of the skills of the internist in supporting the patient through very difficult periods.

The goal of chemotherapy in patients with ALL and AML is cure. As noted in the statistics cited above, steady progress has been made over the past 30 years both in terms of refinements of chemotherapy and in better supportive care. However, further work is necessary for improved responses, an understanding of drug resistance, and a better therapeutic index. The prelude to curing any neoplastic disease is the attainment of a complete clinical remission (complete response, CR). For acute leukemia this can be defined as the reduction of marrow blasts to less than 5%, a return to normal marrow cellularity of the three cell lines, the absence of blasts in the peripheral blood with reappearance of a normal peripheral hemogram, and no evident residual leukemia on physical examination along with restoration of the patient's condition toward normal. With currently available therapies, the transition from florid disease to complete remission of acute leukemia takes approximately 3–5 weeks. This initial period of treatment is termed "induction therapy."

The usage of combinations of drugs is the mainstay of therapy for patients with ALL and AML. Trial and error, rather than unique pharmacological characteristics, have shown that several combinations of drugs are particularly effective for the initial induction of remission for patients with acute leukemia. Drugs with exquisite efficacy in the treatment of ALL (Prednisone, vincristine, asparaginase) are virtually ineffective in AML. Other useful drugs for the treatment of ALL, such as the thiopurines [6-mercaptopurine (6-MP) and 6-thioguanine (6-TG)], standard doses of methotrexate, and cyclophosphamide, are only moderately effective in AML. Today's standard of practice for induction therapy of AML is the combined use of cytosine arabinoside (ara-C) and daunorubicin. Therapy with these drugs produces the remission frequencies and survival statistics noted above. Taken as a whole, i.e., AML and ALL in all age groups, the CR rate ranges from 40% to 95%. There are two main reasons for the failure to achieve a CR. One is the failure of supportive care, i.e., while the leukemia may have been reduced to clinically undetectable levels, the patient succumbs from overwhelming infection and/or bleeding or other organ failure during the period of marrow aplasia. Others may not survive the overwhelming effects of leukemia progression due to the presence of drug-resistant disease. Once in CR, 20%–80% of patients will ultimately relapse; the range in relapse rates reflects the impact of various prognostic factors on the duration of remission. Taken together, initial refractoriness to therapy or subsequent relapse after a period of CR poses an important challenge to the pharmacologist for studies of drug resistance. Such an understanding might suggest alternate therapeutic approaches in an attempt to circumvent drug resistance with the goal to (re)achieve CR.

The following is an overview of the pharmacology of the major drugs used in the treatment of the acute leukemia. The drugs will be grouped in very broad classifications.

B. Antimetabolites

Antimetabolites are essential drugs in the treatment of AML and ALL. Properly used, this drug class plays important roles in the curability of these neoplasms. Antimetabolites are structurally similar analogues of normal metabolites, differing from their natural counterparts in one or more major functional groups. All but one antimetabolite in common usage today has been deliberately designed. Methotrexate, and its predecessor aminopterin, were designed to interfere with folate metabolism. The thiopurines, 6-mercaptopurine and 6-thioguanine, were intended to interfere with purine metabolism. On the other hand, ara-C (cytosine arabinoside, 1-β-D-arabinofuranosylcytosine) was discovered by empirical screening of natural products.

Antimetabolites are transported across the cell membrane and are metabolized like their normal counterparts and interfere with the synthesis of nucleic acids or one of their precursors in neoplastic as well as normal tissues. However, the fact that they display selective cytotoxic effects on leukemia cells relates to some important differences in the metabolism of these drugs in the neoplastic cell vs. the normal cell. Such differences are especially influenced by the dose size, schedule of drug administration, and various drug-drug and/or drug-metabolite interactions. As a group, antimetabolites may be said to display dose-dependent pharmacokinetics (POWIS 1983). This is important not simply for a consideration of the "area under the curve" (AUC) but rather for the shape of the AUC curve in terms of peak concentration vs. duration of exposure. Dose and schedule effects on its shape may cause differential effects on important cellular processes such as membrane transport and cellular accumulation in neoplastic vs. normal cells.

All antimetabolites gain entry to the cell through a carrier protein in the cell membrane. The number of the receptor molecules will influence cellular pharmacokinetics both in terms of influx as well as efflux rates. Cellular pharmacokinetics is further influenced by intrinsic capacities for drug metabolism, both anabolism and catabolism. All antimetabolites are metabolized by the cell. Anabolism to negatively charged molecules, e.g., polyglutamates of methotrexate (MTX) or nucleotides of the purine and pyrimidine analogues, result in retention of the drug metabolites. Differential anabolism and/or catabolism between neoplastic and normal cells affects tissue-distribution pharmacokinetics and is evident in the selectivity of drug action. This selectivity is expressed as the therapeutic index. Because of the narrow therapeutic index and steep dose-response curve for antimetabolites, the optimal use of these drugs requires a detailed understanding of their clinical pharmacology. Unfortunately, information on only two drugs, MTX and ara-C, begins to approximate this goal, although, even for these drugs our clinical information is incomplete.

I. Cytosine Arabinoside (1-β-D-arabinofuranosylcytosine)

1. Chemistry

Ara-C, a pyrimidine antimetabolite, is a close structural analogue of the normal metabolite, deoxycytidine (dCyd). Consequently, the pharmacology of ara-C closely parallels the biochemistry of dCyd. The structural difference between ara-C and dCyd is the presence of an arabinosyl sugar instead of the 2'-deoxyribose of dCyd.

2. Pharmacology

The main features affecting the celular pharmacology of ara-C are sketched in Fig. 1. Ara-C must be administered parenterally; it has virtually no practical oral bioavailability. As ara-C is absorbed by the intestinal mucosa,

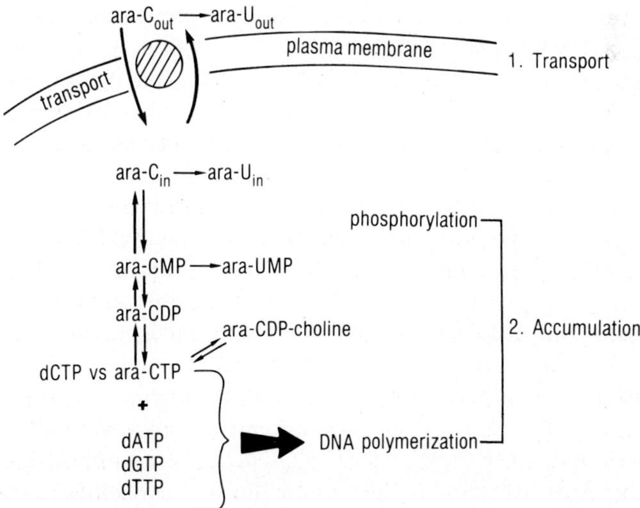

Fig. 1. Pharmacologic determinants of cytosine arabinoside (ara-C) effect

it is rapidly deaminated to uracil arabinoside (ara-U), an analogue with virtually no cytotoxic potential. However, in experimental cell lines, high concentrations of ara-U cause a slowing of cells in S phase (see below).

Ara-C enters the cell by a carrier-mediated facilitated diffusion mechanism common to nucleosides (PLAGEMANN et al. 1978). A clear distinction must be made between the physiological processes termed transport and uptake. For the present discussion, transport will refer to the carrier-mediated membrane translocation of the drug. While "uptake" also invokes "transport," the usual measurements which describe this process primarily apply to cellular accumulation. Thus, in the present discussion, the term "accumulation" will refer to the intracellular metabolism and retention of ara-C and its metabolites. While membrane transport of ara-C in experimental tumor models has been shown to be rapid and not a limiting factor in its metabolism by these cells (KESSEL et al. 1967), it has recently been demonstrated that human leukemia cells taken directly from patients have, in comparison, very low nucleoside transport activity (WHITE et al. 1987).

The number of nucleoside carrier molecules per cell may be directly quantitated by measuring the binding capacity for the high-affinity inhibitor, nitrobenzylmercaptopurine riboside (NBMPR) (CASS et al. 1974). NBMPR is a purine nucleoside analogue which binds tightly to the nucleoside carrier protein (K_d = 0.2 nM) and is not translocated into the cell (CASS et al. 1974). Since NBMPR is a potent inhibitor of transport, relatively moderate concentrations, e.g., 1 μM, will completely block ara-C transport by this route. Since some experimental cell lines may have significant NBMPR-insensitive nucleoside transport capacity, NBMPR is also a useful tool for elucidating alternative transport routes (PLAGEMANN and WOHLHUETER 1984). Transport rates and the number of NBMPR sites, i.e., nucleoside carrier molecules, in human leukemic blasts from patients are contrasted with several murine and human experimental cell lines in Table 3. Consistent with previous studies which indicated that transport was not rate-limiting in ara-C pharmacology, the number of NBMPR sites and ara-C transport rates are high in both murine and human leukemia experimental cell lines, including myeloid (HL-60, ML-1) and lymphoblastic (CCRF-CEM) leukemias. In contrast, the number of NBMPR binding sites (i.e., transport carriers) and ara-C transport rates in leukemic blasts taken directly from patients are strikingly lower (WHITE et al. 1987; WILEY et al. 1982, 1983).

To assess the practical relevance of lower transport activity in human leukemia cells, the transport "control strength" was determined. This, in essence, is an expression of the role of transport as a determinant of the rate of net intracellular accumulation of ara-C metabolites. When transport is in great excess and not a factor of consequence, the control strength is zero. When the rate of transport is slow and is the sole determinant of the rate of net accumulation, control strength is 1 (WHITE et al. 1987). Transport control strength is dependent on the extracellular concentration of ara-C.

Table 3. Ara-C transport rate and nucleoside carrier sites. Reproduced from WHITE et al (1987)

	Rate[a]	NBMPR sites
Patients		
Acute leukemia	14 ± 15 (n = 45)	4223 ± 4334 (n = 61)
Human leukemia in cell culture		
ML-1	805	139 000
HL-60	49	59 000
CCRF-CEM	n.d.	183 000
Mouse ascites tumors		
Ehrlich	272	94 000
L5178Y	105	74 000
P388	n.d.	137 000

[a] pmol/min/10^6 cells at 50 μ*M* [^{3}H] ara-C ± SD
Maximal specific [^{3}H] NBMPR binding sites per cell ± SD
n.d., not determined; ara-C, cytosine arabinoside; NBMPR, nitrobenzylmercaptopurine riboside.

The K_m for ara-C transport is 400 μ*M*, a value that is quite high compared with clinically achievable plasma drug concentrations (see below). Thus, for practical purposes in everyday therapeutics, the transport rate will be approximately proportional to the plasma concentration. In contrast, the rate of ara-C phosphorylation intracellularly approaches a maximal velocity at relatively lower drug levels, in the range of 2–5 μ*M*. Thus, at concentrations below 1 μ*M* which are typical of plasma concentrations achieved during the continuous infusions of standard dose ara-C (SDAC), i.e., 100–200 mg/m^2 daily, transport may be rate-limiting for the cellular effects of ara-C. However, as the concentration is increased and phosphorylation approaches a maximum, the ratio of transport capacity to phosphorylation capacity increases. At high extracellular concentrations, i.e., >10 μ*M*, ara-C transport is in excess. This relationship is illustrated by several examples depicted in Fig. 2. The solid line is based on transport and accumulation data for leukemic blasts taken from 45 patients with AML. This shows that for the majority of patients, membrane transport is the rate-limiting process at ara-C concentrations typical of those achieved during continuous infusion of SDAC (i.e., <1.0 μ*M*). However, as the extracellular concentration of ara-C is increased to the 10–20 μ*M* range, transport becomes less important as a determinant of the cellular accumulation rate. As will be seen below, the extracellular (plasma) concentrations achieved during short-term infusions of high-dose ara-C are in considerable excess of these levels. The dashed and dotted curves illustrate the extremes of this process. Transport is the major rate-determining process for the patient's cells represented by the dashed line up to 8 μ*M* ara-C. For those represented by the dotted line, transport control strength is always less than 0.5, indicating that transport only partially determines the rate of uptake for this patient even at low ara-C concentrations (White et al. 1987).

The practical messages from these studies are that for most patients (illustrated by the solid line) membrane transport is the rate-limiting step in the cellular accumulation of ara-C at plasma concentrations of drug typically achieved with standard dosages and that this impediment may be obviated by a suitable increase in dose which will provide plasma concentrations above 10 μ*M*. At concentrations ≥10 μ*M*, the capacity of the cell to phosphorylate ara-C and the extent of its incorporation into DNA will be the prime determinants of ara-C cytotoxicity. Thus, any means for enhancing these intracellular processes such as the lowering of the competing dCTP pools by biochemical modulation (Danhauser and Rustum 1980; Walsh et al. 1980) or the enhancement of the proportion of cells in S phase by the use of cytostatic agents (Lampkin et al. 1971) may enhance the effects of ara-C. To some extent, these latter mechanisms may be invoked by ara-U/ara-C (Yang et al. 1985; Chandrasekaran et al. 1989), as will be clarified below.

The cellular pharmacokinetics of ara-C described as transport and accumulation are influenced by systemic pharmacokinetics. Plasma drug levels achievable during bolus and continuous infusion of various doses of ara-C are shown in Table 4. Bolus injection of 100 mg/m^2 results in peak plasma levels of approximately 20 μ*M* (Slevin et al. 1981). However, because of the rapid clearance of the drug from the plasma, this drops to 1% of the peak value within 2 h (Slevin et al. 1981). Thus, following a bolus injection, the duration of exposure of the leukemic cells to extracellular concentrations of ara-C capable of overcoming transport deficits would be relatively brief. Continuous infusion of 100 and 200 mg/m^2 (SDAC) results in average plasma steady-state concentrations of 0.2 and 0.4 μ*M*, respectively (Slevin et al. 1981; Weinstein et al. 1982). Again, considering the data relating the impact of transport on cellular metabolism at various drug concentrations, the plasma steady-state values achieved with SDAC would benefit fewer patients, perhaps explaining the observed 25% complete remission rate associated with the use of SDAC (Gale 1979). In contrast, plasma steady-state levels achieved during infusion of 3 g/m^2 for 3 h (as in various high-dose ara-C protocols) average between 50 and 100 μ*M* (Capizzi et al. 1983). This is considerably in excess of that required to

Table 4. Plasma levels of Ara-C

	μ*M*	Reference
100 mg/m^2		
Bolus	20.0 (peak)	Slevin et al. (1981)
Continuous infusion	0.4	Slevin et al. (1981)
200 mg/m^2		
Continuous infusion	0.8	Weinstein et al. (1982)
3000 mg/m^2	100.0	Capizzi et al. (1983)

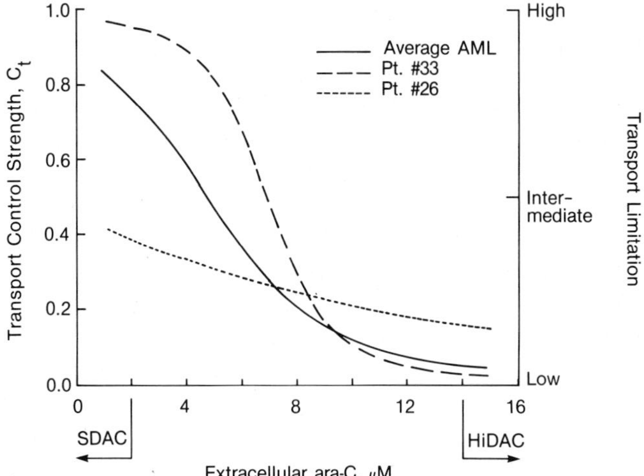

Fig. 2. Concentration dependence of transport control strength as a determinant of the rate of accumulation of ara-C in AML cells from patients. The solid line is based on median kinetic constants (see White et al. 1987). The dashed and dotted lines are derived from kinetic parameters of cells from two patients, which represent extremes of high and low sensitivity to transport capacity as a determinant of the rate of ara-C accumulation. SDAC, standard dose ara-C; HiDAC, high-dose ara-C. (Reproduced from WHITE et al. 1987)

overcome any transport impediment (Fig. 2), and thus the high levels of ara-C should rapidly equilibrate across the cell membrane. The main limitations to ara-C effect with this high dose would be rates of intracellular anabolism and catabolism, the presence of competing pools of dCTP, and incorporation and retention in DNA. The high plasma drug concentrations associated with the use of $3\,g/m^2$ are sufficient to result in therapeutic drug concentrations in the cerebrospinal fluid (CAPIZZI et al. 1983). These levels have been associated with clearance of leukemia cells from the CSF (CAPIZZI et al. 1984) and the regression of intracerebral lymphoma (AMADORI et al. 1984). Repeated administration of high-dose ara-C (8–13 doses in succession) has also resulted in serious neurological toxicity, mostly cerebellar in nature (LAZARUS et al. 1981).

At the conclusion of administration of high-dose ara-C, either bolus or

Table 5. Pharmacokinetic parameters of Ara-C after 3-h constant rate intravenous infusion of $3\,g/m^2$. Reproduced from CAPIZZI et al. (1983)

	$t_{1/2\alpha}$ (min)	$t_{/2\beta}$ (h)	cl (l/h)	vd_β (l)	vd_{ss} (l)	t (h)
Mean ± SD	15.7 ± 2.6	1.81 ± 0.55	86.4 ± 17.7	220.6 ± 33.8	41.4 ± 12.3	0.47 ± 0.07

$t_{1/2}$, half life; cl, clearance; l/hr, liters/hours; vd, volume of distribution; $\bar{t}$, mean residence time.

infusion, the initial plasma clearance rates (α and β half-lives) are fairly comparable with those at other dose levels (Table 5). The plasma clearance of SDAC has been described as a biexponential process (WAN et al. 1974). However, with infusions of high-dose ara-C at 3 g/m^2, most patients display a triexponential process with an additional $\gamma\, t_{1/2}$ of 6 h (Fig. 3) (CAPIZZI et al. 1983). Shortly after the start of infusion, ara-C is rapidly deaminated to ara-U, which is relatively nontoxic. During infusion, the plasma concentration of ara-U is 2–3 times higher than ara-C, ranges between 200 and 300 μ*M*, and displays a monoexponential half-life of 3.75 h (Fig. 3) (CAPIZZI et al. 1983). Clinical and laboratory observations suggest that the extent of this deamination process is dose-dependent (HO and FREI 1971). These data imply that this deamination process is saturable or the presence of a metabolic inhibitor. Studies in vitro (CAPIZZI et al. 1983) and in vivo (CHANDRASEKARAN et al. 1989) indicate that high concentrations of ara-U inhibit Cyd deaminase and thus retard the catabolism of ara-C. This effect of ara-U may explain the altered pharmacokinetics observed with the use of high-dose ara-C (3 g/m^2) in the treatment of patients with acute leukemia.

The most successful clinical reports of the use of high-dose ara-C involve 6–12 consecutive doses at 12-h intervals (CAPIZZI and POWELL 1987). Given the relatively long plasma half-life for ara-U (CAPIZZI et al. 1983), the rapid catabolism of repetitive high doses administered at 12-h intervals mimics, in essence, a continuous infusion of large doses of ara-U. Questions might then

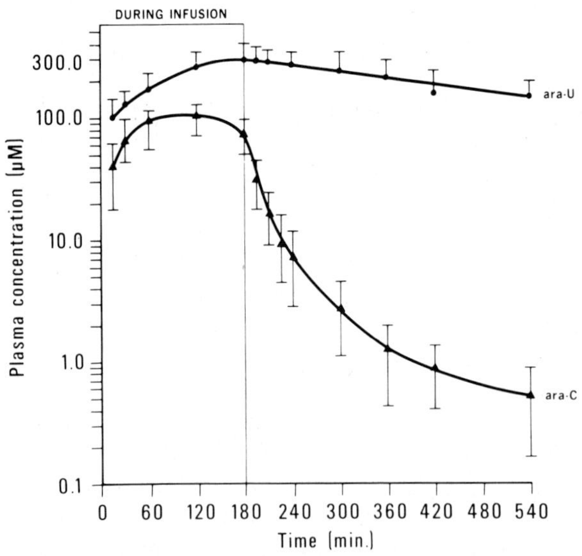

Fig. 3. Plasma ara-C and ara-U concentrations during and after a 3-h infusion of 3 g/m^2 ara-C administered every 12 h for four doses. Points represent the mean ±SD of 20 studies in four patients (*triangle*, ara-C; *circle*, ara-U). (Reproduced from CAPIZZI et al. 1983)

be raised regarding the potential effect of high concentrations of ara-U on the cellular pharmacology of ara-C. When murine leukemia cells are exposed to high concentrations of ara-U, i.e., in the range of 10^{-4}–10^{-3} M, the growth of L5178Y cells was delayed. DNA histogram analysis of these growth-inhibited cells revealed accumulation of the cells in the S phase. There was an *overall* increase in the specific activity of the rate-limiting enzyme for ara-C anabolism, dCyd kinase. Thus, exposure of the leukemia cells to ara-C after ara-U pretreatment for 24–48 h was associated with increased ara-CTP and ara-C-DNA formation with a consequent increase in ara-C cytotoxicity (YANG et al. 1985). Similar effects have been noted in leukemic mice with the continuous infusion of large doses of ara-U followed by ara-C treatment (CHANDRASEKARAN et al. 1989).

These data thus show dose-dependent effects on both the systemic and cellular pharmacokinetics of ara-C. Dose-dependent effects on membrane transport can be critical to the success or failure of therapeutic attempts and undoubtedly contribute to the efficacy of high-dose ara-C therapy in refractory leukemias (CAPIZZI et al. 1985). Dose-dependent changes in the systemic pharmacokinetics which result in a prolonged gamma-phase in the plasma clearance curve provide an increase in the AUC of ara-C above that expected from the dose increase alone. The ara-U generated from the catabolism of high-dose ara-C also has an impact on the cellular pharmacokinetics of the drug by causing an accumulation of cells in S phase, in which anabolism of a subsequent dose of ara-C is increased. These dose-dependent pharmacokinetic and cytokinetic effects could be termed self-potentiation by high-dose ara-C.

There have been a number of studies in murine and human leukemias investigating one or more parameters of ara-C biochemical pharmacology in an attempt to predict the therapeutic outcome or to define the mechanism of drug resistance. These have included (1) decreased membrane transport (KESSEL et al. 1967; CHU and FISCHER 1968; WILEY et al. 1982; WHITE et al. 1987); (2) decreased anabolism to ara-CMP due to low levels of dCyd kinase (KESSEL et al. 1967; CHU and FISCHER 1965; MEYERS and KREIS 1978; DREWINKO et al. 1972); (3) increased catabolism via Cyd deaminase (STEWART and BURKE 1971); (4) expansion of the dCTP pool (TATTERSALL et al. 1974; MOMPARLER et al. 1968); (5) short half-life of cellular ara-CTP (Rustum 1978); (6) possible diminished affinity of DNA polymerase for ara-CTP (BACH 1969; RAMA-REDDY and GOULIAN 1971) and possible excision of ara-CMP from DNA (LECLERC and CHENG 1985). While some studies have linked one or more of the above to the drug's cytotoxic effect, or the lack thereof, others have disputed certain relationships. Given an understanding of these biochemical features, various pharmacologic maneuvers have been employed in an attempt to overcome drug resistance, for example, the use of tetrahydrouridine to inhibit Cyd deaminase (CAMIENER 1968) or of deazauridine (PLAGEMANN et al. 1978; MILLS-YAMAMOTO et al. 1978), high-dose thymidine (HARRIS et al. 1979; DANHAUSER and RUSTUM 1980; ZITTOUN et al. 1985), or hydroxyurea (THEISS and FISCHER 1976; PLAGEMANN et al. 1978; WALSH et al. 1980) to lower the pool size of the competing metabolite, dCTP, a process termed biochemical modulation. While these maneuvers have met with pharmacologic success, the clinical success to date has been limited by a lack of significant improvement in the therapeutic index of ara-C. That is, while cytotoxicity to certain neoplastic cells has been increased, a somewhat parallel increase in toxicity to normal organs has also occurred, resulting in a small net therapeutic gain.

II. 6-Mercaptopurine and 6-Thioguanine

1. Chemistry

6-Mercaptopurine (6-MP) and 6-thioguanine (6-TG) were developed by the Nobel Laureates Elion and Hitchings by substituting a thiol for the 6-hydroxyl group of hypoxanthine (ELION et al. 1952) and guanine (ELION and HITCHINGS 1955), respectively.

2. Pharmacology

Both drugs have similar pharmacology and probably can be used interchangeably. Their clinical use, however, has adhered to oncologic tradition: 6-MP is primarily employed to treat patients with ALL and 6-TG, to treat patients with AML. To date, there is no pharmacological basis for this clinical segregation, especially since 6-MP may be metabolically converted to 6-TG nucleotides in the cell (TIDD and PATTERSON 1974). The bases are inactive and require anabolism to their monophosphate nucleotides to interfere with enzymes involved in the de novo synthesis of the purine structure. Nucleotide triphosphate derivatives may be incorporated into nucleic acids (Table 6).

Table 6. Sites of action for the thiopurines (as nucleotide derivatives)

Affected product	Enzyme inhibited[a]	Reference
Phosphoribosylamine	GlutaminePRPP amidotransferase	HILL and BENNET (1969)
Adenylic acid (AMP)	Adenylosuccinate synthetase	ELION (1967)
Xanthylic acid (XMP) (a precursor of GMP)	Inosinic acid dehydrogenase	ELION (1967)
RNA[b]		MELVIN and KEIR (1979)
DNA[b]		NELSON et al. (1975) CARRICO and SARTORELLI (1977)

[a] Inhibited by negative feedback effect by corresponding thiopurine nucleotide.
[b] Function affected by incorporation of the respective thioguanine nucleotide.

The only commercially available thiopurine products are tablets. While this is certainly convenient, studies indicate erratic oral bioavailability of the drugs; various estimates suggest that only 25%–50% of an oral dose is effectively absorbed (ZIMM et al. 1983a). This relatively poor oral bioavailability is perhaps related to the high concentration of xanthine oxidase in the intestinal mucosa and liver (BRUNCHEDE and KROOTH 1973). Since xanthine oxidase is a major catabolic enzyme for 6-MP, this basically creates a "first pass effect" (ZIMM et al. 1983b). Oral bioavailability may be further impaired by various foodstuffs (BURTON et al. 1986), especially milk and cream which are rich in xanthine oxidase (BURNER and LOW 1985). Additionally, the coadministration of 6-MP with the antibiotic cotrimoxazole may interfere with its absorption and cytotoxicity (REES et al. 1984). These problems would be obviated if a parenteral formulation were commercially available; however, the parenteral form of 6-TG is available only for research purposes.

Following an oral dose, plasma levels are detectable within 15 min, with peak concentrations measured at 1.3 ± 0.6 h. Thereafter, the plasma concentrations decay with a $t_{1/2}$ of 1 ± 0.5 h (LENNARD et al. 1986). Boys appear to tolerate larger doses of 6-MP than girls (LILLEYMAN et al. 1984; LENNARD and LILLEYMAN 1989).

As such, the purine bases 6-MP and 6-TG are inactive and must be anabolized to various nucleotide derivatives in order to exert a cytotoxic effect. The enzyme hypoxanthine: guanine phosphoribosyl transferase (HGPRTase) mediates the anabolism of 6-MP and 6-TG to thioinosinic acid and 6-thioguanylic acid, respectively (BROCKMAN 1963; VAN DIGGELEN et al. 1979; DAVIDSON and WINTER 1964). While deletion of this enzyme is a common mechanism of resistance of these drugs in laboratory cell lines, its occurrence in patient leukemia cells has been disputed (ROSMAN and WILLIAMS 1973). Another proposed mechanism of resistance is increased catabolism of the nucleotides via various alkaline phosphatases (WOLPERT et al. 1971; ROSMAN et al. 1974; SCHOLAR and CALABRESI 1979; LEE et al. 1978a,b). Unfortunately, there are no large scale clinical investigations which address this issue.

Another anabolic step is the conversion of 6-MP and 6-TG to their thiomethyl derivatives via the enzyme thiopurine methyltransferase (TPMT). While these methylated derivatives may be phosphorylated to nucleotides, their cytotoxic capacity has been disputed (ZIMMERMAN et al. 1974; WARNICK and PATERSON 1973). TPMT activity may be inducible during therapy with 6-MP (LENNARD and LILLEYMAN 1987) and may explain a poorer response to therapy (see below).

As mentioned above, 6-MP is metabolized to 6-TG nucleotides in the cell. In an attempt to assess the cellular effect of 6-MP, the concentration of 6-thioguanine nucleotides (6-TGN) can be measured in red blood cells (RBC). In children taking identical doses of 6-MP, wide interpatient variability in RBC 6-TGN has been noted (LENNARD et al. 1986, 1987; LENNARD

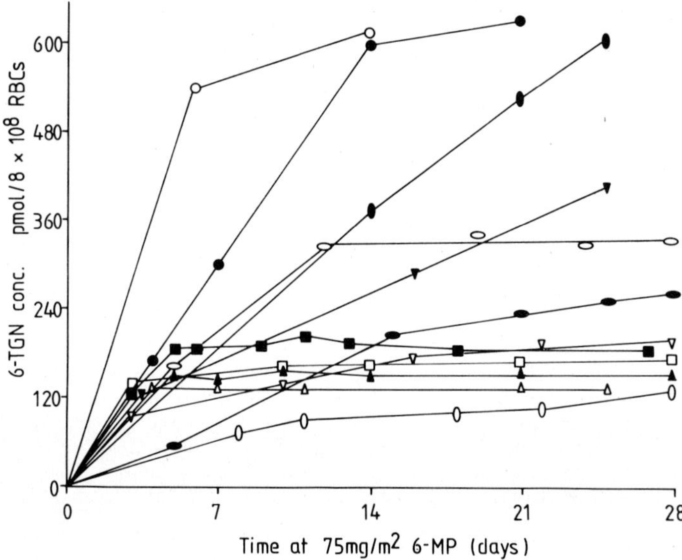

Fig. 4. Interpatient variability of red blood cell (RBC) concentration of 6-thioguanine nucleotides (6-TGN) from the start of 6-mercaptopurine (6-MP) chemotherapy in 12 consecutive children on the UKALL VIII protocol. Six girls (*closed symbols*) and six boys (*open symbols*) were studied. Dose reduction, in response to neutropenia, occurred in four children (○, ●, ●, ▼) before 28 days. Two children (△, ○) subsequently relapsed (Lennard and Lilleyman 1989, p 1816)

and LILLEYMAN 1989). The levels of RBC 6-TGN rather than the dosage of 6-MP most directly correlate with the subsequent myelosuppression (HERBER et al. 1982; LENNARD et al. 1983). Children whose RBC contained low levels of 6-TGN experienced no substantial myelosuppression despite protracted periods of therapy with full doses of 6-MP (LENNARD and LILLEYMAN 1987; LENNARD et al. 1987). The rate and amount of 6-TGN that accumulated in the RBC of 12 children with ALL treated with 75 mg/m^2 daily showed considerable interpatient variability. Five children achieved steady-state concentrations within 4–12 days (median 5 days); the interpatient steady-state concentration varied by about threefold (Fig. 4) (LENNARD and LILLEYMAN 1989). There was no relationship between 6-MP dose or 6-TGN concentration and duration of chemotherapy, age, or WBC count at diagnosis (LENNARD and LILLEYMAN 1989). With a median follow-up of 49 months, 19 of 120 children with ALL had relapsed, and 17 (89%) had 6-TGN below the group median. Figure 5 shows an actuarial difference in relapse-free and event-free survival for 120 children when they are sorted in accordance with RBC 6-TGN levels above and below the median value (LENNARD and LILLEYMAN 1989).

6-MP is catabolized by two enzymes. As mentioned above, xanthine oxidase is present in several organs. It converts 6-MP to 6-thioxanthine and

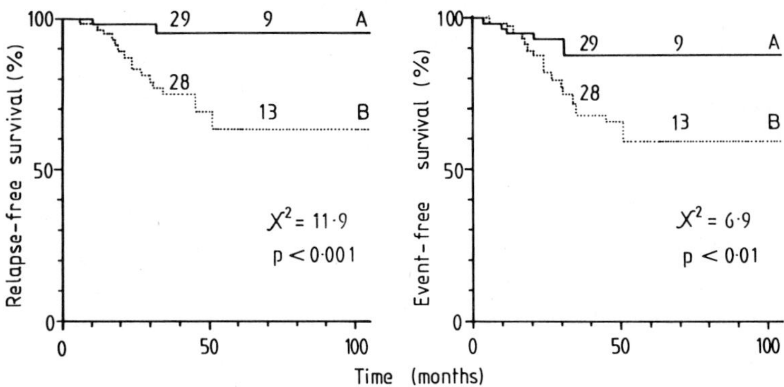

Fig. 5. Actuarial relapse-free survival and event-free survival from the start of 6-mercaptopurine therapy for 120 children in remission when divided at the median red blood cell 6-thioguanine nucleotide concentration (A, $n = 60$ above the median; B, $n = 60$ below). Numbers on the curves indicate the proportion remaining at risk at the time of analysis (LENNARD and LILLEYMAN 1989, p 1816)

then to 6-thiouric acid, which is excreted in the urine. Since many patients treated with 6-MP may also receive concurrent allopurinol, an inhibitor of xanthine oxidase, it has been advised to reduce the dose of 6-MP by at least 25% (some say 50%–75%) and to monitor the blood count carefully (BERNS et al. 1972; ELION et al. 1963a,b). This effect of allopurinol on 6-MP metabolism does not pertain to the intravenously administered drug since this bypasses the first-pass effect of intestinal and liver metabolism (ZIMM et al. 1983b). The 6-TG effect is not increased by allopurinol since 6-TG is converted to 6-thioxanthine by guanase and not xanthine oxidase; thioxanthine is nontoxic (GRANT et al. 1983).

While there is little interindividual or interethnic variation in xanthine orxidase activity, due to genetic polymorphism there can be considerable variability in the activity of a second catabolic enzyme, TPMT (WEINSHILBOUM and SLADEK 1980). An inverse relationship between RBC TPMT and RBC 6-TGN concentrations has been noted, and children with low RBC TPMT appear to be more sensitive to the hematological effects of 6-MP (LENNARD et al. 1987). The selective effects of the thiopurines have been related to differential rates of anabolism and catabolism between tumor tissue and normal organs (MOORE and LEPAGE 1958). Several important schedule-dependent interactions between thiopurines and MTX (BOKKERINK et al. 1988) have been noted in laboratory studies but have not been fully explored clinically.

In summary, while thiopurines have been employed as active anti-leukemia drugs for over 30 years, relatively little is known regarding their precise mechanism of action or of drug resistance and important features of optimal dose and schedule of drug administration. In this regard, progress with these drugs has lagged behind that for other active drugs such as MTX and ara-C.

III. Methotrexate

1. Chemistry

The observation that the vitamin folic acid, then recently discovered, accelerated the growth of leukemia (HEINLE and WELCH 1948) suggested the synthesis of an antifol to chemists at the Lederle Laboratories (SEEGER et al. 1947). The synthesis and clinical trial of aminopterin provided the first rationally synthesized drug, a folate antimetabolite, for the treatment of cancer (FARBER et al. 1948). An analogue, amethopterin (methotrexate, MTX), was then subsequently synthesized (SEEGER et al. 1949) and introduced into clinical trial. While other antifols have since been designed and tested, none have replaced MTX in cancer medicine. The key structural change in folic acid that is responsible for the antitumor effect is the substitution of an amino group for the hydroxyl group at the 4-position of the pteridine ring.

2. Pharmacology

Folic acid exists in many foods, especially leafy vegetables. Intracellularly, folate undergoes extensive biotransformation to the reduced tetrahydrofolate in which form it participates in various one-carbon transfers after undergoing further biotransformation by folate interconverting enzymes (Fig. 6). The three major metabolic functions of the reduced folates are in the synthesis of thymidylate, the purine ring, and the amino acids serine and methionine (HUENNEKENS 1963). The main cellular target of MTX is dihydrofolate reductase (DHFR). By binding to DHFR, MTX reduces the cellular pool of tetrahydrofolates. Studies with various cell lines have linked the cytotoxic effect of MTX to interference with the synthesis of thymidylate (BORSA and WHITMORE 1969) or purines (HRYNIUK et al. 1969). It is highly probable that both effects are active in human neoplasia.

The main cellular determinants of the MTX effect are:

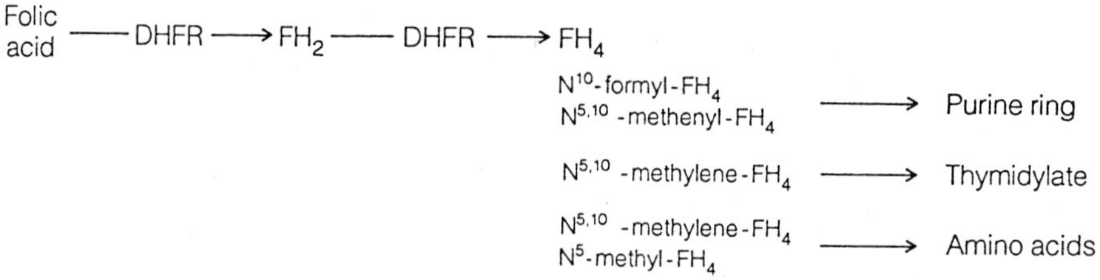

Folic acid —— DHFR ⟶ FH_2 —— DHFR ⟶ FH_4

N^{10}-formyl-FH_4, $N^{5,10}$-methenyl-FH_4 ⟶ Purine ring

$N^{5,10}$-methylene-FH_4 ⟶ Thymidylate

$N^{5,10}$-methylene-FH_4, N^{5}-methyl-FH_4 ⟶ Amino acids

Fig. 6. Transformation pathway of folic acid (FH). Methotrexate inhibits the activity of dihydrofolate reductase (DHFR)

1. Transport.
2. Metabolism to polyglutamates.
3. Level of dihydrofolate reductase (DHFR).
4. Binding to DHFR.

MTX enters the cell by an active, energy-dependent, concentrative process (GOLDMAN et al. 1968). It utilizes the same carrier protein(s) that transport reduced folates into the cell. The K_m for MTX transport in various human and murine cell lines ranges between 1 and 6 μM (GOLDMAN et al. 1968; SIROTNAK and DONSBACH 1976; WARREN et al. 1978; FYFE and GOLDMAN 1973). At very high extracellular drug concentrations, MTX may enter the cell by passive diffusion (WARREN et al. 1978; HILL et al. 1979). This can circumvent presumed "transport resistance" and thus provide part of the rationale for the usage of high-dose MTX protocols.

Once in the cell, MTX is metabolized to polyglutamate forms, adding 1 to 5 glutamate residues in γ-peptide linkage to the glutamate moiety of the MTX structure (GALIVAN 1980; MCGUIRE et al. 1985). The capacity for polyglutamylation varies among different tumor types and organs of the body. Given that the liver is the major storage site for folates, the predominant form found there is the polyglutamate (JACOBS et al. 1977). Metabolism and storage of MTX in the liver may underlie MTX-induced cirrhosis, a consequence of its chronic use. The negative charge of the polyglutamate derivatives of MTX accounts for their cellular retention. Thus, polyglutamylation, in leading to cellular retention, explains the selective antitumor effect of MTX since MTX-sensitive tumor cells polyglutamylate (and retain) MTX better than MTX-sensitive normal tissues such as the intestinal mucosa and bone marrow stem cells. As the polyglutamate form, MTX also affects other enzymes such as thymidylate synthase (ALLEGRA et al. 1985a) and the folate interconverting enzymes (ALLEGRA et al. 1985b).

The enzyme DHFR is the main cellular target for MTX. However, in order to inhibit thymidylate synthesis fully, an excess of "free" or nonDHFR-bound drug is necessary (WHITE et al. 1975). Some tumor cells have been shown to be resistant to MTX due to amplification of the DHFR gene (COWAN et al. 1982; SRIMATKANDADA et al. 1983; KAUFMAN et al. 1978; ALT et al. 1976; TROWSDALE et al. 1980; WOLGEMUTH et al. 1980) or to the synthesis of a DHFR with altered binding affinity to MTX (JACKSON and NIETHAMNER 1977; GOLDIE et al. 1980; FLINTOFF and ESSANI 1980). Unstable MTX resistance (i.e., loss of resistance following serial passage of cells in drug-free medium) has been related to the appearance and subsequent loss of double minute chromosomes containing the DHFR gene (KAUFMAN et al. 1979; CURT et al. 1983). Stable drug resistance corresponds to the appearance of a homogeneously staining region in intact chromosomes (TROWSDALE et al. 1980).

Protracted inhibition of DHFR leads to a cellular buildup of dUMP (FRIDLAND 1974), which in some cells is metabolized to dUTP and incorporated into DNA in place of TTP (GOULIAN et al. 1980; GRAFSTROM et al. 1978). This substitution of uracil for thymine in DNA invokes the activity of a repair enzyme, uracil-DNA glycosylase, which excises the uracil bases, resulting in strand breaks (GRAFSTROM et al. 1978). The relationship of this "DNA damage" to MTX-induced cytotoxicity remains to be determined.

A clinical strategy for the usage of high-dose MTX (gram doses) followed by "leucovorin rescue" is based on various observed possible reasons for MTX resistance:

1. Decreased carrier-mediated transport.
2. Amplification of the DHFR gene.
3. Altered binding affinity of MTX to DHFR.
4. Blood: organ pharmacokinetic barriers (pharmacologic sanctuaries).

As long as leucovorin (folinic acid, ^{5}N-formyltetrahydrofolate) is administered within 36–42 h after MTX administration, vulnerable organs such as the bone marrow and oral and gastrointestinal mucosa can be relatively spared from the cytotoxic effects of MTX (LEVITT et al. 1973). Diminished transport and increased and/or altered binding affinity of DHFR to MTX have been noted. Systemically administered MTX does not gain equal access to all organs of the body; the blood/brain barrier is a well-recognized pharmacologic impediment. The blood/testis barrier may be another. As part of the curative regimen for childhood ALL, intrathecal administration of MTX is important (POPLACK and REAMAN 1988). Alternatively, the administration of gram-doses of MTX followed by leucovorin rescue may provide sufficient drug access so as to eliminate leukemia cells from various pharmacologic sanctuaries (POPLACK and REAMAN 1988).

C. Drugs that Intercalate in DNA

I. Daunorubicin and Doxorubicin

1. Chemistry

Daunorubicin and doxorubicin (Adriamycin) are structurally related anthracycline antibiotics produced from *Streptomyces* species. The two drugs differ chemically by the presence of a hydroxyl function on C-14, in the case of doxorubicin.

2. Pharmacology

Three major mechanisms of action have been advocated: (a) Blockade of DNA and RNA synthesis due to impairment of DNA template activity as a consequence of intercalation of the anthracycline ring between opposing base pairs of nucleotides in the helix (WARING 1970) and interaction with topoisomerase II resulting in increased DNA scission (DEFFIE et al. 1989); (b) alteration in membrane fluidity and ion transport due to the binding of anthracyclines to cell membranes (TRITTON et al. 1978); and (c) formation of semiquinone free radicals (SINHA et al. 1987), catalyzed by cytochrome P-450 reductase in the presence of NADPH, which upon reaction with molecular oxygen can generate superoxide, hydrogen peroxide, and hydroxyl radical. Indeed, superoxide dismutase and catalase have been shown to protect MCF-7 cells from doxorubicin in culture (SINHA et al. 1987). Iron, upon interaction with doxorubicin, has been shown to stimulate the formation of free radicals (MYERS 1976). Doxorubicin binds to iron with a high affinity of 10^{28} to 10^{33}; the resulting iron complex then catalyzes a variety of free radical reactions which may be the basis for anthracycline-induced cardiac toxicity (CHABNER and MYERS 1989). ICRF-187, an iron chelator, has been shown to be selectively cardioprotective against doxorubicin-induced cardiac toxicity (SPEYER et al. 1988). This protection has been achieved without affecting tumor response in animals, suggesting that this mechanism may not be involved with tumor cytotoxicity.

Pleiotropic drug resistance has been shown to occur in cells exposed to anthracyclines. Several mechanisms have been put forward which include (a) increased P-glycoprotein expression through gene amplification (ENDICOTT and LING 1989), (b) decrease in drug-induced, topoisomerase II-mediated DNA cleavage (GANAPATHI et al. 1989; DE JONG et al. 1990), (c) increase in glutathione peroxidase activity (SINHA et al. 1989), and (d) augmented membrane fluidity (BHUSHAN et al. 1989).

Doxorubicin and daunorubicin are administered intravenously. Their pharmacokinetics is complex. Doxorubicin is cleared from plasma in a triphasic mode. The initial $t_{1/2}$ in plasma is 11 min, then an intermediate $t_{1/2}$ of approximately 3 h is followed by a terminal $t_{1/2}$ of 25–28 h (BENJAMIN 1974). It is concentrated in tissues such as the heart, kidney, lung, liver, and spleen. Urinary excretion is low; approximately 4%–5% of the administered dose is eliminated in 5 days. Biliary excretion accounts for 40%–50% of the dose recovered in bile or feces in 7 days (BACHUR 1975). Therefore, impairment of liver function can result in slower excretion and increased retention of anthracyclines in plasma and tissues. Doses of anthracyclines are therefore generally modified, especially in patients with significant elevations of serum bilirubin (>2.5 mg/dl). However, recent studies seem to suggest that the administration of normal doses of doxorubicin in patients with abnormal liver function may not be associated with increased drug toxicity (SULKES and COLLINS 1987).

The anthracyclines are metabolized in liver by the enzyme aldoketo reductase to doxorubicinol and daunorubicinol, which do possess antitumor activity. However, formation of aglycone by hydrolysis leads to an inactive metabolite. Other metabolites include the previously mentioned semiquinone radical formation by the cytochrome P-450 reductase enzyme.

II. Amsacrine

1. Chemistry

Amsacrine is a 9-anilinoacridine derivative developed as a result of structure-activity relationship studies of a large number of acridine analogues as DNA binding agents.

2. Pharmacology

Amsacrine distorts the DNA double helix by intercalation between base pairs of DNA strands and leads to single-stranded and double-stranded breaks. The DNA cleaving enzyme, topoisomerase II, has been shown to form a complex with amsacrine and DNA which then prevents the resealing process of DNA breaks brought about by the normal activity of the enzyme (Pommier et al. 1985; Rowe et al. 1986). Amsacrine-induced and topoisomerase II-mediated DNA strand breaks are maximum during S phase (Markovits et al. 1987), indicating that cells which are not in cycle are relatively less sensitive to the action of amsacrine.

Resistance to amsacrine is perhaps related to an altered topoisomerase II since the enzyme obtained from resistant cells cannot mediate DNA strand breakage in the presence of amsacrine (Pommier et al. 1986).

Amsacrine is administered intravenously. Its plasma clearance is biphasic with a terminal half-life of about 8 h. Approximately 95% of the drug is protein-bound, and thus its penetration through the blood/brain barrier is limited. It is conjugated to glutathione in liver and excreted in bile. Liver impairment can considerably prolong its plasma half-life. A 40% dose reduction is therefore recommended in patients with serum bilirubin greater than 2 mg/100 ml (Chabner and Myers 1989). Urinary excretion of unchanged amsacrine is less than 20%. Renal elimination, although less important, is significant in patients with renal dysfunction and may require a reduction in dosage (Hall et al. 1983).

D. Podophyllotoxin Derivatives

I. Etoposide and Teniposide

1. Chemistry

Podophyllotoxin, an extract of the plant *Podophyllum peltatum* (mandrake or May apple), initially failed as an anticancer drug in clinical trials because of its toxicity. However, two of its semisynthetic glycosides, etoposide (VP-16) and teniposide (VM-26), have shown significant clinical efficacy in the treatment of several types of human cancers including leukemias. The two analogues differ structurally only in a single substitution.

2. Pharmacology

Etoposide and teniposide are similar in their mechanism of action. Both differ from podophyllotoxin which binds to microtubular protein at a site different from that of the vinca alkaloids and causes mitotic arrest (Wilson et al. 1974). The semisynthetic derivatives do not affect microtubular assembly but arrest cells in G_2 phase. They also influence cells in S phase and therefore are only partially cell cycle phase specific. DNA single-strand and double-strand breaks have been shown to occur after intracellular formation of free radical derivatives upon one-electron oxidation due to peroxidase activity (Haim et al. 1986). Recent evidence seems to suggest that these agents induce a ternary complex formation with DNA and topoisomerase II (Glisson and Ross 1987), which is dependent upon the intracellular ionic environment (Lawrence et al. 1989).

Resistance to etoposide and teniposide has been associated with amplification of the multidrug resistance glycoprotein (P-170) pump, which increases drug efflux from the cells (Gupta 1983). Reduced formation of DNA strand breaks due to alterations in topoisomerase II has also been observed in resistant cells (Pommier et al. 1986).

Etoposide is administered either by the oral route or by intravenous infusion, whereas teniposide is usually administered intravenously. Since absorption of etoposide from the oral route is approximately 50%, a twofold increase in dose is required. Plasma clearance of etoposide is biphasic, with a terminal half-life of 11.5 h (Creaven and Allen 1975). The plasma-decay kinetics of teniposide on the other hand is triphasic, with a terminal elimination phase of approximately 20 h. Urinary elimination of both drugs is similar and accounts for about 40% of an administered dose. Approximately 80% of urinary excreted teniposide is in the form of its metabolites, whereas the metabolites of etoposide account for only one-third of the excreted drug. The dosage of etoposide should therefore be adjusted in proportion to changes in creatinine clearance, whereas the dosage of teniposide does not require adjustment for patients with impaired renal function (Sinkule et al. 1984). Both agents are highly protein-bound (>90%), and penetration into the CSF is minimal despite their high lipid solubility.

E. Vinca Alkaloids

I. Vincristine

1. Chemistry

Vincristine and a structurally related compound, vinblastine, have been isolated from the extract of the periwinkle plant (*Vinca rosea*). The two derivatives differ only in a methyl (vincristine) or formyl (vinblastine) side-chain to the parent molecule. Minor changes in the structure of these agents can alter the antitumor activity to a significant extent, such as acetylation of the hydroxyl function, deacetylation, or hydrogenation of the double bond (results in loss of activity).

2. Pharmacology

Both vincristine and vinblastine have a similar mechanism of action, producing mitotic inhibition and metaphase arrest in the cell cycle. Thus, the action of these agents is M phase specific, and therefore they are classified as cell cycle specific agents. The metaphase arrest is caused by a reversible binding of these agents to microtubular protein, tubulin, thus inhibiting its polymerization into microtubules. This action leads to dissolution of the mitotic spindle due to lack of assembly of microtubules (OWELLEN et al. 1976).

Pleiotropic drug resistance arises in cells exposed to vinca alkaloids due to amplification of the membrane glycoprotein P-170 (KARTNER et al. 1983a), which leads to an efflux of the intracellular drug (ENDICOTT and LING 1989). Ca^{2+} channel blockers, such as verapamil, have been shown to reverse this type of resistance (TSUNO 1983). Although vincristine and vinblastine are closely related structurally, cells resistant to vincristine may not be completely cross-resistant to vinblastine (CONTER and BECK 1984). This observation may be related to the specificity in the molecular structure of glycoprotein P-170 induced by each drug.

Vincristine is administered by intravenous bolus injection. It is rapidly cleared from the plasma in a triphasic mode, with a plasma half-life of 0.85, 7.4, and 164 min, followed by a terminal half-life of 24 h (BENDER et al. 1977). Approximately 50% is cleared within 20 min after intravenous administration. Vinca alkaloids bind to plasma proteins and are extensively concentrated in platelets and to a lesser extent in leukocytes and erythrocytes. The major route of excretion (approximately 70% of the administered dose) is via bile into feces (JACKSON et al. 1978). Only about 12% of the administered dose is excreted in urine within 72 h. Vincristine is metabolized in liver, and approximately 50% of the drug excreted in bile is in the form of metabolites. Therefore, a 50% reduction in dosage is indicated in patients with a bilirubin level in plasma greater than 3 mg/dl. Vincristine does not cross the blood/brain barrier in any significant amount.

F. Alkylating/DNA Binding Agents

I. Cyclophosphamide

1. Chemistry

Cyclophosphamide is a derivative of the alkylating agent, mechlorethamine (nitrogen mustard), containing a phosphorus-nitrogen bond, designed for its selective enzymatic hydrolysis in tumor cells leading to release of the active nitrogen mustard moiety. However, cyclophosphamide is extensively metabolized in liver, and the formation of 4-hydroxycyclophosphamide by cytochrome P-450 mixed-function oxidase is a necessary step to produce active metabolites (SLADEK 1988).

2. Pharmacology

The 4-hydroxycyclophosphamide and its tautomeric form, aldophosphamide, are transported to the target cells where they are converted nonenzymatically to active metabolites, phosphoramide mustard and acrolein. The 4-hydroxy metabolite is further oxidized enzymatically to 4-ketocyclophosphamide, an inactive metabolite. The aldophosphamide, on the other hand, is inactivated by aldehyde dehydrogenase to carboxyphosphamide. The phosphoramide mustard is then believed to act as an alkylating agent in a manner similar to other drugs belonging to this class (LUDLUM 1977). The chloroethyl side-chain undergoes cyclization to form a highly reactive ethyleneimmonium intermediate which can then react with the nucleophilic groups through formation of a carbonium ion. Alkylation of the N-7 position of guanine residues in DNA seems to relate to the cytotoxic effects. Following covalent bond formation with one side-chain, the second 2-chloroethyl group undergoes a similar cyclization followed by alkylation with a receptor molecule. The alkylation of DNA leads to interstrand cross-links and DNA-protein cross-links. Acrolein, on the other hand, has been shown to cause single-strand breaks in DNA (CROOK et al. 1986). It has also been implicated in the etiology of hemorrhagic cystitis.

It appears that the cytotoxic effects of cyclophosphamide are related to the total amount of the reactive metabolites produced rather than the rate of production. Therefore, drugs that modify the activity of the hepatic microsomal enzymes do not affect overall therapeutic efficacy, whereas those affecting the rate of inactivation of the reactive metabolites may alter the biological actions. The intracellular concentration of aldehyde dehydrogenase is comparatively lower in tumor cells than in normal cells, which may provide selectivity of cytotoxic action of phosphoramide mustard in tumor cells. In fact, some resistant tumor cells have been shown to contain elevated levels of aldehyde dehydrogenase (HILTON 1984).

Resistance to cyclophosphamide may involve glutathione metabolism. Glutathione depletion has been shown to be a determinant of sensitivity of human leukemic cells to cyclophosphamide and its metabolites (CROOK et al. 1986).

II. Carboplatin

1. Chemistry

Carboplatin (CBDCA, JM-8, Paraplatin) is an analogue of the platinum coordination complex cisplatin, developed as a result of extensive structure-activity relationship studies in an effort to reduce toxicity and retain efficacy of the parent compound. Chemically, it is *cis*-diammine (1,1-cyclobutanedicarboxylato) platinum II and is significantly less reactive than cisplatin.

2. Pharmacology

Carboplatin and cisplatin have similar mechanisms of action. Both require aquation reaction leading to hydrolysis of the parent compounds to form activated species which then bind to DNA. Hydrolysis of carboplatin is slower than that of cisplatin and causes removal of the bidentate cyclobutanedicarboxylato group. After binding to DNA these agents cause equal total cross-links, interstrand cross-links, and cytotoxicity (KNOX et al. 1986). The larger doses of carboplatin required to produce these effects are related to the much faster rate of hydrolysis of cisplatin to produce the activated species. Immunocytochemical techniques have also demonstrated a linear relationship between dose and DNA adduct formation, observed by nuclear staining density, with both carboplatin and cisplatin (TERHEGGEN et al. 1988). The DNA cross-links produced by these agents can be prevented by the presence of other nucleophiles such as sulfhydryl groups. Attempts have been made to administer various thiol-containing compounds along with cisplatin in an effort to reduce the toxicity (ototoxicity and nephrotoxicity). Whether such a rescue process could be utilized with carboplatin to reduce the bone marrow toxicity needs further investigation.

Since the mechanism of action of carboplatin and cisplatin is similar, one would expect cross-resistance between the two drugs. The mechanism of resistancc to these agents is not yet clearly understood. Resistance to cisplatin has been associated with elevated levels of intracellular glutathione or metallothionine (ENDRESSEN et al. 1984), decreased drug uptake, and increased DNA repair (DEGRAEFF et al. 1988).

Carboplatin is administered as an intravenous infusion over 30–60 min. The plasma concentration of total platinum declines in a biexponential fashion, with alpha and beta half-lives of 20–60 min and 450–1200 min, respectively (VANECHO et al. 1989). Most of the drug in plasma is ultrafilterable and is excreted through the kidneys within the first 8 h after drug administration. By 24 h, approximately 50%–70% of the dose is eliminated in the urine. Because of carboplatin's reduced plasma protein binding and extensive renal elimination, dose modification in patients with compromised renal function may be necessary. A direct relationship between the AUC of plasma ultrafilterable platinum and the percentage of reduction in platelets has been demonstrated (VANECHO et al. 1989), suggesting that monitoring of plasma levels may be important in renal insufficiency to prevent thrombocytopenia. Combinations of carboplatin and cisplatin may balance the toxicities of each drug and allow safe administration of therapeutic doses (MUGGIA 1989).

G. Adrenal Glucocorticoids

I. Prednisone

1. Chemistry

Prednisone is a synthetic steroidal congener of the natural adrenal hormone hydrocortisone (cortisol). This group of compounds is known as corticosteroids or glucocorticoids. Prednisone is one of the most important drugs of this class used effectively in combination chemotherapy of lymphocytic leukemias.

2. Pharmacology

Corticosteroids influence a variety of physiological effects such as carbohydrate, protein, and lipid metabolism, mineralocorticoid activity, antiinflammatory activity, and immunological responses. Although their precise mechanism of action is not clearly understood, they are known to bind to a cytosolic receptor protein. The steroid-receptor complex is then translocated to the nucleus and regulates the transcription of specific genes by binding to DNA. The steroid-receptor complex causes the release of a phosphorylated protein, a heat-shock protein (90000 dalton), in the cytosol. This protein may play a significant role in translocation of the complex and/or its interaction with DNA (LITWACK 1988).

The steroid-binding domain in the receptor protein is known to act as a repressor in the promoter region of the genes. The glucocorticoid, after binding to the receptor, inhibits the repressing activity, thus resulting in an enhancement of transcription (GODOWSKI et al. 1988). The presence of significantly higher numbers of glucocorticoid receptors in leukemic lymphoblasts than in normal ones perhaps explains the specificity of the antitumor effects of corticosteroids for lymph-derived neoplasms (LIPPMAN et al. 1978). These studies have directly correlated the number of receptors with the duration of CR after corticosteroid induction therapy.

Prednisone is well absorbed after oral administration and possesses activity of a short duration of less than 24h. Its plasma half-life is 3.5h, whereas the biologic half-life is twice as much. Approximately 75% of its concentration in plasma is bound to plasma proteins, mostly globulin and albumin.

Corticosteroids are extensively metabolized in the liver. Reduction of the 4,5 double bond has been shown to occur at both hepatic and extrahepatic sites. This results in production of an inactive metabolite. Similarly, reduction of the 3-keto function to a 3-hydroxy group in the liver followed by conjugation with sulfate or glucuronic acid results in the formation of water-soluble inactive metabolites which are excreted in urine. Prednisone, however, requires reduction of the 11-keto function to produce a pharmacologically active compound, prednisolone. Reduction of the 20-ketone group, on the other hand, produces an inactive metabolite.

H. Enzymes

I. Asparaginase

1. Chemistry

Asparaginase enzymes catalyze the conversion of the amino acid L-asparagine to aspartic acid and ammonia. Although L-asparagine is commonly considered a nonessential amino acid, some types of leukemia and cancer lack this synthetic capacity and are thus dependent on extracellular sources for protein synthesis. While the enzyme does not enter the cell, it degrades all the circulating asparagine to aspartic acid which, in turn, cannot be converted to asparagine by these cancers. In contrast, most normal cells can synthesize asparagine from aspartic acid. Thus, asparaginase exploits a metabolic difference between normal and cancer cells and provides a relative degree of pharmacologic selectivity.

2. Pharmacology

The possibility of asparaginase treatment stemmed from the observation of KIDD (1953) that certain mouse and rat lymphomas were destroyed by guinea pig serum, a property that was not shared by rabbit or horse serum. In these experiments, the guinea pig serum was used as a source of complement to enhance the antigen-antibody reaction between tumor cells and rabbit antilymphoma antiserum (KIDD 1953). Other unrelated developments during this period provided further intriguing information. Certain experimental neoplasms, the Walker carcinosarcoma 256 and the L5178Y leukemia, were found to require asparagine, an amino acid previously considered nonessential, to support growth in tissue culture (CAPIZZI et al. 1970; COONEY and HANDSCHUMACHER 1970). When BROOME proved that asparaginase was the active antitumor component of guinea pig serum (BROOME 1963), many investigators screened microorganisms for a more practical source of this enzyme. The next major advance came in 1964 when asparaginase from *Escherichia coli* was shown to be as effective as guinea pig serum in treating these tumors (MASHBURN and WRISTON 1964). This finding allowed the production of large quantities of pure enzyme for preclinical and clinical trials (CAMPBELL et al. 1967; HO et al. 1970; ROBERTS et al. 1966; WHELAN and WRISTON 1969). Preparations were sought with the following properties: (1) high activity and stability in blood; (2) low K_m for asparagine since circulating levels of this amino acid are only about 40 μM; (3) selective hydrolysis of asparagine; (4) no inhibition or reversibility by the high concentrations of products of the enzyme reaction that build up in the circulation; (5) slow clearance from the circulation; (6) easy purification and elimination of endotoxin; and (7) no or low antigenicity. While very effective drugs have been discovered, not all of these properties have been universally achieved.

Asparaginase was found to have antitumor activity against more than 50 mouse neoplasms, rat Murphy-Sturm and canine lymphosarcomas, rat fibrosarcoma, Walker carcinosarcoma 256, and Jensen sarcoma (CAPIZZI et al. 1970; CAPIZZI and CHENG 1981; WRISTON 1985; WRISTON and YELLIN 1973). The initial clinical trials in ALL using partially purified guinea pig serum and *E. coli* asparaginase were very promising (DOLOWY et al. 1967; HILL et al. 1967; OETTGEN et al. 1967). Although occasional patients with AML, nonHodgkin's lymphoma, and chronic leukemias responded, most solid tumors are not affected by asparaginase treatment (CLARKSON et al. 1970; CROWTHER 1971; MARMONT and DAMASIO 1970; MATHE et al. 1969). Laboratory observations of the marked sensitivity of T-cell-derived tumor cells relative to the less sensitive B-cell neoplasms (KOISHI et al. 1984; OHNUMA et al. 1982) have not been explored in clinical trials. Extensive monographs detailing the early development of asparaginase are available (CAPIZZI et al. 1970; COONEY and HANDSCHUMACHER 1970).

Although asparaginase enzymes have been isolated and characterized from many gram-negative bacteria, mycobacteria, yeasts, molds, plants, and vertebrates (WRISTON and YELLIN 1973; WRISTON 1985; YUREK et al. 1983), not all were found to have oncolytic activity. Only the asparaginase derived from the serum of the guinea pig and other members of the superfamily Cavioidea and bacterial asparaginase from *E. coli*, *Erwinia chrysanthemi* (formerly called *Erwinia carotovora*), *Vibrio succinogenes*, and *Serratia marcescens* had activity against lymphomas (DISTASIO et al. 1976; WADE et al. 1968). At present, only the enzymes from *E. coli* and *Erwinia chrysanthemi* are used clinically. Their properties are shown in Table 7.

These asparaginases are composed of 4 identical subunits with one active site per subunit. The asparaginases from two *Erwinia chrysanthemi* strains and *E. coli* and *Acinetobacter* glutaminase-asparaginase have been

Table 7. Properies of therapeutic asparaginases. (From CAPIZZI and HOLCENBERG (1991)

	Activity[a] (IU/mg protein)	K_m (μM)		Ratio maximal activity	Molecular weight	pI	Half-life (h)
		l-Asn	l-Gln	l-Gln/l-Asn			
E. coli	280–400	12	3000	0.03	141 000	5.0	8–44
Erwinia	650–700	15	1400	0.10	138 000	8.7	7–13

L-Asn, L-asparagine; L-Gln, L-glutamine; pI, isoelectric point.
[a] One IU hydrolyzes one micromole of asparagine per minute.

sequenced, and their crystallographic structure is being determined (Maita et al. 1974; Minton et al. 1986; Tanaka et al. 1988). The deduced sequence from *Erwinia* asparaginase includes a leader peptide that signals export from the bacteria to the periplasmic space. There is considerable homology between these sequences. The threonine that covalently binds the glutamine analogue DON (6-diazo-5-oxo-L-norleucine) to two glutaminase-asparaginase enzymes lies within an N-terminal, 8-amino-acid segment of 5 different asparaginases and glutaminases (Holcenberg et al. 1978; Tanaka et al. 1988). A threonine at residue 118 of *E. coli* asparaginase that is part of the binding site of the asparagine analogue DONV (5-diazo-4-oxo-L-norvaline) is conserved in the three enzymes that have been sequenced through this region (Peterson et al. 1977).

E. coli and *Erwinia* asparaginases differ greatly in their isoelectric point. Chemical modifications of *Erwinia* asparaginase that decrease the isoelectric point prolong its half-life in animals (Rutter and Wade 1971). The substrate specificity of both enzymes is restricted to 4- and 5-carbon L- or D-amino acids. Enzyme activity does not appear to be affected by high levels of the products of asparagine hydrolysis, aspartic acid and ammonia (Schwartz et al. 1970). The purification (Wriston 1985) and properties of these enzymes have been extensively reviewed (Capizzi et al. 1970; Capizzi and Cheng 1981; Cooney and Handschumacher 1970; Whelan and Wriston 1969; Wriston and Yellin 1973; Wriston 1985). They have most of the ideal properties that were sought: high activity and stability, a low K_m for asparagine, not inhibited by aspartic acid or ammonia (Schwartz et al. 1970), and readily purified and freed from endotoxin. They are similar in size to gamma-globulins. Both enzymes hydrolyze L-glutamine as well as L-asparagine. Although the maximal rate of hydrolysis of L-glutamine is only 3%–9% of that of L-asparagine and the K_m is 100 times greater or more, high doses of these enzymes will deplete circulating glutamine in animals and patients (Miller et al. 1969).

Therapeutic trials of amidohydrolases with high glutaminase and asparaginase activities have revealed a wider spectrum of antitumor activity. *Acinetobacter* glutaminase-asparaginase was chemically modified with succinic anhydride to prolong its half-life in the circulation. This enzyme causes more neurotoxicity and inhibition of protein synthesis than the asparaginase enzymes with low glutaminase activity (Spiers and Wade 1976; Holcenberg et al. 1979; Warrell et al. 1980). Thus, some of the toxicity of these asparaginase enzymes may be caused by glutamine depletion. Furthermore, L-glutamine is a competitive substrate for these asparaginases. Since the plasma levels of L-glutamine are 10 times higher than those of L-asparagine, the relative effect on the plasma asparagine content is greater for those enzymes that hydrolyze both substrates. Thus, an enzyme with no glutaminase activity may have more selectivity and less toxicity. Guinea pig asparaginase has no glutaminase activity, but insufficient quantities are available for clinical trials. *V. succinogenes* asparaginase was originally reported to have very low glutaminase activity, but further studies showed that this was similar to the *E. coli* enzyme activity.

The antitumor activity of asparaginase enzymes is mediated by the depletion of asparagine from the plasma, which, in turn, deprives auxotrophic cells and tissues of their only source of the amino acid. The most prompt biochemical effect of asparaginase is the hydrolysis of plasma asparagine to aspartic acid and ammonia. Plasma asparagine is essentially undetectable throughout the entire period in which asparaginase is present. The plasma level of asparagine is normally tightly controlled by the liver (WOODS and HANDSCHUMACHER 1971, 1973), and there appears to be a rigorous homeostatic control of the plasma concentration of the amino acid in a variety of disease states by endogenous asparaginase activity in the liver and kidneys. Many normal and neoplastic cells concentrate asparagine by an active transport process to levels 2–10 times that in the plasma. Most normal human cells have the ability to synthesize asparagine by induction of the enzyme asparagine synthetase (HASKELL et al. 1969b; PRAGER and BACHYNSKY 1968). Tumors sensitive to asparaginase lack this enzyme activity and are dependent on exogenous sources of L-asparagine. Most tissues have low or undetectable asparagine synthetase activity. This is caused by a feedback control of its synthesis by the high asparagine concentrations in the circulation and in cells. As the circulating levels of asparagine fall following asparaginase treatment, asparagine synthetase activity is induced in normal tissues. Asparagine synthetase activity in asparaginase-resistant tumors may be present before treatment or be induced by treatment. Thus, measurement of asparagine synthetase prior to treatment with asparaginase is usually not predictive of response. Mammalian asparagine synthetase has been cloned and sequenced (ANDRULIS and BARRETT 1989; GRECO et al. 1989). This gene has been identified as one of the causes of temperature-sensitive growth arrest and appears to be regulated in the cell cycle. Methylation of cytosine residues in DNA seems related to the degree of expression of this enzyme. For example, cells with high asparagine synthetase activity have a gene with a 5' region that is less methylated than in those with low activity. 5-Azacytidine, which decreases methylation of cytosine residues in genes, can reactivate asparagine synthetase activity in cells. NYCE (1989) and AVRAMIS and coworkers (CRANE et al. 1989) have recently shown that ara-C and other antitumor drugs increase the methylation of cytosines in DNA. These drugs may be able to lower the activity of asparagine synthetase and thus enhance sensitivity to asparaginase treatment. This effect may relate the observed preclinical (SCHWARTZ et al. 1982) and clinical (CAPIZZI et al. 1988) synergy noted between high-dose ara-C and asparaginase.

BROOME (1968) showed that at 1 and 3 h after treatment, the free asparagine concentration in both asparaginase-sensitive and -resistant murine lymphomas fell to about one-sixth of the normal level. Protein synthesis rapidly decreased, followed by a fall in DNA and RNA synthesis. While these parameters remained suppressed in the asparaginase-sensitive tumors, in asparaginase-resistant tumor cells, the asparagine concentration increased within 1–2 days, and the rate of protein synthesis recovered. This change corresponds to the time course of induction of asparagine synthetase activity (Woods and Handschumacher 1971). Similar effects on macromolecular synthesis occurred in normal tissues; protein synthesis recovered as asparagine synthetic activity increased.

Half-maximal growth of an asparaginase-sensitive lymphoma occurred at extracellular asparagine concentrations of about 1 μM. This is 3% of the normal circulating level and the lower level of detection by most methods of amino acid analysis (Uren and Handschumacher 1977). It is not known how much lower asparagine levels must be for optimal kill of circulating cells. The concentration of asparagine in the intercellular spaces may be of even greater importance. Since asparaginase is largely confined to the vascular space, asparagine is primarily depleted in the interstitial spaces by diffusion of the amino acid into the circulation. Because of the intrinsic glutaminase activity of asparaginase, plasma levels of glutamine are temporarily depressed or eliminated, and the levels of glutamic acid are correspondingly elevated (Cooney and Handschumacher 1970).

In man, asparaginase enzymes from *E. coli* and *Erwinia chrysanthemi* have a wide range of circulating half-lives (7–44 h). The current commercial *E. coli* preparation from Merck has a longer half-life (mean 23 h) than earlier *E. coli* preparations from Bayer (mean 11 h) or the *Erwinia chrysanthemi* enzyme (mean 10 h) (Capizzi et al. 1971; Capizzi and Cheng 1981; Haskell et al. 1970, 1972, 1969a; Ho et al. 1970; Ohnuma et al. 1970; Schwartz et al. 1970). The half-life is independent of the dose administered, age, sex, disease status, and extent of hepatic or renal function (Schwartz et al. 1970; Wriston and Yellin 1973). Various chemical modifications have been employed in order to alter the half-life in the circulation and mask the antigenic determinants. The most extensively studied altered enzyme is PEG-asparaginase. This is formed by covalent attachment through succinate linkages of monomethoxypolyethylene glycol (PEG) to *E. coli* asparaginase. PEG-asparaginase has similar kinetic properties to the native *E. coli* enzyme but has decreased immunogenicity and a prolonged serum half-life (Abuchowski et al. 1984; Ho et al. 1986; Viau et al. 1986). Initial clinical trials show that it is safe and effective even in patients with a prior allergy to the native enzyme (Jurgens et al. 1988; Kurtzberg et al. 1990). The prolonged half-life of PEG-asparaginase allows lower doses and less frequent administration.

Some 18–24 h after intravenous injection of 10, 200, 1000, and 5000 IU/kg of the *E. coli* enzyme, plasma levels of 0.1–0.4, 2–6, 14–27, and 57–70 IU/ml are achieved, respectively (Capizzi et al. 1971; Schwartz et al. 1970). Daily administration of the same dose achieves a sustained or slightly cumulative plasma level, and after cessation of therapy, measurable plasma levels may persist for 10 or more days. If administered intramuscularly, the peak plasma level is about one-half that following intravenous administration (CAPIZZI and CHENG 1981). The volume of distribution is slightly greater than the plasma volume. The enzyme activity in lymphatic fluid is 5%–20% that in plasma; in interstitial fluid it is about 10% and in cerebrospinal fluid, less than 0.5% of that in plasma (HO et al. 1971).

J. Multidrug Resistance

The acute leukemias in approximately 5%–10% of patients display resistance to standard induction therapy: prednisone, vincristine, and daunorubicin for ALL; ara-C and daunorubicin for AML. This drug resistance is evident at the outset as a failure to achieve CR. Of those patients who do enter CR, 20%–80% will eventually relapse. While second or third remissions may be achieved with the same or different chemotherapy, the remissions are usually of short duration (weeks to months), and the leukemias subsequently display resistance to further therapy. Thus, de novo or acquired drug resistance is a major obstacle to the cure of the acute leukemias. Specific biochemical mechanisms involved in this resistance have been discussed above with each drug group.

Recent studies of drug resistance in various cell culture lines have revealed a multidrug resistance (MDR) phenotype, a phenomenon of substantial clinical interest (BEIDLER and RIEHM 1970; LING and THOMPSON 1973). In this situation, the development of resistance to one drug automatically conferred cross-resistance to unrelated drugs with divergent chemical structures. The feature these drugs share in common is that they are all natural products either derived from fermentation of various bacterial species or extracted from plants.

The MDR phenotype has been related to the presence of a 170-kDa glycoprotein in the plasma membrane (P-glycoprotein) (JULIANO and LING 1976; KARTNER et al. 1983b). It functions as an active, ATP-dependent pump which effects the outward efflux of various drugs from cells. A number of reviews have recently appeared in the literature on P-glycoprotein (JURANKA et al. 1989) and on the pharmacology of drugs that alter MDR in cancer cells (FORD and HAIT 1990).

Multidrug-resistant cells have been shown to contain an amplified gene (*mdr* gene) that codes for the P-glycoprotein (SCOTTO et al. 1986). The sequence of the cDNA that codes for human P-glycoprotein has been analyzed (CHEN et al. 1986), and the cDNAs that code for different P-glycoproteins have also been identified (VANDER BLICK et al. 1987). The structure of P-glycoprotein consists of two homologous halves, each containing a hydrophobic and a hydrophilic domain. Each half has a nucleotide binding region in the hydrophilic domain. The single polypeptide chain contains about 1280 amino acids (JURANKA et al. 1989).

The calcium channel blocker verapamil is prototypic of various drugs that can compete with the cytotoxic drug for the binding site on P-glycoprotein and in so doing can reverse MDR (Ford and Hait 1990). These agents which reverse the MDR phenotype have been referred to as "chemosensitizers." Although there has been a rapid emergence of information related to MDR and the drugs capable of reversing the effects of P-glycoprotein, the role of P-glycoprotein in determining a patient's overall response to chemotherapy is still unknown. Recent studies have shown raised levels of P-glycoprotein in different forms of human cancers such as leukemias, lymphomas, sarcomas, and carcinomas. This is especially evident in tumor biopsies obtained after relapse from chemotherapy. However, increased P-glycoprotein levels were also observed in certain tumor specimens even before the initiation of chemotherapy (Goldstein et al. 1989). The possibility of using "chemosensitizers" in patients refractory to chemotherapy who have an increased P-glycoprotein concentration is under active investigation. Other biochemical features related to the MDR phenotype have been described and constitute areas of fruitful investigation in pharmacology and drug development (Ross et al. 1989).

References

Abuchowski A, Kazo GM, Verhoest CJ Jr et al. (1984) Cancer therapy with chemically modified enzymes: I. Antitumor properties of polyethylene glycol-asparaginase conjugates. Cancer Biochem Biophys 7:175–186 (Abstract)

Allegra CJ, Chabner BA, Drake JC, Lutz R, Robard D, Jolivet J (1985a) Enhanced inhibition of thymidylate synthase by methotrexate polyglutamates. J Biol Chem 260:9720–9726

Allegra CJ, Drake JC, Jolivet J, Chabner BA (1985b) Inhibition of phosphoribosylaminoimidazolecarboxamide transformylase by methotrexate and dihydrofolic acid polyglutamates. Proc Natl Acad Sci USA 82:4881–4885

Alt FW, Kellems RE, Schimke RT (1976) Synthesis and degradation of folate reductase in sensitive and methotrexate-resistant lines of S180 cells. J Biol Chem 251:3063–3074

Amadori S, Papa G, Avvisati G (1984) Sequential combination of systemic high-dose ara-C and asparaginase for the treatment of central nervous system leukemia and lymphoma. J Clin Oncol 2:98–101

Andrulis IL, Barrett MT (1989) DNA methylation patterns associated with asparagine synthetase expression in asparagine-overproducing and -auxotrophic cells. Mol Cell Biol 9:2922–2927

Bach M (1969) Biochemical and genetic studies of a mutant strain of mouse leukemia L1210 resistant to 1-β-D-arabinofuranosylcytosine (cytarabine) hydrochloride. Cancer Res 29:1036–1044

Bachur NR (1975) Adriamycin (NSC 123127) pharmacology. Cancer Chemother Rep 6:153

Beidler JL, Riehm H (1970) Cellular resistance to actinomycin D in Chinese hamster cells in vitro: cross-resistance, radioautographic, and cytogenetic studies. Cancer Res 30:1174–1184

Bender R, Castle M, Martiletter D, Oliverio V (1977) The pharmacokinetics of H-vincristine in man. Clin Pharmacol Ther 22:430–438

Benjamin RS (1974) Pharmacokinetics of adriamycin in patients with sarcomas. Cancer Chemother Rep 58:271–273

Berns A, Rubenfeld S, Rymzo WT (1972) Hazard of combining allopurinol and thiopurine. N Engl J Med 286:730–731

Bhushan A, Kermode JC, Posada J, Tritton TR (1989) Anthracycline resistance. Kluwer, Boston, pp 55–72

Bokkerink JPM, Bakker MA, Hulscher TW, De Abreu RA, Schretlen DAM (1988) Purine de novo synthesis as the basis of synergism of methotrexate and 6-mercaptopurine in human malignant lymphoblasts of different lineages. Biochem Pharmacol 37:2321–2327

Borsa J, Whitmore GF (1969) Studies relating to the mode of action of methotrexate: II. Studies on sites of action on L cells in vitro. Mol Pharmacol 5:303–317

Brockman RW (1963) Mechanism of resistance to anticancer agents. Adv Cancer Res 7:129–234

Broome JD (1963) Evidence that the L-asparaginase of guinea pig serum is responsible for its antilymphoma effects. J Exp Med 118:99–120

Broome JD (1968) Studies on the mechanism of tumor inhibition by L-asparaginase. J Exp Med 127:1055–1072

Brunchede H, Krooth RS (1973) Studies on the xanthine oxidase activity of mammalian cells. Biochem Genet 8:341–350

Burner RC, Low PS (1985) Identification and partial characterization of xanthine oxidase transitions of the milk fat globule membrane. Arch Biochem Biophys 240:60–69

Burton NK, Barnett MJ, Aherne G, Evans J, Douglas I, Lister TA (1986) The effect of food on the oral administration of 6-mercaptopurine. Cancer Chemother Pharmacol 18:90–91

Camiener GW (1968) Studies of the enzymatic deamination of ara-cytidine-V. Inhibition in vitro and in vivo by tetrahydrouridine and other reduced pyrimidine nucleosides. Biochem Pharmacol 17:1981–1991

Campbell HA, Mashburn LT, Boyse EA, Old LJ (1967) Two L-asparaginase from *E. coli* B., their separation, purification and antitumor activity. Biochem Genet 6:721–730

Capizzi RL, Cheng YC (1981) Therapy of neoplasia with asparaginase. In: Holcenberg JS, Roberts J (eds) Enzymes as drugs. Wiley, New York, pp 1–24

Capizzi RL, Holcenberg JS (1991) Asparaginase. In: Holland JF, Frei E (eds) Cancer medicine. Lea and Febiger, Philadelphia

Capizzi RL, Powell BL (1987) Sequential high dose ara-C and asparaginase versus high dose ara-C alone in the treatment of patients with relapsed and refractory acute leukemias. Semin Oncol 14[Suppl 1]:40–50

Capizzi RL, Bertino JR, Handschumacher RE (1970) L-asparaginase. Ann Rev Med 21:433

Capizzi RL, Bertino JR, Skeel RT et al. (1971) L-Asparaginase: clinical, biochemical, pharmacological and immunological studies. Ann Intern Med 74:893–901

Capizzi RL, Yang JL, Cheng T et al. (1983) Alteration of the pharmacokinetics of high dose araC by its metabolite, high araU in patients with acute leukemia. J Clin Oncol 1:763–771

Capizzi RL, Poole M, Cooper MR et al. (1984) Treatment of poor risk acute leukemia with sequential high dose ara-C and asparaginase. Blood 63:694–700

Capizzi RL, Yang JL, Rathmell JP et al. (1985) Dose-related pharmacologic effects of high dose ara-C and its self-potentiation. Semin Oncol 12[Suppl 3]:65–75

Capizzi RL, Davis R, Powell B et al. (1988) Synergy between high-dose cytarabine and asparaginase in the treatment of adults with refractory and relapsed acute myelogenous leukemia – a cancer and leukemia group B study. J Clin Oncol 6:499–508

Carrico CK, Sartorelli AC (1977) Effects of 6-thioguanine on macromolecular events in regenerating rat liver. Cancer Research 37:1868–1875

Cass CE, Gaudette LA, Paterson ARP (1974) Mediated transport of nucleosides in human erythrocytes. Specific binding of the inhibitor nitrobenzythioinosine to nucleoside transport sites in the erythrocyte membrane. Biochim Biophys Acta 345:1–10

Chabner BA, Myers CE (1989) Clinical pharmacology of cancer chemotherapy. Lippincott, Philadelphia, p 377

Chandrasekaran B, Capizzi RL, Kute TE, Morgan T, Dimling J (1989) Modulation of the metabolism and pharmacokinetics of 1-β-D-arabinofuranosylcytosine by 1-β-D-arabinofuranosyluracil in leukemic mice. Cancer Res 49:3259–3266

Chen CJ, Chin JE, Veda K et al. (1986) Internal duplication and homology to bacterial transport proteins in the *mdr* (P-glycoprotein) gene from multidrug-resistant human cells. Cell 47:381–389

Chu MY, Fischer GA (1965) Comparative studies of leukemic cells sensitive and resistant to cytosine arabinoside. Biochem Pharmacol 14:333–341

Chu MY, Fischer GA (1968) The incorporation of ^{3}H-cytosine arabinoside and its effects on murine leukemia cells. Biochem Pharmacol 17:753–767

Clarkson B, Krakoff I, Burchenal J et al. (1970) Clinical results of treatment with *E. coli* L-asparaginase in adults with leukemia, lymphorma, and solid tumors. Cancer 25:279

Conter V, Beck WT (1984) Acquisition of multiple drug resistance by CCRF-CEM cells selected for different degrees of resistance to vincristine. Cancer Treat Rep 68:831–836

Cooney DA, Handschumacher RE (1970) L-Asparaginase and L-asparagine metabolism. Ann Rev Pharmacol 10:421–440

Cowan KH, Goldsmith ME, Levine RM et al. (1982) Dihydrofolate reductase gene amplification and possible rearrangement in estrogen responsive methotrexate-resistant human breast cancer cells. J Biol Chem 257:15079–15086

Crane LR, Jackson R, Avramis VI (1989) DNA hypermethylation studies in CEM/O cells after treatment with therapeutic and sub-therapeutic concentrations of cytosine arabinoside (ara-C). Proc Am Assoc Cancer Res 30:496 (abstr)

Creaven PJ, Allen LM (1975) EPEG, a new antineoplastic epipodophyllotoxin. Clin Pharmacol Ther 19:221–226

Crook TR, Souhami RL, McLean AEM (1986) Cytotoxicity, DNA cross-linking and single strand breaks induced by activated cyclophosphamide and acrolein in human leukemic cells. Cancer Res 46:5029–5034

Crowther D (1971) L-asparaginase and human malignant disease. Nature 229:168–171

Curt GA, Carney DN, Cowan KH et al. (1983) Unstable methotrexate resistance in human small-cell carcinoma associated with double-minute chromosomes. N Engl J Med 308:199–202

Danhauser LL, Rustum YM (1980) Effect of thymidine on the toxicity, antitumor activity, and metabolism of 1-β-D-arabinofuranosylcytosine in rats bearing a chemically induced colon carcinoma. Cancer Res 40:1274–1280

Davidson JD, Winter TS (1964) Purine nucleotide pyrophosphorylases in 6-mercaptopurine-sensitive and -resistant human leukemias. Cancer Res 24:261–267

Deffie AM, Batra JK, Goldenberg GJ (1989) Direct correlation between DNA topoisomerase II activity and cytotoxicity in Adriamycin-sensititive and -resistant P388 leukemia cell lines. Cancer Res 49:58–62

DeGraeff A, Slebos RJC, Rodenhuis S (1988) Resistance to cisplatin and analogues: mechanisms and potential clinical implications. Cancer Chemother Pharmacol 22:325–332

De Jong A, Zijlstra JG, De Vries EGE, Mulder NH (1990) Reduced DNA topoisomerase II activity and drug-induced DNA cleavage activity in an Adriamycin-resistant human small cell lung carcinoma cell line. Cancer Res 50:304–309

Distasio JA, Niederman RA, Kafkewitz D, Goodman D (1976) Purification and characterization of L-asparaginase with anti-lymphoma activity from *Vibrio succinogenes*. J Biol Chem 251:6929–6933

Dolowy WC, Elrod LM, Ammeraal RN, Schrek R (1967) Toxicity of L-asparaginase to resistant and susceptible lymphoma cells in vitro. Proc Soc Exp Biol Med 125:598–601

Drewinko B, Ho DHW, Barranco SC (1972) The effects of arabinosylcytosine on cultured human lymphoma cells. Cancer Res 32:2737–2742

Elion GB, Hitchings GH (1955) The synthesis of 6-thioguanine. J Am Chem Soc 77:1676

Elion GB, Burgi E, Hitchings GH (1952) Studies on condensed pyrimidine systems: IX. The synthesis of some 6-substituted purines. J Am Chem Soc 74:411–418

Elion GB (1967) Biochemistry and pharmacology of purine analogs. Fed Proc 26:898–904

Elion GB, Callahan S, Nathan H, Bieber S, Rundles RW, Hitchings GH (1963a) Potentiation by inhibition of drug degradation: 6-substituted thiopurines and xanthine oxidase. Biochem Pharmacol 12:85–93

Elion GB, Callahan S, Rundles RW, Hitchings GH (1963b) Relationship between metabolic fates and anticancer activities of thiopurines. Cancer Res 23:1207–1217

Ellison RR (1982) Acute myelocytic leukemia. In: Holland JF, Frei E (eds) Cancer medicine. Lea and Febiger, Philadelphia, pp 1407–1446

Endicott JA, Ling V (1989) The biochemistry of P-glycoprotein-mediated multidrug resistance. Annu Rev Biochem 58:137–172

Endressen L, Schjerven L, Rugstad HE (1984) Tumours from a cell strain with a high content of metallothionein show enhanced resistance against cisdichlorodiammineplatinum. Acta Pharmacol Toxicol 55:183–187

Farber S, Diamond LK, Mercer RD, Sylvester RF Jr, Wolff JA (1948) Temporary remissions in acute leukemia in children produced by folic acid antagonist, 4-aminopteroyl-glutamic acid (Aminopterin). N Engl J Med 238:787

Flintoff WF, Essani K (1980) Methotrexate-resistant Chinese hamster ovary cells contain a dihydrofolate reductase with an altered affinity for methotrexate. Biochemistry 19:4321–4327

Ford JM, Hait WN (1990) Pharmacology of drugs that alter multidrug resistance in cancer. Pharmacol Rev 42:155–199

Fridland A (1974) Effect of methotrexate on deoxynucleotide pools and DNA synthesis in human lymphocyte cells. Cancer Res 34:1883–1888

Fyfe MJ, Goldman ID (1973) Characteristics of the vincristine-induced augmentation of methotrexate uptake in Ehrlich ascites tumor cells. J Biol Chem 248:5067–5073

Gale RP (1979) Advances in the treatment of acute myelogenous leukemia. N Engl J Med 300:1189–1199

Galivan J (1980) Evidence for the cytotoxic activity of polyglutamate derivatives of methotrexate. Mol Pharmacol 17:105–110

Ganapathi R, Grabowski D, Ford J, Heiss C, Kerrigan D, Pommier Y (1989) Progressive resistance to doxorubicin in mouse leukemia L1210 cells with multidrug resistance phenotype: reductions in drug-induced topoisomerase II-mediated DNA cleavage. Cancer Commun 1:217–224

Glisson BS, Ross WE (1987) DNA topoisomerase II: a primer on the enzyme and its unique role as a multidrug target in cancer chemotherapy. Pharmacol Ther 32:89–106

Godowski PJ, Picard D, Yamamoto KR (1988) Signal transduction and transcriptional regulation by glucocorticoid receptor-LexA fusion proteins. Science 241:812–816

Goldie JH, Krystal G, Hartley D, Andauskas G, Dedhar S (1980) A methotrexate-insensitive variant of folate reductase present in two lines of methotrexate-resistant L5178Y cells. Eur J Cancer 16:1539–1546

Goldman ID, Lichtenstein NS, Oliverio VT (1968) Carrier-mediated transport of the folic acid analogue, methotrexate, in the L1210 leukemia cell. J Biol Chem 243:5007–5017

Goldstein LJ, Galski H, Fojo A et al. (1989) Expression of a multidrug resistance gene in human tumors. J Natl Cancer Inst 81:116–124

Goulian M, Bleile B, Tseng BY (1980) Methotrexate induced misincorporation of uracil into DNA. Proc Natl Acad Sci USA 77:1956–1960

Grafstrom RH, Tseng BY, Goulian M (1978) The incorporation of uracil into animal cell DNA in vitro. Cell 15:131–140

Grant DM, Tang BK, Kalow W (1983) Variability in caffeine metabolism. Clin Pharmacol Therapeut 33:591–602

Greco A, Gong SS, Ittmann M, Basilico C (1989) Organization and expression of the cell cycle gene, ts11, that encodes asparagine synthetase. Mol Cell Biol 9:2350–2359

Gunz FW, Henderson ES (1983) Leukemia 4th edn. Grune & Stratton, New York

Gupta RS (1983) Genetic, biochemical, and cross-resistance studies with mutants of Chinese hamster ovary cells resistant to the anticancer drugs VM-26 and VP16-213. Cancer Res 43:1568–1574

Haim N, Roman J, Nemec J (1986) Peroxidative free radical formation and demethylation of etoposide (VP-16) and teniposide (VM-26). Biochem Biophys Res Commun 135:215–220

Hall SW, Friedman J, Legha SS, Benjamin RS, Gutterman JU, Loo TL (1983) Human pharmacokinetics of a new acridine derivative, 4'-(9-acridinylamino) methanesulfon-*m*-anisdide (NSC 249992). Cancer Res 43:3422–3426

Harris AW, Reynolds EC, Finch LR (1979) Effect of thymidine on the sensitivity of cultured mouse tumor cells to 1-β-D-arabinofuranosylcytosine. Cancer Res 5:67–82

Haskell CM, Canellos GP, Leventhal BG, Carbone PP, Block JB (1969a) L-Asparaginase: therapeutic and toxic effects in patients with neoplastic disease. N Engl J Med 2810:1028–1034

Haskell CM, Canellos GP, Leventhal BG, Carbone PP, Block JB (1969b) L-Asparaginase resistance in human leukemia-asparagine synthetase. Biochem Pharmacol 18:2578–2580

Haskell CM, Canellos GP, Cooney DA, Hansen HH (1970) Biochemical and pharmacologic effects of L-asparaginase in man. J Lab Clin Med 75:763–770

Haskell CM, Canellos GP, Cooney DA, Hardesty CT (1972) Pharmacologic studies in man with crystallized L-asparaginase. Cancer Chemother Rep 56:611–614

Heinle RW, Welch AD (1948) Experiments with pteroylglutamic acid and pteroylglutamic acid deficiency in human leukemia. J Clin Invest 27:539

Herber S, Lennard L, Lilleyman JD, Maddocks JL (1982) 6-Mercaptopurine: apparent lack of relation between prescribed dose and biological effect in children with leukemia. Br J Cancer 46:138–141

Hill BT, Bailey BD, White JC, Goldman ID (1979) Characteristics of transport of 4-amino antifolates and folate compounds by two lines of L5178Y lymphoblasts, one with impaired transport of methotrexate. Cancer Res 39:2440–2446

Hill DL, Bennett LL Jr (1969) Purification and properties of 5-phosphoribosyl pyrophosphate amidotransferase from adenocarcinoma 758 cells. Biochemistry 8:122–130

Hill JM, Roberts J, Loeb E, Khan A, MacLellan A, Hill RB (1967) L-Asparaginase therapy for leukemia. JAMA 202:882–888

Hilton J (1984) Role of aldehyde dehydrogenase in cyclophosphamide-resistant L1210 leukemia. Cancer Res 44:5156–5160

Ho DHW, Frei E (1971) Clinical pharmacology of 1-β-D-arabinofuranosylcytosine. Clin Pharmacol Ther 12:944–954

Ho DHW, Thetford B, Carter CJK, Frei E III (1970) Clinical pharmacologic studies of L-asparaginase. Clin Pharmacol Ther 11:408–417

Ho DHW, Carter CJK, Thetford B, Frei E III (1971) Distribution and mechanism of clearance of L-asparaginase (NSC-109229). Cancer Chemother Rep 55:539–545

Ho DH, Brown NS, Yen A et al. (1986) Clinical pharmacology of polyethylene glycol-L-asparaginase. Drug Metab Disp 14:349–352

Holcenberg JS, Ericsson L, Roberts J (1978) Amino acid sequence of the diazo-oxo-norleucine binding site of *Acinetobacter* and *Pseudomonas* 7-A glutaminase-asparaginase enzymes. Biochemistry 17:411–417

Holcenberg JS, Borella LD, Camitta BM, Ring BJ (1979) Human pharmacology and toxicology of succinylated *Acinetobacter* glutaminase-asparaginase. Cancer Res 39:3145–3151

Huennekens FM (1963) The role of dihydrofolic reductase in the metabolism of one-carbon units. Biochemistry 2:151

Jackson DV, Castle MC, Bender RA (1978) Billiary excretion of vincristine. Clin Pharmacol Ther 24:101–107

Jackson RC, Niethamner D (1977) Acquired methotrexate resistance in lymphoblasts resulting from altered kinetic properties of dihydrofolate reductase. Eur J Cancer 13:567–575

Jacobs SA, Derr CJ, Johns DG (1977) Accumulation of methotrexate diglutamate in human liver during methotrexate therapy. Biochem Pharmacol 26:2310–2313

Juliano RL, Ling V (1976) A surface glycoprotein modulating drug permeability in Chinese hamster ovary cell mutants. Biochem Biophys Acta 455:152

Juranka PF, Zastawny RL, Ling V (1989) P-glycoprotein: multidrug-resistance and a superfamily of membrane-associated transport proteins. FASEB J 3:2583–2592

Jurgens H, Schwamborn D, Korholz D, Wahn V, Gobel U (1988) Klinische Erfahrungen mit polyathylenglykol-gekoppelter *E. coli*-L-asparaginase bei Patienten mit ALL-Mehrfachrezidiv. Klin Padiatr 200:184–189

Kartner N, Shales M, Riordan JR (1983a) Daunorubicin-resistant Chinese hamster ovary cells expressing multidrug resistance and a cell-surface P-glycoprotein. Cancer Res 43:4413–4419

Kartner N, Riordan JR, Ling V (1983b) Cell surface P-glycoprotein as associated with multidrug resistance in mammalian cell lines. Science 221:1285–1288

Kaufman RJ, Bertino JR, Schimke RT (1978) Quantitation of dihydrofolate reductase in individual parental and methotrexate-resistant murine cells: use of a fluorescence activated cell sorter. J Biol Chem 253:5852–5860

Kaufman RJ, Brown PC, Schimke RT (1979) Amplified dihydrofolate reductase genes in unsteady methotrexate-resistant cells are associated with double minute chromosomes. Proc Natl Acad Sci USA 76:5669–5673

Kessel D, Hall TC, Wodinsky I (1967) Transport and phosphorylation as factors in the antitumor action of cytosine arabinoside. Science 156:1240–1241

Kidd JG (1953) Regression of transplanted lymphomas induced in vivo by means of normal guinea pig serum. J Exp Med 98:565–582

Knox RJ, Friedlos R, Lydall DA, Roberts JJ (1986) Mechanism of cytotoxicity of anticancer platinum drugs: evidence that *cis*-diamminedichloroplatinum (II) and *cis*-diammine (1,1-cyclobutanedicarboxylato) platinum (II) differ only in the kinetics of their interaction with DNA. Cancer Res 46:1972–1979

Koishi T, Minowada J, Henderson ES, Ohnuma T (1984) Distinctive sensitivity of some T-leukemia cell lines to L-asparaginase. Gann 75:275–283

Kurtzberg J, Friedman H, Asselin B et al. (1990) The use of polyethylene glycol-conjugated L-asparaginase in pediatric patients with prior hypersensitivity to native L-asparaginase. Proc Am Soc Clin Oncol 9:219 (abstr)

Lampkin BC, Nagao T, Mauer AM (1971) Synchronization and recruitment in acute leukemia. J Clin Invest 50:2204–2214

Lawrence TS, Canman CE, Maybaum J, Davis MA (1989) Dependence of etoposide-induced cytotoxicity and topoisomerase II-mediated DNA strand breakage on the intracellular ionic environment. Cancer Res 49:4775–4779

Lazarus HM, Herzig RH, Herzig GP, Phillips GL, Roessmann U, Fishman DJ (1981) Central nervous system toxicity of high-dose systemic cytosine arabinoside. Cancer 48:2577–2582

Leclerc JM, Cheng YC (1985) Purification and characterization of a human myeloblast DNA exonuclease activity which could remove 1-β-D-arabinofuranosylcytosine (ARAC) from DNA with ARAC at 3'terminal. Proc Am Assoc Cancer Res 26:52 (abstr)

Lee MH, Huang YM, Sartorelli AC (1978a) Alkaline phosphatase activities of 6-thiopurine-sensitive and -resistant sublines of sarcoma 180. Cancer Res 38:2413–2418

Lee MH, Huang YM, Sartorelli AC (1978b) Immunological studies on alkaline phosphatases of 6-thiopurine-sensitive and -resistant sublines of sarcoma 180. Cancer Res 38:2419–2423

Lennard L, Lilleyman JS (1987) Are children with lymphoblastic leukaemia given enough 6-mercaptopurine? Lancet 3:785–787

Lennard L, Lilleyman JS (1989) Variable mercaptopurine metabolism and treatment outcome in childhood lymphoblastic leukemia. J Clin Oncol 7:1816–1823

Lennard L, Rees CA, Lilleyman S, Maddocks JL (1983) Childhood leukaemia: a relationship between intracellular 6-mercaptopurine metabolites and neutropenia. Br J Clin Pharmacol 16:359–363

Lennard L, Keen D, Lilleyman JS (1986) Oral 6-mercaptopurine in childhood leukemia: parent drug pharmacokinetics and active metabolite concentration. Clin Pharmacol Ther 40:287–292

Lennard L, Van Loon JA, Lilleyman JS, Weinshilboum RM (1987) Thiopurine pharmacogenetics in leukaemia: correlation of erythrocyte thiopurine methyltransferase activity and 6-thioguanine nucleotide concentration. Clin Pharmacol Ther 41:18–25

Levitt M, Mosher MB, DeConti RC et al. (1973) Improved therapeutic index of methotrexate with "leucovorin rescue". Cancer Res 33:1729–1734

Lilleyman JS, Lennard L, Rees CA, Morgan G, Maddocks JL (1984) Childhood lymphoblastic leukaemia: sex difference in 6-mercaptopurine utilization. Br J Cancer 49:703–707

Ling V, Thompson CH (1973) Reduced permeability in CHO cells as a mechanism of resistance to colchicine. J Cell Physiol 83:103–116

Lippman ME, Yarbro GIK, Leventhal BG (1978) Clinical implications of glucocorticoid receptors in human leukemias. Cancer Res 38:4251–4256

Litwack G (1988) The glucocorticoid receptor at the protein level. Cancer Res 48:2636–2640

Ludlum DB (1977) Alkylating agents and the nitrosoureas. In: Becker FF (ed) Cancer: a comprehensive treatise, 5th edn. Plenum, New York, pp 285–307

Markovits J, Pommier Y, Kerrigan D (1987) Topoisomerase II-mediated DNA breaks and cytotoxicity in relation to cell proliferation and the cell cycle in NIH 3T3 fibroblasts and L1210 leukemia cells. Cancer Res 47:2050–2055

Marmont AM, Damasio EE (1970) Recent results in cancer research. Cancer Res 33:296 (abstr)

Mashburn LT, Wriston JC (1964) Tumor inhibitory effect of L-asparaginase from *Escherichia coli*. Arch Biochem Biophys 105:451–452

Mathe G, Amiel JL, Schwarzenberg L et al. (1969) Essai de traitment de la leucemie aigue lymphoblastique par la L-asparaginase. La Presse Med 77:461–463 (Abstract)

McGuire JJ, Mini E, Hsieh P, Bertino JR (1985) Role of methotrexate polyglutamates in methotrexate and sequential methotrexate-5-fluorouracil-mediated cell kill. Cancer Res 45:6395–6400

Melvin WT, Keir HM (1979) Interaction of 6-thiopurines and thiol containing RNA with a cellulose mercurial. Analytical Biochemistry 92:324–330

Meyers MB, Kreis W (1978) Comparison of enzymatic activities of two deoxycytidine kinases purified from cells sensitive (P815) or resistant (P815/ara-C) to 1-β-D-arabinofuranosylcytosine. Cancer Res 38:1105–1112

Miller HK, Salser JS, Balis ME (1969) Amino acid levels following L-asparaginase amidohydrolase (EC.3.5.1.1) therapy. Cancer Res 29:183–187

Mills-Yamamoto C, Luzon GJ, Paterson ARP (1978) Toxicity of combinations of arabinosylcytosine and 3-deazuridine toward neoplastic cells in culture. Biochem Pharmacol 27:181–186

Minton NP, Bullman HMS, Scawen MD, Atkinson T, Gilbert HJ (1986) Nucleotide sequence of the *Erwinia chrysanthemi* NCPPB 1066 L-asparaginase gene (recombinant DNA; M13 phage vector; amino acid sequencing; signal peptide, codon utilization; NIF sequence). Gene 46:25–35

Momparler RL, Chu MY, Fischer GA (1968) Studies on a new mechanism of resistance of L5178Y murine leukemia cells to cytosine arabinoside. Biochim Biophys Acta 161:481–493

Moore EC, LePage G (1958) The metabolism of 6-thioguanine in normal and neoplastic tissues. Cancer Res 18:1075–1083

Muggia FM (1989) Overview of carboplatin: replacing, complementing, and extending the therapeutic horizons of cisplatin. Semin Oncol 16:7–13

Myers CE (1976) Role of iron in anthracycline action. In: Hacker MP, Lazo JS, Tritton TR (eds) Organ-directed toxicities of anticancer drugs. Nijhoff, Boston, pp 17–30

Nelson JA, Carpenter JW, Rose LM et al. (1975) Mechanisms of action of 6-thioguanine, 6-mercaptopurine and 8-azaguanine. Cancer Research 35:872

Nyce J (1989) Drug-induced DNA hypermethylation and drug resistance in human tumors. Cancer Res 49:5829–5836

Oettgen HF, Old LJ, Boyse EA et al. (1967) Inhibition of leukemias in man by L-asparaginase. Cancer Res 27:2619–2631

Ohnuma T, Holland JF, Freeman A, Sinks LF (1970) Biochemical and pharmacological studies with asparaginase in man. Cancer Res 30:2297–2305

Ohnuma T, Arkin H, Takahashi I, Andrejczuk A, Roboz J, Holland JF (1982) Biochemical bases of the differential susceptibility of malignant immune cells to asparaginase and to cytosine arabinoside. In: Arnott MS, van Eys J, Wang YM (eds) Molecular interrelations of nutrition and cancer. Raven, New York, pp 105–121

Owellen RJ, Hartke CA, Dickerson RM (1976) Inhibition of tubulin-microtubule polymerization by drugs of the vinca alkaloid class. Cancer Res 36:1499–1502

Peterson RG, Richardson FF, Handschumacher RE (1977) Structure of peptide from active site region of *Escherichia coli* L-asparaginase. J Biol Chem 252:2072–2076

Plagemann PGW, Wohlhueter RM (1984) Inhibition of the transport of adenosine, other nucleosides and hypoxanthine in Novikoff rat hepatoma cells by methylxanthines, papaverine, N_6-cyclohexyladenosine and N^6-phenylisopropyladenosine. Biochem Pharmacol 33:1783–1788

Plagemann PGW, Marz R, Wohlhueter RM (1978) Transport and metabolism of deoxycytidine and 1-β-D-arabinofuranosylcytosine into cultured Novikoff rat hepatoma cells, relationship to phosphorylation, and regulation of triphosphate synthesis. Cancer Res 38:978–989

Pommier Y, Minford JK, Schwartz RE (1985) Effects of the DNA intercalators 4'-(9-acridinylamino) methanesulfon-*m*-anisidide and 2-methyl-9-hydroxyellipticinium on topoisomerase-II-mediated DNA strand cleavage and strand passage. Biochemistry 24:6410–6416

Pommier Y, Kerrigan D, Schwartz R, Swack JA, McCurdy A (1986) Altered DNA topoisomerase II activity in Chinese hamster cells resistant to topoisomerase II inhibotors. Cancer Res 46:3075–3081

Poplack DG, Reaman GH (1988) Acute lymphoblastic leukemia in childhood. In: Poplack DG (ed) Pediatric clinic of north america, the Leukemias. WB Saunders, Philadelphia, pp 903–932

Powis G (1983) Metabolism, therapeutic effect, on toxicity of anticancer drugs in man. Drug Metab Rev 14:1145–1163

Prager MD, Bachynsky N (1968) Asparagine synthetase in normal and malignant tissues; correlation with tumor sensitivity to asparaginase. Arch Biochem Biophys 127:645–654

Rama-Reddy GV, Goulian M (1971) Inhibition of *E. coli* DNA polymerase II by ara-CTP. Nature 234:286–288

Rees CA, Lennard L, Lilleyman JS, Maddocks JL (1984) Disturbance of 6-

mercaptopurine metabolism by cotrimoxazole in childhood lymphoblastic leukaemia. Cancer Chemother Pharmacol 12:87–89

Roberts J, Prager MD, Bachynsky N (1966) The antitumor activity of *Escherichia coli* L-asparaginase. Cancer Res 26:2213–2217

Rosman M, Williams HE (1973) Leukocyte purine phosphoribosyl transferases in human leukemia sensitive and resistant to 6-thiopurines. Cancer Res 33:1202–1209

Rosman M, Lee ML, Creasey WA (1974) Mechanisms of resistance to 6-thiopurines in human leukemia. Cancer Res 34:1952

Ross WE, Sullivan DM, Chow KC (1989) Altered function of DNA topoisomerases as a basis for anti-neoplastic drug action. In: DeVita VT, Hellman S, Rosengerg SA (eds) Important advances in oncology, 5th edn. Lippincott, Philadelphia

Rowe TC, Chen GL, Hsiang YH (1986) DNA damage by antitumor acridines mediated by mammalian DNA topoisomerase-II. Cancer Res 46:2021–2026

Rustum YM (1978) Metabolism and intracellular retention of 1-β-D-arabinofuranosylcytosine as predictors of response of animal tumors. Cancer Res 38:543–549

Rutter DA, Wade HE (1971) The influence of isoelectric point of L-asparaginase upon its persistence in the blood. Br J Exp Pathol 52:610–614

Scholar EM, Calabresi P (1979) Increased activity of alkaline phosphatases in leukemic cells from patients resistant to thiopurines. Biochem Pharmacol 28:445–446

Schwartz MK, Lash ED, Oettgen HF, Tomao FA (1970) L-Asparaginase activity in plasma and other biological fluids. Cancer 25:244–252

Schwartz SA, Morgenstern B, Capizzi RL (1982) Schedule-dependent synergy and antagonism between high-dose 1-β-D-arabinofuranosylcytosine and asparaginase in the L5178Y murine leukemia. Cancer Res 42:2191–2197

Scotto KW, Biedler JL, Mclora PW (1986) Amplification and expression of genes associated with multidrug resistance in mammalian cells. Science 232:751–755

Seeger DR, Smith JM Jr, Hultquist ME (1947) Antagonist for pteroylglutamic acid. J Am Chem Soc 69:2567

Seeger DR, Cosulich DB, Smith JM Jr, Hultquist MD (1949) Analogs of pteroylglutamic acid: III. 4-amino derivatives. J Am Chem Soc 71:753

Sinha BK, Katki AG, Batist G (1987) Differential formation of hydroxyl radicals by adiramycin in sensitive and resistant MCF-7 human breast cells: implication for the mechanism of action. Biochemistry 26:3776–3781

Sinha BK, Mimnaugh EG, Rajagopalan S, Myers CE (1989) Adriamycin activation and oxygen free radical formation in human breast tumor cells: protective role of glutathione peroxidase in adriamycin resistance. Cancer Res 49:3844–3848

Sinkule JA, Stewart CF, Crom WR, Melton ET, Dahl GV, Evans WE (1984) Teniposide (VM-26) disposition in children with leukemia. Cancer Res 44:1235–1237

Sirotnak FM, Donsbach RC (1976) Kinetic correlates of methotrexate transport and therapeutic responsiveness in murine tumors. Cancer Res 36:1151–1158

Sladek NE (1988) Metabolism of oxazaphosphorines Pharmacol Ther 37:301

Slevin ML, Piall EM, Aherne GW, Johnston A, Sweatman MC, Lister TA (1981) The pharmacokinetics of subcutaneous cytosine arabinoside in patients with acute myelogenous leukemia. Br J Clin Pharmacol 12:507–510

Speyer JL, Green MD, Ward C (1988) A trial of ICRF-1878 to selectively protect against chronic adriamycin cardiac toxicity: rationale and preliminary result of a clinical trial. In: Hacker MP, Lazo JS, Tritton TR (eds) Organ directed toxicities of anti-cancer drugs. Nijhoff, Amsterdam, pp 64–76

Spiers ASD, Wade HE (1976) Bacterial glutaminase in treatment of acute leukemia. Br Med J 1:1317–1319

Srimatkandada S, Medina WD, Cashmore AR et al. (1983) Amplification and organization of dihydrofolate reductase in a human leukemic cell line, K-562, resistant to methotrexate. Biochemistry 22:5774–5781

Stewart CD, Burke PJ (1971) Cytidine deaminase and development of resistance to arabinosyl cytosine. Nature 233:109–110

Sulkes A, Collins JM (1987) Reappraisal of some dosage adjustment guidelines. Cancer Treat Rep 71:229–233

Tanaka S, Robinson EA, Appella E et al. (1988) Structure of amidohydrolases. Amino acid sequence of a glutaminase-asparaginase from *Acinetobacter glutaminasificans* and preliminary crystallographic data for an asparaginase from *Erwinia chrysantemi*. J Biol Chem 263:8583–8591

Tattersall MHN, Ganeshaguru K, Hoffbrand AV (1974) Mechanisms of resistance of human acute leukemia cells to cytosine arabinoside. Br J Haematol 27:39–46

Terheggen PMAB, Dijkman R, Begg AC et al. (1988) Monitoring of interaction products of *cis*-diammine-dichloroplatinum (II) and *cis*-diammine (1,1-cyclobutamedicarboxylato) platinum II with DNA in cells from platinum-treated cancer patients. Cancer Res 48:5597–5603

Theiss JC, Fischer GA (1976) Inhibition of intracellular pyrimidine ribonucleotide reduction by deoxycytidine, arabinosylcytosine and hydroxyurea. Biochem Pharmacol 25:73–79

Tidd DM, Patterson ARP (1974) A biochemical mechanism for the delayed cytotoxic reaction of 6-mercaptopurine. Cancer Res 34:738–7460

Tritton TR, Murphree SA, Sartorelli AC (1978) Adriamycin: a proposal on the specificity of drug action. Biochem Biophys Res Commun 84:802

Trowsdale J, Hoch JA, Francke U (1980) A methotrexate-resistant subline of mouse L1210 leukemia cells containing high levels of dihydrofolate reductase and with a homogenously staining region on chromosome 4. Oncodev Biol Med 1:369–374

Tsuno T (1983) Reversal of acquired resistance to vinca alkaloids and anthracycline antibiotics. Cancer Treat Rep 67:889–893

Uren JR, Handschumacher RE (1977) Enzyme therapy. In: Becker FF (ed) Cancer – comprehensive treatise. Plenum, New York, pp 457–487

VanDer Blick AM, Baas F, Ten Houte de Lange T (1987) The human *mdr*3 gene encodes a novel P-glycoprotein homologue and gives rise to alternatively spliced mRNAs in liver. EMBO J 6:3325–3331

Van Diggelen OP, Donahue TF, Shin SL (1979) Basis for differential cellular sensitivity to 8-azaguanine and 6-thioguanine. J Cell Physiol 98:59–72

VanEcho DA, Egorin MJ, Aisner J (1989) The pharmacology of carboplatin. Semin Oncol 16:1–6

Viau AT, Abuchowski A, McCoy JR, Kazo GM, Davis FF (1986) Toxicologic studies of a conjugate of asparaginase and polyethylene glycol in mice, rats, and dogs. Am J Vet Res 47:1398–1401

Wade HE, Elsworth R, Herbert D, Keppie J, Sargeant K (1968) A new L-asparaginase with antitumor activity. Lancet 2:776–777

Walsh CT, Craig RT, Agarwal RP (1980) Increased activation of 1-β-D-arabinofuranosylcytosine by hydroxyurea in L1210 cells. Cancer Res 40:3286–3292

Wan SH, Hoffman DH, Azarnoff DL (1974) Pharmacokinetics of 1-β-D-arabinofuranosylcytosine in humans. Cancer Res 34:392–397

Waring M (1970) Variation of the supercoils in closed circular DNA by binding of antibiotics and drugs: evidence for molecular models involving intercalation. J Mol Biol 54:247

Warnick CT, Paterson ARP (1973) Effect of methylthioinosine on nucleotide concentrations in L5178Y cells. Cancer Res 33:1711–1715

Warrell RP, Chou TC, Gordon C, Tan C, Roberts J (1980) Phase I evaluation of succinylated *Aotinobacter* glutaminase-asparaginase in adults. Cancer Res 39:3145–3151

Warren RD, Nichols AP, Bender RA (1978) Membrane transport of methotrexate in human lymphoblastoid cells. Cancer Res 38:668–671

Weinshilboum RM, Sladek SL (1980) Mercaptopurine pharmacogenetics: monogenic

inheritance of erythrocyte thiopurine methyltransferase activity. Am J Hum Genet 32:651–662
Weinstein HJ, Griffin TW, Feeney J, Cohen HJ, Propper RD, Sallan SE (1982) Pharmacokinetics of continuous intravenous and subcutaneous infusions of cytosine arabinoside. Blood 59:1351–1353
Whelan HA, Wriston JC Jr (1969) Purification and properties of asparaginase from *Escherichia coli* B. Biochemistry 8:2386–2393
White JC, Loftfield S, Goldman ID (1975) The mechanism of action of methotrexate: III. Requirement of free intracellular methotrexate for maximal suppression of [^{14}C]formate incorporation into nucleic acids and protein. Mol Pharmacol 11:287–297
White JC, Rathmell JP, Capizzi RL (1987) Membrane transport influences the rate of accumulation of cytosine arabinoside in human leukemia cells. J Clin Invest 79:380–387
Wiley JS, Jones SP, Sawyer WH, Paterson ARP (1982) Cytosine arabinoside influx and nucleoside transport sites in acute leukemia. J Clin Invest 69:479–489
Wiley JS, Jones SP, Sawyer WH (1983) Cytosine arabinoside transport by human leukemia cells. Eur J Cancer Clin Oncol 19:1067–1074
Wilson L, Bamburg JT, Mizel SB, Grisham LM, Crewell KM (1974) Interaction of drugs with microtubule proteins. Fed Proc 33:158–166
Wolgemuth DJ, Biedler JL, Melera PW (1980) Repetitive DNA sequences in methotrexate- and methasquin-sensitive and -resistant Chinese hamster cell lines. Biochem Genet 18:655–667
Wolpert MK, Damle SP, Brown JE, Sznycer E, Argrawal KC, Sartorelli AC (1971) The role of phosphohydrolases in the mechanism of resistance to 6-thiopurines. Cancer Res 31:1620–1626
Woods JS, Handschumacher RE (1971) Hepatic homeostasis of plasma L-asparagine. Am J Physiol 221:1785–1790
Woods JS, Handschumacher RE (1973) Hepatic regulation of plasma L-asparagine. Am J Physiol 224:740–745
Wriston JC Jr (1985) Asparaginase. Methods Enzymol 113:608–617
Wriston JC Jr, Yellin TO (1973) L-Asparaginase: a review. Adv Enzymol 39:185–248
Yang JL, Cheng EH, Capizzi RL, Cheng YC, Kute T (1985) Effect of uracil arabinoside on metabolism and cytotoxicity of cytosine arabinoside in L5178Y murine leukemia. J Clin Invest 75:141–146
Yurek E, Peru D, Wriston JC Jr (1983) On the distribution of plasma L-asparaginase. Experientia 39:383–385
Zimm S, Collins JM, Riccardi R et al. (1983a) Variable bioavailability of oral 6-mercaptopurine: is maintenance chemotherapy in acute lymphoblastic leukaemia being optimally delivered? N Engl J Med 308:105–109
Zimm S, Collins JM, O'Neill D, Chabner BA, Poplack DG (1983b) Inhibition of first-pass metabolism in cancer chemotherapy: interaction of 6-mercaptopurine and allopurinol. Clin Pharmacol Ther 34:810–817
Zimmerman TP, Chu LC, Bugge CJL, Nelson DJ, Lyon GM, Elion GB (1974) Identification of 6-methylmercaptopurine ribonucleoside 5'-diphosphate and 5'-triphosphate as metabolites of 6-mercaptopurine in man. Cancer Res 34:221–224
Zittoun R, Zittoun J, Marquet J, Rustum Y, Creaven P (1985) Modulation of 1-β-D-arabinofuranosylcytosine metabolism by thymidine in human acute leukemia. Cancer Res 45:5186–5192

Subject Index

Handbook of Experimental Pharmacology

Volume 57
Tissue Growth Factors

Volume 58
Cyclic Nucleotides

Part 1: **Biochemistry**

Part 2: **Physiology and Pharmacology**

Volume 59
Mediators and Drugs in Gastrointestinal Motility

Part 1: **Morphological Basis and Neurophysiological Control**

Part 2: **Endogenous and Exogenous Agents**

Volume 60
Pyretics and Antipyretics

Volume 61
Chemotherapy of Viral Infections

Volume 62
Aminoglycoside Antibiotics

Volume 63
Allergic Reactions to Drugs

Volume 64
Inhibition of Folate Metabolism in Chemotherapy

Volume 65
Teratogenesis and Reproductive Toxicology

Volume 66
Part 1: **Glucagon I**

Part 2: **Glucagon II**

Volume 67
Part 1: **Antibiotics Containing the Beta-Lactam Structure I**

Part 2: **Antibiotics Containing the Beta-Lactam Structure II**

Volume 68
Antimalarial Drugs

Part 1: **Biological Background, Experimental Methods and Drug Resistance**

Part 2: **Current Antimalarias and New Drug Developments**

Volume 69
Pharmacology of the Eye

Volume 70
Part 1: **Pharmacology of Intestinal Permeation I**

Part 2: **Pharmacology of Intestinal Permeation II**

Volume 71
Interferons and Their Applications

Volume 72
Antitumor Drug Resistance

Volume 73
Radiocontrast Agents

Volume 74
Antieliptic Drugs

Volume 75
Toxicology of Inhaled Materials

Volume 76
Clinical Pharmacology of Antiangial Drugs

Volume 77
Chemotherapy of Gastrointestinal Helminths

Volume 78
The Tetracyclines

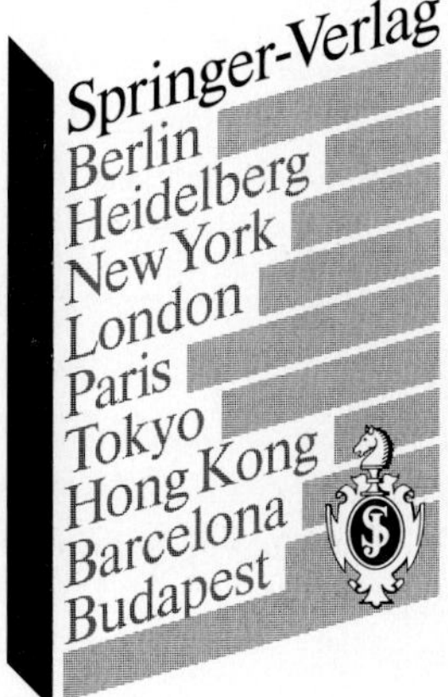

Handbook of Experimental Pharmacology

Volume 79
New Neuromuscular Blocking Agents

Volume 80
Cadmium

Volume 81
Local Anesthetics

Volume 82
Radioimmunoassay in Basic and Clinical Pharmacology

Volume 83
Calcium in Drug Actions

Volume 84
Antituberculosis Drugs

Volume 85
The Pharmacology of Lymphocytes

Volume 86
The Cholinergic Synapse

Volume 87
Part 1: **Pharmacology of the Skin I**
Part 2: **Pharmacology of the Skin II**

Volume 88
Drugs for the Treatment of Parkinson's Disease

Volume 89
Antiarrhythmic Drugs

Volume 90
Part 1: **Catecholamines I**
Part 2: **Catecholamines II**

Volume 91
Microbial Resistance to Drugs

Volume 92
Insulin

Volume 93
Pharmacology of Antihypertensive Therapeutics

Volume 94
Part 1: **Chemical Carcinogenesis and Mutagenesis I**
Part 2: **Chemical Carcinogenesis and Mutagenesis II**

Volume 95
Part 1: **Peptide Growth Factors and Their Receptors I**
Part 2: **Peptide Growth Factors and Their Receptors II**

Volume 96
Chemotherapy of Fungal Diseases

Volume 97
Histamine and Histamine Antagonists

Volume 98
Pharmacology of Asthma

Volume 99
Pharmacology of Peptic Ulcer Disease

Volume 100
Targeted Drug Delivery

Volume 101
Biochemical Pharmacology of Blood and Blood-Forming Organs

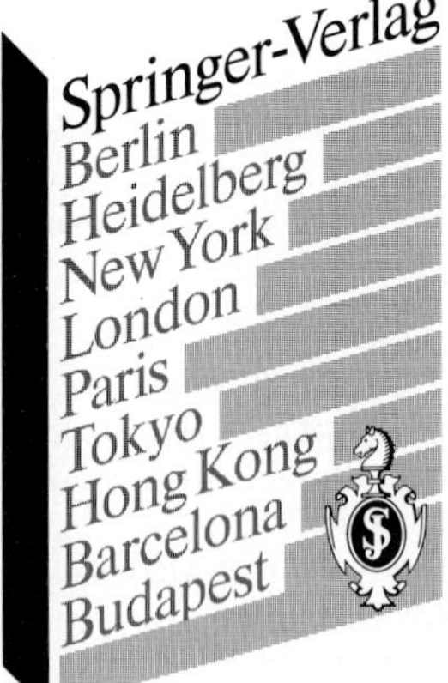